Lecture Notes on Pathology

To the memory of Sheila
and to Andrew,
Richard, David and Matthew

Lecture Notes on Pathology

PRINCIPALLY BY

R.E. COTTON MD, FRCPath

Emeritus Consultant Pathologist,
City Hospital, Nottingham;
Formerly Special Professor of
Diagnostic Oncology,
University of Nottingham

FOURTH EDITION

OXFORD

BLACKWELL SCIENTIFIC PUBLICATIONS

LONDON EDINBURGH BOSTON

MELBOURNE PARIS BERLIN VIENNA

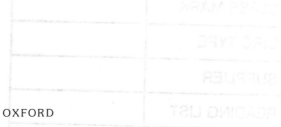

© 1962, 1968, 1983, 1992 by
Blackwell Scientific Publications
Editorial Offices:
Osney Mead, Oxford OX2 0EL
25 John Street, London WC1N 2BL
23 Ainslie Place, Edinburgh EH3 6AJ
238 Main Street, Cambridge
   Massachusetts 02142, USA
54 University Street, Carlton
   Victoria 3053, Australia

Other Editorial Offices:

Librairie Arnette SA
2 rue Casimir-Delavigne
75006 Paris
France

Blackwell Wissenschafts-Verlag
Meinekestrasse 4
D-1000 Berlin 15
Germany

Blackwell MZV
Feldgasse 13
A-1238 Wien
Austria

First published 1962
Reprinted 1963, 1965, 1967
Second edition 1968
Reprinted 1970, 1974, 1976
Third edition 1983
Fourth edition 1992
Four Dragons edition 1992

Set by Semantic Graphics, Singapore
Printed and bound in Great Britain at
The Alden Press, Oxford

DISTRIBUTORS

Marston Book Services Ltd
PO Box 87
Oxford OX2 0DT
(*Orders*: Tel: 0865 791155
         Fax: 0865 791927
         Telex: 837515)

USA
Blackwell Scientific Publications, Inc.
238 Main Street
Cambridge, MA 02142
(*Orders*: Tel: 800 759-6102
         617 876-7000)

Canada
Times Mirror Professional Publishing, Ltd
5240 Finch Avenue East
Scarborough, Ontario M1S 5A2
(*Orders*: Tel: 800 268-4178
         416 298-1588)

Australia
Blackwell Scientific Publications
   (Australia) Pty Ltd
54 University Street
Carlton, Victoria 3053
(*Orders*: Tel: 03 347-0300)

A catalogue record for this book is
available from the British Library

ISBN 0–632–03355–X (BSP)
ISBN 0–632–03397–5 (Four Dragons)

Contents

Contributors

I.D. ANSELL MA, MB, FRCPath, *Consultant Histopathologist, City Hospital, Nottingham* Chapter 10, Section E, Kidney Tumours; Chapter 11, Diseases of the Genito-Urinary Tract

R.E. COTTON MD, FRCPath, *Emeritus Consultant Pathologist, City Hospital, Nottingham* Chapter 1, Diseases Due to Infections and Infestations; Chapter 2, Diseases of the Alimentary System Sections A and B; Chapter 4, Diseases of the Cardiovascular System; Chapter 6, Soft Tissue Tumours; Chapter 7, Diseases of the Ear; Chapter 8, Endocrine Gland Diseases; Chapter 9, Diseases of the Eye; Chapter 10, Diseases of the Genito-Urinary System—Kidney; Chapter 17, Diseases of the Musculo-Skeletal System Sections B–G

I.O. ELLIS BMedSci, BM, MRCPath, *Consultant Histopathologist, City Hospital, Nottingham* Chapter 15, Diseases of the Lymphoreticular System

C.W. ELSTON MD, FRCPath, *Consultant Histopathologist, City Hospital, Nottingham* Chapter 3, Diseases of the Breast

S.G. HÜBSCHER MB, MRCPath, *Senior Lecturer in Pathology, University of Birmingham* Chapters 13 and 14, Diseases of the Liver and Biliary Tract; Chapter 19, Diseases of the Pancreas

J. JOHNSON BSc, MB, FRCPath, *Consultant Histopathologist, City Hospital, Nottingham* Chapter 12, Female Genital Tract

N. KIRKHAM MB, MRCPath, *Consultant Histopathologist, Royal Sussex County Hospital, Brighton* Chapter 21, Diseases of the Skin

J.S. LOWE BMedSci, BM, MRCPath, *Reader and Honorary Consultant in Neuropathology, University of Nottingham* Chapter 17, Section A Non-Neoplastic Muscle Disorders; Chapter 18, Diseases of the Nervous System

R.J. POWELL MB, MRCP, *Consultant and Senior Lecturer in Clinical Immunology, University of Nottingham* Chapter 5, Connective Tissue Diseases

M. STEPHENS MB, MRCPath, *Consultant Histopathologist, Central Pathology Laboratory, Stoke-on-Trent* Chapter 16, Diseases of the Mediastinum; Chapter 20, Diseases of the Respiratory System

J.I. WYATT MB, MRCPath, *Consultant Histopathologist, St James's University Hospital, Leeds* Chapter 2, Sections C–G, Diseases of the Alimentary System

Contributors to previous editions

Though very extensively rewritten, this fourth edition does contain some relatively unaltered parts contributed by Drs W. Jeffcoate and P. B. Schofield and illustrations prepared by Professor J. S. P. Jones, to whom, with grateful thanks, I acknowledge their past help.

To my previous co-author Dr A. D. Thomson goes the credit for the lecture notes on which the original book was based. His contribution to the first edition and, to a lesser extent, the second and third revisions were inestimable and my profound thanks to him are hereby recorded.

List of Illustrations

Preface to the Fourth Edition

Though identified as a fourth edition, this book is so different in content from its predecessors that for practical purposes it should be regarded as a new work. After most of a much-enjoyed career in pathology and many generations of undergraduate and postgraduate students, a 'new look' was essential for so many reasons, and retirement from hospital and university duties have given me the time, energy and motivation to rewrite the book. This time, however, a substantial part has been rewritten by invited contributors; all are enthusiasts for their chosen specialty, and all have great in-depth knowledge of the special areas of interest about which they have written. My grateful thanks to each of them for their excellence and cooperation.

During the 'life span' of this book, pathology has seen a remarkable and welcome resurgence as a group of disciplines increasingly important to scientific progress and clinical relevance. Paramount in this is a much more dynamic and functional approach to study of disease and its processes, a much enhanced clinical involvement, and a will and skill to incorporate new techniques including ultrastructural studies, immunocytochemistry, cytopathology and molecular biological methods.

As well as producing a wealth of new information about both 'old' and more recently discovered diseases, new concepts have emerged and have given a philosophical impetus to this science. Multidisciplinary cooperative studies have been consolidated and expanded with great benefit to all.

The basic type of presentation of the work is largely unchanged except for reorganization of chapters and reduction of their synopses of contents, but the content is much altered by the decision to leave out the general pathology and haematology sections which were previously incorporated. As a major science in its own right, haematology could no longer be sensibly retained, though due reference is made at appropriate places. The study of the processes of pathology, which is what 'general pathology' is about, is probably the most important bridging science between preclinical and clinical undergraduate courses in medicine, and requires study in depth at an early stage in the curriculum. This edition assumes successful learning of those dynamic processes and is aimed at correlation of pathological knowledge in individual clinical disease entities. It is therefore particularly addressed to the clinical student near the end of the undergraduate medical school course and to those in postgraduate specialist training in clinical disciplines where an up-to-date and extensive knowledge of pathology is so essential.

In terms of travel and communication, the world shrinks (though not its population). Diseases increasingly do not respect geographical boundaries and therefore it has been policy to incorporate additional material of worldwide significance. Where at all possible, internationally acceptable nomenclature and classifications have been utilized.

It is a great pleasure to record grateful thanks to many colleagues and friends, and for wonderful support at family level, now including another generation. Yet again Ann Booth has achieved the impossible in producing manuscript from illegible scrawl, difficult enough to identify even as writing, and to her and the secretaries of the individual contributors my warmest thanks.

That another *Lecture Notes on Pathology* has been published is a tribute to the continued persuasiveness of Per and Peter Saugman and their splendid team at Blackwell Scientific Publications in Oxford, with whom it has been my good fortune to work for 30 years. I am full of admiration and gratitude for them.

R.E. COTTON
Northfield Farmhouse
Wysall
Nottingham

Preface to the First Edition

This book is based on lectures in pathology which we give to the students at the Middlesex Hospital Medical School, London.

Appreciating the already heavily burdened curriculum of medical students, we have endeavoured to present a comprehensive and yet concise account of the important pathological features of disease and to link, where possible, the pathological changes with the effects on the patient.

With a view to clarity, liberal use of headings and subheadings has been employed in the layout of the book and the text is purposely written in a didactic manner for brevity. Some abbreviations, e.g. polymorphs for polymorphonuclear leucocytes, have been used in an attempt to limit the length of the text; we apologize to those who may find this a source of annoyance. Each chapter starts with a tabulated summary sheet of the entire contents of the section which lays out the subject matter in a classified form for clarity of presentation, ease of understanding and speed of revision. We have endeavoured to give a figure in respect of the incidence and/or prognosis of many of the commoner clinical diseases. The incidence figures, many of which are derived from the Registrar-General's statistics for England and Wales, are designed to act as a general guide and it should not be implied that these are necessarily universally applicable in all geographical areas. The figures for results are approximately the average of reported series.

It is hoped that this method of presenting the subject of pathology will prove to be of value to undergraduate students studying for their final examinations and to postgraduate students preparing for higher qualifications in medical and surgical specialities. It is for these groups that this book has been primarily designed.

After some hesitation we decided not to include references, but a list of books for additional reading is appended in many of which lists of references are to be found for the benefit of those seeking further information.

A.D. THOMSON
R.E. COTTON

Books for Additional Reading and Reference

Adams J.H. & Graham D.I. (1988) *Introduction to Neuropathology*. Churchill Livingstone, Edinburgh.

Ansell I.D. (1985) *Atlas of Male Reproductive Pathology*. MTP Press, Lancaster.

Anthony P.P. & MacSween R.N.M. (Eds) (1992) *Recent Advances in Pathology*, vols 11–15. Churchill Livingstone, Edinburgh.

Dail D.N. & Hammar S.P. (Eds) (1988) *Pulmonary Pathology*. Springer-Verlag, New York.

Davies M.J. (1986) *Colour Atlas of Cardiovascular Pathology*. Oxford University Press, Oxford.

Dieppe P.A., Doherty M., Macfarlane D.G. & Maddison P.J. (1985) *Rheumatological Medicine*. Churchill Livingstone, Edinburgh.

Esiri M.M. & Oppenheimer D.R. (1989) *Diagnostic Neuropathology*. Churchill Livingstone, Edinburgh.

Heptinstall R.H. (1991) *Pathology of the Kidney*, 4th edn. Little Brown, Boston.

Katzenstein L. & Askin F. (1990) *Surgical Pathology of Non-Neoplastic Lung Disease*, 2nd edn. Saunders, Philadelphia.

Kovacs K. & Asa S. (1990) *Functional Endocrine Pathology*. Blackwell Scientific Publications, Oxford.

Kurman R. (Ed.) *Blaustein's Pathology of the Female Genital Tract*, 3rd edn. Springer-Verlag, New York.

MacSween R.N.M., Anthony P.P. & Sheur P.J. (1987) *Pathology of the Liver*, 2nd edn. Churchill Livingstone, Edinburgh.

Morson B.C., Dawson I.M.P., Day D.W., Jass J.R., Price A.B. & Williams G.T. (1990) *Gastrointestinal Pathology*, 3rd edn. Blackwell Scientific Publications, Oxford.

Murphy W.M. (1989) *Urological Pathology*. Saunders, Philadelphia.

Page D.L. & Anderson T.J. (Eds) (1987) *Diagnostic Histopathology of the Breast*. Churchill Livingstone, Edinburgh.

Rubin E. & Farber J.L. (1988) *Pathology*. Lippincott, Philadelphia.

Sherlock S. (1992) *Diseases of the Liver and Biliary System*, 9th edn. Blackwell Scientific Publications, Oxford.

Stansfeld A.G. (Ed.) (1992) *Lymph Node Biopsy Interpretation*, 2nd edn. Churchill Livingstone, Edinburgh.

Talbot I.C. & Price A.B. (1987) *Biopsy Pathology in Colorectal Disease*. Chapman and Hall, London.

Walter J.B. & Israel M.S. (1987) *General Pathology*, 6th edn. Churchill Livingstone, Edinburgh.

Chapter 1
Diseases due to Infections and Infestations

Introduction

In spite of modern antibiotic therapy and progress in creating improvements in hygiene and social circumstances, deaths from bacterial, viral, protozoal, fungal and helminthic diseases remain hugely numerous, particularly in developing countries. The accelerating pandemic of AIDS has served to remind health professions of just how much still needs to be achieved in the prevention of unnecessary death and disease in the human race from infecting agents.

Patterns of infection have changed markedly in the past 10–20 years, some diseases almost or actually disappearing and others becoming more frequent or, like AIDS, being new and very alarming in global terms.

Many such infective conditions relate to specific geographical or climatic situations and many have a specific affinity for particular tissues and organ systems. In this book many are described in relation to those sites which are maximally involved or are clinically predominant.

There remain, however, many important systemic or otherwise non-localized infections and infestations which are more appropriately considered separately in this chapter.

Infective conditions described in other chapters

These agents and their points of reference are as follows:

Bacteria

1 Pyogenic organisms, e.g. streptococci, staphylococci, Gram-negative cocci and cocco-bacilli are recorded relevant to the lesions which they cause in respect of individual anatomical sites.
2 Cholera, bacillary dysentery, *Salmonella* infections (see gastrointestinal tract, p. 32 and p. 40).
3 Gonorrhoea, granuloma inguinale, chancroid, chlamydial infections (see genito-urinary tract, pp. 196, 203 and 207).
4 Meningococcal infections (see nervous system, p. 324 and adrenal glands, p. 116).
5 *Campylobacter* and *Helicobacter* (see stomach and intestine, p. 26 and p. 40).
6 Leptospirosis (see liver, p. 235 and eye, p. 150).
7 *Yersinia* (see lymph nodes, p. 268).
8 Diphtheria (see larynx, p. 362).
9 *Legionella*, *Haemophilus influenzae* (see lung, pp. 370–371).
10 *Listeria* (see nervous system, p. 325).
11 Tuberculosis (see lung, p. 374 and bones, p. 295; kidney, p. 165 and intestine, p. 33).

Viruses

1 Human papilloma virus (see skin, p. 415, cervix, p. 210, penis, p. 204 and larynx, p. 362).
2 Hepatitis viruses (see liver, p. 231).
3 Infectious mononucleosis (see lymph nodes, p. 268).
4 Influenza and *Mycoplasma* (see lung, p. 371).
5 Measles (see lung, p. 371 and mouth, p. 12).
6 Mumps (see testis, p. 119 and salivary glands, p. 19).
7 Poliomyelitis (see nervous system, p. 326).
8 Herpes simplex (see mouth, liver, nervous system and cervix, pp. 11, 234, 326 and 210).
9 Cytomegalovirus (see liver, lymph nodes and lung, pp. 234, 265 and 397).

Fungi

1 Actinomycosis (see lung, liver and jaw, pp. 399, 235 and 12).
2 *Candida* (see mouth, lung, oesophagus and genital tract, pp. 12, 399, 22 and 207).
3 Aspergillosis (see lung, p. 398).

Protozoa

1 Amoebic dysentery (see intestine, p. 41).
2 Pneumocystis (see lung, p. 372).

Helminths

1 Hydatid disease (see liver, p. 236).
2 Liver fluke and *Fasciola hepatica* (see liver, p. 237).

Bacterial infections

Tetanus and gas gangrene

These conditions are caused by anaerobic clostridia which gain entrance through wounds by contamination with their spores. They are particularly important in penetrating military wounds and other injuries where there is soft tissue devitalization. Tetanus produces a very powerful exotoxin which affects the spinal cord and medullary nerve cells resulting in muscle spasms, respiratory difficulty and death unless antitoxin is administered early enough. In gas gangrene, necrosis and putrefaction lead to gas formation with further separation of tissues from their blood supply, spreading infection and severe toxaemia from the enzymes and toxins produced by the organisms, septicaemia and a high mortality rate.

Brucellosis

This is a chronic febrile disease of insidious onset and protean clinical manifestations caused by *Brucella abortus*, *B. melitensis* or *B. suis*.

Infection is by ingestion of infected cow's or goat's milk with rapid dissemination by the blood stream and invasion of the lymphoreticular cells of many organs, particularly spleen, lymph nodes, liver and bone marrow. The organisms cause a granulomatous reaction usually small and discrete.

Antibiotic therapy is curative but the course may be very chronic.

Anthrax

Infection by *Bacillus anthracis*, a Gram-positive sporing organism, occurs by contact with infected animals or their products—sheep, cattle, horses, pigs.

The most frequent lesion is a '*malignant pustule*' in skin at the site of an injury, with local spreading oedema and vesicle and pustule formation.

Occasionally inhaled spores can produce a highly lethal haemorrhagic pulmonary consolidation—'*wool-sorter's disease*'.

Syphilis

Incidence

Because of widespread availability of antibiotic drugs to which *Treponema pallidum* is sensitive, this formerly extremely important disease is now less frequently seen, particularly in its later stages.

Infection

This is usually sexually transmitted through minor abrasions of the skin or mucosal surfaces and rapidly disseminates from the primary lesion—*chancre* which is usually genital, i.e. cervix (see p. 207) or penis (see p. 202), but may be extragenital, e.g. rectum, anus, mouth.

Course

The primary lesion heals without treatment but may be followed by *secondary syphilis* 1–3 months after the chancre if no treatment is given. The manifestations are protean, affecting skin—rashes, lymph nodes—enlargement, mucous membranes—ulcers, eyes—retinitis or iridocyclitis (see p. 149), etc.

In one-third of untreated cases *tertiary* manifestations may occur 3–25 years after primary infection and affect the cardiovascular system (see p. 81), central nervous system (p. 328) or may produce gummas which can be in many organs (see p. 235).

Congenital syphilis

The spirochaetes can cross the placenta from an infected mother and produce a wide range of debilitating and deforming lesions at birth or in childhood or adolescence. Routine serological testing, e.g. Venereal Disease Research Laboratory (VDRL) or Wasserman reaction, has largely eliminated this condition in developed countries.

Leprosy

Incidence

This infection with *Mycobacterium leprae*, an acid-but not alcohol-fast bacillus, is still common in Asian and African countries, though its incidence is steadily declining due to therapeutic and public health measures.

Course

Studies of the disease have been hampered by its extremely long incubation period and clinical course, but it appears to spread by case-to-case contact through abrasions in skin or mucous membranes which, together with peripheral nerves, are the site of lesions.

Types

1 *Lepromatous—nodular*. A rash becomes nodular; it may then ulcerate, spread and cause great disfigurement, particularly on the nose, face and mucous membranes of the upper respiratory tract. Numerous organisms can be seen with modified Ziehl–Nielsen stains in macrophages in the granulomatous lesions.

2 *Tuberculoid—maculo-anaesthetic*. This develops in more resistant hosts with a macular skin rash and progressive involvement of local and then more proximal peripheral nerves, which become thickened with functional loss leading to anaesthesia, trauma, trophic changes and contractures. Histologically the granulomas become very fibrotic and organisms are very scanty indeed.

Viral infections

HIV infection—acquired immunodeficiency syndrome—AIDS

Organism

Two strains of the human immunodeficiency retrovirus—HIV I and HIV II, are presently known. The viruses are not very pathogenic, are very susceptible to drying and temperature change and infection is acquired mostly through sexual activity via seminal fluid, vaginal secretions, saliva or through contaminated infected blood or blood products.

The virus causes disease by destroying T lymphocytes with a marked selectivity for the 'helper' cells.

Geographic distribution

It now appears certain that the virus developed in Africa where HIV infection is currently most prevalent. Countries and societies where promiscuity (either homosexual or heterosexual) is of high incidence show the highest levels of HIV positivity and of cases of AIDS, with low levels of promiscuity producing comparable 'protection' from the infection.

Epidemiology

HIV infection is frequently asymptomatic for a time interval which may be many years. During this period blood tests are positive and the person can transmit the infection to others.

As a predominantly sexually transmitted infection it is thus most frequently found in sexually active persons, originally largely homosexual but increasingly heterosexuals or bisexuals. Drug addicts and other persons coming into contact with infected blood products, e.g. haemophiliacs, who in the past accidentally received contaminated clotting factor preparations or where used syringes were re-used without re-sterilization, are further groups at risk.

Course

After the asymptomatic HIV-positive phase a variable proportion over differing periods of time develop clinical manifestations which are of three main types:

1 Disease directly due to virus infection of tissues, e.g. generalized lymphadenopathy (see p. 265), HIV enteropathy (see p. 33), pulmonary lesions (see p. 397), nervous system lesions (see p. 329).

2 Opportunistic infections due to the immunodeficient state including:

    (a) viruses: cytomegalovirus;

    (b) bacteria: *M. tuberculosis*, atypical mycobacteria (see pp. 374–377);

    (c) fungi: cryptococcosis, invasive aspergillosis, candidosis (see pp. 398–399);

    (d) protozoal: *Pneumocystis carinii* (see p. 372);

    (e) helminthic: hyperinfection with *Strongyloides*.

3 Development of tumours—particularly Kaposi's sarcoma (see p. 419) and non-Hodgkin's lymphoma (see p. 265). The main manifestations are described in individual systems or organs.

Prognosis

It is not yet possible to predict when the change from HIV-positive but asymptomatic to clinical AIDS will occur, or how inevitable it actually is. At present about 30% become symptomatic within 10 years.

Once AIDS appears then, at present, death occurs relatively rapidly—usually from pulmonary infection by *Cryptococcus*, *Pneumocystis* or *Mycobacteria*, or through spread of malignant lymphoma or Kaposi's sarcoma.

Herpes—pox virus diseases

Though smallpox—*variola*—appears to have been globally eliminated, other viruses of this group are important causes of morbidity.

Chickenpox

Nature
A usually mild common highly contagious disease in childhood caused by the varicella virus and with an incubation of about 14 days.

Lesions
A vesicular skin eruption appearing in successive crops starting on the trunk and spreading outwards. The vesicles may become pustules and secondary infection may lead to disfiguring scars. Cytopathic changes and inclusion bodies are seen in epithelial cells in and around the vesicles.

Course
In the absence of pyogenic infection the skin lesions heal with minimal scarring. In immunocompromised patients, and very occasionally in the immunocompetent, systemic lesions, notably in lung and brain, may cause death.

Herpes zoster
This disease is also caused by the varicella virus and usually affects older persons. The virus localizes in the dorsal root or cranial nerve ganglia causing segmental skin lesions over the sensory distribution of affected nerves. Pain is a prominent feature and may persist for months or years—*post-herpetic neuralgia*.

Herpes simplex
There are several strains of this virus which affect the mouth and lips (see p. 11), female genital tract (see p. 210), nervous system (see p. 326) and liver (see p. 234). Usually clinical manifestations are mild, but in all these sites recurrent attacks are common, alternating with episodes of continued presence but dormancy of the virus in epithelial cells. Herpes encephalitis (see p. 326) can be fatal in the immunocompetent and severe symptoms can result from infection in the immunocompromised, especially in the mouth associated with chemotherapy for haematological malignancies, particularly leukaemias.

Fungal infections

Cryptococcosis—European blastomycosis

Organism
Cryptococcus neoformans, a worldwide round or oval 5–10 μm diameter organism which reproduces by budding and has a distinctive gelatinous capsule.

Sites
1 Superficial: skin and subcutaneous abscesses.
2 Lungs: solitary or scanty pulmonary granulomas, which are usually asymptomatic but in the immunosuppressed a disseminated pneumonic process which is a frequent cause of death in AIDS (see p. 397).
3 Meninges: a chronic meningitis which can be very serious but which evokes very little inflammatory reaction (see p. 325).

Results
In immunocompetent persons the course is very protracted and self-limiting but rather resistant to therapy. Death usually follows in the immunocompromised from pulmonary or meningitic lesions.

North American blastomycosis

Organism
Blastomyces dermatitidis, a pathogenic round or oval 5–15 μm diameter budding fungus with a double-contoured wall. It occurs in the North American continent.

Sites
1 Skin: spreading irregular papule with microabscesses in the raised margins.
2 Lung: numerous abscesses or occasionally solid granulomas.
3 Disseminated: many organs affected, particularly bone.

Results
Even in the immunocompetent the disseminated disease responds poorly to treatment and in immunosuppressed persons fatalities are frequent. The cutaneous form is disfiguring but benign.

Histoplasmosis

Organism
Histoplasma capsulatum—a small budding oval fungus 1–5 μm diameter with a thick capsule producing a clear surrounding halo. Most common in central regions of the USA but worldwide in its distribution.

Sites

1 Lung:

(a) localized granuloma (see p. 406);

(b) disseminated.

2 Lymphoreticular. Diffuse involvement of spleen, liver, intestine and lymph nodes.

Results

The primary lung granuloma—*histoplasmoma*—usually remains localized but may become reactivated in a manner similar to *M. tuberculosis* (see p. 397) with local or distant spread and significant mortality. This process is accelerated by acquired immunosuppression.

The disseminated lymphoreticular and pulmonary lesions also have a high mortality, but may be controlled by amphotericin B.

Coccidioidomycosis

Organism

Coccidioides immitis: a large thick-walled spherule which reproduces by endosporulation. It is largely confined to the southwestern parts of the USA.

Sites

1 Localized:

(a) skin;

(b) lung; granuloma resembling tuberculosis, less commonly multiple cavitating pneumonic lesions.

2 Disseminated. Involvement of spleen, liver, lymph nodes, bone, nervous system, in less than 1% of cases.

Results

The localized lesions are largely self-limiting and heal by fibrosis and calcification. Sixty per cent are asymptomatic but can reactivate with immunosuppression producing fatal disseminated disease.

Paracoccidioidomycosis—South American blastomycosis

Organism

Coccidioides brasiliensis: a budding endosporulating fungus often intracellular and confined to Brazil, Colombia and Central America.

Sites

1 Lung: nodules or infiltrates which frequently cavitate.

2 Disseminated: lymphoreticular, cutaneous and mucous membrane involvement.

Results

A pathogenic organism with substantial fatality rate but usually responsive to amphotericin B and ketoconazole.

Protozoal diseases

Malaria

Incidence

This is still one of the most important infective conditions causing severe morbidity and mortality around the world. Though most common in tropical and subtropical areas it is frequently exported to many other regions.

Organisms

The disease is transmitted through the bite of various species of anopheline mosquitoes: *Plasmodium falciparum*—malignant malaria; *P. viva* and *P. ovale*—tertian malaria; *P. malariae*—quartan malaria.

Life cycle

1 In mosquito: sexual cycle, 7–12 days. Female mosquito bites humans (natural reservoir)—blood contains male and female gametocytes—mature in stomach forming a zygote—penetrates wall of stomach forming oocyst in which sporozoites develop—rupture of sporocyst into body cavity—release of sporozoites and migration to salivary gland thence to saliva and, following a bite, introduction to new host.

2 In humans: asexual cycle.

(a) Exoerythrocytic phase—7 days: sporozoites from mosquito bite enter blood—drain to liver and develop into merozoites—invade blood and enter erythrocytes.

(b) Erythrocytic phase—36–72 hours depending on species: maturation of merozoites in erythrocytes to trophozoites which develop into schizonts and these divide into numerous merozoites—rupture of infected cells—release into blood—destroyed by defence mechanisms or enter fresh red cells—after about five such cycles in humans, merozoites change to gametocytes which can infect mosquitoes and so continue the cycle.

Effects

1 *Red cells*: trophozoites show as ring forms 10–14

days after the bite. Destruction of cells leads to a haemolytic anaemia and pigment production—*haemazoin*.

2 *Lymphoreticular system*: splenomegaly (see p. 279) and lesser degrees of hepatomegaly (see p. 235) and lymphadenopathy.

3 *Brain*: in infection with *P. falciparum*, cerebral vessels may become plugged with infected red cells causing ischaemia (see p. 328).

Results

1 *Acute*:

(a) Benign malaria: spontaneous or therapeutic remission of a severe febrile illness with repeated attacks possible over many years.

(b) Malignant malaria: rapidly progressive to death unless urgent treatment is given.

2 *Chronic*. In high-incidence areas some resistance occurs in the populations with progressive debilitating ill-health, chronic anaemia and severe progressive hepatosplenomegaly.

Toxoplasmosis

Organism

Toxoplasma gondii, an intracellular round or crescent-shaped organism 5 μm by 2.5 μm with basophilic cytoplasm and a prominent nucleus. It is worldwide in distribution and common in all domestic animals.

Congenital toxoplasmosis

Infection *in utero* causes lesions in the central nervous system (CNS)—hydrocephalus, calcified necrotic granulomas (see p. 328) and choroidoretinitis (see p. 150): focal necrotic areas in heart and other viscera. Skin rash, low-grade fever, jaundice and hepatosplenomegaly may also occur.

Adult toxoplasmosis

The most common presentation is a benign febrile lymphadenopathy with small ill-defined histiocytic granulomas (see p. 268) and choroidoretinitis and uveitis (see p. 150). Atypical pneumonia and disseminated granulomas of lungs and cerebrum are less common.

Results

In the congenital form the predominant serious feature is hydrocephalus, and in adults the only serious effect is in the disseminated type. Otherwise the infection is usually self-limiting.

Leishmaniasis

Three clinical patterns of disease caused by three different species.

Cutaneous—oriental sore

Organism

Leishmania tropica, a round or oval organism 2 μm diameter, with central nucleus and usually intracellular in macrophages. It is found in the Near, Middle and Far East.

Infection is transmitted by a sandfly bite.

Effects

Skin papule later ulcerated and encrusted, persisting for weeks or months before healing. Macrophages filled with organisms are present.

Mucocutaneous—Espundia

Organism

Leishmania brasiliensis, morphologically similar to *L. tropica* and found in Central and South America.

Effects

In addition to cutaneous lesions the mucous membranes of mouth, nose and larynx are involved and constitutional symptoms may develop.

Visceral—kala-azar

Organism

Leishmania donovanii, which has an additional rod-like structure extending from the nucleus and terminating in a blepharoplast. Wide prevalence in Mediterranean countries, India, Russia, China and parts of Africa.

Infection is from humans, the chief reservoir, via the bite of *Phlebotomus* sandflies.

Effects

This is a systemic infection of the lymphoreticular system involving spleen (see p. 279), liver (see p. 236), lymph nodes, bone marrow and the lymphoid elements of other organs.

This is a disease with significant mortality often after a prolonged course.

Trypanosomiasis

Organisms
1 *Trypanosoma gambiense*: Gambian sleeping sickness (Africa).
2 *T. rhodesiense*: Rhodesian sleeping sickness (Africa).
3 *T. cruzi*: Chagas' disease (Central and South America).

All are flagellated, slender and spindle-shaped, 15 μm by 1.3 μm.

The vector in Africa is the tsetse fly and in the South American type the cone-nosed bug.

Effects
1 *T. cruzi*: produces a necrotizing myocarditis (see p. 66).
2 *T. rhodesiense and gambiense*: lymphadenopathy, cerebral and meningeal oedema, inflammatory reaction with ischaemic effects, variable hepatosplenomegaly.

In all sites organisms can be identified.

Results
The course is variable with a predominant neurological illness in the African types, sometimes with rapid progression to death, or as a chronic disease of several years duration. Chagas' disease is rarely fatal but may produce a chronic slow progression with heart failure.

Helminthic infestations

Nematodes
The whole life cycle of nearly all members of this class of worms occurs without the need for an intermediate host.

Ascariasis—roundworm

Parasite
Ascaris lumbricoides largely resembles the common earthworm and is about 15–35 cm long with both ends pointed. It is of worldwide distribution.

Life cycle
Completed in 1 month.

Embryos enter the blood stream from the jejunum where ingested ova hatch. They pass through liver to hepatic veins thence to heart, lungs, bronchi and trachea to oesophagus. Passing down the intestinal tract they mature and produce ova in the faeces.

Auto-infection is common, with contaminated water or vegetation as alternative sources.

Effects
These are usually relatively mild with some growth retardation and weight loss in children. Slight intestinal inflammatory reaction may produce eosinophilia and asthmatic symptoms or a pneumonitis may occur.

Oxyuriasis—threadworm

Parasite
Enterobius vermicularis—the male is 0.4 cm long with coiled tail and the female 1.0 cm long with a pointed tail. Distribution is worldwide.

Life cycle
Fertilized females deposit ova around the anus. These are transferred to new hosts by faecal contamination or by auto-infection via fingers to the mouth. The mature worms attach themselves to ileal, appendicular or caecal mucosa.

Effects
Usually insignificant but may occasionally cause an inflammatory reaction with eosinophils or a chronic granuloma within tissues.

Trichiniasis—muscle worm

Parasite
Trichinella spiralis—an adult worm 0.2–0.6 cm long. Encysted larvae are seen in voluntary muscle. Distribution is worldwide.

Life cycle
The chief source for humans is from infected pig, by ingestion of inadequately cooked pork.

The fertilized female in the intestine lays eggs in the submucosa and hatched larvae enter lymphatics or capillaries, pass through lung in systemic blood and reach striated muscle, heart and nervous system, where they coil up and become encysted but can remain viable for many years.

Effects
Severe muscular pain with fever, heart failure if cardiac involvement is severe, and fits or encephalitic picture with nervous system involvement.

Ancylostomiasis—hookworm

Parasite
Ancylostoma duodenale, a small cylindrical worm 1.0–1.3 cm long with a large mouth containing two pairs of hook-shaped teeth.

Most commonly found in India and Ceylon but present in all tropical and subtropical areas, where infestation is extremely common.

Life cycle
This takes 7 weeks.

Embryos hatch from ova in warm wet soil, penetrate human skin and, via veins, lungs and air passages, reach the oesophagus and intestine where they mature and produce ova.

Effects
The worm attaches itself to the mucosal villi with resulting inflammatory reaction with oedema and ulceration. Severe anaemia caused by extraction of blood by the parasite is common.

Trichuriasis—whipworm

Parasite
Trichuris trichiura, a worm 3–5 cm long with thin anterior portion but thick posteriorly, hence 'whip'

Distribution is worldwide; most common in the tropics.

Life cycle
This is similar to oxyuriasis (see p. 7).

Effects
Minimal or no clinical effects from the superficially implanted adult worms in the caecum.

Filariasis

Parasites
Wuchereria bancrofti, a hair-like worm 4–10 cm long found in the thoracic duct, lymphatics and lymph nodes. The motile microfilariae are only 0.3 mm long by 7 μm wide and can pass through capillaries. They inhabit peripheral blood at night.

Geographically filariae are found in the Middle and Far East, Hungary, Turkey, Central and South America, Pacific Islands and northern Australia.

Life cycle
This takes 12–30 days to complete.

An infected *Culax fatigans* mosquito injects microfilariae into a bite and, after penetrating skin lymphatics, they disseminate in lymph and blood vessels, localize and mature in lymphatics and lymph nodes where the fertilized female discharges microfilariae into blood. A mosquito then bites the subject, restarting the cycle.

Cestodes
These are hermaphrodite tapeworms which require the interposition of an intermediate host for the completion of their life cycles.

Humans are the *definitive host* of the adult worm of:

1 *Taenia solium*: pork tapeworm—pig intermediate host.
2 *Taenia saginata*: beef tapeworm—cattle intermediate host.
3 *Diphyllobothrium latum*: fish tapeworm—freshwater fish (perch and pike) and species of *Cyclops* intermediate hosts.

Humans are the *intermediate host* of *Taenia echinococcus* (*Echinococcus granulosus*)—hydatid disease, rarely of *T. solium*—cysticercosis.

Parasites
Humans infected by eating flesh of intermediate hosts which contain the cystic stage of the parasite. *T. solium* and *saginata* are flat, multisegmented and 300 and 600 cm long respectively. The fish tapeworm is even longer, 900 cm.

All have small heads and 1–3000 hermaphrodite segments which discharge ova into the faeces. There is species variation in characteristics of the head which is essential for survival of the worms.

Life cycle

Human definitive host
Pig (or cattle) ingest ova, embryos develop in intestine, pass into blood and become encysted in muscles, brain or liver. Humans eat infected inadequately cooked pork or beef and in the intestine the encysted stage matures into adult worms.

Human intermediate host
Human self-contamination or ingestion of ova occurs

with hatching in intestine, entry to the blood stream and the cysticercus stage in humans.

Effects

1 Adult worm: variable gastrointestinal disturbances, loss of weight and anaemia, sometimes macrocytic.
2 Cysticercus stage: an inflammatory reaction occurs followed by a granuloma around the dead encysted parasite which is commonly in the brain.

Hydatid disease

This infestation of humans with the cystic stage of *Echinococcus granulosus* produces cysts, often of enormous size, in liver (see p. 236), lung and less commonly other organs, e.g. spleen, kidney, brain.

Adult worms inhabit the intestines of dogs and many other domestic animals and are themselves only 2.5–6 mm long.

Trematodes

Schistosomiasis—bilharziasis

Parasites and life cycle

Three species:
1 *Schistosoma haematobium*—bladder involvement (see p. 190).
2 *S. mansoni*
3 *S. japonicum* } intestinal and visceral (see p. 33).

The male is 11–15 μm long by 1 mm wide with sides curved to form a gynaecophoric canal in which the long filamentous female lies. The adult worms mature in the portal or mesenteric veins and then migrate to deposit ova in the small veins of bladder, intestine or liver as appropriate. The ova traverse the tissues to the lumen and are excreted in urine or faeces.

In water the ova hatch to produce a *miracidium*, which is ingested by a snail which releases *cercariae* into water. These can penetrate human skin and enter the blood. The life cycle takes 6 weeks to complete.

Geographical

1 *S. haematobium*: Africa, Egypt and other parts of Middle East, Greece, Cyprus, Portugal.
2 *S. mansoni*: Africa, Central and South America, Caribbean.
3 *S. japonicum*: Far East.

Effects

1 Liver: fibrosis around ova and 'pipe-stem cirrhosis' (see p. 236).
2 Rectum: acute then chronic inflammation of granulomatous type around ova and worms with ulceration, necrosis, fibrosis and polyp formation and stricture (see p. 33).
3 Bladder: chronic cystitis, fibrosis, metaplasia, fistula formation, carcinoma (see p. 190).

Other trematodes

1 Intestinal fluke. *Fasciolopsis buski*, a common fluke in China producing diarrhoea and anaemia. Intermediate hosts are a snail and a water plant which is eaten raw in salads.
2 Liver flukes:
  (a) *Fasciola hepatica*, only rarely parasitic to humans in sheep-raising areas.
  (b) *Clonorchis sinensis*—Chinese liver fluke, found in the Far East only.
Both these cause biliary tract inflammation, obstructive jaundice and hepatic abscesses (see p. 237).
3 Lung fluke—*Paragonimus westermani*, limited to the Orient: two intermediate hosts—snail and crayfish or crabs, from which humans are infected. Consolidation of lung with abscess formation and fibrosis result.

Chapter 2
Diseases of the Alimentary System

A/MOUTH, LIPS, TONGUE, GUMS

Congenital
Lips
Oral inflammations
Miscellaneous mouth lesions
Leukoplakia
Carcinoma of tongue
Carcinoma floor of mouth
Carcinoma pharynx and tonsil
Verrucous carcinoma
Gums

Congenital

Hare lip
An abnormality due to failure of fusion of the nasal and maxillary processes which form the upper lip and maxilla. There may be only a slight indentation in the outer part of the middle third of the upper lip, or a fissure may extend to the anterior nares. The condition may be unilateral or bilateral.

There are genetic and environmental factors in the aetiology: risks to children are one in 30 with one affected parent.

Cleft palate
This may be associated with hare lip and is also of variable degree. It may affect both the hard and soft palates in complete cases. The fissure then forms a direct communication between mouth and nose and requires urgent operative closure to avoid inhalation of food into the respiratory tract.

Stomal abnormalities
Lip development may extend too far towards the midline—microstomia, or conversely, a failure of development—macrostomia, shows as a fissure extending towards the ear. The lips may be the site of a congenital lymphangioma—macrocheilia.

Jaw abnormalities
These are rare but include absence of the jaw—agnathia; underdevelopment of the mandible or maxilla—micrognathia; failure of formation of the condyle.

Lips

Infections
The lip is usually involved secondarily from infections of the oral cavity (see below).

Tumours
Benign tumours, e.g. haemangioma, lymphangioma, fibroma, squamous cell papilloma, rarely occur in the lip. Benign non-neoplastic retention mucous gland cysts are common.

Carcinoma of lip

Age
This tumour is very rare in the young and usually occurs in the 50–70 age group.

Sex
Male:female, 20:1.

Sites
The lower lip is involved in 90% of cases.

Predisposing factors
In many cases there is no definite predisposing factor but one or more of the following may be operative:
1 *Leukoplakia.*
2 *Betel chewers.*
3 *Clay pipe smoking*: the main factor is repetitive thermal injury. This raises the incidence in women who smoke pipes.

4 *Sunlight*: actinic carcinoma—outdoor workers, e.g. sailors, farmers, fishermen and fair-skinned people in sunny climates, have an increased incidence.

5 *Tar*: repeated contact with tar in fish net menders.

Macroscopical

The tumour may be nodular, papillary, fissured or ulcerated and approximately 50% of the patients have cervical or submandibular lymph node metastases at the time of diagnosis.

Microscopical

Squamous cell carcinomas usually with well-marked keratin formation.

Spread

Direct spread to adjacent structures, e.g. gum and bone; lymphatic spread to the submandibular and cervical lymph nodes. Blood spread to many organs may occur but is a late manifestation.

Prognosis

There is an 80% 5-year survival without nodal involvement; 40% with lymph node metastases.

Inflammations of the oral cavity

Vincent's infection—trench mouth

Nature

An ulcerating infection, maximal on the gums around the teeth. It does not occur in edentulous mouths.

Aetiology

The organisms are Vincent's spirochaetes and fusiform bacilli, which are frequently present as commensals in normal mouths. The factors leading to their pathogenicity remain unknown but a symbiotic effect of the two organisms is apparent.

Appearances

Widespread, irregular, painful ulceration with slough formation, involving the gum margins and resulting, in untreated cases, in progressive destruction of gum tissues and much necrosis.

Results

The condition rapidly clears with antibiotic therapy but repeated relapses are common.

Herpetic stomatitis

Aetiology

The virus of herpes simplex.

Pathogenesis

The lesions are very commonly associated with infections of the upper respiratory tract and pneumonia. It is believed that the virus is present in a dormant state in the squamous cells of many individuals and is activated by febrile illnesses.

Macroscopical

Multiple, small, clear, discrete vesicles on the lips, gums and oral mucosa, which after 24 hours rupture to form shallow ulcers. These become encrusted and are frequently secondarily infected.

Microscopical

Intra-epidermal vesicle formation with swelling and enlargement of the squamous cells in some of which nuclear inclusions may be seen.

Results

Locally these painful lesions heal spontaneously. The virus may also affect the cornea, brain and genital tract (see p. 210).

Aphthous stomatitis

Aetiology

Unknown.

Appearances

Multiple, small, painful, shallow ulcers on the tip of the tongue, floor or elsewhere in the mouth. Histological appearances are of non-specific inflammation.

Results

Often resistant to treatment, these ulcers pursue a chronic course but have no significant sequelae.

Oral moniliasis

Aetiology
The disease is due to *Candida albicans*, but the precise pathogenesis remains obscure. Many cases occur in children but, when adults are infected, they are frequently debilitated or the condition follows antibiotic, immunosuppressive or steroid administration.

Appearances
Multiple white patches on the mucosal surfaces, particularly the tonsils, which leave a bleeding surface on scraping—*thrush*. There is an acute inflammatory reaction with the yeasts visible on direct examination or on culture.

Results
This usually remains a superficial infection which is commonly difficult to eradicate. Spread to the oesophagus or respiratory tract may occur (see p. 22) and occasionally systemic infection follows.

Tuberculosis
A rare buccal manifestation due to infection from a tuberculous pulmonary focus. A tuberculous ulcer may be present on the lip, tongue or tonsil and produces a painful, watery, irregular ulcer with slightly undermined edges. Biopsy is the usual method of diagnosis, but when suspected, smears and cultural methods may demonstrate the organisms.

Actinomycosis

Incidence
Cervicofacial actinomycosis accounts for at least 50% of all cases of infection by *Actinomyces israeli*.

Macroscopical
The mouth or jaw, commonly a tooth socket, is the primary site, with direct extension to involve the skin surface. This becomes red–blue with multiple hard nodules and marked surrounding very firm induration. Multiple sinuses of face, mouth, jaw or neck develop, from which the pathognomonic 'sulphur granules' may be expressed.

Microscopical
An intense polymorph infiltration around colonies of the fungus, surrounded by dense fibrosis.

Results
From this cervicofacial site the process may remain localized, spread to the lungs, or become disseminated by the blood stream (see p. 399). Local deformity is usually marked unless treated by appropriate antibiotics.

Cancrum oris

Aetiology
A rare gangrenous condition of the mouth, usually in children in whom it is preceded by a debilitating illness or malnutrition. The organisms involved are the normal commensals of the area and sometimes additionally anaerobic streptococci which have a synergistic effect.

Appearances
A rapidly spreading necrotizing or frankly gangrenous inflammation with only a sparse inflammatory cell response.

Syphilis

Primary
A chancre may occur on the lip, tongue, or even tonsil.

Secondary
Linear superficial ulcers with irregular margins occur on the mucous membranes—'snail-track' ulcers.

Tertiary
Three lesions of tertiary syphilis may affect the tongue.
1 *Leukoplakia* (see p. 13).
2 *Gumma*: a typical punched-out ulcer with a wash-leather slough in the base, most common on the dorsum of the tongue.
3 *Chronic interstitial inflammation*: the tongue may be hard and involved by a diffuse syphilitic inflammatory granulomatous reaction.

Congenital
Rhagades at the angle of the mouth or occasionally a gumma.

Miscellaneous lesions in the mouth

Infections
1 *Measles*: Koplik's spots on the buccal mucosa.
2 *Chickenpox*: small vesicles or a papular eruption.

3 *Diphtheria*: a grey membrane on the mucosa of the oropharynx.

4 *Scarlet fever*: 'strawberry tongue' with prominence of papillae, is associated with this infection by erythrogenic strains of β-haemolytic streptococci.

Blood diseases

1 *Iron deficiency anaemia*: atrophic glossitis with a smooth pale tongue—Plummer–Vinson syndrome (see p. 24).

2 *Pernicious anaemia*: smooth red tongue with pallor of mucous membranes (see p. 27).

3 *Leukaemia*: the lymphoid tissue of the oropharynx may enlarge or ulcerate, especially in acute leukaemia. Hyperplastic ulcerative gum lesions may be a presenting feature of the disease.

4 *Agranulocytosis*: pharyngeal ulceration is a common feature.

5 *Infectious mononucleosis*: pharyngeal ulceration with the membrane mimicking diphtheria is frequent in the 'anginose' type (see p. 268).

6 *Polycythaemia*: reddish blue discoloration of the tongue.

7 *Osler's familial telangiectasia*: multiple small spider-like vascular dilatations of mucosal blood vessels.

8 *Thrombocytopenic purpura*: multiple petechial haemorrhages of skin and mucosae.

Vitamin deficiency diseases

1 *Vitamin B complex*—angular cheilosis.
 (a) Nicotinic acid—angular cheilosis and a red beefy tongue with atrophy of papillae.
 (b) Riboflavine—atrophic glossitis, angular cheilosis and gingivo-stomatitis.

2 *Vitamin C*: gingivitis, with swollen haemorrhagic gums and loose teeth, occurs in scurvy (see p. 298).

Pigmentations

1 *Metals*: prolonged industrial or therapeutic exposure to metals may produce pigmentation and gingivitis: arsenic—black line; bismuth—black line; lead—blue–grey line; mercury—grey–violet line; silver—grey line.

2 *Addison's disease*: patches of brown–black melanotic pigmentation of the buccal mucosa.

3 *Haemochromatosis*: bronze colour.

4 *Peutz–Jegher's syndrome*: mouth and lip melanin pigmentation associated with congenital polyposis of the intestinal tract (see p. 43).

Leukoplakia

Nature
Hyperplasia of the squamous epithelium with hyperkeratosis producing raised white plaques. Related conditions also occur on the vulva (p. 208) and in the larynx.

Age
Rare under 30, the majority occur at about 50 years of age.

Sites
The most common site is the tongue, but the lips, gums, cheeks and floor of mouth may also be involved.

Aetiology
A small percentage are syphilitic in origin, but otherwise the aetiology is obscure. Dental sepsis, pipe smoking, trauma from teeth and dental plates, electrical currents from fillings of dissimilar metals, vitamin A deficiency and hormonal factors, may all be contributory.

Macroscopical
The process starts as an area of surface thickening which is white and raised. At a later stage, multiple foci may coalesce to form a large area which becomes rough, white and fissured—'coat of white paint'. Carcinoma may subsequently develop, usually in one of the fissures.

Microscopical
The white appearance is due to surface keratin and hyperplasia of the prickle and basal cell layers to form atypical thickened rete pegs which extend downwards into the underlying tissues. There is also increased fibrosis and a lymphocyte and plasma cell infiltrate in the dermis. Varying grades of epithelial dysplasia give prognostic assistance in respect of the risk of malignancy.

Results
Leukoplakia should be regarded as precancerous since carcinoma will ultimately develop in approximately 5% of cases. The time interval, however, is very variable.

Carcinoma of tongue

Incidence
Tumours of the mouth, including tongue, lip and pharynx, account for about 2% of malignant tumours in Caucasians but very much higher in Asians.

Age
Average 55 years of age.

Sex
Male : female, 9 : 1.

Sites
Sixty-five per cent arise on the lateral borders of the tongue; approximately 70% on the anterior two-thirds.

Predisposing factors
Leukoplakia predisposes to tongue cancer and is present in many cases. Betel chewers have a high incidence and the Plummer–Vinson syndrome predisposes in women.

Macroscopical
The tumours may be papillary, nodular, diffuse, fissured or ulcerated, with an area of leukoplakia frequently visible at the periphery.

Microscopical
Usually keratinizing squamous cell carcinoma but poorly differentiated types, including a lymphoepithelioma, do occur, especially in the posterior third (see below).

Spread
Direct spread through the tongue results in fixation to adjacent structures, e.g. floor of mouth. Approximately 50% of patients have evidence of lymph node metastases in the cervical glands when first diagnosed and, at death, 40% have evidence of blood-borne metastases in lungs, liver or other viscera.

Prognosis
This is poor; tumours of the anterior two-thirds have a 5-year survival of 20%; of the posterior third 12%. Most of the long-term survivors are stage 1 cases, i.e. growth restricted to the tongue.

Carcinoma of floor of mouth, cheek, palate

Age
Average age is about 60 years.

Predisposing factors
As for tongue (see above).

Structure
The tumours are keratinizing squamous cell carcinomas; only rarely are they undifferentiated.

Prognosis
Five-year survival figures are: floor of mouth, 17%; cheek, 14%; palate, 14%.

Carcinoma of pharynx and tonsil

Types
The commonest tumours are keratinizing squamous cell carcinomas, but in addition in this region there are undifferentiated types.

'Transitional cell' carcinoma
Composed of sheets and strands of undifferentiated epithelial cells with a palisade arrangement at the periphery mimicking to some extent the true transitional epithelial tumours seen in the urinary tract. There are no prickle cells and keratin formation is not seen.

Lymphoepithelioma
A tumour in which there are sheets of undifferentiated tumour cells intermingled with a diffuse lymphocytic infiltrate. These tumours present at a younger age (30–40), usually with enlarged regional lymph nodes. The primary lesion in the nasopharynx or tonsil is usually very small and readily missed clinically. They are extremely radiosensitive tumours but are rarely radiocurable.

'Transitional cell' carcinoma and lymphoepithelioma are variants of squamous cell tumours.

Spread
Direct spread plays an important part at this site due to the close proximity of the base of the skull which is invaded at an early stage. The tumours frequently, therefore, cause cranial nerve palsies. Lymphatic and blood dissemination occur early, consequently the prognosis is poor.

Prognosis
Pharynx and tonsil—10% 5-year survival.

Verrucous carcinoma
This variant of squamous cell carcinoma usually shows a surface type of papillary mucosal spread and little pleomorphism or mitotic activity. Histological diagnosis on small superficial biopsies may be very difficult. Change to an aggressive spindle cell carcinoma may be radiation-induced.

Gums

Inflammation
Any of the inflammatory processes described on p. 11 may involve the gums. In addition there is the condition of pyorrhoea.

Pyorrhoea

Nature
A progressive inflammatory gingivitis involving the periodontal tissues, resulting in bone destruction, loss of the tooth-bearing tissues and eventual loss of teeth. The condition is often associated with poor dental hygiene.

Appearances
Starts as a non-specific gingivitis which then involves the gingival sulcus to produce a periodontal pocket. Suppuration occurs in the pocket and destroys the gum margin. Underlying bone is also destroyed, resulting in exposure of the tooth roots and loss of tooth-holding tissues. Eventually the tooth is loosened and falls out.

Swellings

Epilepsy therapy
Swellings of the gums occurs in many epileptic patients treated by diphenylhydantoin sodium.

Scurvy
Vitamin C deficiency with spongy scorbutic gums.

Epulis
Localized swellings of the gum which are of different histological types.
1 *Myeloid or giant cell epulis—peripheral giant cell granuloma*: a squamous-covered nodule of cellular fibroblastic tissue containing many giant cells. These are of foreign-body type and are smaller than osteoclasts. The lesion is reactive.
2 *Fibrous epulis*: a squamous-covered nodule of benign, but often vascular, fibrous tissue.
3 *Haemangiomatous epulis*: this squamous-covered nodule is composed of extremely vascular tissue and commonly arises during pregnancy—'pregnancy tumour'. Sometimes there is ulceration of the epithelium with an inflammatory reaction and the nodule is then called 'granuloma pyogenicum'.
4 *'Myoblastoma' epulis*: a rare epulis composed of pink-staining granular cells which form small lumps in children. The tumours may occur on the tongue, gum or elsewhere in the body. They are frequently associated with thickening of the overlying squamous epithelium. The 'myoblasts' are of uncertain origin, but are probably derived from Schwann cells. The lesions are benign and excision is curative.

B/JAW, SALIVARY GLANDS

Jaw
    Tumours of dental tissues
    Inflammations
    Tumours of the jaw
Salivary glands
    Inflammations
    Benign lymphoepithelial lesion
    Mucous gland tumours

Jaw

Normal tooth development
A tooth is derived from two germ layers:
1 The ectodermal dental lamina derived from oral squamous epithelium forms a downgrowth to produce the bell-shaped enamel organ (see Fig. 1). The enamel organ has an inner layer of cells which form the enamel—ameloblasts. The remainder of the organ, including the stellate reticulum forming the bulk of the structure, does not form enamel but persists as the sheath of Hertwig in the periodontal membrane around the fully formed tooth. Small epithelial foci may persist as the rests of Malassez. In addition, the cells of the dental lamina may not completely disappear but may remain as the epithelial islands of Serres.
2 The mesodermal dental papilla forms the dentine, cementum and pulp of the tooth (see Fig. 1).

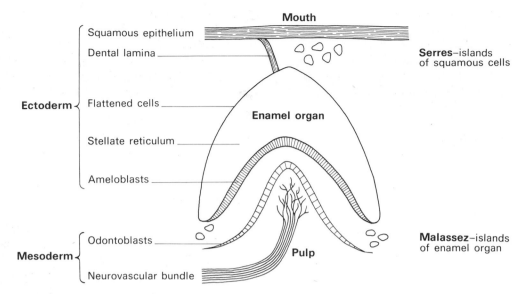

Fig. 1 Development of a tooth.

Tumours of dental tissues

Due to inductive changes exerted by dental tissues on each other, this is a very complex group. Many of the lesions are not true tumours in the neoplastic sense but are developmental anomalies or overgrowths. The term odontogenic tumours is used here in its broadest sense. Many are very rare and incompletely documented in respect of natural history but the WHO classification is, at present, the most logical, in that it groups the various lesions according to their structural characteristics.

Lesions consisting of odontogenic epithelium

Ameloblastoma—adamantinoma

This relatively common true tumour accounts for 1% of all oral tumours; average age 33 years and 80% in the mandible. There is wide geographical variability in incidence which is much greater in Africans. The tumour is slow growing, may reach a very large size and is commonly polycystic. There is a very common association with an unerupted tooth and it is widely believed that the tumour may arise in a pre-existing dentigerous cyst. Histological appearances are of epidermal epithelial cells resembling ameloblasts surrounding a central core of stellate reticulum which forms microcysts due to degeneration. Histogenetically, the tumour almost certainly arises from the

enamel organ. Whilst largely expansile in growth, local invasion can occur but metastasis is exceptionally rare. Recurrence after curettage is frequent but permanent cure is usually achieved by formal resection.

Adenomatoid odontogenic tumour

A variably cystic/solid, benign, truly neoplastic tumour mostly in the maxilla of young persons in the second or third decade and with an epithelial duct-like histological appearance which probably represents abortive attempts to form enamel organs.

Calcifying epithelial tumour—Pindborg tumour

A potentially recurrent, locally destructive true tumour, consisting of sheets of polyhedral epithelial cells of epidermal characteristics in an eosinophilic matrix in which extensive calcium deposition occurs in a concentric manner. The lesions usually contain an unerupted tooth, present at an average age of 42 years, and probably develop from the residual enamel epithelium of this associated tooth.

Lesions consisting of odontogenic epithelium and mesenchyme

Ameloblastic fibroma and ameloblastic sarcoma

The fibroma is a soft solid mass expanding bone but

non-invasive. Ameloblastic-like epithelium is embedded in an abundant fibroblastic stroma resembling the dental papilla. In the rare sarcoma this stroma shows frank malignant appearances.

Lesions consisting of odontogenic epithelium and calcified dental tissues

Odonto-ameloblastoma
A mixture of odontogenic epithelium with mature enamel and dentine.

Lesions consisting of calcified dental tissues but without odontogenic epithelium

Complex odontome
A tumour-like mass of enamel, dentine and cementum deposited in a irregular manner.

Compound odontome
More highly organized, the enamel and dentine forming recognizable tooth-like structures.

Dens invaginatus
A developmental malformation in which an invagination of enamel is formed in a tooth.

Enameloma
A malformation consisting of ectopic deposits of enamel on a tooth.

Dentinoma
A tumour-like lesion composed of dentine.

Cementoma
A fibrous lesion containing cementum.

Lesions consisting of odontogenic mesenchyme

Fibroma and myxoma
These resemble similarly named lesions elsewhere in the body.

Cysts of odontogenic origin
1 *Odontogenic keratocyst*: this term largely replaces the use of '*primordial cyst*', though some true examples of this developmental condition in childhood in which no tooth remains, only degenerate stellate reticulum, do occur.

2 *Calcifying odontogenic cyst*: a benign intraosseous or gingival cystic lesion showing histological similarity to ameloblastoma but with characteristic keratinous ghost cells and masses with accompanying foreign-body giant cells and focal calcification. Though often poorly circumscribed the consensus view is that this is not a neoplasm.

3 *Dentigerous cyst*: an epithelial-lined cyst around an unerupted tooth and which may be associated with development of ameloblastoma or of a calcifying epithelial tumour.

Non-odontogenic cysts
1 *Radicular cysts*: these common periapical cysts are the end-result of caries and pulp death with production of granulation tissue.
2 *Fissured cysts*: these probably arise from entrapped epithelium at suture lines.

Inflammations
Both acute and chronic osteomyelitis may occur in the jaw bones, in the mandible usually associated with tooth infection, and in the maxilla with either tooth or sinus infection.

Leontiasis osseum—'lion face'
This deformity of the maxilla and nose may be caused by a low-grade chronic inflammation of the bone or by fibrous dysplasia, although Paget's disease of bone may produce an identical clinical picture. Also see leprosy, p. 3.

Tumours of the jaw
Tumours of jaw are infrequent but, in addition to the tumours of dental tissues mentioned above, the following types may be found:
1 *Skeletal tissues*:
   (a) *Bone tumours*: osteoma; osteosarcoma.
   (b) *Cartilaginous tumours*: chondroma; chondrosarcoma.
   (c) *Giant cell lesions*: giant cell variants; reparative granuloma.
2 *Soft tissues within bone*:
   (a) *Fibrous tissue*: fibroma; ossifying fibroma; fibrosarcoma.
   (b) *Blood vessels*: haemangioma; angiosarcoma.
   (c) *Nerve tissue*: neurofibroma; neurofibrosarcoma.
   (d) *Marrow cells*: myeloma; Ewing's tumour; lymphoma.

Thus, any tumour which is encountered elsewhere in the skeleton may occur in the jaws and detailed descriptions will be avoided, except where they are pertinent to the jaw lesion (see p. 302–309).

Skeletal tissues

Bony tumours
The osteoma is usually of the ivory type and the osteosarcoma is frequently associated with Paget's disease of bone.

Cartilaginous tumours
Chondromas occur in the lower jaw but are rare. Chondrosarcoma may also be associated with Paget's disease.

Giant cell lesions
It was formerly stated that giant cell tumours frequently arose in the jaw. This true tumour entity is in fact an extreme rarity in the jaw bones, but 'giant cell variants', all of which are benign, are common. A giant cell epulis has to be distinguished from the true osteoclastoma and there is also the condition of 'reparative granuloma'—central giant cell granuloma. This is a destructive osteolytic lesion in the jaws of young adults consisting of a cellular fibroblastic stroma in which there are red cells and haemosiderin, some foam cells and giant cells which simulate osteoclasts but which are phagocytic. This lesion, which mimics a giant cell tumour, is probably a reactive process and is benign. Other giant cell variants may occur in the jaw and are considered on p. 306.

Soft tissues

Fibrous lesions
'Fibromas', many of which show ossification, are common in the jaw and various names have been attached to the lesions. They form radiotranslucent swellings with a mottled appearance due to new bone formation. Histologically, they are composed of fibrous tissue in the pure fibroma, with osteoid tissue or bone in the ossifying fibromas. Most authorities regard them all as variants of fibrous dysplasia (see p. 296).

Blood vessels
Haemangioma and its malignant counterpart, angiosarcoma are rare in the jaw.

Nerve tissue
The inferior dental nerve is incorporated within the mandibular canal and from this nerve, neurofibromas or malignant nerve sheath tumours may arise.

Marrow cells
The jaw may occasionally be the site of involvement by malignant marrow cell tumours, e.g. myeloma, lymphoma and Ewing's tumour (see p. 307).

Salivary glands

Introduction
Mucous glands are widespread throughout the upper alimentary and respiratory tracts. Large aggregations occur in the major salivary glands—parotid, submandibular and sublingual; minor collections are numerous in the mouth, palate, lip, cheek, nose, larynx, pharynx, whilst the trachea and major bronchi and the lacrimal glands contain similar mucous glands.

Whilst most attention is usually focused on the major salivary glands, diseases affecting these organs commonly produce similar changes in any mucous gland at any site.

Congenital
Congenital abnormalities are rare, but include atresias and anomalies of the ducts. Occasionally, one or more glands may be absent.

Inflammations—sialodenitis

Non-specific

Acute suppurative
This usually occurs in debilitated individuals, particularly children. The exact pathogenesis is obscure but there seems little doubt that the pyogenic organisms gain access to the glands via the duct from the mouth. In severe cases, frank suppuration with abscess formation may occur with destruction of the gland.

Chronic
This is usually associated with duct calculi but occasionally can arise de novo as necrotizing sialometaplasia, a condition of obscure origin where florid metaplastic changes lead to diagnostic difficulties.

Specific

Mumps

The diffuse interstitial parotid inflammation in mumps is usually bilateral but occasionally unilateral. In 20% the submandibular and other salivary glands are involved (see p. 199).

Granulomatous

Tuberculosis or actinomycosis may rarely involve salivary glands. Salivary gland involvement by sarcoidosis is rather more frequent.

Cytomegalovirus

Nature

A rare disease of infancy and childhood characterized by the presence of inclusion bodies in the nucleus and cytoplasm of the epithelial cells of salivary glands, renal tubules, septal cells of the lungs and less commonly in other sites. Infection may also become established in any age group in patients receiving immunosuppressive therapy.

Aetiology

The cytomegalovirus.

Appearances

The affected cells, particularly in the salivary glands, are grossly swollen and contain large inclusion bodies in the nucleus and cytoplasm.

Effects

The clinical pattern and course are extremely variable, the usual manifestations being of a blood dyscrasia and hepatomegaly. When the salivary glands only are affected, the disease is of no significance, but when of widespread distribution, death may result.

Sialolithiasis

Stone formation in the duct results in acute or chronic sialoadenitis with eventual atrophy of the salivary gland acini. The submandibular duct is the most common site. The pathogenesis of the calculi is obscure.

Benign lymphoepithelial lesion—Sjögren's syndrome

Nature

Salivary gland enlargement characterized histologically by atrophy of glandular parenchyma and lymphocytic infiltration with epimyothelial islands replacing the intralobular ducts.

Types

Primary—an exocrine destructive lesion without associated evidence of a connective tissue disease and leading to destruction of glandular tissue with resulting mucosal dryness—*sicca complex*. This is a lymphocyte-mediated disorder. *Secondary*—there is associated connective tissue disease (lupus erythematosus or rheumatoid disease) with presence of auto-immune antibodies and hyperglobulinaemia.

Incidence

Largely in the middle-aged with a female preponderance.

Macroscopical

Affected glands are painless and have usually progressively enlarged. One or more parotid, submandibular and lacrimal glands are most typically involved. The lesion may be diffuse or discretely nodular with a rubbery whitish cut surface and retention of the normal lobular pattern.

Microscopical

Glandular atrophy, lymphocytic infiltration usually without follicle formation and duct proliferation forming the epimyothelial islands.

Course

Slowly progressive benign course with a significant risk of development of lymphoma.

Cysts

Non-neoplastic cysts of retention type are common in minor glands but rare in the major where occasionally they can be clinically mistaken for tumours.

Mucous gland tumours

Epithelial tumours

Adenomas

Pleomorphic adenoma—'mixed tumour'
Incidence. The most common tumour of salivary glands. About 70% of parotid gland tumours are of this type and it is 10 times more frequent in the parotid gland than in the submandibular.

Age
Increasing with age from 25 years onwards.

Sex
Male : female, 3 : 4.

Macroscopical. A lobulated, firm circumscribed tumour within the salivary gland. The cut surface often glistens and appears semi-translucent.

Microscopical. A very variable appearance of differing arrangements of epithelial cells in ductular or acinar patterns with associated myoepithelial cell proliferation and the presence of luminal mucin and areas of cartilage in the stroma which is probably produced by the myoepithelial cells. There is a thin fibrous capsule through which extensions of new lobules of tumour grow, rendering complete excision by enucleation impossible.

Results. Growth is slow and by expansion and if surgical excision is performed with a margin of salivary gland tissue, cure results. Local recurrence is quite frequent following enucleation and may be subsequently very troublesome and difficult to effect a cure without severe mutilation. Malignant change can infrequently occur (see p. 21).—*Carcinoma ex mixed tumour.*

Monomorphic adenomas
Adenolymphoma
1 *Incidence*—about 8% of parotid gland tumours, rare in the submandibular and minor salivary glands.
2 *Age*—35–80 years.
3 *Sex*—Male : female, 5 : 1.
4 *Macroscopical*—variably cystic, smooth surfaced, ovoid and moderately firm, usually situated near the gland surface and not uncommonly multiple.
5 *Microscopical*—the cystic spaces are lined by papillary adenomatous tissue with variable amounts of lymphocytic infiltration, including follicles, in the stroma. The epithelium is double-layered with a tall, very regular, characteristic eosinophilic inner layer.
6 *Results*—these tumours are benign. Similar lesions are occasionally found within lymph nodes adjacent to the parotid gland and in the upper cervical groups. These also behave innocently.

Oxyphilic adenoma. This benign, encapsulated, uncommon tumour is composed of regular acini of large eosinophilic cells—*oncocytes*. It is nearly always in the parotid where it forms 1% of tumours of this gland.

Other adenomas. Rare benign epithelial tumours include: tubular, clear-cell, basal-cell, trabecular and sebaceous adenomas.

Mucoepidermoid tumour

Incidence
About 8% of major salivary gland tumours, 90% in the parotids and nearly all the remainder in the submandibular gland.

Age
Most 20–60 years but occasionally in children.

Sex
Male : female equal.

Macroscopical
Solitary, locally infiltrative, solid or partially cystic.

Microscopical
A mixture of mucus-secreting and squamous epithelial cells with cysts containing thick mucin.

Results
Radical removal leads to cure in 85%. In some patients growth and local infiltration is rapid and in others cervical lymph node or visceral metastatic spread may occur.

Acinic cell tumour
This rather rare tumour accounts for about 2% of parotid gland tumours and is even less common in the submandibular. More frequent in males (3 : 1) they may occur at almost any age. The tumour is composed of epithelial cells resembling the salivary serous cells and with basophilic granular cytoplasm. Results of surgical removal are good with 80% 5-year survival, but local recurrence and, in 5–10% of patients, local lymph node or distant metastases, indicate the malignant potential.

Carcinomas

Adenoid cystic carcinoma—cylindroma—
adenocystic carcinoma
An infiltrative malignant tumour of characteristic

cribriform pattern composed of two cell types, duct-lining cells and myoepithelial cells. The fibrous stroma is commonly very hyaline and marginal and perineural lymphatic invasion is usually prominent. The tumour is more common in females in the 40–60 age group and forms 4% of parotid gland tumours. It is relatively more common in submandibular gland (10%) and forms 60–70% of malignant tumours of minor salivary glands, e.g. palate, lip, tongue and respiratory tract. Growth is slow and lymphatic and blood-borne metastases are late, with 5-year survival figures of 70% but 20-year survival of 13%. The best results occur in patients in whom the tumour is widely locally excised at the first attempt.

Other carcinomas
Adenocarcinoma, squamous cell and undifferentiated carcinomas arise *de novo* or on the basis of a pre-existing pleomorphic adenoma. They are obviously infiltrative and of poor prognosis with 5-year survival of only 25% and 50% of these patients die from distant metastases.

Non-epithelial tumours
Connective tissue tumours within the glands are uncommon with the exception, in young children, of haemangioma and lymphangioma; lipomas and neurofibromas occasionally occur.

C/GASTROINTESTINAL TRACT, OESOPHAGUS

Oesophagus
  Oesophagitis
  Barrett's oesophagus
  Tumours
  Carcinoma
  Disorders of wall

Structure of gut wall
The gut from the oesophagus to the anal canal is composed of the same four layers. The type of mucosa varies with the site and is related to the function of the gut at each level; the other layers are similar at all sites (see Fig. 2).

Basic classification of disorders
In all parts of the gastrointestinal tract, most pathological conditions can be divided into:

1 Mucosal diseases—most of which are:
  (a) Inflammations—which may be due to: (i) microbial agents, (ii) chemical injury, (iii) idiopathic.
  (b) Tumours—benign, malignant.
2 Diseases of the wall—including stricture, perforation, hernia, diverticula, neoplasms.
3 Motility disorders.
4 Vascular abnormalities.

Functions
1 Propulsion and storage of contents.
2 Secretion of enzymes.
3 Digestion of food material within the lumen.
4 Absorption of water, electrolytes and digested food.
5 Maintenance of mucosal integrity, including cell proliferation and immunological defences.
6 Regulation of the above functions, hormonal and neurological.
  Throughout the gastrointestinal tract, the clinical effects of pathology are related to the function of the part of the tract affected.

Development of gastrointestinal pathology
Knowledge of gastrointestinal pathology has grown in stepwise fashion following advances in techniques for investigation of the gastrointestinal tract.
1 *Pre-1940s.* Pathology study was restricted to surgical and autopsy specimens. Detailed descriptions of peptic ulcer disease, gastric and large bowel cancers were made, and inflammatory conditions of stomach and large bowel recognized. Infective conditions, e.g. TB, typhoid were relatively common, and their morphology described from autopsy material.
2 *1940s–1970s.* Rigid endoscopes were introduced allowing direct visualization and biopsy of oesophagus, gastric corpus, sigmoid colon and rectum. This allowed the microscopic features of some gastric and rectal disorders to be determined. Capsule biopsy of small intestinal mucosa was developed in the 1960s–1970s, allowing the diagnosis of coeliac disease. Investigation of other sites was still dependent on radiology.
3 *Mid-1970s—present.* Introduction of flexible, fibre-optic endoscopes enabled the whole stomach, duodenum, and colon to be visualized and biopsied, with increasing use of biopsy for diagnostic purposes in, e.g. inflammatory bowel disease, and malignancy. Prevention of malignancy by surveillance of patients with premalignant conditions (e.g. familial adenomatous

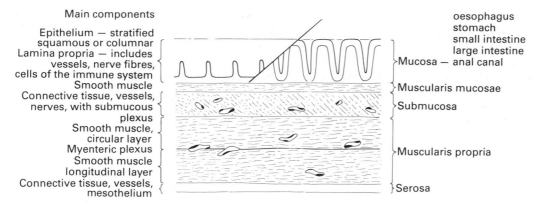

Main components

Epithelium — stratified
squamous or columnar
Lamina propria — includes
vessels, nerve fibres,
cells of the immune system
Smooth muscle
Connective tissue, vessels,
nerves, with submucous
plexus
Smooth muscle,
circular layer
Myenteric plexus
Smooth muscle
longitudinal layer
Connective tissue, vessels,
mesothelium

oesophagus
stomach
small intestine
large intestine
Mucosa — anal canal

Muscularis mucosae

Submucosa

Muscularis propria

Serosa

Fig. 2 Structure of the wall of the gastrointestinal tract.

polyposis, Barrett's oesophagus, ulcerative colitis) can be undertaken. Video-endoscopy now being introduced improves endoscopic visualization of the mucosa, and images can be recorded for comparison with subsequent examination and for training purposes.

Oesophagus
(See Fig. 3)

Oesophagitis
Inflammation in the oesophagus may be caused by:
1 *Acid reflux* through the gastro-oesophogeal junction, the most common (see below).
2 *Ingestion of irritants.*
3 *Infections*:
  (a) Fungal—Candida ⎫ occur in immuno-
  (b) Viral—CMV, HSV ⎭ compromised hosts.
  (c) Bacterial—rare.
4 *Physical*—radiation.
5 Association with skin disease, e.g. pemphigoid, pemphigus (see p. 414), lichen planus.
6 *Graft-versus-host disease.*

Reflux oesophagitis
Reflux of gastric contents into the distal oesophagus is a common physiological occurrence. When this happens to a pathological degree in terms of frequency and duration, reflux oesophagitis results.

Diagnosis
1 pH monitoring—the gold standard.
2 Endoscopy and biopsy.

Appearances
Histological changes are as follows:
1 Thickened basal zone of epithelium.
2 Elongated lamina propria papillae.
3 Vasodilatation.
4 Inflammatory cell infiltrate.
In practice the correlation of these with reflux as measured by pH monitoring is variable; a thickened basal zone is often present in normal people.

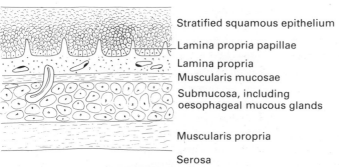

Stratified squamous epithelium

Lamina propria papillae

Lamina propria
Muscularis mucosae
Submucosa, including
oesophageal mucous glands

Muscularis propria

Serosa

Fig. 3 Oesophageal histology.

Complications

1 Ulceration—a type of peptic ulceration.
2 Scarring, leading to stricture formation.
3 Barrett's oesophagus.

Barrett's oesophagus

This is a metaplastic change of the lower oesophageal epithelium from squamous to columnar in type, first described by Barrett in 1957. It is diagnosed by endoscopy with biopsy > 3 cm above the gastro-oesophageal junction.

Frequency

Ten per cent of patients with symptomatic reflux oesophagitis

Appearances

Three types of columnar epithelium are recognized:
1 Gastric body.
2 Gastric cardia.
3 Intestinal—analogous to 'incomplete' type of intestinal metaplasia in the stomach (see p. 27).

Important as a marker of gastro-oesophageal reflux and as a premalignant condition.

Risk of malignancy

Patients with Barrett's oesophagus have an increased risk of developing adenocarcinoma. This arises following a series of changes from metaplastic glandular epithelium—particularly 'intestinal' type, through dysplasia to intramucosal and finally invasive adenocarcinoma. The risk of developing adenocarcinoma is not considered sufficient to screen regularly for this complication by endoscopy. However, if high-grade dysplasia is found by endoscopy, oesophagectomy should be considered.

Tumours

Benign

These are uncommon, and may be:
1 *Derived from epithelium*—squamous papilloma.
2 *Derived from oesophageal wall*—lipoma, leiomyoma, neurofibroma, haemangioma.

Malignant

1 Squamous cell carcinoma.
2 Adenocarcinoma.
3 Rare types—carcinosarcoma, melanoma, adenocarcinoma of middle third, derived from oesophageal glands, including adenoid cystic carcinoma and mucoepidermoid carcinoma, malignant stromal tumours, e.g. leiomyosarcoma.

Squamous cell carcinoma

Epidemiology

This is one of the gastrointestinal malignancies which shows a remarkable geographic variation in its incidence—up to 500 times variation in incidence between high- and low-risk areas.
1 *High-risk areas*—include parts of China, Iran and Africa.
2 *Low-risk areas*—most of Europe and North America.

Such variation implies the presence of environmental risk factors for the disease.

In the UK, major risk factors are: age, male sex, alcohol, smoking. In high-incidence countries abroad, proposed additional aetiological factors include: fungal contamination of diet and low vitamin intake.

Appearances

Although squamous cell carcinoma develops from a sequence of changes through dysplasia and carcinoma *in situ*, most are diagnosed at a late stage, when there is already invasion of muscle.

Macroscopical

1 The carcinoma may be polypoid, ulcerated or diffusely infiltrative.
2 Many are inoperable due to direct infiltration of the adjacent mediastinal structures.
3 Metastases to lymph nodes are common, including mediastinal and cervical groups.

Microscopical

Tumours may be well differentiated and keratinizing, or poorly differentiated, where intercellular bridges and keratin formation are difficult to find.

Submucosal infiltration beyond macroscopic tumour is common, therefore examination of resection margins in surgical specimens is important to determine completeness of excision.

Adenocarcinoma

Incidence

These tumours account for 10% of oesophageal malignancies and develop from Barrett's oesophagus as described above. They occur in the distal oeso-phagus, and spread by direct infiltration into medias-tinal structures. Lymph node metastases are common.

Prognosis of oesophageal carcinoma
This is poor for any type of carcinoma, with 5% 5-year survival.

Disorders of the oesophageal wall

Achalasia

Nature
Failure of relaxation of the lower oesophageal sphinc-ter, resulting in progressive dilatation of the oeso-phagus.

Appearances
1 Loss of ganglion cells in dilated segment.
2 Secondary changes in oesophageal wall—ulceration, fibrosis and carcinoma in up to 5%.
3 May be caused by *Trypanosoma cruzi* in South America (see p. 7).

Hiatus hernia
This herniation of part of stomach, through the oesophageal hiatus in the diaphragm, may be congen-ital (see below) or acquired, of which two types are recognized:
1 Sliding—90%.
2 Para-oesophageal—rolling, in 10%.

The diagnosis is commonly by radiology. Many cases so demonstrated are asymptomatic but may be associated with complications of gastro-oesophageal reflux—sliding type.

Hiatus hernias are difficult to identify at post mortem following the relaxation of muscular struc-tures.

Diverticulum
There are two types of oesophageal diverticula:
1 *'Pulsion' type*: pressure from within the oeso-phagus creates a diverticulum through a weakness in the cricopharyngeus muscle.
2 *'Traction' type*: formed by tension on the oeso-phageal wall from adherent inflammatory lesions, classically tuberculous lymph nodes.

Oesophageal webs and rings
These are localized constrictions of the oesophagus, due to mucosal folds/muscular contractions. The classical example of *Plummer–Vinsen syndrome*—the association of upper oesophageal web with iron deficiency anaemia in women, is now rarely seen.

Oesophageal perforation
This is rare, caused by:
1 Traumatic rupture, usually associated with vomit-ing. Lesser degrees may cause mucosal tearing—'Mallory–Weiss tear'—resulting in haemorrhage.
2 Impaction of sharp foreign body.
3 Intubation of strictures.

Oesophageal stricture

Causes
1 Any oesophageal tumour.
2 Stricture following oesophagitis (see p. 22).
3 Achalasia (see above).
4 Scleroderma (see p. 98).

Vascular disorders

Oesophageal varices

Nature
These are varicose, dilated, submucosal veins in the distal oesophagus.

Aetiology
In patients with liver disease which has caused portal hypertension (see p. 230), the existing portosystemic anastomoses in the oesophagus, distal rectum and umbilical veins provide a pathway for shunting high-pressure portal vein blood away from the liver. This is most evident in the distal oesophagus, where the submucosal veins become dilated and engorged.

Appearances
1 Varices are visible by endoscopy, but may be difficult to detect at post mortem.
2 Distended thin-walled vessels are susceptible to rupture resulting in severe haemorrhage; this is the cause of death in 50% of patients with advanced liver disease.

D/GASTROINTESTINAL TRACT, STOMACH

Structure and functions
Gastritis
Intestinal metaplasia
Peptic ulceration
Tumours

Structure and functions
(See Fig. 4)
1 The mucosa of the cardia and the antrum produce mucus and alkaline secretion. The fundus and body secrete acid, vitamin B_{12} produced by parietal cells and pepsin from chief cells, as well as mucus.
2 The sack-like configuration of the stomach is capable of considerable distension to act as a reservoir for ingested food.
3 The digestive process begins in the stomach with the activity of acid and pepsin.
4 'Mucosal protection': the gastric mucosal lining is able to withstand the corrosive effects of a luminal pH below 2.5.
5 Neuroendocrine cells in the mucosa secrete hormones including gastrin and somatostatin with regulatory functions.

Gastritis

Nature
Gastritis is a commonly used word by:

1 Patients to indicate dyspeptic symptoms.
2 Endoscopists to describe reddened, 'inflamed' gastric mucosa.
3 Pathologists to describe the presence of excess inflammatory cells in the gastric mucosa.

The correlation between dyspeptic symptoms or endoscopic reddening with histological inflammation is far from complete. 'Gastritis' is used here to refer only to the histopathological changes.

Acute gastritis
Acute inflammation of the gastric mucosa is rarely encountered in gastric biopsies. Suggested causes include:
1 Alcohol.
2 Drugs.
3 Acute *Helicobacter pylori* infection (see below).

Acute haemorrhagic/erosive gastritis

Nature
This is the breakdown of superficial gastric mucosa with bleeding. If severe it develops into gastric erosions (see below). Inflammatory cells are sparse or absent.

Aetiology
Develops in association with:
1 Stress of burns/trauma.
2 Shock.

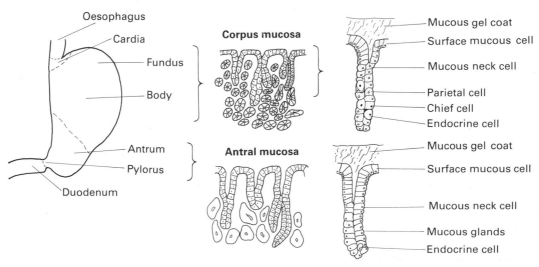

Fig. 4 Stomach—anatomy and histology.

3 Drug ingestion—aspirin, non-steroidal anti-inflammatory drugs (NSAIDs), cancer chemotherapy.
4 Heavy alcohol consumption.

Pathogenesis

1 *Mucosal ischaemia* is important in stress and shock when blood is shunted away from the superficial mucosa.
2 *Direct damage* to the surface is caused by alcohol or drugs, which impairs resistance to 'autodigestion'.

Results

When severe, acute gastric erosions develop, which may result in severe bleeding. Gastric erosions are defined as destruction of part of the thickness of the gastric mucosa, as distinct from gastric ulcers in which the full thickness of the mucosa/muscularis mucosae is destroyed.

Chronic gastritis

Nature

Chronic inflammation of the gastric mucosa is very common in the general population; its prevalence increases with age to over 50% in persons over 50 years old in developed countries. It is present in over 90% of patients with duodenal ulceration, about 70% with gastric ulceration and is also common in those with gastric cancer. However, in most people with chronic gastritis there is no other gastric pathology, and this condition is commonly asymptomatic.

Classification

Chronic gastritis can be divided into:
1 The commonest type, previously 'non-specific', which is now known to be associated with *Helicobacter pylori* infection.
2 Rare specific types, with characteristic histology.

Helicobacter-associated gastritis

Nature

The bacterium *H. pylori* was first cultured and characterized in 1982, and is now recognized to be present in > 90% of people with chronic gastritis. It is a curved, microaerophilic organism which is able to attach to the gastric surface epithelium, and persist in the stomach beneath the mucus layer where the pH is near neutral. Its presence results in an immune response in the gastric mucosa. *H. pylori* produces

enzymes, including a powerful urease, which may damage the epithelium and gastric mucus, but it does not invade the tissue. Once established, the infection persists for years but the mechanism by which the bacteria is able to evade the host's immune response is not yet understood.

Human ingestion of *H. pylori* results in gastritis, and eradication of *H. pylori* by antibacterial treatment results in resolution of gastritis, demonstrating its causal role.

Appearances

1 A mixed inflammatory cell infiltrate in mucosa, including neutrophils within the epithelium.
2 A variable degree of mucin depletion and damage to the surface epithelial cells.
3 The inflammation involves antral and body/fundic mucosa or antrum alone.
4 There may be any degree of atrophy of gastric glands and intestinal metaplasia (see p. 27)—both these features are commoner in older subjects.

Diagnosis

Helicobacter pylori may be detected by:
1 *Non-invasive techniques*
(a) *Urea breath test*: the urease enzyme produced by *H. pylori* splits the ingested dose of radiolabelled urea (containing carbon-13 or carbon-14) to produce labelled carbon dioxide which can be detected in the breath soon after the urea has been ingested.
(b) *Serology*: specific antibodies to *H. pylori* are present in the serum of infected individuals.
2 *Invasive techniques*:—requiring endoscopy and biopsy:
(a) *Microbiology*: *H. pylori* requires culture in microaerophilic conditions for 3–5 days. Culture is important for determining antibiotic sensitivity.
(b) *Histology*: *H. pylori* has a very characteristic appearance in gastric biopsies—numerous, monomorphic curved bacteria adjacent to the surface epithelium.
(c) *Biopsy urease test*: a biopsy is added to medium containing urea and an indicator. If urease produced by *H. pylori* is present the indicator changes colour due to the release of ammonia.

Course

The clinical importance of *H. pylori* infection is still much debated. Treatment by two or three antimicrobial agents—usually including a bismuth-containing compound, may be used for duodenal ulcer, some adults with 'non-ulcer dyspepsia' or children with epigastric pain.

Autoimmune chronic gastritis

Nature
This is an example of an organ-specific autoimmune disease. It is much less common than *Helicobacter*-associated gastritis, and affects mainly older women. In addition to autoantibodies to parietal cells and intrinsic factor, other autoantibodies may be present, and there is an increased incidence of autoimmunity in patients' relatives.

Appearances
1 The inflammation involves the fundic/body mucosa.
2 Autoantibodies against parietal cells and intrinsic factor are detectable in the blood—in 90% and 60% respectively.
3 The disease progresses to atrophy of the glands of the fundic mucosa with consequent loss of acid secretion and intrinsic factor production.

Effects
1 Both achlorhydria and pernicious anaemia due to vitamin B_{12} deficiency result. This vitamin cannot be absorbed from the terminal ileum unless it has been bound to intrinsic factor derived from the fundic gastric glands.
2 Malignancy: atrophic gastritis is associated with an increased risk of developing gastric carcinoma. One suggested mechanism for this is the formation of nitrosamines—which are potent animal carcinogens in the gastric lumen, by bacterial breakdown of nitrites in the food. The achlorhydria of atrophic gastritis allows the growth of these faecal bacteria which are not normally able to survive in the stomach.

Other types of chronic gastritis

'Reflux gastritis'
Chemical injury to mucosa from refluxed bile/duodenal contents may occur following partial gastrectomy or gastroenterostomy. The histology of this is characterized by mucosal oedema and an increased depth of the gastric pits, but little or no inflammatory cell infiltration.

A similar pattern of mucosal histology is seen in some patients without duodenogastric reflux, and may result from other chemical injury, e.g. ingestion of NSAIDs.

Granulomatous gastritis
Inflammation of the gastric mucosa with granuloma formation occurs in Crohn's disease (see p. 33), sarcoidosis (see p. 394), tuberculosis (see p. 374), 'food granulomas' which are foreign-body granulomas forming around fragments of food material embedded in the mucosa, or 'idiopathic', when the other causes are excluded.

Rare forms of gastritis
1 *Lymphocytic gastritis*: characterized by an excess of lymphocytes in the surface epithelium, of unknown aetiology.
2 *Eosinophilic gastritis*: believed to be allergic in aetiology.
3 *Hypertrophic gastritis—Menetrière's disease*: this condition of unknown cause results in gross hyperplasia of gastric pits and a protein-losing gastropathy.

Intestinal metaplasia
Metaplasia of the gastric epithelium to intestinal type occurs in chronic gastritis of any type. Small foci of intestinal metaplasia around the mid-lesser curve gradually increase until large areas of the stomach are affected. This increases with age, and may be related to healing of microerosions. It is important in relation to gastric carcinogenesis (see p. 29) and has been classified into different types:
1 *Type I or 'complete'*—where the epithelium exactly mimics that of the normal small intestine.
2 *Type II or 'incomplete'*—which resembles large bowel mucosa; in type IIB sulphomucins are demonstrable by histochemistry in some cells.

Peptic ulceration
This is defined as ulceration resulting from acid/peptic damage to the mucosa.

Acute peptic ulcer
Acute ulceration may follow acute erosions; such ulcers are usually large, shallow and often bleed. Those associated with shock occur in the proximal stomach, those with ingestion of irritants are more distal and on the greater curve. They may heal without scarring, or progress to chronic ulcers.

Chronic peptic ulcer

Chronic peptic ulcers develop when the aggressive actions of acid and pepsin are not opposed by adequate mucosal protection mechanisms.

Sites

Always related to acid-secreting gastric mucosa:
1 Duodenum ⎱ 98%.
2 Stomach ⎰
3 Oesophagus—associated with reflux oesophagitis.
4 Distal duodenum—in patients with severe acid hypersecretion.
5 Distal to gastroenterostomy site.
6 Meckel's diverticulum—when heterotopic gastric fundic mucosa is present.

Aetiology

Many factors show an association with peptic ulceration:
1 Acid hypersecretion.
2 *Helicobacter*-associated gastroduodenitis.
3 Male sex, genetic factors.
4 Ingestion of non-steroidal anti-inflammatory drugs.
5 Smoking and perhaps alcohol.
6 Diet and perhaps stress.

Disease associations:
1 Uraemia.
2 Hyperparathyroidism and hypercalcaemia (see p. 138).
3 Chronic obstructive airways disease (see p. 377).

Pathogenesis

A disturbance of the balance of aggressive/protective factors at the mucosal surface leads to the breakdown in mucosal protection mechanisms. Normally the healthy gastroduodenal surface epithelium secretes bicarbonate, and a pH gradient is formed across the 1 mm thick mucus gel which covers the epithelial surface and shields it from acid. Deficiencies in this mucus coat allow damage of the mucosa by back-diffusion of acid.

Factors interfering with this mucosal protection are:
1 *Helicobacter*-associated gastritis.
2 Ingestion of NSAIDs.

Peptic ulcers characteristically develop in specific sites in the duodenum and stomach (see below). The explanation for this localization is not known, but it may be an effect of the microcirculation; functional 'end-arteries' supply the mucosa at these sites, predisposing to limitation of ulcer healing due to ischaemia.

Appearances

Macroscopical
Characteristic sharply defined, clean-based area of ulceration, on the lesser curve at the pylorus or incisura of the stomach, or the anterior or posterior wall of first part of the duodenum. Usually < 2 cm diameter but can be much larger. Scarring causes mucosal folds to radiate to the edge of the ulcer and there is no elevation of mucosa at the margin.

Microscopical
The ulcer base shows zones on histology (see Fig. 5).

Course

Healing occurs naturally, but is hastened by acid-inhibiting agents or mucosal protectants. Ulcers usually develop in adulthood, and have a natural history of repeated healing and relapse over many years.

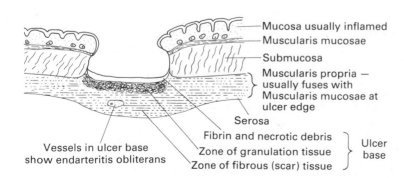

Fig. 5 Microscopical appearance of chronic peptic ulcer.

Complications
1 *Scarring*: resulting in pyloric stenosis.
2 *Bleeding*: due to erosion of a vessel in the ulcer base.
3 *Adherence and erosion* into underlying tissues, e.g. pancreas, liver.
4 *Perforation*: resulting in peritonitis.
5 *Malignant change*: rarely *if ever* occurs.

Tumours of stomach

Benign

Polyps
A polyp is a focal lesion which projects above the surface; a number of different types of polyp may occur, and all require endoscopic removal and histology to determine their nature, since malignancy cannot be excluded from the macroscopic appearance.
1 *Regenerative/hyperplastic polyps*. These form 90% and are single or multiple, may be at the margin of an ulcer, and are composed of elongated glands lined by regular epithelium, in an oedematous stroma.
2 *Fundic gland polyps*: these are multiple small polyps composed of cystic glands in the fundus, usually in middle-aged women.
3 *Neoplastic polyps*: adenomatous polyps with the same features as large bowel adenomas (see p. 44) or polypoid adenocarcinomas. There is a high risk of malignant transformation in gastric adenomas.
4 *Other rare polyps*:
   (a) *Hamartomatous polyps*: may occur in Peutz–Jeghers syndrome (see p. 43).
   (b) *Juvenile polyps*.
   (c) *Inflammatory fibroid polyps*.
   (d) *Cronkhite–Canada syndrome*.

Malignant

Gastric adenocarcinoma

Epidemiology
This tumour shows a wide variation in incidence between countries:
1 *High incidence*: Japan, parts of South America, Eastern Europe, Iceland.
2 *Intermediate*: Western Europe, North America.
3 *Low incidence*: Parts of Africa, Philippines.
   In most countries the incidence has been declining steadily during this century, but until recently this was still the commonest malignant tumour worldwide, a position now held by lung cancer.
   Immigrants from high- to low-incidence areas, e.g. Japanese to America, retain their high incidence, but second and later generations acquire the incidence of the adopted country.

Aetiology
1 *Dietary Factors*: low salt, high unrefined carbohydrate, nitrate preservatives, low animal fat and proteins, low fresh vegetables.
2 *Genetic factors*: association with blood group A, racial factors, but only 4% of gastric cancer patients have a family history of the disease.

Pathogenesis
Gastric cancer is believed to develop by a sequence of pathological changes:

normal mucosa
|
chronic gastritis
|
intestinal metaplasia, especially incomplete type
|
dysplasia
|
intramucosal carcinoma
|
invasive gastric cancer

   Chronic gastritis with atrophy and intestinal metaplasia (see p. 27) are common in populations with high gastric cancer risk.
   Conditions with increased risk of gastric cancer:
1 Achlorhydria—due to chronic gastritis (see p. 27)—autoimmune, *Helicobacter*-associated.
2 Following partial gastrectomy.
3 Menetrière's disease.

Appearances

Macroscopical
Polypoid or ulcerated tumours or infiltrative with diffuse thickening of gastric wall—'linitis plastica'. Most are > 2 cm diameter.

Site
Fifty per cent are in the pylorus, commoner on lesser curve, but can be in any site.

Twenty-five per cent are in the cardia. These tumours are less often associated with chronic gastritis and may have different aetiological factors to more distal carcinomas. Unlike other gastric cancers these are increasing in incidence.

Ulceration

Many gastric cancers show surface ulceration, and it is very important to distinguish these from benign ulcers. Malignancy should be suspected if an ulcer has:
1 Raised/irregular edges, surrounding tissue indurated.
2 Necrotic, shaggy base.
3 Site other than distal lesser curve.
4 Larger size.
5 Lack of radiating folds.

It is not possible to distinguish benign from malignant ulcers with certainty without microscopy. Multiple biopsies should be taken from any gastric ulcer, and endoscopy repeated after treatment to ensure healing has occurred.

Microscopical

Gastric adenocarcinomas vary greatly in the degree of glandular formation and mucin production, and large tumours are often histologically heterogeneous. There are several different classifications:
WHO: Papillary, tubular, mucinous, signet-ring cell types.
Ming: Expansile or infiltrative depending on the nature of the invading margin.
Lauren: Intestinal—with a glandular pattern resembling colonic carcinoma, or diffuse—extensive infiltration by individual cells, often of signet ring type, without formation of glands.

The 'intestinal' type of adenocarcinoma is believed to arise from the metaplasia → dysplasia → carcinoma sequence described above, and is more frequent in areas of high incidence for gastric cancer. Diffuse gastric carcinomas have a similar incidence in different countries.

Spread

1 *Direct*: through gastric wall into adjacent organs—omentum, pancreas, liver, colon. The extent of spread cannot be determined by the gross appearances, and microscopy of resection margins of operative specimens is essential.
2 *Lymph nodes*: metastases are commonly present; the nodes affected depend on the site of the primary tumour.
3 *Blood-borne*: metastases to liver and elsewhere.
4 *Transcoelomic*: to omentum, peritoneum and ovaries—'*Krukenberg tumour*' (see p. 227).

Staging

Stage I: invasion confined to mucosa or submucosa—known as '*early gastric cancer*'.
Stage II: invasion of muscle wall of stomach.
Stage III: metastases present but all tumour removable by surgery.
Stage IV: unresectable tumour.

Prognosis

Many gastric cancers do not present until the tumour has spread to become inoperable; if removal by gastrectomy is possible, 5-year survival, except in early gastric cancer, is less than 30%.

Early gastric cancer is defined as cancer limited to mucosa or to mucosa and submucosa. The prognosis is good—> 90% cure if the cancer is removed at this stage.

In Japan, where the incidence of gastric cancer is high, population based screening results in about 50% of the gastric cancers resected being at this early stage. In countries without screening, most gastric cancers do not cause symptoms until they are advanced, i.e. invading the muscularis propria and beyond.

In the UK, where early gastric cancer is rarely diagnosed, the overall 5-year survival is 10%.

Other malignant tumours

Carcinoid tumours

These tumours are derived from neuroendocrine cells—a population of mucosal cells which secrete hormones, e.g. gastrin and somatostatin, and are now believed to be derived from epithelial stem cells (see p. 36). Tumours derived from these cells are found in all parts of the gastrointestinal tract, though rare in the stomach.

Multiple very small carcinoid tumours may occur in pernicious anaemia—these develop on a background of neuroendocrine cell hyperplasia and behave in a benign fashion.

Large, biologically malignant tumours are rare, and are distinguished from adenocarcinomas by histology.

Gastric carcinoid tumours may rarely produce symptoms due to hormone release.

Lymphoma

The concept of mucosa-associated lymphoid tissue—
MALT (see also p. 32).

The gastrointestinal tract contains more lymphoid tissue—present in Peyer's patches and the lamina propria, than do the lymphoreticular organs—spleen, lymph nodes, thyroid, bone marrow. The immune cells of MALT comprise a population distinct from the 'systemic' immune system. For example the memory B cells in the lamina propria respond to antigenic stimulation by entering the circulation, maturing and 'homing' back to the mucosa as plasma cells.

Lymphomas derived from MALT may remain localized to their organ of origin for long periods, and when dissemination occurs this tends to be to other mucosal sites rather than to systemic lymph nodes and spleen.

Secondary involvement of the gastrointestinal tract by disseminated lymphoma occurs frequently in primarily node-based disease. Primary gastrointestinal lymphomas are distinguished from such secondary involvement by:
1 The absence of superficial lymphadenopathy.
2 No mediastinal enlargement.
3 Normal white cell count.
4 Predominantly a gut lesion at laparotomy, with or without local lymph node enlargement.

Primary gastric lymphoma

Incidence
Between 2% and 4% of gastric maligancies, 60% of primary gastrointestinal lymphomas occur in the stomach. These are usually derived from B cells and spread relatively late to local lymph nodes and to other mucosal sites.

Macroscopical
Various appearances, including polyps, ulcers or diffuse thickening of the rugal folds.

Microscopical
1 Sheets of monomorphic lymphoid cells, with or without follicular structures.
2 Destruction of mucosal glands by these cells—
lympho-epithelial lesions.

Prognosis
After treatment with surgery and/or chemotherapy this is better than for gastric carcinoma.

Tumours of connective tissue

Benign
Lipoma, leiomyoma, haemangioma, neurofibroma, etc. usually present as incidental findings but larger leiomyomas may elevate and ulcerate the overlying mucosa, and bleed.

Sarcomas
These spindle cell tumours are rare—2% of gastric malignancies, and are derived from smooth muscle, nerves, vessels, etc. Smooth muscle tumours are the most frequent; the malignant potential of these tumours can be difficult to predict by microscopy—features suggestive of malignant behaviour are:
1 Large size.
2 Necrosis/cystic degeneration.
3 Infiltrative margin.
4 Cellular pleomorphism.
5 Presence and numbers of mitotic figures.
Epithelioid smooth muscle tumours—'leiomyoblastoma', are composed of smooth muscle cells which resemble epithelial cells on microscopy, and are often vacuolated (see p. 107).

E/GASTROINTESTINAL TRACT, SMALL INTESTINE

Structure and functions
Infections
Crohn's disease
Malabsorption syndromes
Tumours
Vascular
Mechanical

Normal mucosa
This is illustrated in Fig. 6.

Mucosal villi are covered by goblet cells producing mucus and absorptive cells with a brush border.

Mucosal crypts contain the proliferating cell compartment of the epithelium, Paneth cells and endocrine cells.

The lamina propria includes lymphatics and capillaries which carry away absorbed nutrients, and lymphoid tissue.

Functions
1 Brush border enzymes—saccharidases, complete the digestion of carbohydrates.
2 Dietary nutrients are absorbed across the

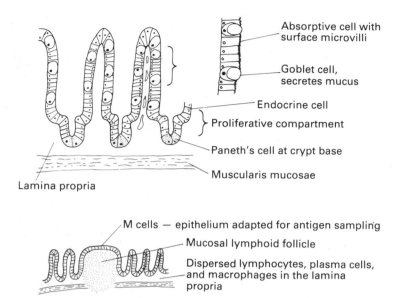

Fig. 6 Structure of small intestine.

epithelium, and transported into lymphatics and blood capillaries.

3 The smooth muscle mixes and propels bowel contents.

4 The mucosa-associated lymphoid tissue responds to dietary antigens.

5 The neuroendocrine system regulates the function of the small bowel and related organs.

Infective conditions

These mostly present as diarrhoeal diseases; the small and large bowel are often both involved.

Pathogenesis

There are two main pathogenetic mechanisms:

1 Bacteria which *invade* the mucosal surface, leading to exudation of blood and pus cells into the lumen, and abdominal pain. Bacteria which cause invasive enterocolitis include *Campylobacter jejuni*, *Eschericia coli*, *Salmonella*.

2 Infective agents producing *toxins* which leave the mucosal surface intact. These usually cause watery diarrhoea. Organisms which cause toxigenic enterocolitis include *E. coli*, *Vibrio cholerae*, viruses, e.g. rotavirus and adenovirus, protozoa.

Diagnosis

This depends on the isolation of the pathogenic organism from stool samples, or its recognition in mucosal biopsies. All invasive organisms result in an acute inflammatory reaction histologically; non-invasive agents cause little morphological change.

Typhoid fever—Salmonella typhi

Pathogenesis

1 This organism is spread by poor hygiene and by asymptomatic 'carriers', and is still widespread in hot and developing countries.

2 After ingestion the organisms invade and proliferate in the lymphoid tissue of the small bowel for 10 days.

3 Septicaemic phase follows with generalized infection, accompanied by the development of 'rose spots' on the skin.

4 Organisms then localize in the reticuloendothelial system, causing inflammation, and at other sites, e.g. the gallbladder, bone (see p. 295).

Appearances

At 2–3 weeks there is small bowel ulceration over Peyer's patches; ulcers are typically longitudinally orientated—cf. tuberculosis, p. 33.

Microscopically the inflammatory infiltrate consists mainly of mononuclear cells.

Dissemination of infection occurs to many organs, including the liver, bone marrow, gall bladder.

Results
Though curable with appropriate antibiotics it still carries a high mortality in developing countries.

Other Salmonella infections
1 *Enteric fever group*: S. *paratyphae* and S. *cholerae-suis*; these cause a less severe enteric fever.
2 Food poisoning group: S. *typhimurium*, S. *enteritidis*, etc.; these cause either an acute gastroenteritis—incubation 8–24 hours, or septicaemia without apparent enteritis.

Other bacterial infections which involve the gut, affect predominantly the colon, and will discussed in that section under 'infective colitis' (see p. 40).

Tuberculosis

Incidence
In Western countries this occurs most often in immigrant patients, and may be with or without active pulmonary infection. In developing countries it remains common, increasingly so in HIV-infected patients.

Macroscopical
Ulcers—usually transverse, and strictures, most frequently in the terminal ileum and with serosal tubercles. It may mimic Crohn's disease or malignancy.

Microscopical
Confluent caseating granulomas in which acid-fast bacilli may be demonstrable, with prominent fibrosis and absence of fissure—ulcers—cf. Crohn's disease, see below.

Other infections
The following agents may also cause small bowel infection/infestation:
1 *Fungi*. Mainly in immunocompromised patients and including *Candida*, *Cryptococcus*, *Histoplasma* and *Mucor*.
2 *Helminths*. Mostly in tropical countries and including: ankylostoma—hookworm, ascaris, *Schistosoma mansonii* and S. *japonicum* and *Strongyloides stercoralis*.
3 *Protozoans*. Cryptosporidia, isospora, microsporidia, *Giardia lamblia*.

Giardiasis
Giardia lamblia is a protozoan which may colonize the small bowel in great numbers and lead to malabsorption, although there is little histological abnormality of the mucosa. *Giardia* are easily recognized by microscopy in biopsies from infested patients.

Intestinal infections in the immunocompromised host
Many immunocompromised patients, especially those with HIV infection and AIDS, have diarrhoea and weight loss. This may be due to infection with agents not normally pathogenic to humans, but in some cases no causal organism can be found, and it is likely that infection of the mucosa by the HIV virus itself results in an enteropathy (see p. 3).
1 *Viral*—cytomegalovirus, herpes virus, HIV-enteropathy.
2 *Bacteria*—these are a less common problem, the same organisms are involved as in non-immunocompromised subjects.
3 *Fungi*—*Cryptococcus neoformans*, *Candida*.
4 *Parasites*—*Giardia lamblia*, *Cryptosporidia*, *Isospora belli*, *Micrococcus*.

Crohn's disease

Nature
This is a chronic inflammatory condition of unknown cause which affects the alimentary canal at any site from mouth to anus, but most characteristically the terminal ileum, which is involved in about 70% of cases.

Epidemiology
Crohn's disease is more common in Northern European countries, less in Japan, South America.

Aetiology and pathogenesis
This remains unknown despite years of intensive research. Hypotheses include:
1 *An infection*. Proposed agents include mycobacteria, chlamydia, viruses. There is no firm evidence for any of these.
2 *Abnormal immune mechanisms*. Differences in cell-mediated and humoral immunity can be demonstrated between Crohn's disease patients and controls; there may be an abnormal immune response to normal gut antigens.
3 *Vascular*. Focal small vessel narrowing has been

claimed to precede the development of inflammatory lesions.

4 *Miscellaneous.* Food antigens, reaction to toothpaste, psychosomatic factors and others have been proposed.

Appearances

Macroscopical
1 Segmental involvement by disease, with 'skip' lesions of normal-appearing bowel.
2 The small bowel is classically involved, but any part of the gastrointestinal tract may be affected.
3 The involved bowel shows:
  (a) thickening of the wall, which becomes rubbery and rigid;
  (b) encroachment of mesenteric fat over the serosal surfaces;
  (c) mucosal ulceration which tends to be linear;
  (d) a 'cobble-stone' pattern of islands of surviving mucosa;
  (e) deep linear ulceration, typically *'fissure-shaped'* leading to adhesions to adjacent structures, and development of fistulous tracks into adherent organs.

Microscopical
1 Granulomas. Non-caseating, 'sarcoid-like' granulomas are present in the inflamed bowel wall, in the mucosa at non-ulcerated sites, and in mesenteric lymph nodes. Granulomas are only found in 60% of cases.
2 Discontinuous mucosal inflammation and ulceration; normal mucosa is seen in uninvolved segments.
3 Inflammation which extends deeply into the submucosa, muscle wall and serosa. This forms the basis of fissure ulcers and adhesions.
4 Lymphoid aggregates which develop deep in the bowel wall.
5 Lymphatic dilatation.
6 Neural hypertrophy.

When Crohn's disease involves the colon—25% of cases—its distinction from ulcerative colitis is very important for clinical management. The relevant features for making this distinction are summarized under ulcerative colitis (p. 41).

Complications
1 *Intestinal obstruction*: due to stenosis or adhesions.
2 *Fistulae*: to other loops of bowel, bladder.

3 *Abscess formation.*
4 *Poor healing*: of surgical sites with fistula formation.

Other effects
Extra-gastrointestinal manifestations develop in a minority of patients with Crohn's disease, and include polyarthritis, sacroiliitis, ankylosing spondylitis (see p. 103), erythema nodosum, finger clubbing, uveitis (see p. 149), pericholangitis, gallstones, amyloid.

Eosinophilic gastroenteritis
Inflammation of the gut of presumed allergic aetiology, characterized by predominantly submucosal oedema and infiltration by eosinophils. It may cause pyloric or small intestinal obstruction.

Malabsorption syndromes
Since the absorption of nutrients is the main function of the small bowel, many of its diseases present as a malabsorption syndrome.

Classification
1 *Luminal defects*:
  (a) pancreatic insufficiency;
  (b) bacterial overgrowth in blind loops, postgastrectomy, multiple strictures, jejunal diverticula;
  (c) bile salt deficiency.
2 *Abnormality of mucosa*:
  (a) brush-border enzyme deficiency, e.g. disaccharidases, monosaccharidases;
  (b) coeliac disease;
  (c) tropical sprue;
  (d) Whipple's disease;
  (e) Crohn's disease;
  (f) allergic gastroenteritis;
  (g) parasitic infections.
3 *Lymphatic obstruction*:
  (a) primary lymphangiectasia;
  (b) tuberculosis;
  (c) radiation enteritis.
4 *Extensive small bowel resection.* Also jejunal-ileal bypass procedures.

Coeliac disease

Nature
A sensitivity to gliadin, a constituent of wheat protein, resulting in small bowel mucosal damage with loss of mucosal villi, crypt hyperplasia, and an excess of inflammatory cells in the mucosa.

Aetiology

1 *Hereditary factors*: strongly linked with HLA-B8 and HLA-DR3 and DR7—90% of cases.
2 *Possible virus association*: this remains unproven.

Pathogenesis

Gluten, which contains gliadin, is present in grains of wheat, barley and rye.

Affected patients have humoral and cell-mediated immunity to this protein; withdrawal of gluten from the diet results in improvement of the mucosal lesion, with a return to a near-normal mucosal architecture. The subsequent reintroduction of gluten as a 'challenge' results in relapse of the coeliac disease. Most gastroenterologists believe that this challenge must be undertaken to prove the diagnosis.

Microscopical

Total or partial villous atrophy with crypt hyperplasia, mucosal inflammation and damage to surface epithelium (see Fig. 7). Milder, possibly early, forms of the disease may be patchy.

Differential diagnosis

Other small bowel diseases may cause similar changes, although usually of a lesser degree; crypt hyperplasia and villous atrophy are non-specific responses to injury.

1 *Dermatitis herpetiformis*: partial villous atrophy associated with a blistering skin disease (see p. 415); also responds to gluten withdrawal.
2 *Tropical sprue*: due to bacterial overgrowth in the small bowel, responds to treatment with tetracycline and folate.
3 *Other food-sensitive enteropathies*, e.g. cow's milk intolerance in children.

4 *Unknown*: a few patients have histological changes of coeliac disease not responding to gluten withdrawal.

Whipple's disease

Whipple's disease is an extremely rare multisystem disease characterized by accumulation of PAS-positive macrophages in the lamina propria of the small bowel, and in many other organs.

Electron microscopy shows accumulation of an unknown bacterium within these macrophages. The condition responds to antibiotic therapy.

Brush-border enzyme deficiencies

The commonest is *lactase deficiency* which may be congenital or acquired—following infective gastroenteritis. This presents with malabsorption symptoms after drinking milk.

The mucosa is normal on light microscopy but the enzyme deficiencies can be demonstrated by histochemical techniques.

Tumours of small intestine

Tumours in the small bowel are curiously rare, accounting for approximately 5% of all gastrointestinal malignancies. Adenocarcinomas, which are so common in the stomach and large bowel, are particularly unusual in the small bowel except in the region of the ampulla of Vater. Elsewhere carcinoid tumours and lymphomas are more frequently encountered than adenocarcinomas.

Polyps

Small bowel polyps may be:
1 *Hamartomas*, including polyps in Peutz–Jegher's syndrome.

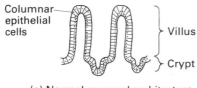
(a) Normal mucosal architecture villus : crypt ratio > 3 : 1

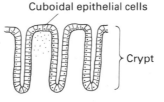
(b) Total villous atrophy, with crypt hyperplasia, increase in inflammatory cells in lamina propria, characteristic of coeliac disease

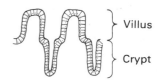
(c) Partial villous atrophy with crypt hyperplasia

Fig. 7 Normal and atrophic small intestinal mucosa.

2 *Juvenile polyps*.

3 *Adenomatous polyps*: in familial adenomatous polyposis and Gardner's syndrome.

4 *Inflammatory fibroid polyp*.

Adenocarcinoma

Incidence
Adenocarcinomas account for < 1% of gastrointestinal carcinomas, but are slightly more common in the small intestine than endocrine cell tumours.

Macroscopical
Usually annular and constricting.

Microscopical
Resemble large bowel adenocarcinoma.

Prognosis
Poor, due to late presentation.

Neuroendocrine cell tumours—carcinoid tumours

Origin
These tumours arise from cells of the *diffuse neuroendocrine system* (see also p. 30).

Neuroendocrine cells are scattered singly in the mucosal crypts throughout the gastrointestinal tract. These cells secrete gut hormones which, in the small intestine, include *somatostatin*, *cholecystokinin*, *pancreatic polypeptide* and *vasoactive intestinal polypeptide—VIP*. Tumours derived from these cells are characterized by the presence of neurosecretory granules within their cell cytoplasm; specific peptides can often be demonstrated in these granules by immunohistochemistry, and secretion of the peptide by the tumour may cause clinical syndromes as in carcinoid syndrome, vipoma and somatostatinoma.

Sites
The small bowel is the commonest site for carcinoid tumours; these tumours have characteristic histological patterns, but their biological behaviour—benign or malignant, is difficult to predict by microscopy. The commonest site for such tumours is in the appendix, but it is extremely rare for these to give rise to metastases. By comparison the majority of similar tumours elsewhere in the small bowel behave in a malignant fashion.

Macroscopical
Solid yellow or grey tumour. The overlying mucosa may be intact and there is diffuse infiltration of muscle wall, often with stricturing at the site of the tumour.

Microscopical
Characteristically composed of islands and trabeculae of cells which have regular round nuclei and finely granular cytoplasm, with little nuclear pleomorphism or mitotic activity. Electron microscopy demonstrates the typical membrane-bound neurosecretory granules.

Histochemistry
1 *Argentaffin reaction*: granules containing 5-hydroxytryptamine reduce silver salts to a granular precipitate, e.g. diazo stain.

2 *Argyrophil reaction*: neuroendocrine granules containing other substances which can reduce silver salts in the presence of a reducing agent, e.g. Grimelius stain.

3 *Immunohistochemistry*: includes the demonstration of the presence of neuroendocrine granules, e.g. by chromogranin, and demonstration of the specific peptide product, e.g. somatostatin.

Course
The biological behaviour of neuroendocrine tumours cannot be reliably predicted from their histological appearances, and all carcinoids should be regarded as potentially malignant.

Malignant behaviour is more likely if:
1 The tumour is of large size—over 2 cm.
2 There is vascular invasion.
3 There is nuclear pleomorphism.
4 Lymph node metastases are present.
5 The tumour is of goblet cell type (see p. 39).

The carcinoid syndrome
Serotonin—5-hydroxytryptamine (5-HT)—released from liver metastases of carcinoid tumours results in this clinical syndrome which includes facial flushing, diarrhoea, hypotension and wheezing. It is diagnosed on finding high levels of the metabolite 5-HIAA in the urine.

5-HT produced by the primary tumour is inactivated in the liver and therefore does not produce carcinoid syndrome unless there are metastases.

Many carcinoid tumours are multihormonal, producing a variety of peptides.

Lymphomas

The small bowel is a common site for primary lymphoma of the gastrointestinal tract. Three types are recognized; these are all examples of lymphomas of the mucosa-associated lymphoid tissue—MALT (see p. 31).

Classification

1 *Western—sporadic, type*: derived from B cells of the lamina propria.

2 *Lymphoma associated with coelic disease*: derived from T cells and associated with villous atrophy of the surrounding mucosa, although a history of preceding coeliac disease is not available in many cases.

3 *Mediterranean type—alpha heavy chain disease*: a plasmacytoid lymphoma which produces alpha heavy chains of immunoglobulin, not conjugated with light chains. This shows a geographic restriction to Mediterranean and North African countries.

Connective tissue tumours

Benign

Including lipoma, neurogenic tumours, leiomyoma and haemangioma. These usually present as incidental findings or with obstruction, intussusception or bleeding.

Malignant

Smooth muscle tumours may be benign or malignant and are discussed under tumours of the stomach (see p. 31).

Vascular lesions

The vascular supply is by a series of arterial arcades, filled from the superior mesenteric artery.

Ischaemia

Mechanisms

Reduction in blood supply may be due to vascular narrowing/occlusion, severe hypotension, or a combination of both. When the circulation falls below that required to maintain mucosal integrity, mucosal defence is impaired, allowing bacterial invasion from the lumen.

Causes

1 *Vessel disease*. Atherosclerosis, embolism, thrombosis associated with clotting disorders—affecting arteries or veins, vasculitic syndromes, e.g. polyarteritis nodosa, Henoch–Schönlein purpura, systemic lupus erythematosus (see p. 83). Partial occlusion combined with hypotensive shock.

2 *Mechanical*: ischaemic damage is also important in the pathogenesis of damage to the intestine in mechanical disorders causing intestinal obstruction: obstructed hernia, volvulus, intussusception and adhesions.

3 *Shunting*: when the blood supply to the bowel is reduced blood is shunted preferentially away from the superficial mucosa, which is therefore the layer of the wall most susceptible to injury due to its high metabolic requirements.

Results

1 Haemorrhagic mucosal necrosis with oedema of the bowel wall—the lesion appears haemorrhagic because of the flow of blood into the area from vascular anastomoses, which then escapes through damaged vessel walls.

2 Full-thickness necrosis of bowel wall—gangrene rapidly develops due to secondary infection from gut bacteria.

3 Stricture secondary to chronic vascular insufficiency.

Mechanical obstruction

Causes

1 Luminal factors:
   (a) *Meconium ileus*—thick viscid mucus in infants with cystic fibrosis (see p. 351).
   (b) *Obstruction*—by gallstones, foreign bodies, polypoid tumours.

2 *Disease of the bowel wall*:
   (a) *Strictures*—due to Crohn's disease, infiltrating tumours, ischaemia.
   (b) *Strictures following ulceration*, e.g. from non-steroidal anti-inflammatory agents, potassium tablets.
   (c) *Intussusception*.

3 *Obstruction from the serosal aspect*: intestinal adhesions, hernias and volvulus.

Small bowel perforation

Obstruction and ischaemia occurring in any of the above conditions may result in perforation if unrelieved.

Additional causes of perforation are:

1 Perforation by foreign body.
2 *Salmonella typhi* infection.
3 Perforation of congenital diverticula, including Meckel's.
4 Perforating tumour, especially lymphoma.

Bowel obstruction, perforation and ischaemia present as surgical emergencies generally requiring laparotomy with removal of the damaged segment of bowel.

Hernias

Nature
A hernial sac is formed when a portion of peritoneum protrudes through a defect in the structures of the abdominal wall.

Sites
1 Inguinal.
2 Femoral.
3 Incisional—postoperative.
The sac may contain omentum or bowel wall.

Results
If the hernia becomes irreducible—contents fail to return to abdominal cavity on pressure—the contained bowel may develop increasing oedema resulting from compromise of the venous and lymphatic flow, followed by impaired arterial flow resulting in ischaemic injury as described on p. 37.

Volvulus
This is the twisting of a loop of bowel on its mesentery. The entire small bowel can twist, especially if the mesentery has a short insertion on the posterior abdominal wall. As the bowel twists, venous return and then arterial supply become obstructed.

Intussusception
Due to the action of peristalsis a portion of bowel is propelled into the lumen of more distal bowel (as if closing a telescope).

There is usually some mass lesion at the head of the intussusception, either enlarged lymphoid tissue in children or a tumour in adults. As the intussusception progresses, the vascular supply to the intussusceptum is gradually compromised.

Adhesions
Band adhesions which are either congenital, or follow inflammation or surgery, constrict the bowel, resulting in impairment of its blood supply.

All these mechanical conditions present as surgical emergencies, requiring removal of ischaemic bowel.

Non-obstructive stasis

Acute—paralytic ileus
Occurs due to peritoneal irritation from peritonitis, trauma, surgery, metabolic disturbances, e.g. hypokalaemia, uraemia, diabetic ketoacidosis and spinal injuries.

Chronic intestinal pseudo-obstruction
A very rare condition causing recurrent pain, distension, nausea and vomiting. This may be due to:
1 *Disorders of smooth muscle*—inherited visceral myopathy, collagen diseases, muscular dystrophy, amyloid.
2 *Neurological disorders*: inherited visceral neuropathy, diabetes, hypothyroidism, drugs—psychotropic, antineoplastic.

F/GASTROINTESTINAL TRACT, APPENDIX, LARGE INTESTINE

Appendix
   Inflammations
   Tumours
Large intestine
   Structure and functions
   Colitis
   Miscellaneous mucosal
   Tumours
   Vascular
   Diverticular disease

Appendix
The mucosa of the appendix is colonic in type, but lymphoid follicles are very prominent, especially in young persons.

Inflammation—acute appendicitis

Incidence
Acute appendicitis is the commonest surgical emergency in Western countries, but is rare in the rural Third World.

Aetiology

Related to Western-style low-fibre diets and may be associated with obstruction in the lumen of the appendix by inspissated faecal material—*faecolith*—but this is by no means invariably present.

Macroscopical

1 Serosal congestion, mucosal inflammation.
2 Acute suppurative appendicitis—serosa covered by purulent exudate.
3 Gangrenous appendicitis—with full-thickness necrosis of the appendix wall, often leading to perforation.
4 Appendix mass—localized walled-off abscess around an inflamed and perforated appendix.

Microscopical

1 Early appendicitis is present when the acute inflammation is limited to the mucosa; this progresses to:
2 Full-thickness inflammation with mucosal ulceration and necrosis of muscle wall.

Other infections

Tuberculosis, actinomycosis, schistosomiasis of the appendix are all uncommon or rare.

Crohn's disease

Features of Crohn's disease including fissure-ulcers and granulomas are occasionally seen in appendicectomy specimens. Some patients later develop clinical Crohn's disease.

Ulcerative colitis

The appendix is frequently inflamed in colectomy specimens, whether or not the adjacent caecal mucosa is involved.

Tumours

Carcinoid tumours

The appendix is the commonest site for these tumours (*see* p. 36).

Macroscopical

These are yellow solid tumours associated with hypertrophy of the muscle wall. They are usually < 2 cm diameter, and detected as an incidental finding in appendices removed for symptoms of acute appendicitis.

Microscopical

Carcinoid tumours have a typical insular/trabecular arrangement of regular cells which infiltrate through the muscle wall. Nearly all carcinoids in the appendix are argentaffin- and argyrophil-positive due to their content of 5-hydroxytryptamine.

Prognosis

The great majority of carcinoid tumours behave in a benign fashion. Appendicectomy alone is considered adequate treatment unless:
1 The tumour extends to the resection margin.
2 There is vascular invasion.
3 There are lymph node metastases.

Goblet cell carcinoid

This is a rare type of carcinoid tumour in which the cells contain both neuroendocrine granules and mucin. It is more likely to metastasize than other carcinoid tumours in the appendix, and may spread by the transcoelomic route.

Mucocoele

Distension of the lumen of the appendix by mucus, sometimes leading to rupture of the appendix with release of mucus into the peritoneal cavity. Mucocoeles are due to:
1 *Mucinous cystadenoma*—a benign tumour equivalent to a villous adenoma of the appendix.
2 *Mucinous cystadenocarcinoma*—the malignant counterpart of mucinous cystadenoma. Rupture of the mucocoele in this case leads to transcoelomic spread of tumour cells within the peritoneal cavity; these cells continue to produce mucin, which becomes surrounded by fibrosis, resulting in *myxoma peritonei* (see also p. 49).

Large intestine

Large bowel structure

This is illustrated in Fig. 8. The mucosa has a flat surface of absorptive surface epithelium covered with small microvilli. Mucosal crypts open on to the surface and secrete mucus.

The ascending and descending colon are retroperitoneal. The transverse and sigmoid colon are covered by visceral peritoneum and have a mesentery. The rectum is retroperitoneal. *N.B.*: these factors are important when considering the spread of tumours.

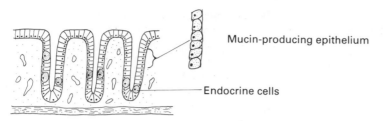

Mucin-producing epithelium

Endocrine cells

Normal crypts are regular and straight

Fig. 8 Normal large bowel mucosa.

Colitis

Inflammation of the colon may be due to:

1 *Infective agents*:
(a) *Bacterial—Shigella, Campylobacter, E. coli. Vibrio cholerae*, toxic effect of *Clostridium difficile*—pseudomembranous colitis.
(b) *Viruses*.
(c) *Protozoa*—amoebic dysentery.
(d) Helminths—Schistosomiasis (*see* p. 9).
2 *Drugs*.
3 *Idiopathic inflammatory bowel disease*:
(a) Ulcerative colitis.
(b) Crohn's disease.

Infective agents

Infective causes of colitis result in self-limiting episodes of diarrhoea, with or without pain and passage of blood. Diagnosis depends on demonstration of pathogen in faecal material; the morphological changes in the bowel wall are non-specific, and only point towards an infective cause of the colitis, as opposed to a chronic inflammatory bowel disease.

Shigella *infection—bacillary dysentery*

Pathogenesis

Shigella dysenteriae, S. flexneri, S. boydii and *S. sonnei* are the four species of *Shigella*. The infection is spread by the faecal–oral route, and the organisms invade the colonic mucosa, proliferate in the lamina propria, and release endotoxin which damages the mucosa. This results in severe diarrhoea, with mucus, blood and pus cells in the stool. The patient may become severely ill.

Appearances

The mucosal surface is covered by yellowish exudate, and appears red and inflamed.

Histologically there is mucosal inflammation with prominent oedema and congestion. Necrotic mucosa sloughs, leaving ulcers lined by fibrin and granulation tissue.

Later regeneration occurs, with restitution of the normal mucosa.

Campylobacter jejuni *colitis*

Nature

Organisms of the *Campylobacter* genus, first distinguished from *Vibrio* in the mid-1970s, are now known to be one of the most frequent causes of bacterial colitis in Western countries. They cause a self-limiting enterocolitis, often associated with severe abdominal pain, general malaise and blood in the stool. *Campylobacter* require micro-aerophilic culture at 42°C for detection.

Pathogenesis

C. jejuni invades the mucosal surface, and produces a toxin which damages the mucosa.

Appearances

A mainly acute inflammatory cell infiltrate in the mucosa, with crypt abscesses, mucosal haemorrhages and some ulceration. The colitis is usually less severe than *Shigella*.

Cholera

Pathogenesis

Caused by water-borne, non-invasive, toxigenic strains of *Vibrio cholerae*; the toxin enters the enterocytes where it irreversibly activates adenylate cyclase, stimulating secretion of water and electrolytes from the cell. This causes severe diarrhoea with passage of watery stools flecked with mucus, resulting in life-threatening dehydration.

Appearances

Although the organism itself may not damage the mucosa there may be non-specific effects, e.g. lymphocytic infiltrate of the mucosa, lymphatic dilatation, desquamation of enterocytes.

Amoebic dysentery

Organism

The causative organism, *Entamoeba histolytica*, is a small amoeba which resembles a macrophage on microscopy; pathogenic strains in humans are recognizable because they contain ingested red blood cells. There are several non-pathogenic amoebae, found particularly in immunosuppressed subjects as incidental findings.

In unfavourable conditions, amoebae form cysts with four nuclei which can survive outside the gut. Asymptomatic carriage is much more common than symptomatic infection, but symptoms of dysentery may develop years after foreign travel.

Pathogenesis

The organism damages host cells by lysis, resulting in localized necrosis with little inflammatory reaction.

Appearances

Colitis, often most severe in the ascending colon. Organisms enter the crypts, and destroy the surrounding tissue resulting in 'flask-shaped' ulceration. Organisms are usually numerous and readily identified, with relatively little surrounding inflammation.

Complications

Dissemination of amoebae via the blood stream occurs in about 40% of cases, and may be to the liver, brain, lung or kidney. This results in an *'amoebic abscess'*, which is a collection of brown tissue debris said to resemble the appearance of anchovy paste; there is characteristically little surrounding inflammatory reaction (see p. 236).

Diagnosis

Diagnosis is by recognition of parasites or cysts in stools and biopsies. Serological tests are positive only in invasive amoebiasis. Correct diagnosis is very important, since erroneous treatment of presumed ulcerative colitis with corticosteriods would result in colonic perforation.

Antibiotic-associated diarrhoea

The use of antibiotics disturbs the normal balanced flora of commensal colonic bacteria, and may result in diarrhoea. The following situations are distinguished:
1 *Antibiotic-associated diarrhoea*: symptoms that are not associated with pathological changes in the bowel wall; the diarrhoea is attributed to an imbalance of gut commensal organisms
2 *Antibiotic-associated colitis*: colonic inflammation following the use of antibiotics, which may be due to the opportunist growth of *E. coli*, or a mild infection with *Clostridium difficile*.
3 *Pseudomembranous colitis*: caused by toxin-producing strains of *C. difficile*, which proliferate in patients treated with broad-spectrum antibiotics, especially clindomycin and lincomycin.

Macroscopical

Pseudomembranous colitis shows characteristic discrete areas of shaggy mucosal exudate surrounded by a hyperaemic rim dotted over the colonic mucosal surface.

Microscopical

Classical 'volcano' lesion of superficial erosion covered with exudate of fibrin, mucus, neutrophils and inflammatory debris.

Collagenous colitis and microscopic colitis

These are rare causes of diarrhoea, where the mucosa is macroscopically normal but shows histological changes of deposition of collagen beneath surface epithelium or excess of mononuclear cells in the lamina propria.

Ulcerative colitis

Nature

This is a chronic relapsing inflammatory disorder of the colonic and rectal mucosa, of unknown cause.

Aetiology

Like Crohn's disease, the cause of ulcerative colitis is unknown, and similar aetiological factors have been suggested, in particular:
1 Abnormal immune response to gut microorganisms.
2 Autoimmunity with antibodies against colonic epithelial cells.

3 Genetic factors—25% of patients have a family member with inflammatory bowel disease.
4 Geographic factors—much commoner in Western countries than in the developing world.

Macroscopical

The disease affects the large bowel in a continuous pattern extending for a variable distance proximally from the rectum. Thus there may be:
1 *proctitis*: inflammation limited to the rectum;
2 *varying extent of colitis*, up to:
3 *total colitis*, with or without *backwash ileitis*.

The affected mucosa is red and inflamed with areas of flat ulceration; in severe cases inflammatory pseudopolyps develop from hyperplastic surviving islands of mucosa. Since only the mucosa is affected, the bowel wall does not become thickend, and fistulae do not occur.

Microscopical

Acute or chronic inflammation affects the mucosa but rarely extends deep to the muscularis mucosae. Characteristic features are:
1 A diffuse mixed inflammatory cell infiltraté in the lamina propria.
2 Crypt abscess formation.
3 Distortion of the glandular architecture, with shortened and branched crypts.
4 Epithelial mucin depletion.
5 Flat-based mucosal ulceration.

During exacerbations, severe inflammation may lead to sloughing of the mucosa and confluent areas of ulceration.

Complications

1 *Toxic dilatation—megacolon*: in fulminant ulcerative colitis and requiring urgent surgical resection.
2 *Risk of malignant change* (see below).
3 *Sclerosing cholangitis*: over 70% of cases of this condition are associated with ulcerative colitis (see p. 244).

Differential diagnosis

Ulcerative colitis must be distinguished from:
1 *Acute self-limiting—infective colitis*, by the short clinical history, together with stool culture, and rectal biopsy histology.
2 *Crohn's disease*, by clinical, radiological and pathological features. Table 2.1 contrasts the pathological characteristics of ulcerative colitis and Crohn's disease.

Colitis indeterminate

In about 10% of cases the distinction between ulcerative colitis and Crohn's disease is difficult or impossible to make. These cases are typically patients who have had colectomy for fulminant colitis with toxic megacolon, and show:
1 Inflammation extending more deeply than the submucosa, but continuous in pattern.
2 Hyperaemia and lysis of muscularis propria.
3 Absence of granulomas, but deep lymphoid aggregates may be present.

Risk of malignancy

Ulcerative colitis patients, particularly those with *total colonic involvement for over 10 years*, are at risk of developing large bowel adenocarcinoma. The presence of epithelial dysplasia is an additional marker for patients at risk. Surveillance screening programmes are recommended by some, using colonoscopy and multiple biopsy to detect dysplasia and early malignancy. High-grade dysplasia is considered an indication for colectomy.

Miscellaneous conditions of the mucosa

Melanosis coli

Grey discoloration of the colonic mucosa due to accumulation of ceroid pigment in lamina propria macrophages; attributed to the use of certain laxatives.

Stercoral ulceration

Ulceration of the mucosa proximal to an obstructing lesion, or in severe constipation, due to pressure on the mucosa from hard faecal material.

Pneumatosis coli

Presence of nitrogen-containing gas cysts in the submucosa, of uncertain aetiology.

Mucosal prolapse

Large bowel mucosa may prolapse:
1 At colostomy sites.
2 With haemorrhoids.
3 Prolapsed rectum.
4 *Solitary rectal ulcer syndrome*. Where the anterior rectal wall prolapses—a misnomer since there may be no ulcer.

Table 2.1 Pathological features distinguishing ulcerative colitis and Crohn's disease .

	Ulcerative colitis	Crohn's disease
Macroscopical		
Site of involvement	Large bowel, extends proximally from rectum	Most commonly terminal ileum, may be any part of GI tract
Distribution	Continuous	Discontinuous, with skip lesions
Bowel wall	Not thickened	Thickened, serosal fat encroachment, strictures, adhesions, deep ulcers and fistulae
Mucosal surface	Diffusely inflamed, small flat-based ulcers, or confluent ulceration with inflammatory polyps	Oedematous, aphthous or linear ulcers, cobblestone appearance
Microscopical		
Inflammation	Diffuse infiltrate confined to mucosa, crypt abscesses, vascular congestion	Patchy infiltrate extends deep into gut wall, many lymphoid aggregates, granulomas in 60%
Ulcers	Flat-based, do not extend to submucosa	Deep knife-like fissures, form the basis of fistulae
Crypt pattern	Distorted, branched atrophy in long-standing disease	Little distortion
Mucin depletion	Prominent in inflamed areas	Less depletion in inflamed areas
Other features		Oedema, lymphatic dilatation, neural hypertrophy

Microscopical

In all of these situations the mucosa has the same characteristic histology:

1 Smooth muscle fibres extend up into lamina propria.

2 Fibrosis of lamina propria.

3 Hyperplastic glandular epithelium, with or without ulceration.

Tumours of large bowel

Epithelial polyps

There are several types of large bowel polyp arising from the mucosa: see also Fig. 9 on p. 44.

1 *Non-neoplastic*: hyperplastic, hamartomatous or juvenile and regenerative 'pseudo'-polyps in ulcerative colitis.

2 *Neoplastic*: tubular adenoma, villous adenoma and tubulovillous adenoma.

Non-neoplastic polyps

Hyperplastic polyps—metaplastic polyps

These are very common and occur at increasing frequency with age. They are more frequent in populations which have a high incidence of colorectal carcinoma, but are not themselves considered premalignant.

Appearances

Usually small, <5 mm, sessile pale polyps, often multiple and with elongated glands lined by mature epithelium, with a serrated appearance near the surface.

Hamartomatous polyp

A hamartoma is a non-neoplastic tumour composed of tissues native to the site of origin but of abnormal arrangement.

Types

Hamartomatous polyps occur in:

1 Peutz–Jegher's syndrome.

2 Cronkhite–Canada syndrome—commoner in small than large bowel but extremely rare.

3 Juvenile polyps—these may be multiple in juvenile polyposis syndrome of autosomal dominant inheritance.

4 Sporadic.

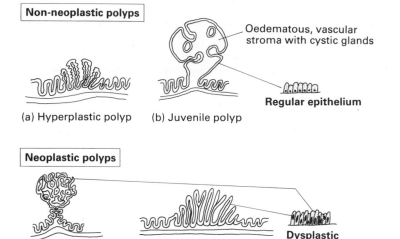

Fig. 9 Polyps of large bowel.

Non-neoplastic polyps

(a) Hyperplastic polyp   (b) Juvenile polyp

Oedematous, vascular stroma with cystic glands

Regular epithelium

Neoplastic polyps

(c) Tubular adenoma   (d) Villous adenoma

Dysplastic epithelium

Microscopical

1 Peutz–Jegher's type show a fronded arrangement of elongated and dilated glands around a branching muscular stalk.

2 Juvenile type show cystic glands in excess oedematous stroma but without a muscular stalk.

Inflammatory pseudo-polyps

Tags of regenerative mucosa which remain between areas of flat ulceration in ulcerative colitis.

Adenomas and adenomatous polyps

Epidemiology

Small adenomatous polyps are very common in older subjects from countries with high incidence of colorectal carcinoma (see below), where they are present in up to 50% of persons aged over 60:

1 Male:female ratio 2:1.

2 Commoner in left side of colon.

3 Immigrants to high incidence areas acquire a high incidence within one generation, indicating environmental—presumed dietary, aetiological factors.

Macroscopical

Pedunculated—i.e. on a stalk or sessile polyps, size variable, rarely up to several cm.

Tubular adenomas are round/lobulated, often pedunculated.

Villous adenomas are sessile, velvety lesions.

Microscopical

1 Glands are crowded together, elongated and branched.

2 The epithelium shows dysplastic features:

    (a) increased nuclear:cytoplasmic ratio,

    (b) stratification of nuclei,

    (c) cellular pleomorphism,

    (d) increased mitotic figures.

    The degree of dysplasia is subjectively graded as mild, moderate or severe.

Malignant change—the polyp → cancer sequence

Adenomatous polyps are premalignant lesions—the risk of adenocarcinoma developing in a polyp depends on:

1 Size: polyps <1 cm, 1% malignant; polyps 1–2 cm, 12% malignant; polyps > 2 cm, 30% malignant.

2 Villous component—villous adenomas are more likely to undergo malignant transformation.

3 Presence of severe dysplasia.

    All large bowel polyps should be removed, and examined microscopically to determine:

1 The type of polyp—whether adenomatous or non-neoplastic.

2 If adenomatous:

    (a) the type and degree of dysplasia;

    (b) completeness of excision;

    (c) evidence of malignant invasion of the muscularis mucosae.

Multiple polyps

Sporadic adenomas are often multiple; 30% of patients have more than one and 15% have more than five.

Patients with multiple polyps are at increased risk of developing colorectal carcinoma: removal of polyps is important to establish their nature and reduce the subsequent risk of malignancy.

Familial adenomatous polyposis

An autosomal dominant inherited mutation on the long arm of chromosome 5. In this condition more than 100 adenomatous polyps (usually well over 1000) develop at a young age—during teens or 20s. Adenomas begin as 'unicryptal' lesions, which develop into typical tubular adenomas. If the colon is not removed, carcinoma—often multiple, invariably develops. Therefore prophylactic colectomy or proctocolectomy is performed in family members once the presence of adenomas has been confirmed.

Gardner's syndrome

The combination of adenomatous polyposis with connective tissue tumours—osteomas, desmoid tumours, and ectodermal abnormalities—epidermoid cysts, dental changes. This is a variant of familial adenomatous polyposis and is autosomal dominant with variable penetrance.

Malignant

Adenocarcinoma of large intestine

Epidemiology
1 Adenocarcinomas account for 98% of large bowel malignancies.
2 Second commonest (non-skin) malignancy in Western countries.
3 Rare in Africa—but increasing in urban centres there.

Aetiology
1 All adenocarcinomas are believed to develop from adenomas, except in patients with ulcerative colitis, where they usually arise in areas of flat dysplasia.
2 The same dietary factors—low-residue, high-carbohydrate high-fat diet, are implicated in the aetiology of:
  (a) adenomas, carcinoma;
  (b) diverticular disease;
  (c) appendicitis;
  (d) possibly inflammatory bowel disease.
3 Hereditary factors—when the polyposis syndromes described above are excluded, about 10% of colorectal cancer patients have one or more close relatives with colorectal cancer. This includes patients with the Lynch syndromes:
  (a) type I, associated with tumours at other sites;
  (b) type II, inherited risk for colorectal cancer only.

Macroscopical
Polypoid, elevated, ulcerated, or diffusely infiltrative tumours.

Right-sided carcinomas tend to be exophytic—cauliflower-like, or form tight strictures; left-sided ones to be ulcerated, often circumferential and stricturing.

Left-sided carcinomas present with change in bowel habit, bleeding, or obstruction, due to mechanical effects on the passage of faeces, and so tend to present earlier than right-sided carcinomas.

Right-sided carcinomas which develop where faecal material is soft tend to present later with weight loss, anaemia, and a right-sided abdominal mass.

Microscopical
Most are moderately or well-differentiated adenocarcinomas, forming recognizable glandular structures. Poorly differentiated carcinomas have a poorer prognosis.

There are two rarer types of undifferentiated carcinoma:
1 *Small cell carcinoma*, which resembles oat cell carcinoma of lung (see p. 404).
2 *Signet ring cell carcinoma*, which resembles diffuse gastric cancer (see p. 30).

Spread
1 *Direct*—into adjacent bowel wall and adherent structures. Unlike gastric cancer, colorectal cancer rarely extends far along the bowel wall beyond the macroscopic limits of the tumour.
2 *Lymphatic*—to lymph nodes.
3 *Blood*—to liver and then elsewhere.
4 *Transcoelomic*—if the primary tumour has invaded through the peritoneum.

Staging
The extent of spread of the adenocarcinoma is described by its Dukes' stage, which can then be

related to the prognosis:

	5-year survival
Stage A: invasive adenocarcinoma, not extending through the full thickness of the muscularis propria.	> 90%
Stage B: carcinoma invading through the muscularis propria; no lymph node metastases.	> 70%
Stage C: lymph node mestastases present	30%

    C1: metastases in local nodes

    C2: metastasis in highest lymph node resected.

Recent additions to this staging system which give additional prognostic information include:

1 Features related to the likelihood of distant micro-metastases at the time of surgery:

  (a) pattern of the invasive edge (expansile or infiltrative);

  (b) presence/absence of inflammatory infiltrate at the invasive edge;

  (c) number of lymph node metastases.

2 Presence of carcinoma at the circumferential margin of excision of rectal tumours; this indicates a high risk of local recurrence.

Carcinoid tumours

Small carcinoid tumours, < 1 cm diameter, occur as incidental findings in the rectum and have a good prognosis.

Large carcinoid tumours of the large bowel are rare and usually do not produce functioning hormones, although they are often multihormonal by histochemistry. About 50% will have metastasized at the time of diagnosis.

The histological pattern and demonstration of neuroendocrine nature of the tumour is as described under small intestinal tumours, on p. 36.

Lymphomas

Very uncommon in the large bowel. Are usually of B cell type, or represent secondary involvement by generalized lymphoma. Two patterns of primary lymphoma are recognized:

1 Single plaque-like or exophytic tumour.

2 Multiple lymphomatous polyposis.

Metastatic tumours

These are unusual and generally from primary tumours of stomach, breast, ovary, kidney or melanoma.

Connective tissue tumours

Lipomas, smooth muscle tumours, haemangiomas and neurofibromas all occur occasionally, usually as incidental findings or at post mortem. They are seldom responsible for symptoms.

Vascular

Blood supply

The ascending and transverse colon are supplied from the superior mesenteric artery, the rest of colon and rectum from inferior mesenteric artery and rectal arteries.

Ischaemia

Features as described on p. 37 for small bowel chronic ischaemia may cause stricturing, typically at the splenic flexure.

Angiodysplasia

Nature

This is an abnormal dilatation of the mucosal and submucosal veins, usually present in the right side of the colon in elderly patients, and sometimes associated with valvular heart disease. The lesions are a cause of colonic blood loss which is often difficult to diagnose. This is best demonstrated by angiography, but visible by colonoscopy; it is very difficult to see in the resected colon unless the vessels have first been injected with a material such as barium/gelatin.

Appearances

In specimens in which the vascular tree has been injected prior to opening, the dilated vessels appear as small spider-like lesions. Microscopically there are widely dilated, thin-walled, vascular channels within the mucosa and submucosa.

Pathogenesis

The development of angiodysplasia is associated with hypertension and left-sided valvular heart disease. Predilection for the right side of the colon is attributed to greater tension in the bowel wall at this site, due to the larger diameter of the right colon.

Diverticular disease

Nature

A diverticulum—literally 'wayside house of ill repute',

is an out-pouching of the colonic mucosa through a defect in the muscle wall of the colon.

Diverticular disease is extremely common in 'Western' civilisations, and is attributed to low-fibre diet. It is rare in tropical countries and in Japan.

Pathogenesis

Diverticula are believed to form due to increased intraluminal pressure forcing the mucosa to herniate through the muscle wall, typically at the site of weakness where arteries penetrate the muscularis propria.

Distribution

Most diverticula, 90%, occur in the sigmoid colon, but the more proximal or even the entire colon are occasionally affected.

Macroscopical

There are two lesions:

1 The diverticula themselves, which are flask-shaped mucosal herniations about 5 mm diameter, may contain faecal material, visible as protrusions from the serosal surface. They typically occur along the line of the appendices epiploicae.

2 A marked thickening of the muscularis propria with hardening of the taenia coli, and shortening of the sigmoid colon.

Microscopical

Uninflamed diverticula have a normal colonic mucosal lining and wall composed of muscularis mucosae and a thin line of muscle derived from muscularis propria.

Diverticulitis

Stasis of faecal material within the diverticula predisposes to inflammation and ulceration of the diverticular mucosa, followed by rupture with pericolic abscess formation, or free perforation.

Complications

1 *Diverticulitis*—with pericolic abscess and risk of spread to liver (see p. 234).
2 *Perforation*.
3 *Bleeding*.
4 *Stricture*—scarring around the healing diverticular abscess may cause narrowing of sigmoid colon. This can closely mimic carcinoma macroscopically; a malignant stricture can be excluded only by histological examination.

Sigmoid volvulus

Twisting of the sigmoid loop on its mesentery rarely occurs in elderly patients in Western countries, but is more common in the developing world.

'Irritable bowel syndrome'

By definition, these patients with gastrointestinal symptoms have no demonstrable pathological abnormality.

G/GASTROINTESTINAL TRACT, ANAL CANAL, PERITONEUM, PAEDIATRIC GASTROINTESTINAL DISEASES

Anal canal
  Inflammations
  Tumours
Peritoneum
  Peritonitis
  Tumours
  Paediatric gastroenterology

Anal canal

This is lined below the pectinate line by squamous epithelium, and is therefore subject to different tumours than those affecting the rectum.

Inflammation

Perianal sepsis with fissure, sinus, abscess and fistula formation is a common surgical problem. Histology of excised tissue is important to exclude malignancy and Crohn's disease. Venereal diseases including syphilis (see p. 2), herpes simplex and chancroid (see p. 203) may also present with perianal ulceration.

Tumours of the anal canal

Benign

Condyloma—squamous cell papilloma

These are warty growths associated with infection by human papilloma virus (HPV), and are sexually transmitted (see p. 211). Microscopy shows features of virus infection including koilocytosis as occurs in condylomas in the female and male genital tracts. The lesions may become very large—'*giant condyloma of Buschke and Lowenstein*'—which as in the vulva or penis are now usually regarded as verrucous carcinomas (see p. 15).

Dysplasia or carcinoma *in situ* may be seen in the squamous epithelium either in flat areas or in the epithelium of a condyloma. As in other areas, this may represent the precursor or pre-invasive stage of squamous cell carcinoma.

Malignant

Squamous cell carcinoma

This has macroscopical and microscopical features identical to squamous carcinoma at other sites, e.g. skin, oesophagus. Squamous carcinoma arising in the anal canal is distinguished from that arising at the anal verge. Anal canal carcinomas tend to grow upwards beneath the rectal mucosa, and are commoner, more frequently seen in women, non-keratinizing and have a poorer prognosis than those of the anal verge. 'Cloacogenic'—'basaloid', *carcinoma* of the anal canal microscopically resembles basal cell carcinoma of the skin, but has a more aggresive clinical behaviour.

Other rare tumours

1 Paget's disease in the perianal region, with or without associated adenocarcinoma (see p. 208).
2 Adenocarcinoma of anal glands.
3 Mucoepidermoid carcinoma (see p. 20).
4 Adenoid cystic carcinoma (see p. 20).
5 Malignant melanoma (see p. 417).

Vascular

Haemorrhoids—'piles'

Nature
These are dilated, varicose veins forming in the anal canal, either below the anorectal margin—external haemorrhoids, or more proximally from the superior haemorrhoidal plexus—internal haemorrhoids. They commonly occur following constipation and straining, or pregnancy, but are occasionally an indication of portal hypertension.

Complications
Haemorrhoids prolapse, bleed, ulcerate, become thrombosed and may strangulate.

Peritoneum

The serous membrane covering the abdominal organs may be involved in inflammatory and neoplastic processes.

Peritonitis

Inflammation of the peritoneum is nearly always secondary to disease in the gastrointestinal tract, with or without perforation of a viscus. Necrosis of the bowel wall may allow gut organisms to pass through it in the absence of perforation. There may be:
1 *Chemical injury*—from pancreatic enzymes, bile, or gastric acid/pepsin, occurring in acute pancreatitis, leakage from the biliary tree, and perforated peptic ulcer respectively. This is usually followed by bacterial contamination.
2 *Bacterial injury*—following appendicitis, diverticulitis, cholecystitis, bowel ischaemia, salpingitis or secondary infection of above 'chemical' causes.
3 *Infected peritoneal dialysis fluid*—common in continuous ambulatory peritoneal dialysis (CAPD) management of chronic renal failure.

Primary bacterial peritonitis

Peritoneal infection without any of the above causes occurs very rarely, usually in patients with cirrhosis and ascites.

Complications of peritonitis

1 Severe toxaemia from absorbed bacterial products which may be fatal.
2 Localization of purulent exudate as subphrenic, subhepatic or paracolic abscesses.
3 Organization of exudate with formation of fibrous adhesions.
4 Spread via the portal vein to the liver—*portal pylophlebitis* and abscess formation (see p. 234).

Tuberculous peritonitis

Represents spread from abdominal tuberculosis, and results in numerous tiny white nodules over the peritoneum (see p. 33).

Tumours of peritoneum

Tumours of the peritoneum must be distinguished from reactive changes of the mesothelial cells, which may be:
1 Hyperplastic in response to nearby inflammatory lesions.
2 Metaplastic as in endometriosis, and more rarely endosalpingiosis (see p. 219).

Mesothelioma

Diffuse malignant mesothelioma is rare in the peritoneum but corresponds to the much commoner pleural mesothelioma. It is also associated with exposure to asbestos (see p. 388).

Appearances

Sheets of white tumour tissue encase the abdominal organs, forming dense adhesions between them. Histologically there is a variable appearance including papillary and spindle cell patterns (see p. 409).

Secondary tumours

Spread of intra-abdominal malignancy to the peritoneum with subsequent transcoelomic dissemination to peritoneal surfaces is a common late occurrence, particularly in carcinoma of stomach, ovary, pancreas, colon and breast.

Appearances

Ascites associated with multiple tiny white nodules which coalesce to form tumour sheets over the surface of the viscera, with adhesions. This may mimic tuberculous peritonitis or mesothelioma.

Paediatric gastroenterological pathology

Gastrointestinal disorders presenting in infancy and childhood are frequently developmental abnormalities, although some such abnormalities present at birth may not become apparent until adult life. Other conditions specific to infancy are also included in this section.

Congenital malformations

Abnormal embryonal or fetal development may result in the following anomalies at any level of the gastrointestinal tract:

1 Atresia—failure of recanalization of the viscus involved.
2 Stenosis.
3 Fistula.
4 Duplication.
5 Congenital diverticulum.
6 Cysts.
7 Malrotation.
8 Heterotopic tissue.
9 Congenital hernia—hiatus hernia and omphalocele.

These are all very uncommon, except for oesophageal atresia, atresia of the anal canal—imperforate anus, Meckel's diverticulum and minor malrotations.

Oesophageal atresia

Defective separation of the oesophagus from the trachea during foregut development results in oesophageal atresia, with or without *tracheo-oesophageal fistula* (see p. 402).

Anorectal anomalies

Various degrees of anorectal atresia occur, with or without fistula formation to bladder or vagina, due to abnormal development of cloacal structures.

Meckel's diverticulum

A diverticulum formed by persistence of the proximal vitello-intestinal duct is present in 1–4% of the population, but rarely causes symptoms. The diverticulum is lined by small intestinal mucosa, often with heterotopic gastric or pancreatic tissue present.

Complications

1 *Peptic ulceration*: if acid-secreting gastric mucosa is present.
2 *Volvulus or obstruction*: if linked to umbilicus by a fibrous cord.
3 *Intussusception*.
4 *Diverticulitis*.
5 *Tumours*: adenocarcinoma.

Congenital pyloric stenosis

Incidence

Up to four per 1000 births and commoner in males, first-born, patients with affected family members.

Appearances

A band of hypertrophic muscle results in narrowing of the pyloric canal, probably due to an underlying abnormality of the myenteric plexus. Treatment is by surgical splitting of the muscle band.

Meconium ileus

Neonatal intestinal obstruction due to plugging of the ileum by thick viscid contents occurs in 10% of babies with cystic fibrosis (see p. 35). Histologically, mucosal glands are distended by inspissated mucus.

Neonatal necrotizing enterocolitis

A disorder of premature infants in which necrosis of

the ileocaecal mucosa is associated with gas-filled cysts in the bowel wall. This develops after the introduction of enteral feeding and may be attributed to clostridial infection.

Hirschsprung's disease

Nature
A variable length of rectum and distal colon is narrowed due to a disturbance of innervation in which ganglion cells of both submucosal and myenteric plexuses are absent. The bowel wall becomes greatly dilated above the aganglionic segment.

Patterns
1 Rectum and sigmoid narrowed—50%.
2 'Short segment' disease in distal rectum—25%.
3 Proximal colon with or without small bowel involvement in continuity—25%.

Appearances
The abnormal, narrowed portion shows:
1 Absence of ganglion cells in both plexuses.
2 Hypertrophy of cholinergic nerve fibres in nerve plexuses, and extending into the lamina propria.

Chapter 3
Diseases of the Breast

The normal breast

In humans the breasts are paired organs situated on the chest wall. They are modified apocrine sweat glands arising from the 'milk line'. Before puberty the structure of male and female breast tissue is identical, composed of a rudimentary branching duct system which discharges onto the surface at the nipple. At puberty, under the coordinated action of a number of hormones including prolactin, oestrogen and progesterone, the *female* breast enlarges due both to an increase in the amount of stromal connective and adipose tissue and to a proliferation of the duct system. Breast lobules bud from subsegmental ducts to form functional terminal duct lobular units. The ducts and acini have a two-layered structure composed of inner secretory epithelial cells and outer myoepithelial cells, bounded by a basement membrane.

During *pregnancy* the breasts enlarge due to physiological hyperplasia, with increased secretory activity. At the onset of *lactation* secretory activity becomes more pronounced, with marked distension of acini. Involution of breast lobules occurs with increasing age, especially after the menopause. Lobules become atrophic due to a reduction in the amount of glandular tissue, with stromal hyalinization.

In the *male* the stucture of the breast remains unchanged throughout adult life, and lobular development never occurs.

Disorders of growth

Congenital

These are rare and unimportant, with the exception of *polymastia* and *polythelia*—accessory breasts and nipples. These may occur anywhere along the 'milk line' from the chest to the groin and are subject to the same disorders as normally situated breasts.

Failure of growth

Failure of the development of the breasts at puberty is distinctly uncommon, and when it occurs is usually associated with ovarian agenesis as in Turner's syndrome (see p. 206).

Precocious development

The breasts may develop early as part of the syndrome of precocious puberty. Although a small proportion of cases is associated with a granulosa cell or other ovarian tumour (see p. 224) in most cases no cause is found. Surgical intervention is not indicated.

Adolescent hypertrophy

This is the commonest form of true hypertrophy of the female breast. The breasts may enlarge so greatly that they become a *severe physical and psychological* burden. Occasionally the hypertrophy is unilateral. The cause is unknown and the only effective treatment is surgical.

Microscopical

The breast tissue consists of normal epithelial elements with an increase in connective and adipose tissue.

Inflammatory

Acute mastitis and breast abscess

Most *breast abscesses* are associated with lactation when staphylococci or streptococci gain entry into the breast tissue through a cracked nipple. The whole of the breast may be enlarged and painful or a more localized abscess may form.

Microscopical

Acute suppurative inflammation is centred on breast ducts and lobules. Rapid resolution nearly always occurs with appropriate antibiotic therapy, although some fibrous scarring may follow abscess formation. Incomplete resolution may be followed by a true chronic mastitis.

Chronic mastitis

True chronic inflammation of the breast due to bacterial infection is extremely uncommon. Most cases are due to incomplete resolution of an acute mastitis. Persistent chronic mastitis occurring in older women should raise the possibilty of deliberate self-mutilation.

Chronic granulomatous mastitis is an uncommon condition of unknown aetiology. It usually occurs in parous premenopausal women and is characterized by painful lumpiness in the breast, usually unilaterally.

There are discrete non-caseating granulomata composed of neutrophils, eosinophils, histiocytes and giant cells, confined to breast lobules. No organisms can be identified. Complete surgical excision may be curative if the process is localized, but the condition may be recurrent and require corticosteroid therapy.

Tuberculosis

In the Western hemisphere tuberculosis of the breast is very rare and is due either to lymphatic or haematogenous spread from intrathoracic foci.

Traumatic fat necrosis

Although a convincing history of a specific injury is obtained in under half the patients there is good evidence that the lesion results from trauma to an area of adipose tissue sufficient to disrupt the fat cells and allow the escape of fat globules into adjacent tissue. The lesion usually presents as a firm nodule in the breast, sometimes with skin tethering and local fixity, and it may be difficult to exclude a carcinoma on clinical grounds.

Microscopical

There is an area composed of fat spaces, foamy macrophages, foreign-body giant cells and neutrophils. Healing by fibrosis occurs in the later stages, leaving a residual contracted scar.

Fibrocystic change

A wide range of terms has been used for this condition, including *fibroadenosis*, *cystic hyperplasia*, *chronic* *mastitis* and *mammary dysplasia*. None is entirely satisfactory, but fibrocystic change has now become widely accepted throughout the world. Fibrocystic change is the commonest of all breast conditions, and produces clinical symptoms in at least 10% of women. The peak frequency is in the premenopausal decade and after the menopause there is a sharp decline in symptomatic cases. The lesion usually presents as a discrete palpable lump in the breast or as a more diffuse 'lumpiness' which occasionally may be bilateral. The introduction of the National Health Service Breast Screening Programme (NHS BSP) is likely to reveal an increased number of impalpable but mammographically visible cases.

Aetiology

The underlying cause of the morphological entities which are grouped together as fibrocystic change is poorly understood. The lesion is not, as some of the descriptive terms used would imply, inflammatory in nature, but almost certainly has a hormonal basis. The cyclical activity of the ovaries, with its complex interactive secretion of oestrogens and progesterone, produces effects on the breasts as well as the endometrium. Subtle proliferative changes occur in the acini and stroma of the lobules during the menstrual cycle, and it is likely that these become exaggerated and abnormal in the premenopausal era due to hormonal imbalance related to diminishing ovarian function.

Microscopic components

A wide range of histological appearances may be seen, and, apart from cystic change, there is no correlation with the gross findings. Any of the microscopic components may occur in a focal or diffuse distribution and are present in variable amounts in one or both breasts. There is considerable variation from case to case.

Cystic change

It is the presence of cysts, with associated fibrosis, which most frequently produces clinical symptoms in the form of a palpable lump. They may be single or multiple, and usually contain clear or yellow fluid. Cysts are frequently only detectable histologically— the so-called *microcysts*. All cysts develop from dilated lobular acini and are normally lined by cuboidal or flattened epithelium. Cyst walls may be thickened due to reactive inflammation and fibrosis.

Adenosis

The broad terms 'adenosis' and 'fibroadenosis' are greatly overused by pathologists, often when no definite pathological lesion is present, and they should be abandoned. In *blunt-duct adenosis* there is an organoid hypertrophy of lobules with dilatation of acini and an increase in intralobular stroma. *Sclerosing adenosis* is considered below.

Epithelial hyperplasia

The epithelial lining of lobular acini and cysts frequently undergoes metaplasia to columnar cells with abundant eosinophilic cytoplasm resembling those of normal apocrine sweat glands, the so-called pink cell change or *apocrine metaplasia*. The degree of proliferation varies and papillary structures may be seen.

In about a quarter of cases a significant degree of epithelial proliferation is seen within ductular structures. This is termed epithelial hyperplasia of *usual* type. The duct spaces are lined by several layers of large epithelial cells having abundant cytoplasm and the lumen may be obliterated by a solid proliferation. Nuclei are regular, and although occasional mitoses may be seen they are of normal configuration. Cell necrosis is not present. Care must be taken to distinguish this benign epithelial hyperplasia from ductal carcinoma *in situ*. In cases where abnormal features are present and the epithelial proliferation has some but not all of the morphological and cytological changes of *in situ* malignancy, the term *atypical ductal hyperplasia* is used. The commonest pattern is that of an irregular lacy network resembling the cribriform type of ductal carcinoma *in situ*, but a micropapillary pattern may also be seen.

Lobular proliferations are considered below, on p. 57.

Sclerosing lesions

Sclerosing adenosis

Although frequently found microscopically as part of the spectrum of fibrocystic change, sclerosing adenosis may also present in the nodular form as a palpable mass in an otherwise normal breast.

Microscopical

The normal configuration of lobules is distorted by a disorderly proliferation of epithelial, myoepithelial and intralobular stromal cells. The nuclei are regular and mitoses infrequent. Sclerosing adenosis may be mistaken for carcinoma radiologically because of the presence of microcalcifications resembling those seen in ductal carcinoma *in situ*, and histologically because the presence of microtubular structures can mimic tubular carcinoma.

Complex sclerosing lesion—radial scar

These terms are applied to stellate lesions with a dense fibroelastic core and a varying degree of epithelial proliferation in ductules within the radiating connective tissue arms. The term *radial scar* is used for lesions which measure up to 1 cm in maximum extent, and *complex sclerosing lesion* for those measuring more than 1 cm. They were once thought to be uncommon, largely because they are usually impalpable, but with the greater use of mammography they are now known to occur relatively frequently. The exact pathogenesis is unknown, but most evidence suggests that they are associated with the spectrum of fibrocystic change. The great majority are benign, but both *in situ* and invasive carcinoma may develop within the lesion.

Mammary duct ectasia

This is the term given to the progressive dilatation of a group of large or intermediate breast ducts. It affects one or more segments of the breast and is often subareolar in location. Periductal inflammation is a hallmark of this condition, and it is now thought that the process begins with such a change, and proceeds by destruction of the elastic network to dilatation and periductal fibrosis.

Macroscopical

There is an area of firmness in which numerous ducts distended by creamy material are seen.

Microscopical

The dilated lumina contain lipid-rich amorphous material and foamy macrophages. The epithelium is thinned and there is periductal chronic inflammation and fibrosis. There is no association with malignancy, but the presence of a firm mass, and nipple retraction may simulate carcinoma.

Fibroadenoma and related lesions

Fibroadenoma

Although these lesions are by convention classed as

benign tumours of fibrous and epithelial elements there is considerable evidence to support the view that they are not true neoplasms, but rather focal areas of lobular hyperplasia. They develop after puberty, and although they may be found at any age, occur most commonly between 20 and 35 years. They present clinically as a small, well-defined firm mobile nodule, which may occasionally be multiple.

Microscopical

They are composed of proliferating ductules and stroma with characteristic cleft-like spaces—intracanalicular pattern and periacinar connective tissue whorls—pericanalicular pattern. They are circumscribed but not encapsulated.

At operation fibroadenomas are easily enucleated and if completely excised do not recur, although further nodules may develop in either breast. There is an increasing tendency amongst clinicians not to intervene surgically once a benign preoperative diagnosis has been established (see p. 59); if left in this way fibroadenomas become sclerotic with age. Neoplastic change is exceedingly rare.

Juvenile fibroadenoma

Considerable terminological confusion has been produced by inconsistent use of the terms 'juvenile' and 'giant' fibroadenoma. For example, the latter has been used to describe both large fibroadenomas *and*, incorrectly, benign phyllodes tumour (see p. 55). In practice all juvenile fibroadenomas are large. The term is used to denote fibroadenomas which occur in adolescents, grow rapidly and reach a size which is often at least double that of the opposite breast, stretching the skin and distorting the nipple.

Microscopical

They do not differ significantly from the typical fibroadenoma.

Hamartoma

These are uncommon lesions which may occur at any age after puberty, the majority presenting around the age of 40. It appears that with the increasing use of mammography they may be detected more frequently in the future. Grossly they have a similar circumscribed appearance to fibroadenomas, but are usually larger.

Microscopical

Numerous lobular structures are present with associated stroma but lacking the cleft-like spaces of a fibroadenoma. There is no association with carcinoma.

Benign breast lesions and risk of malignancy

It has now been established that the risk of subsequent carcinoma in patients who have had breast biopsies showing benign lesions is related to the degree of epithelial hyperplasia present. If no epithelial hyperplasia is seen (this includes fibroadenoma and sclerosing adenosis) there is no increase in risk; because this category accounts for about 70% of all benign biopsies the majority of women can be reassured and do not require follow-up. The presence of epithelial hyperplasia of usual type, present in about 25% of biopsies, increases the risk of carcinoma by twofold. The most significant increase in risk—of four times—occurs in patients whose biopsies show *atypical hyperplasia*, and this doubles in the presence of a family history of breast cancer. However, atypical hyperplasia is found in only 4% of biopsies, and atypia with a family history in 1%. Long-term follow-up is advisable for the very small group of patients with epithelial atypia; they should be taught breast self-examination and offered biennial mammography, but further surgical intervention at the time of the original biopsy is not appropriate.

Benign tumours

Adenoma

The existence of a true mammary adenoma has only recently been established, most cases previously termed adenomas being in reality cellular fibroadenomas. They are very uncommon and usually occur only in younger women.

Microscopical

Tubular adenomas are composed of closely packed ductules with little intervening stroma. There is no significant risk of subsequent carcinoma.

Adenoma of the nipple

A rare benign tumour arising from the main nipple ducts which may mimic Paget's disease of the nipple (see p. 56). Complete local excision is curative.

Papilloma

Duct papillomas are uncommon tumours which occur predominantly in middle-aged patients and occasionally in younger women. They are usually single and located in one of the large central ducts near to the nipple. More rarely they are peripheral and multiple. In most cases the presenting symptom is single duct discharge from the nipple which may be blood-stained.

The great majority of papillomas pursue a benign course, and this is particularly true for the solitary central lesion. There is an increased risk of subsequent invasive carcinoma in patients with multiple peripheral papillomas; risk appears to be related to the degree and type of associated epithelial hyperplasia.

Microscopical

Papillomas are composed of a fronded fibrovascular core covered by a two-layered duct-type epithelium. Occasionally the duct becomes cystically dilated, resulting in an *intracystic papilloma*; this may present as a palpable nodule.

Other benign tumours

Benign connective tissue tumours are uncommon but include lipoma, leiomyoma and angioma.

Phyllodes tumour

Several conflicting terms have been applied to this lesion, including cystosarcoma phyllodes and giant fibroadenoma. Neither of these is appropriate since most tumours behave in a benign way whilst a minority are malignant. For this reason the designation phyllodes tumour benign or malignant, is preferable.

Phyllodes tumours are uncommon. Although they may occur at any age after puberty, they are most frequent in middle-aged or elderly patients. They form large, lobulated circumscribed masses. Ulceration of the skin may occur by pressure necrosis due to the rapid growth and large size. Grossly they are firm and lobulated with a whorled cut surface which resembles a compressed leaf bud—*phyllo = leaf* (Greek).

The great majority of phyllodes tumours are benign and complete excision is curative. Approximately 10% recur locally after enucleation, due to incomplete excision, and less than 10% are truly malignant with sarcomatous change in the stroma. Features which are associated with malignant change are an infiltrative edge, overgrowth of the stroma and an increased mitotic count.

Microscopical

Elongated cleft-like spaces are lined by duct-type epithelial cells and there is a cellular stroma. The epithelial cells are regular and benign, but nuclear abnormalities may be present in the stromal cells and mitoses may be increased in number.

Carcinoma of the breast

Epidemiology

Carcinoma of the breast is still the commonest malignant tumour in women—25% in Western Europe, although it is closely followed by carcinoma of the bronchus. The frequency is increasing worldwide and this is not entirely due to the increase in the 'at-risk' population. The annual mortality in the UK is in excess of 15 000. Breast cancer may occur at any age, but is rare below 25 years and most frequent between 40–70 years. It is commoner in women than men by a factor of more than 200 : 1, and male breast cancer is relatively rare.

Predisposing factors

The aetiology of breast cancer is obscure although a number of risk factors have been identified. The strongest of these, are of course, age and sex (see above). Other predisposing factors are:

1 *Geographical*: there is marked geographical variation in frequency, which increases as follows; Asia, eastern Europe, western Europe, North America. This is almost entirely due to socioeconomic rather than racial factors, e.g. Japanese migrants to the United States acquire the higher incidence rate prevalent in North America after two or three generations.

2 *Reproductive experience*: the risk is 50% greater for nulliparous than parous women. There is a slight protection if the first pregnancy takes place early in the reproductive period. Breast feeding may be protective against premenopausal breast cancer.

3 *Ovarian activity*: the enormous difference in frequency between women and men points to a hormonal role in the aetiology of breast cancer, but data are inconclusive. Early natural or artificial menopause is slightly protective. Prolonged oral contraceptive use may increase the risk in younger women. Approximately one-third of breast cancers are 'hormone-dependent' and patients may undergo remission if given anti-oestrogenic therapy. Response to therapy is better in patients whose tumour cells contain oestrogen receptor protein (ER). Evidence from a number of clinical trials suggests that the most effective form of treatment is adjuvant tamoxifen which acts by blocking the effect of circulating oestrogens on cancer cells.

4 *Genetic and familial factors*: molecular biological techniques have identified sequence deletions on chromosomes 11 and/or 17 in some cases; this is clearly an area for more extensive study. Risk is increased 2–3 times in first-degree female relatives of women with breast cancer. In addition there are rare 'breast cancer families' affecting several generations, e.g. grandmother, mother, daughter.

5 *Diet*: there is an increased risk from obesity in premenopausal women, but no convincing link has been demonstrated with high fat intake. Increased alcohol intake appears to increase the risk for all women.

6 *Benign breast lesions*: risk of subsequent breast cancer in women who have had a previous biopsy for a benign lesion is related to the degree and type of epithelial hyperplasia (see p. 53).

Experimental

'High' and 'low' breast cancer strains of mice have been developed, which breed true. However, it has been shown that in addition to the hereditary element, an RNA virus, transmitted by suckling, is also important. The third factor is hormonal activity, removal of the ovaries preventing the development of breast cancer in female mice and administration of exogenous oestrogens inducing carcinomas in males of 'high' risk strain. However, no convincing evidence has yet been produced to implicate a virus in human breast cancer.

Classification

Breast cancer is not a single entity, but is made up of a number of different malignant processes. There is a fundamental division into *in situ* and invasive carcinoma and within these two broad categories further subtypes are recognized. Carcinomas may arise in any part of the breast which contains epithelium, including the axillary tail. The upper outer quadrant is the most frequent site of origin.

Carcinoma *in situ*

By definition the term carcinoma *in situ* is used when the cytological changes of malignancy are present in the epithelium of an organ or structure, but the basement membrane is intact and no evidence of invasion into adjacent tissues is seen.

It has been conventional to divide carcinoma in situ of the breast into two types, ductal and lobular. Paget's disease of the nipple is included with ductal carcinoma in situ because of their close association. Lobular carcinoma in situ is now considered as a separate entity, together with atypical lobular hyperplasia, under the umbrella of *lobular neoplasia* (see p. 57).

Ductal carcinoma in situ

This accounts for up to 5% of symptomatic cases of carcinoma of the breast, but between 15% and 20% in breast screening programmes. This is due to the identification of impalpable lesions mammographically, usually because of the presence of microcalcification. A variable number of ducts or ductular structures is involved. In the great majority of cases a single contiguous focus is present, although more rarely there may be diffuse involvement of the whole breast. The ductular structures are the site of a proliferation of abnormal epithelial cells, and several *microscopical* patterns are recognized. In the *solid* type the cells are usually large and vary in size and shape, filling the entire lumen. When there is extensive central necrosis the term *comedo* is applied—the yellow necrotic material can be expressed from the ducts on pressure like a comedone. In the *cribriform* type there is a proliferation of smaller cells which form a lacy network with geometric punched-out spaces around the periphery of the ductules. The *micropapillary* type is characterized by small peripheral papillary projections.

The prognosis of ductal carcinoma *in situ* is excellent. Mastectomy is curative, but conservation therapy may result in local recurrence in the comedo or solid large cell types.

The term *microinvasive carcinoma* is applied to those cases in which the dominant lesion is ductal carcinoma *in situ* but one or more foci of invasion are present, none of which amounts to more than 1 mm diameter. Available data suggest that the prognosis is no different from that of the comedo type of ductal carcinoma *in situ*.

Paget's disease of the nipple

Paget's disease presents as a red scaly eczematous rash involving the nipple and areola. Biopsy shows thickening of the squamous epithelium with elongation of the rete pegs and an underlying chronic inflammatory infiltrate. Within the epidermis there is an infiltrate of large pale cells with aypical nuclei—

Paget's cells. Although the nature of these cells was in dispute for many years, modern immunostaining techniques have established that they are carcinoma cells which have migrated up the duct system from an *in situ* carcinoma of the underlying mammary ducts. The ductal carcinoma *in situ* may be impalpable and is usually situated deep in one of the breast quadrants, but in a small minority of cases is confined to the nipple ducts. In up to 40% of cases, particularly if the nipple lesion has been present for some time, the ductal carcinoma *in situ* is also associated with an invasive carcinoma.

The *prognosis* in Paget's disease is that of the asssociated underlying mammary carcinoma. If this is *in situ* then long-term survival is excellent. However, if an asssociated invasive carcinoma is present survival may be less satisfactory (see p. 58). Conservation therapy is not appropriate and mastectomy is the treatment of choice.

Lobular neoplasia

This term encompasses both *atypical lobular hyperplasia* and *lobular carcinoma in situ*, because these entities are now regarded as risk factors for subsequent invasive carcinoma rather than established malignancies which require treatment. Lobular neoplasia is an incidental finding seen in less than 5% of breast biopsies. When present it is frequently multifocal, usually involving more than one quadrant of the breast, and bilateral.

Microscopical

In lobular carcinoma *in situ* lobular units are enlarged and the acini distended by a solid proliferation of small darkly staining epithelial cells of uniform appearance. Basement membranes remain intact and the acinar lumina are obliterated. In atypical lobular hyperplasia the changes are less developed. Lobules may not be enlarged and the epithelial proliferation does not fill the acini, so some lumina are preserved.

Results

The risk of subsequent invasive carcinoma is equal for both breasts. In atypical lobular hyperplasia there is a fourfold increase in risk, and this rises to 10-fold for lobular carcinoma *in situ*. In the presence of a family history of breast cancer these relative risks are doubled. The greatest absolute risk, for a woman with lobular carcinoma *in situ* and a positive family history is 20% after 15 years follow up.

Invasive carcinoma

In the absence of breast screening most invasive carcinomas are detected because a palpable lump is present in the breast. These vary in size from one to several centimetres in diameter, are firm or hard, and the edge may be poorly or well defined. In advanced cases fixity to deep fascia and skin is observed.

Histological type

Invasive carcinoma of the breast arises from a pre-existing *in situ* carcinoma, although by the time the tumour has presented clinically the *in situ* element may no longer be detectable histologically. The following morphological subtypes are recognized:

1 *Infiltrating ductal (no special type)*: over 50% of cases fall into this category in a symptomatic series. They are composed of sheets and cords of large epithelial cells which infiltrate a cellular or hyalinized connective tissue stroma in a disorganized way without a specific morphological pattern.

2 *Infiltrating lobular*: this type accounts for about 10% of symptomatic cases. Classically, linear cords of small, regular epithelial cells infiltrate diffusely within connective tissue, giving a so-called 'Indian file' pattern. The infiltrate of tumour cells often assumes a concentric 'targetoid' arrangement around preserved normal ducts or acini.

3 *Medullary*: these uncommon tumours have a sharply demarcated edge and are composed of anastomosing sheets of epithelial cells forming syncytial masses. No tubule formation is seen and the epithelial cells exhibit marked nuclear atypia with a high mitotic count. There is an associated intense lymphoplasmacytoid infiltrate in the stroma.

4 *Tubular*: these tumours are seen infrequently in symptomatic patients—less than 3% of invasive carcinomas, but are much more common in the prevalent round of breast screening—15–20%, where impalpable tumours are detected mammographically. They are small—usually less than 1.5 cm diameter, firm, and have an irregular stellate outline. As the name implies they are composed of tubular structures with a clear central lumen, lined by a single layer of small regular epithelial cells. Mitoses are rarely seen. Only tumours in which 90% or more of the lesion shows clear tubule formation are included as tubular carcinomas. Tumours in which a tubular structure is present centrally but more than 10% of the periphery has other morphological features (e.g. no special type, infiltrating lobular) are designated as *tubular mixed carcinomas*.

5 *Invasive cribriform*: this rare tumour is composed of infiltrating ductular structures in which the epithelial cells are arranged in the 'lacy network' pattern also seen in the cribriform type of ductal carcinoma *in situ*.

6 *Mucoid*: these may also be termed mucinous or colloid carcinomas. They are uncommon tumours— 2% of invasive carcinomas, which have a sharply defined pale soft gelatinous appearance. Microscopically they are composed of clumps and nests of regular epithelial cells lying in lakes of mucin.

7 *Papillary*: these are rare tumours, accounting for less than 1% of breast carcinomas. A small proportion arises from a pre-existing duct or intracystic papilloma, but the majority occur *de novo*. Microscopically the tumour is composed of papillary structures with central fibrovascular cores lined by epithelial cells of variable atypia.

8 *Miscellaneous*: very rare subtypes include adenoid cystic, metaplastic (spindle cell), squamous and secretory.

Histological grade

In addition to the morphological pattern, carcinomas of the breast may be subdivided according to their degree of differentiation. In the commonest system used three variables are assessed: the amount of tubule formation, variation in the size and shape of nuclei, and mitotic count. Three grades of differentiation are recognized: grade 1, well differentiated; grade 2, moderately differentiated; grade 3, poorly differentiated. This method of histological grading has an important bearing on prognosis (see below).

Routes of spread

1 *Local*: if a tumour remains undetected it will continue to grow and may eventually invade the overlying skin or the deep muscle and chest wall— '*locally advanced primary*'.

2 *Lymphatic*: thorough histological studies have shown that the axillary lymph nodes contain metastatic tumour deposits in approximately 50% of patients with apparently 'operable' breast cancer. The internal mammary lymph nodes may also be involved, especially if the primary tumour is located in the inner quadrants. Careful examination of the breast tissue at the periphery of the primary tumour reveals carcinoma cells in lymphatics in up to 20% of cases.

3 *Blood*: this is the route through which distant metastases occur. Unfortunately, about 75% of women with breast cancer have bloodstream spread at the time of initial diagnosis. Many organs may be involved but the commonest sites are lung, bone and liver.

Assessment of prognosis

Long-term follow-up studies have shown that in women with primary operable breast cancer—stage I and II, i.e. tumours measuring less than 5 cm clinically and without skin fixity, approximately 60% will be alive 5 years after diagnosis, 40% after 10 years and only 20% after 25 years. The prognosis for advanced carcinoma is much worse.

The pathological features of breast cancer described above can be used to predict the prognosis for an individual patient. They can be divided into two broad categories, *time-dependent*—tumour size, lymph node stage and vascular invasion, and *tumour dependent*—morphological type and histological grade.

Pathological *tumour size* correlates well with prognosis, and survival worsens as tumour size increases. This fact forms the basis of mammographic screening in which it is hoped to detect very small tumours at a stage when they are impalpable. *Involvement of locoregional lymph nodes*, confirmed histologically, is one of the most powerful prognostic factors available. Patients with nodal metastases have a significantly poorer survival than patients whose nodes are uninvolved—30% compared with 75% at 10 years. Peritumoral lymphatic invasion correlates strongly with lymph node status, but its presence also indicates a poorer survival in patients who are lymph node negative.

The *morphological types* of breast cancer carry differing prognoses. The special types such as tubular and invasive cribriform carcinoma are associated with excellent long-term survival closely similar to that of an age-matched population without breast cancer. Tubular mixed and mucoid carcinomas have a good prognosis—75% 10-year survival. Medullary and infiltrating lobular carcinoma have an intermediate prognosis compared with that of infiltrating ductal carcinoma—40% at 10 years. *Histological grade*, assessed by the method described above, provides powerful prognostic information, and there is a highly significant correlation between grade and survival— grade 1, 85%, grade 2, 60%, grade 3, 45% survival at 10 years.

Prognostic index

The value of these pathological prognostic factors is enhanced by their combination into a composite prognostic index. The Nottingham Prognostic Index, based on tumour size, lymph node stage and histological grade, divides patients into three groups with survival at 15 years follow-up, as follows:

Good: 32% of cases—80% survivors.

Moderate: 52% of cases—45% survivors.

Poor: 16% of cases—10% survivors.

Such an index can be used to compare treatment groups and, more importantly, to stratify patients for appropriate therapy.

Other malignant tumours

Primary *sarcomas* of the breast are exceedingly rare. They include angiosarcoma, liposarcoma and fibrosarcoma. Primary *lymphomas* are also very rare, and are usually of non-Hodgkin's B cell type.

Male breast lesions

In comparison with the female breast, lesions of male breast are rare. The commonest is *gynaecomastia*, in which there is enlargement of the breast which may be unilateral or bilateral. Microscopically there is a proliferation of branching ducts surrounded by a loose cellular, occasionally myxoid, connective tissue stroma.

Carcinoma of the breast is at least 200 times less frequent in males than females. The prognosis is thought to be poorer but definite statistical evidence is lacking. *Sarcomas* are exceptionally rare.

Diagnostic methods

In the absence of specific screening programmes using mammography most patients with breast cancer present with a lump in the breast. However, numerous other pathological processes, such as fibroadenoma, fibrocystic change and fat necrosis, may also give rise to a lump in the breast, and a definite tissue diagnosis must be established before surgical treatment such as mastectomy is carried out. Two main types of preoperative technique have become established for symptomatic breast disease: a wide-bore cutting needle (e.g. Trucut) which gives a histological preparation, and fine-needle aspiration (FNA) which provides a cytological smear. A high level of diagnostic accuracy can be achieved with both methods, but FNA is simple, less traumatic and more successful in small lesions. Using the 'triple' criteria of clinical examination, imaging—ultrasonography and mammography, and FNA, a positive diagnosis of carcinoma can be achieved in over 95% of cases. Preoperative frozen section, previously the method of choice, should never be used as an 'open-ended' procedure, even in symptomatic women. It is now appropriate only in patients whose palpable lump is thought clinically to be malignant but in whom preoperative needle biopsy has proved unhelpful. Many surgeons are now prepared to avoid excision biopsy in cases where a lump is thought to be benign on all three criteria, e.g., fibroadenoma.

The advent of mammographic screening for breast cancer has resulted in the development of methods for evaluation of impalpable lesions. Stereotactic devices localize a lesion by computer-based plotting of co ordinates from two mammographic views taken at different angles. A thin needle for FNA is then inserted through a guide needle and samples aspirated for cytology. If this method fails to achieve a definite diagnosis, then excision biopsy is performed following localization of the lesion by insertion of a hooked wire under mammographic control—*marker biopsy*. Frozen section plays *no* part in the diagnosis of impalpable lesions.

Chapter 4
Diseases of the Cardiovascular System

A/HEART DISEASES

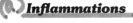
Pericardium

Inflammations

Acute pericarditis

Nature
Primary pericarditis is rare. Most cases are due to direct involvement from myocardial or endocardial disease, or by extension from neighbouring tissues, e.g. lungs.

Aetiology
1 *Bacterial*, e.g. staphylococci, streptococci, pneumococci; septicaemic or pyaemic; tuberculous.
2 *Viral—acute benign pericarditis*: virus infections are probably the most common cause now of acute pericarditis and follow upper respiratory tract infections or mumps, infectious mononucleosis, etc.
3 *Aseptic*: rheumatic; uraemic; secondary to myocardial infarction; tumour infiltration; systemic lupus erythematosus.

Appearances
The usual inflammatory phenomena occur, with hyperaemia, loss of lustre and exudates of varying appearance.

Types
1 *Serous*: occurs particularly with non-bacterial inflammations. The fluid is clear, straw-coloured, protein-rich and has a relative density of 1.020 or more, with small numbers of polymorphs, lymphocytes and shed mesothelial cells. The volume is usually small (50–200 ml) and when formed slowly, produces little effect on cardiac function. With remission of the underlying disease, the fluid reabsorbs with minimal adhesion formation.
2 *Sero-fibrinous or fibrinous*: this is the most frequent type and occurs with rheumatic fever, myocardial infarction and in uraemia. There is an abundant fibrin-rich exudate with variable amounts of fluid and the 'bread and butter' appearance on separating the parietal and visceral layers. With remission of the underlying cause there is:
  (a) Resolution with digestion of the fibrin.
  (b) Organization with variable obliteration of the pericardial sac which may result in an adherent pericardium.
The condition only rarely leads to embarrassment of cardiac action or to other sequelae.
3 *Purulent or suppurative*: the cause is almost always pyogenic bacterial invasion:
  (a) Direct extension from neighbouring inflammations, e.g. empyema, pneumonia.
  (b) Blood spread from other sites in septicaemia or pyaemia.

(c) Lymphatic spread from neighbouring sites, including subdiaphragmatic inflammation, e.g. subphrenic or hepatic abscesses.

(d) Penetrating injuries which become infected.

There may be large volumes of watery turbid fluid or thick creamy pus from which the organisms can be cultured. Variable amounts of fibrin are present on the surfaces and the inflammatory process may extend into the myocardium. Death may occur, but in survivors, complete resolution is unusual; more commonly, organization and an adherent pericardium ensue.

4 *Haemorrhagic*: this is blood mixed with inflammatory exudate and has to be differentiated from haemopericardium. It is usually due to invasion by tumour but sometimes occurs in fulminating bacterial infections. When due to tumour, malignant cells may be identified in aspirated fluid.

Tuberculous pericarditis

Origin

1 Miliary spread, i.e. blood-borne.

2 Extension from pulmonary disease or from mediastinal lymph nodes.

Appearances

Fibrinous exudate with granulation tissue covering the pericardial surfaces, visible tubercles and sometimes areas of caseation. It may occasionally be haemorrhagic with copious amounts of fluid. Microscopically, tuberculous caseating giant cell systems are seen.

Results

Resolution does not occur and the process heals by gross fibrosis often followed by calcification. Not only is the pericardial sac obliterated, but the dense fibrous tissue layer contracts and restricts filling of the heart in diastole—*constrictive pericarditis*.

Constrictive pericarditis—Pick's disease

Aetiology

Most cases are due to healed tuberculous pericarditis but a few may follow suppurative bacterial disease or connective tissue diseases.

Macroscopical

There is a thick, firm layer of fibrous tissue obliterating the pericardium and completely ensheathing the heart. The tissue frequently contains plaques of calcification and may be firmly adherent internally to the myocardium and externally to the lung, anterior chest wall or diaphragm. In addition, there is often a particularly dense fibrous area around the orifices of the inferior and superior vena cavae as they enter the right atrium.

Microscopical

Hyaline fibrous tissue with plaques of calcium in which there is rarely any significant inflammatory cell infiltration. Only occasionally is there histological evidence of residual active tuberculosis.

Effects

The fibrous tissue impedes venous return, resulting in an enlarged liver, ascites and distended neck veins. In addition, direct mechanical embarrassment to cardiac action may occur.

Results

Excision of the constricting fibrous and partially calcified tissues leads to relief, but this may be technically exceptionally difficult.

Hydropericardium

Nature

Accumulation of a transudate with a low relative density of 1.012, low protein content and usually containing only very scanty mesothelial cells.

Aetiology

1 Cardiac failure.

2 Chronic renal disease.

3 Hypoproteinaemia.

Appearances

The pericardial surfaces remain smooth and glistening and the fluid is clear and faintly straw-coloured.

Effects

There may be very large amounts of fluid which eventually interfere with the heart's action.

Results

Absorbs with removal of the cause, leaving a normal pericardium.

(c) *Haemopericardium*

Nature
Pure blood in the pericardial sac.

Aetiology
1 Rupture of the heart:
  (a) traumatic—e.g. stab wound;
  (b) spontaneous—e.g. myocardial infarct.
2 Rupture of the intrapericardial portion of the aorta;
  (a) dissecting aneurysm;
  (b) syphilitic aneurysm;
  (c) traumatic.
3 In haemorrhagic diatheses—e.g. purpura, scurvy, hypoprothrombinaemia, anticoagulant therapy.

Effects
In most cases, death occurs rapidly due to cardiac tamponade, as little as 200–300 ml commonly being sufficient.

(d) *Pneumopericardium*
Air in the pericardial sac due to:
1 Trauma.
2 Perforation of the lung or the oesophagus into the pericardium.
3 Pericarditis due to gas-forming organisms.

(e) *Tumours of the pericardium*

Primary
Extremely rare—lipoma, fibroma, mesothelioma.

Secondary
Fairly common.
1 Direct extension from adjacent organs—e.g. lung, oesophagus, etc.
2 Blood-borne or lymphatic metastases—e.g. malignant melanoma, malignant lymphomas, etc.

2. Myocardium

(a) *Myocardial metabolism*
The myocardium requires basic high-energy production with the capacity to increase this rapidly by demands for increased cardiac output, particularly in exercise. Oxygen-dependent aerobic metabolism is essential to convert glucose, lactate and fatty acids to high-energy phosphates, particularly adenosine triphosphate (ATP). At rest oxygen utilization and extraction from blood is almost maximal, so increased requirements have to come from increased coronary artery blood flow. Inadequacy creates anaerobic metabolism which, if not rapidly corrected, causes irreversible myocardial cell damage.

(b) *Ischaemic heart disease—IHD*

Nature
This term is applied to the effects of a reduction or cessation of the blood supply of the myocardium. With the exception of rare cases of coronary embolism, arteritis or ostial obstruction the cause is atherosclerosis—*atheroma* (see p. 79).

Some degree of atheroma is virtually inevitable in Caucasians, but IHD is not identifiable until complications occur causing clinical symptoms and/or myocardial damage.

Clinical
Ischaemic changes, whether reversible or irreversible, cause angina which may be of two main types:
1 *Stable angina*: this is predictable at a fixed exercise level and is due to fixed arterial obstruction which limits any increase in coronary blood flow. It probably requires stenosis of at least 75% of cross-sectional areas of the arteries to produce angina on exercise. Prognosis in these circumstances depends on how many of the major coronary artery branches have stenotic segments of this degree. Stenosis may be due directly to concentric or eccentric atheromatous plaques or to 'silent' previous thrombosis which has organized and partially recanalized.
2 *Unstable angina*: the pain is unpredictable and not related to exercise. It reflects reversible ischaemia due to variability of luminal stenosis of some segments—*dynamic* stenosis. Some cases are due to variations in vasomotor tone in segments markedly stenosed by eccentric plaques, others to active fissuring or rupture of plaques with intimal surface thrombus deposition, microembolization and occlusion.

(c) *Acute myocardial infarction*

Nature
Necrosis of myocardial cells caused by cessation, reduction or interference with their blood supply.

Incidence
Extremely common, though recently with a 10–15%

fall in incidence. This condition causes about 60% of sudden unexpected deaths and is directly responsible for 10–15% of all deaths.

Sex
Under 50 years the male : female ratio is 5 : 1, increasing incidence in women post-menopausally but there is a 'time-lag' of 10–20 years between the sexes.

Age
Predominantly middle-aged between 50 and 60 years, but 10% occur in the younger age groups, 35–50. The average age of onset appears to be decreasing.

Types
The pattern of distribution of the necrosis is of great importance:
1 *Regional*: infarction occurs in the territory supplied by one major common artery.
2 *Diffuse*: this relates to problems of overall myocardial perfusion rather than to thrombotic occlusion in any one artery.

Regional infarction
Nearly all such infarcts are related to thrombi or atheromatous plaques undergoing fissuring. Clinical coronary angiography has demonstrated that, within 1 hour of onset of original pain, 90% of arteries supplying a regional infarct are occluded. Subsequently a proportion of these vessels reopen spontaneously or the flow can be restored by angioplasty or use of fibrinolytic agents. Thrombi form before infarction but propagate progressively and particularly distally. In fatal cases the vast majority of patients with regional full-thickness transmural regional infarcts show complete occlusion of an artery at autopsy.

When the regional necrosis is *subendocardial* only, fewer cases show a complete arterial occlusion. This relates to the presence of previous collateral flow or to spontaneous fibrinolysis.

Diffuse infarction
The distribution of necrosis varies from being confined to centres of papillary muscles to loss of the inner third of the wall of the entire left ventricular circumference—*diffuse subendocardial necrosis*. It can occur independently from coronary atheroma in shock, in high diastolic pressure—as in aortic valve stenosis (see p. 72), and in patients with hypertrophied or dilated ventricles. Likewise it can follow severe prolonged left ventricular failure.

Sites of occlusion
First 1–2 cm of the main left and right arteries—less common. Next 2–3 cm—frequent.

Branches: 1, anterior descending, left—most common; 2, circumflex branch, left—common; 3, main trunk, right—common; 4, other branches—rare.

Sites of regional infarction
Almost always involves the left ventricle; the right ventricle and both atria are very rarely affected. The sites within the left ventricular myocardium correspond to the distribution of the artery occluded:
1 Anterior descending, left—anterior wall and anterior part of the interventricular septum.
2 Circumflex branch, left—left border of the heart and left side of the posterior surface.
3 Main trunk, right—posterior wall of the left ventricle and posterior part of the interventricular septum.

Appearances
Changes are not uniform over the whole area of infarction.
0–12 hours. *Macroscopical*. Largely normal but slight pallor and flabbiness with early oedema. Margin indistinct. *Microscopical*. The earliest changes are of 'contraction bands' and oedema. Cytoplasmic evidence of cell death is seen with Picro–Mallory stains and by 6 hours polymorphs start to infiltrate at the margins. Nuclear evidence of myocardial fibre death follows with karyolysis and karyorrhexis.
12–24 hours. *Macroscopical*. The area is still indistinctly defined but there is friability and pallor. *Microscopical*. Cytoplasmic and nuclear changes of cell death are more apparent, oedema is marked and polymorphs are more numerous.
2–4 days. *Macroscopical*. Well-defined hyperaemic irregular border with the necrotic tissue soft and yellow–grey in colour. *Microscopical*. The marginal inflammatory response is well developed and the myocardial fibres are amorphous with progressive loss of nuclei.
4–10 days. *Macroscopical*. The dead tissue is structureless, yellow and very soft—*myomalacia cordis*. Foci of streaky haemorrhage are seen and there is intense marginal hyperaemia. *Microscopical*. Macrophages, lymphocytes, plasma cells and fibroblasts extend into the necrotic area from the periphery together with proliferated new blood vessels.
10 days–6 weeks. *Macroscopical*. Progressive fibrous replacement from the margin to give a greyish

coloration. This organization is largely or entirely completed by 6 weeks. *Microscopical*. Fibroblasts lay down collagen, the histiocytes and other inflammatory cells progressively disappear and the new vessels become less prominent leading to a hyalinized avascular scar by 6 months.

Effects and sequelae

1 Sudden death: virtually all patients have angiographic evidence of actively fissuring atheromatous plaques and mural thrombus but not all are necessarily occlusive, though about 30% will have demonstrable platelet microemboli in the myocardium. The vast majority of these deaths are due to ventricular fibrillation. If this is successfully reversed about 30% will develop regional infarcts.

2 Death from cardiogenic shock or pulmonary oedema in the first few days, particularly with large areas of necrosis.

3 Rupture:
(a) *External*. Leading to haemopericardium, tamponade and death. The risk is maximal at 5–7 days in the central areas of infarcts and much earlier when it occurs at the junction between normal and necrotic myocardium.
(b) *Internal*. Ruptures can cause an acquired septal defect, or loss of papillary muscles with resulting acute torrential regurgitation.

4 Mural thrombosis: about 30% of fatal cases show laminated thrombus over the infarcted area with consequential high risk of emboli—e.g. cerebral, renal, splenic, mesenteric, limbs.

5 Ventricular aneurysm: the weakened fibrotic ventricular wall progressively stretches with thrombus formation, embolism or severe functional deficit.

6 Arrhythmias: if the conducting tissue is involved, heart block supervenes.

7 Chronic congestive cardiac failure: the loss of contractile myocardium may lead to inability to maintain satisfactory cardiac output. This most commonly occurs with multiple or very large infarcts.

Results

Emergency treatment markedly reduces the acute mortality and is particularly aimed at reversing arrhythmias and re-establishing blood flow in the occluded arteries—e.g. by coronary angioplasty or fibrinolytic agents both local and systemic, though restoration of *flow–re-flow*, can cause complications, particularly arrhythmias, by releasing hydrogen ions and other products of anaerobic metabolism into the circulation. Urgency is imperative also to reduce the incidence of non-fatal infarction and other sequelae. Of the survivors of episodes of myocardial infarction at least 25% live for 10 years.

Disabling angina due to multiple narrowed arterial segments may respond symptomatically extremely well to coronary artery bypass grafts using lengths of vein, though prolongation of life by this procedure is less predictable.

Degenerations and infiltrations

Brown atrophy

Aetiology
Unknown, but is frequently associated with wasting diseases and old age.

Appearances
The heart is small and the surface wrinkled with loss of epicardial fat, tortuous coronary vessels and brown friable muscle.

Microscopical
The muscle fibres are shrunken and contain brownish pigment at the nuclear poles—*lipofuscin*.

Cloudy swelling

Aetiology
Infections and many toxic states, e.g. typhoid, influenza, septicaemia, etc.

Macroscopical
Soft, pale and friable myocardium.

Microscopical
The muscle fibres are swollen with granular fragmentation of the cytoplasmic mitochondria.

Fatty infiltration
Increased epicardial deposition of fat associated with generalized adiposity. This may extend into the fibrous septa and between the muscle fibres but the myocardial fibres are normal.

Fatty degeneration

Nature
Represents damage to myocardial cells, as a result of which there is accumulation of fatty material within the cell cytoplasm. It may be due to any of the many causes of cell damage.

Appearances
There is a pale mottling of the muscle, particularly of the subendocardial fibres and especially in the left ventricle—'thrush-breast' or 'tabby-cat' appearance. There are fine fatty droplets in the muscle fibres, most marked in those situated furthest from the blood vessels and therefore at the sites of maximal anoxia.

Cardiomyopathy

Nature
A heterogeneous group of diseases each of which may present as different syndromes but which have in common abnormality in structure and/or function of the myocardium. By common consent, however, the term excludes disease of the heart due to hypertension, coronary insufficiency, valvular malfunction or rheumatism.

Cardiomyopathies may be present in families or be sporadic. The cardiac lesion may be the only demonstrable abnormality or many other systems may be affected. The illness may arise associated with a particular disease, after or during the main presenting factor, e.g. in haemochromatosis, occur in an alcoholic or in malnourishment or pregnancy. It may occur in a family with a known illness, e.g. a myopathy, and thus be classifiable. More often, however, the patient presents with the cardiac illness without any clue to the aetiology, and this may not be determinable even at post-mortem examination; in the present stage of knowledge regarding treatment, this is of little importance.

Types

Dilated (congestive) cardiomyopathy

Nature
Functional abnormalities of the myocardium causing poor systolic contraction and with dilatation of the ventricular cavities associated with reduced wall thickness.

Macroscopical
In addition to dilatation of chambers and thinning of their walls, mural thrombus in ventricles and atrial appendages is frequently seen.

Microscopical
There is a non-specific rather diffuse interstitial fibrosis with tiny foci of individual cell necrosis with localized and usually slight inflammatory cell response. The features are non-specific and do not point to any particular aetiology.

Pathogenesis
This is the end-stage of myocardial damage for many causes including viral myocarditis and the more identifiable causes included in 'specific heart muscle disease' (see p. 66). Mostly the aetiology is not identifiable.

Hypertrophic (obstructive) cardiomyopathy

Nature
Systolic function is hyperkinetic with marked reduction in systolic volume and difficulty in diastolic filling.

Macroscopical
The ventricular wall appears grossly thickened and weight is commonly but not invariably increased. The thickening may be septal, bilateral or unilateral, symmetrical or asymmetrical. There may appear to be obstruction to the outflow tract by muscle bulk, but whether this is truly obstructive is debatable.

Microscopical
There are consistent and fairly specific histological abnormalities with interstitial fibrosis and a whorling or mal-arrangement of myocardial fibres. On electron microscopy there is myofibrillary disarray.

Pathogenesis
This is probably always familial and may result from an abnormal myocardial sensitivity to catecholamines leading to changes in fibre shape.

Restrictive (obliterative) cardiomyopathy

Nature
Abnormal stiffness of myocardium or endocardium causing ventricular filling to be restricted to diastole only at high pressures. Systolic function and cavity size are normal.

Aetiology

In its pure form this occurs in amyloid deposition and the earlier stages of endomyocardial fibrosis (EMF) both in its tropical and non-tropical forms.

Endomyocardial fibrosis (EMF)

In the acute phase thrombotic material is deposited on the endocardial surfaces and becomes organized with increasing fibrosis which starts apically and extends to involve the ventricular mural endocardium and atrioventricular valves. It seems likely that the non-tropical type is related to degranulation of circulating eosinophils, which produces an endocardial damaging factor. Tropical EMF has no consistent association with eosinophilia but the findings in the heart are identical.

Specific heart muscle disease

Nature

'Cardiomyopathies' associated with or caused by a systemic disease—secondary cardiomyopathy.

Causes

1 Amyloidosis: small amounts of AL amyloid in over 80-year-old hearts—*senile amyloid*, are seldom clinically significant.
2 Haemochromatosis and haemosiderosis.
3 Alcohol.
4 Muscular dystrophies and hereditary neuromyopathy syndromes particularly Friedreich's ataxia and myotonic dystrophy (see p. 337).
5 Glycogen storage disease (see p. 249)—Von Gierke's disease, a systemic derangement of glycogen metabolism.
6 Mucopolysaccharidosis—of all types, e.g. gargoylism.
7 Nutritional—starvation and deficiencies, e.g. beriberi from lack of vitamin B_1.

Endocardial fibroelastosis

A primary condition presenting in infancy which characteristically shows endocardial thickening in the left atrium and ventricle with a smooth glossy surface. Histologically the thickened areas show collagenous tissue with numerous parallel elastic laminae. Some cases may be due to foetal virus infection but otherwise the aetiology is obscure. Secondary fibroelastosis occurs in cases in left-sided congenital heart defects.

Myocarditis

Nature

The presence of inflammatory cells in the myocardium. Clinical features are due to ventricular electrical irritability with rhythm and conduction abnormalities manifest by electrocardiography.

Causes

1 Toxic or metabolic damage, e.g. typhoid fever, streptococcal infections—particularly if β-haemolytic, diphtheria; chemical poisons including arsenic, phosphorus, chloroform; metabolic abnormalities including hypokalaemia and hyperkalaemia, magnesium deficiency and excess catecholamines, either iatrogenic or endogenous. In these conditions the predominant histological feature is of focal necrosis of myocardial cells and an inflammatory cell infiltrate is seldom marked.
2 Microbial organisms.
   (a) *Pyogenic bacteria*: suppurative myocarditis is rare except as a terminal event in debilitating illnesses or immune deficiency states complicated by septicaemia.
   (b) *Viruses*: Coxsackie virus infections are the best-documented both as sporadic fatal cases and in known epidemics, particularly in neonates. Other viruses causing myocarditis are poliomyelitis, mumps and ECHO.
   (c) *Protozoa*: of importance are toxoplasmosis, usually as a congenital infection in the neonatal period and, in South America (particularly Brazil), Chagas' disease due to *Trypanosoma cruzi* (see p. 7).
   (d) *Syphilis*: the aortitis (see p. 81) causes aneurysm and aortic valve incompetence. Gummas affecting the myocardium, particularly the conducting system in the upper intraventricular septum.
3 Sarcoidosis: seldom clinically important but granulomas are commonly found in the generalized disease.
4 Rheumatic fever (see below).
5 Giant cell myocarditis: an acute fulminating form of fatal acute myocarditis with foci of necrosis, at the margins of which there are numerous elongated multinucleated cells. Whether these cells are of myocardial or histiocytic origin is debatable. The pathogenesis has not been established.

Rheumatic fever

Rheumatic affection of the heart involves the pericardium, myocardium and endocardium—*pancarditis*.

Nature
A systemic inflammatory process of connective tissues affecting joints, tendons, serosal membranes, skin, respiratory system and blood vessels in a comparatively transient or benign manner, but with common and frequently fatal sequelae in the heart.

Incidence
Rheumatic heart disease forms a significant but decreasing proportion of cases of organic heart disease. The incidence of acute rheumatic fever is impossible to establish, as many cases, severely debilitated in later life by the heart complications, give no clear history of a previous acute attack.

Aetiology
Epidemiological, clinical and experimental evidence suggests that the disease is closely related to group A haemolytic streptococcal infections. Organisms are not present in the lesions and the evidence points to an indirect immunological response on the part of the affected tissues to the presence of circulating streptococcal toxins. Other factors which may predispose are:
1 Climate: increased frequency in temperate, damp climates.
2 Social: more common in urban than in rural areas and in those with poor living conditions and inadequate nutrition.

Age
Ninety per cent of the first attacks occur between the ages of 5 and 15, and a first attack of acute rheumatic fever is rare above the age of 20.

Sex
Male : female equal.

Clinical
Insidious onset of fever 2–3 weeks after a sore throat or other streptococcal infection. Symptomatic evidence of involvement of several systems follows:
85% have a migratory polyarthritis, usually of large joints.
65% have pancarditis.
30% have chorea.
Subcutaneous nodules and pulmonary symptoms less commonly occur. This initial acute attack subsides after a few weeks and may remain quiescent, but clinical exacerbations may occur at intervals, usually within the first 5 years. With each exacerbation the risk of carditis increases, so that eventually 75% of all patients show evidence of cardiac involvement.

Heart

Pericardium
Diffuse fibrinous inflammation with adhesion of the two layers and a 'bread and butter' appearance. Little fluid is present. This may resolve by fibrinolysis, but is more commonly organized to produce relatively thin fibrous plaques on the visceral layer but little adhesion formation.

Myocardium

Macroscopical
There may be little or no gross abnormality visible. Occasionally, scattered pin-head-sized pale grey foci may be seen.

Microscopical
The characteristic Aschoff nodes are seen in the connective tissues of the atrial and ventricular myocardium, particularly in the subendocardial fibrous tissue and around blood vessels in the intermuscular fibrous septa.

Aschoff node

Exudative phase
There is focal mucoid degeneration of the collagen with surrounding polymorphs, plasma cells and histiocytes. This histological appearance is seen only transiently in the early stages.

Proliferative phase
The characteristic Aschoff node consists of:
1 Central focus of fibrinoid collagen necrosis.
2 Surrounding granulomatous reaction with:
   (a) Fibroblasts.
   (b) Plasma cells and lymphocytes but scanty polymorphs.
   (c) Multinucleate giant cells—Aschoff cells, composed of two to five centrally arranged nuclei and a basophilic cytoplasm.
   (d) 'Anitschkow' myocytes. These cells are characteristically oval with a central chromatin bar from which fine projections are visible, mimicking the legs of a caterpillar—'caterpillar cells'. Their origin

is disputed, being either modified fibroblasts or altered muscle cells.

Healed phase

Progressive hyalinization and fibrosis with disappearance of Aschoff and Anitschkow cells. The last elements to disappear are the plasma cells and lymphocytes at the periphery.

The Aschoff node is diagnostic of rheumatic myocarditis. It is present in a recognizable form in 40–50% of atrial appendages removed from patients at mitral valvotomy for mitral stenosis, in whom there has been no clinical or laboratory evidence of rheumatic activity for many years. This paradox raises problems which are at present unanswerable as to the exact significance of Aschoff nodes in relation to the disease process as a whole.

Effects

The scarring from the healed lesions causes a diffuse fibrosis and injury to adjacent myocardial fibres. Death may occur in the acute stage due to this myocarditis or, in the later stages, the heart's action may be impeded. Generally, however, the endocardial sequelae overshadow those of the myocardium.

Endocardium

Mural

Patchy involvement of the atrial endocardium with subendocardial Aschoff nodes leads to scarring and to MacCallum's patch, usually situated just above the posterior cusp of the mitral valve.

Valvular

Sites. The valve lesions are distributed as follows: mitral alone—40%; mitral and aortic—40%; aortic alone—10%; mitral, aortic and tricuspid—5%; tricuspid alone—rare; pulmonary alone—very rare.

Appearances. Sequence. Similar for all valves:
1 Red, swollen and thickened, particularly at the free margins.
2 Vegetations form due to erosion of the inflamed surfaces at the lines of closure and on the chordae tendinae. Small (1–2 mm), firmly adherent, rubbery, low, warty nodules are seen along the lines of closure and on the surfaces exposed to blood flow. They consist of platelets and fibrin.

3 The valve cusps show mucoid degeneration or fibrinoid necrosis of the ground substance, with occasional Anitschkow myocytes and mononuclear inflammatory cells, but well-formed Aschoff nodes are rare.
4 Organization with vascularization of the valve cusps. The valves are thickened, deformed, opaque and inflexible with thickening at the sites of the vegetations. Fibrous tissue bridges across the commissures, resulting in fusion of the valve cusps. In the mitral valve this commissural fusion produces the slit-like, 'buttonhole' type of mitral stenosis. In addition the chordae tendinae are thickened and fused.
5 Contracture of fibrous tissue increases the deformity of the valves. At the mitral valve, the fibrous contraction of the chordae tendinae results in anchoring of the valve cusps on the ventricular aspect and produces the 'funnel-shaped' type of mitral stenosis, when viewed from the atrial aspect.
6 Deposition of calcium in the damaged valves further increases the deformity and inelasticity.

Effects. The later stages progress slowly over many years, either as recurrent subclinical attacks or as passive secondary change in a damaged valve. The two main effects of the valvular deformities result in:
1 Stenosis of the orifice.
2 Incompetence of valve cusps causing regurgitation. There is a variable mixture of one or both effects in individual cases and in individually affected valves (see p. 71).

Joints

The lesions are transient and only rarely give rise to residual disability.

Macroscopical. Swelling, redness and heat with subsidence in a few days. The larger joints are usually involved and arthritis is often multiple and symmetrical. The synovium is thickened, red and granular, later resolving to normal.

Microscopical. Aschoff nodes, or alternatively mucoid or fibrinoid degeneration, are seen in the connective tissues and similar changes are found in the joint capsules, affected tendons, fascia and muscle sheaths, frequently accompanied by a lymphocytic infiltrate.

Skin—rheumatic nodule

Sites. Subcutaneous tissues, particularly over bony prominences of wrist, elbow, ankle, knee or occiput.

Macroscopical. Circumscribed mobile subcutaneous nodules of firm consistency with erythema but no ulceration of the overlying skin.

Microscopical. Massive central area of fibrinoid necrosis with a palisade of radially arranged histiocytes at the margin and a surrounding inflammatory cell infiltration.

Fate. Gradually replaced by dense fibrous tissue which may subsequently calcify.

Blood vessels
An acute vasculitis, confined to the intima, may rarely occur and is usually inconspicuous with little or no effect on the involved organ. It may be widespread and affect the coronary, pulmonary, renal, mesenteric and cerebral arteries and the aorta.

Lungs
A few cases show focal areas of interstitial inflammation with fibrinous exudate into the alveoli and histiocytic and lymphocytic infiltration of the alveolar septa. The affection is mostly mild, transient and of doubtful specificity.

Brain—chorea—Sydenham's chorea

Clinical
Nearly 30% of patients with acute rheumatism show clinical evidence of cerebral irritability or sudden, involuntary, irregular, rapid movements with muscular incoordination and weakness—St Vitus' dance. Only very rarely are these manifestations serious and the majority recover completely, usually in a few months.

Appearances
Variable and inconspicuous lesions are found in the rare fatal cases in the corpus striatum and cerebral cortex. Perivascular lymphocyte infiltration, hyperaemia and, rarely, Aschoff nodes, may be seen.

Results of rheumatic fever
Functional derangements of the valves are by far the most important sequelae but can now nearly always be surgically corrected by insertion of prostheses. There are mechanical types—ball valve, tilting disc or double-hinged plates—or grafts of human or animal tissues, e.g. fascia lata, bovine pericardium, porcine aortic valve. Results are usually extremely good.

Complications of prosthetic valves
The most frequent are infection, thrombus formation and embolization, but mechanical factors can include dehiscence of the valvular ring, paravalvular leak, disproportion, turbulent flow and red cell haemolysis. Fracture of mechanical components is uncommon.

Hypertensive heart disease
The effect of sustained systemic hypertension on the heart is to produce hypertrophy of the left ventricle. As long as the cardiac reserve is not exhausted, and the hypertrophic myocardium maintains a normal output, a compensated state exists. Eventually, the reserve may be exhausted when the ventricle will dilate and congestive heart failure supervenes.

The disease is commonly associated with coronary atherosclerosis, depriving the thickened cardiac muscle of essential oxygen, and myocardial infarction is a common complication.

Death in 50–70% of hypertensive patients is due to heart failure from myocardial or coronary insufficiency. There is commonly a sudden fatal termination with ventricular fibrillation (see p. 92).

Endocardium

Endocarditis
When used as an unqualified term this implies inflammation of the valves. Mural endocarditis is inflammation of the lining of the heart chambers.

Rheumatic endocarditis
See p. 68.

Infective endocarditis

Organisms

Bacteria
1 Pathogenic: staphylococci, β-haemolytic streptococci, pneumococci, meningococci, *Escherichia coli*, etc.
2 Low-grade pathogens: *Streptococcus viridans*, *S. faecalis*, *Haemophilus*, *Brucella*, mycobacteria, various Gram-negative organisms.

Rickettsiae
Coxiella burnetti (Q fever).

Fungi

Candida, *Aspergillus*, etc. Particularly in drug addicts and debilitated persons, those immunosuppressed or on valve prostheses.

Age and sex

Almost any age with an increasing number in the more elderly. Male : female, 3 : 1.

Predisposing factors

1 Previous valve damage by rheumatic fever, congenital abnormalities or floppy valve (see p. 71).
2 Bacteraemia and septicaemia of low-grade pathogens, particularly *S. faecalis* and *E. Coli* with urinary tract catheterization and *S. viridans* with tooth extraction.
3 Valve prostheses.
4 Intravenous drug abusers and immunocompromised.

Appearances

There may be evidence of previous structural abnormality. Vegetations are present on the valve cusps, usually at site of contact, and vary from small lowish friable polypoid detachable fibrinous masses when the lesser pathogens are the cause, to larger very friable soft vegetations when infection is from pyogenic bacteria. With the latter, extension on to the mural surface or adjacent endocardium is common, as is ulceration, perforation or rupture of cusps or chordae.

Sites

1 Mitral valve only, 40%.
2 Aortic valve only, 20%.
3 Mitral and aortic valves, 20%.
4 Tricuspid or pulmonary valve endocardial infection is rare.

Effects

1 *Valves*: functional disturbances due to failure of closure, perforation, distortion.
2 *Embolism*: pyogenic bacteria produce septic infarction and abscess. The lower-grade pathogens give rise to non-suppurative infarcts in brain, spleen, kidney, etc. Splinter haemorrhages and Osler's nodes in the skin and a similarly immune-complex-induced focal proliferative glomerulonephritis (see p. 168) may occur.
3 *Mycotic aneurysm*: emboli containing low-grade pathogens may cause aneurysmal weakening of the wall at the site of impaction. These occur mostly in the cerebral, renal and limb arteries.

Diagnosis

1 *Blood culture*: the responsible organisms can usually be recovered from blood cultures though multiple specimens may be necessary. They should preferably be taken whilst pyrexia is rising, or during embolic episodes and before antibiotics are administered.
2 *Blood*: there is always a high sedimentation rate, a variably marked leucocytosis and anaemia. The latter can be severe.

Atypical verrucous endocarditis—Libman–Sacks endocarditis

Nature

The endocardial manifestations of systemic lupus erythematosus (SLE; see p. 96).

Sites

Seen in 50% or more of fatal cases of SLE. The mitral and tricuspid valves are commonly affected and the pulmonary valve only occasionally.

Macroscopical

Small warty excrescences, firmly adherent anywhere on the valve cusps. They are usually multiple and on either aspect of the cusp, whilst frequently they extend on to the atrial or ventricular endocardium.

Microscopical

The vegetations are composed of fibrin with necrotic debris, fibrinoid material and entangled fibroblasts with mononuclear cells. The valves show fibrinoid necrosis of the ground substance with vascularization, fibroblastic proliferation and scanty mononuclear and polymorph inflammatory cell infiltration. Haematoxyphil bodies may be found in the fibrinoid material (see p. 168).

Effects

Clinical evidence of cardiac involvement is common, but the valvular changes seldom give rise to any appreciable functional deficiency.

Carcinoid syndrome

Nature

Some cases of carcinoid tumour, usually of the small intestine and with metastases in the liver, have a symptom complex associated with secretion of excessive amounts of 5-hydroxytryptamine. In such cases, endocardial lesions of the tricuspid and pulmonary valves are commonly present (see p. 36) as thickened, fibrotic and distorted cusps resulting in stenosis or incompetence.

Floppy valve syndrome

Nature
This '*floppy valve*' lesion results from myxoid degeneration of the ground substance of cardiac valves, usually and most severely the mitral cusps. Chordae are also affected and may rupture. The condition is increasingly seen with advancing years but also occurs associated with Marfan's syndrome and in some congenital cardiac lesions.

Appearances
The affected valve cusps are thickened, opaque, slightly nodular and stretched with irregular free margin. Stretching or rupture of chordae may cause prolapse into the left atrium—*parachute deformity*. Histologically there is cystic degeneration of the collagen rich in acid mucopolysaccharides.

Effects
Mildly affected valves are very commonly found in the elderly and usually appear to have little effect. Less often mitral regurgitation, which may be severe and intractable, results.

Calcific aortic stenosis

Types
Though calcification may occur in valves damaged by rheumatic disease, and show characteristic features, it is usually more marked in two other types of calcific valve disease.
1 *Bicuspid calcific aortic valve stenosis*: this is of congenital origin and is quite common, usually manifest by 40–50 years of age.
2 *Senile calcific aortic valve stenosis*: the valve is tricuspid and the calcification increasingly frequent with advancing years, usually over 70.

Appearances
In severe cases there is marked fibrous thickening of the valve cusps with deformity and rigidity. Large nodular masses of calcium may be found subendothelially within the sinuses of Valsalva behind the aortic cusps. Ulceration over the calcified areas may occur, and some adhesion of the cusps at the commissures may increase the rigidity and the degree of stenosis. Calcified material is also found in the valve ring. The congenital bicuspid appearance is readily identifiable when present.

Results
1 Left ventricular hypertrophy.
2 Coronary insufficiency.
3 Syncopal attacks or sudden death due to acute heart failure.

Valvular lesions

Stenosis and incompetence (regurgitation)
Both may be present together, but one is usually dominant. The mitral and aortic valves are the most frequently affected; the tricuspid and pulmonary valves only infrequently.

Mitral valve
In 40% this is the only valve affected; in 40% there are combined mitral and aortic lesions.

Stenosis
Causes:
1 Rheumatic.
2 Infective endocarditis.

Effects:
1 Dilated, slightly hypertrophied left atrium which may be grossly distended—giant left atrium. Thrombus commonly forms in the left atrial appendage.
2 Normal-sized left ventricle, unless mitral incompetence is also present.
3 Right ventricular hypertrophy.
4 Chronic passive congestion of the lungs—*brown induration*.
5 Pulmonary hypertension.
6 Functional tricuspid incompetence.
7 'Nutmeg' liver and congested kidneys, etc.

Regurgitation
Causes. As for stenosis above together with myxomatous degeneration—floppy valve and ischaemic papillary muscle damage.

Effects:
1 Dilated, hypertrophied left ventricle.

2 Dilated left atrium.
3 Chronic passive venous congestion of the lung.
4 Pulmonary hypertension and right ventricular hypertrophy, but less marked than in mitral stenosis.

Results of mitral disease
Death from:
1 Congestive heart failure.
2 Emboli from left atrial thrombus.
The results of mitral valve surgery by prosthetic replacement are good in selected patients.

Aortic valve

Forty per cent show aortic and mitral involvement; 10% aortic alone.

Stenosis
Causes:
1 Congenital—bicuspid calcific.
2 Calcific aortic stenosis.
3 Rheumatic—common.
4 Infective endocarditis.

Effects:
1 Hypertrophy of left ventricle.
2 Coronary artery insufficiency.
3 Cerebral vascular insufficiency—syncopal attacks.
4 Sudden death, probably due to ventricular fibrillation.

Regurgitation
Causes:
1 As for stenosis above.
2 Aortic root disease.
  (a) Aortitis. Due to syphilis, ankylosing spondylitis (see p. 103), Reiter's syndrome, psoriatic aortitis and giant cell aortitis similar to the more common temporal artery disease (see p. 84).
  (b) Idiopathic aortic root dilatation.

Effects:
1 Left ventricular dilatation.
2 Later left ventricular hypertrophy.

Results of aortic disease
Death from acute heart failure with pulmonary oedema. The results of surgery in aortic valve disease by prosthetic replacement are good when the cause is valvar.

Tricuspid valve

Stenosis
This is rare.

Causes. Rheumatic and the carcinoid syndrome.

Effects:
1 Right atrial dilatation.
2 Right heart failure.

Regurgitation
Uncommon.

Causes:
1 Functional: distortion of the valve ring in mitral stenosis.
2 Structural:
  (a) rheumatic—nearly always associated with mitral and aortic involvement;
  (b) atypical verrucous endocarditis (SLE).

Effects:
1 Right atrial dilatation.
2 Right-sided heart failure.
3 Chronic venous congestion with a pulsatile liver and 'nutmeg' appearance leading to cardiac fibrosis and derangement of function.

Results of tricuspid disease
Death from right-sided heart failure. Prosthetic replacement is usually successful.

Pulmonary valve

Stenosis
Causes:
1 Congenital:
  (a) isolated valvular stenosis;
  (b) Fallot's tetralogy (see p. 76).
2 Rheumatic, very rare.
3 Carcinoid syndrome (see p. 70).

Effects:
1 Right ventricular hypertrophy.
2 Pulmonary oligaemia with cyanosis.

Incompetence
Causes:
1 Functional: distortion of the valve in mitral stenosis—Graham Steell murmur.

2 Structural—very rare—congenital with superimposed endocarditis.

Effects:
1 Right ventricular dilatation and hypertrophy.
2 Pulmonary hypertension.

Results of pulmonary valve disease
Right-sided heart failure. Surgical correction may be possible particularly in the true valvular type.

Myocardial hypertrophy

Nature
Increase in size of individual myocardial fibres as a result of prolonged increased work.

Types

Concentric
Thickening of the wall, the lumen of the chamber appearing decreased in size.

Eccentric
Thickening of the wall and dilatation of the chamber.

Left ventricle—'cor bovinum'

Causes

Obstruction to outflow
1 Structural: aortic stenosis, coarctation of aorta.
2 Functional: systemic hypertension.

Increased output
1 Aortic incompetence.
2 Mitral incompetence.
3 Hypermetabolic states, e.g. thyrotoxicosis.
4 Vascular anomalies including shunts, e.g. in Paget's disease of bone.

Right ventricle—'cor pulmonale'

Causes

Pulmonary hypertension
1 Mitral stenosis.
2 Left to right shunts—mostly congenital (see p. 76).
3 Pulmonary fibrosis, e.g. pneumoconioses (see p. 387).
4 Emphysema (see p. 381).

5 Thromboembolic pulmonary disease.
6 Idiopathic—primary pulmonary hypertension (see p. 94).

Pulmonary stenosis
1 Valvular stenosis.
2 Fallot's tetralogy.

Tricuspid incompetence

Atria
Although hypertrophy of the atria occurs in mitral and tricuspid stenosis, this is overshadowed by the gross degree of atrial dilatation in each case.

Effects
1 Very considerable degrees of hypertrophy occur and may be present for long periods. The hypertrophic myocardium is, however, more likely to fail due to relative insufficiency of the coronary blood flow.
2 Sudden death due to the development of arrhythmias, notably ventricular fibrillation, are common in hypertensive patients and particularly so in cases of pulmonary hypertension which is less well tolerated than the systemic type.
3 Relief of the causative factors may result in a diminution of the size of the myocardial fibres and a return to normal chamber size.

Dilatation of the heart

Nature
Increased capacity of the chambers which may be associated with hypertrophy or occur alone.

Causes

Inability to expel all the blood it receives
1 Myocarditis—including rheumatic carditis.
2 Ischaemic heart disease.
3 The atria in mitral or tricuspid stenosis.

Reflux
1 Left ventricle in aortic regurgitation.
2 Left atrium in mitral regurgitation.
3 Right atrium in tricuspid regurgitation.

Other conditions—cardiomyopathies
See p. 65.

Lesions of the conducting tissue

Interruption of the conducting tissue gives rise to arrhythmias, complete or partial heart block.

Causes

Myocarditis
1 Acute, e.g. diphtheria, influenza, pyaemic abscesses, rheumatic fever.
2 Chronic: rheumatic carditis, syphilis.

Ischaemic heart disease

Digitalis
Overdosage.

Tumours
Usually secondary.

Tumours

Benign

Connective tissues
Fibroma, lipoma and angioma are all very rare.

Myxoma

Incidence
The commonest primary heart tumour but even this is rare.

Macroscopical
A globular or polypoid mass arising from the endocardial surface of the left atrium, usually from the limbus of the foramen ovale. It projects into the chamber and is commonly pedunculated, having a soft and gelatinous appearance. Some may attain a large size and even extend through the mitral valve orifice.

Microscopical
Myxomatous fibrous tissue containing thin-walled blood vessels and clumps, cords or gland-like masses of 'lepidic' cells (said to resemble the scales on butterfly wings).

Nature
The histogenesis is thought to be related to undifferentiated mesenchymal cells sequestered in the formation of the foramen ovale. Local recurrence after surgical removal may occur unless the cuff of muscle around the base is excised or destroyed by diathermy.

Effects
May cause interference with the blood flow or act as a 'ball-valve' obstruction, especially in the mitral valve.

Rhabdomyoma
A rare hamartomatous malformation of cardiac muscle fibres, usually associated with tuberose sclerosis (see p. 332).

Malignant

Primary
Rhabdomyosarcomas, angiosarcomas and fibrosarcomas exist but are extremely rare.

Secondary

Direct
Extension of tumours from adjacent structures, e.g. lung, oesophagus, etc.

Metastatic
Malignant melanoma, carcinomas from any site, lymphomas. However, secondary tumours in the heart are surprisingly uncommon.

B/CONGENITAL HEART DISEASE

Introduction
Disorders of whole heart
Defects of septum
Great vessel abnormalities
Valvular
Patent ductus
Coarctation of aorta
Veins
Coronary vessels
Others
Dangers
Results

Introduction
Many of these disabling congenital abnormalities of the heart and blood vessels are now surgically correctable and thus the subject is no longer of mere academic interest.

Incidence

Two per cent of all organic heart disease. Ten per cent of all heart disease in children.

Aetiology

Definitive development of the heart from a simple tube occurs in the fifth to eighth weeks of intrauterine life and it is in this period that most of the congenital abnormalities are produced. The precise causation is unknown but factors include the following.

Intrinsic

Heredity—a genetic defect; 20% show congenital lesions in other organs.

Extrinsic

1 Virus infections—rubella during the first 3 months of pregnancy carries a 25–50% risk of congenital heart disease or cataracts. Other maternal virus infections have come under suspicion, including influenza, but positive proof is still lacking.
2 Vitamin deficiency in pregnancy.
3 Foetal endocarditis and other intrauterine infections.
4 Heavy metals—especially lead.
5 Syphilis.

With the exception of rubella infection, however, there is little evidence to support any of the other postulated extrinsic factors.

Classification

The lesions vary in severity, from those which are incompatible with life to those completely asymptomatic and which cause no appreciable interference with a normal life span.

Most of the simpler defects are shunts left to right or right to left, or are due to obstructions in the regions of valves or aorta. There are also highly variable and complex abnormalities which are not considered here.

Disorders of the whole heart

Ectopia cordis

Failure of development of the anterior chest wall, the heart lying outside the chest or subcutaneously. This is incompatible with life and is fortunately extremely rare.

Dextrocardia

1 Complete mirror image with transposition of all viscera—*situs inversus*. The incidence is 1 in 5000 births and causes no significant disability.
2 Partial transposition of the viscera. This is associated with other serious congenital heart abnormalities.
3 Isolated dextrocardia with normally positioned viscera. This is usually associated with other grave cardiac abnormalities.

Defects of the septum

Interatrial septal defect—ASD

Patent foramen ovale

Functionally, the foramen ovale normally closes within a few hours following birth, but structurally may not be completely fused for a year. Minor degrees of probe-patency at one margin of the membrane are extremely common, but these are non-functional, and are clinically insignificant.

Ostium secundum type

This is persistence of the foramen ovale and is of variable size and always functional. This type is readily closed by sutures without recourse to a 'patch'.

Ostium primum type

The defect is large and involves the lower portions of the septum. It is commonly associated with abnormal attachments of the septal cusps of the mitral and tricuspid valves, or with a deficiency of the membranous portion of the inverventricular septum. Surgical correction requires interposition of a 'patch' of foreign material and may be technically extremely difficult owing to the associated valvular abnormalities.

Lutembacher' s syndrome

Atrial septal defects of the secundum type associated with congenital or acquired mitral stenosis and gross dilatation of the pulmonary artery.

Interventricular septal defect—VSD

As a solitary lesion

There may be single or multiple defects in the muscular part of the septum, but more commonly there is a solitary defect restricted to the upper membranous portion. When the defect is very large—*trilocular heart*.

Associated with other abnormalities

For example Fallot's tetralogy.

Abnormalities of the great vessels

Truncus arteriosus

The abnormalities vary in degree from common pulmonary and aortic trunks to fistulous communications between the two.

Transposition

Complete

The aorta and pulmonary arteries arise from the right ventricle and the left ventricle respectively and the ventricles are also transposed, i.e. the bicuspid mitral valve is on the right side and the tricuspid valve is on the left. Unless a septal defect is present or the great veins are also transposed, the condition is incompatible with life.

Partial

The great vessels are transposed but the ventricles are normally situated.

Abnormalities of valves and outflow tracts

Supernumerary cusps

Extra aortic or pulmonary cusps.

Missing cusps

Bicuspid aortic or pulmonary valves.

Aortic stenosis

1 Valvular.
2 Subvalvular.

Pulmonary stenosis

1 Isolated valvular stenosis.
2 Fallot's tetralogy.

Fallot's tetralogy

Incidence

This is the commonest (70%) of the congenital heart lesions causing cyanosis at rest.

Lesions

1 *Pulmonary stenosis*: this is usually of the subvalvular type with muscular thickening of the narrowed infundibulum; rarely it may be valvular as a diaphragm formed by fusion of the cusps.
2 *Ventricular septal defect*: the defect is in the upper membranous part of the septum.
3 *Dextraposition and overriding of the aorta*: the aorta overrides the VSD and receives blood from both ventricles.
4 *Right ventricular hypertrophy*: the right ventricular hypertrophy, with a concavity along the left border of the heart due to the absence of the pulmonary conus, produces the 'boot-shaped' deformity seen radiologically.

Effects

Most of the blood from the right ventricle passes into the aorta and the pulmonary blood flow is diminished. The aortic blood is thus mixed and unsaturated and cyanosis is therefore marked in all but the very mildest cases.

Eisenmenger complex

This is Fallot's tetralogy without the pulmonary stenosis—*trilogy*. The blood from the left ventricle passes through the VSD into the pulmonary circulation resulting in pulmonary hypertension.

Tricuspid atresia

Failure of development of one or more cusps of the tricuspid valve, sometimes associated with a complete septum across the valve orifice and a rudimentary right ventricle. In such cases a VSD is usually present, otherwise the lesion is incompatible with life.

Patent ductus arteriosus

Nature

In intrauterine life the blood passes from the pulmonary circulation through the ductus arteriosus into the aorta. In the normal infant, contraction of smooth muscle very soon after birth produces functional occlusion of the lumen of the ductus followed by permanent obliteration, usually by about 8 weeks. Failure of occlusion leads to a patent ductus arteriosus.

Results

A patent ductus arteriosus is compatible with life but, as the aortic systemic pressure is higher than the pulmonary pressure, there is a persistent left to right shunt through the ductus which produces the 'machinery' murmur. In cases with a large ductus, there follows hypertrophy of the left ventricle and left atrium, with engorgement of the pulmonary vessels and pulmonary hypertension.

If untreated, the majority of patients (about 70%) will succumb to either cardiac failure or to *Streptococcus viridans* infection at the site of the ductus. Operative ligation of the patent vessel obviates both serious sequelae and carries only a small mortality.

Coarctation of the aorta

Nature
A segmental area of narrowing of the aortic lumen between the left subclavian artery and the site of the ductus arteriosus.

Results
The stenosis of the aorta jeopardizes the blood supply below the area but compensation occurs by:
1 Left ventricular hypertrophy producing a raised systemic pressure.
2 Opening up of collateral vessels thus by-passing the obstruction, e.g. via the subscapular to the intercostal arteries thus reaching the thoracic aorta and producing radiological 'rib notching'; via the internal mammary artery to anastomose with the epigastric vessels.

These two mechanisms occur in the 'adult' form of coarctation when there has been closure of the ductus arteriosus.
3 In the 'foetal' type of coarctation there is a patent ductus arteriosus and this allows a by-pass of the coarctation by permitting a flow of blood from the pulmonary artery to the aorta below the level of the obstruction. However, this pulmonary arterial blood is unsaturated.

Effects
The defect produces:
1 An increased blood pressure in the arms, head and neck.
2 Prominence of collateral blood vessels.
3 Diminished pulses and blood pressure in the legs.
   These abnormalities predispose to:
1 Severe hypertension in the head and neck with heart failure or cerebral haemorrhage.
2 *Streptococcus viridans* infection at the site of the coarctation.

3 Aneurysm formation above or just below the coarcted segment.
4 Rupture or dissecting aneurysm of the aorta.

These sequelae can be avoided by the surgical removal of the narrowed aortic segment and re-anastomosis or interposition of a graft of human aorta or of synthetic material.

Veins

Persistent left superior vena cava
Usually opens into the coronary sinus or left atrium.

Abnormal pulmonary veins
Usually all four are present, but one or more may open into the right atrium, particularly if an ASD is also present.

Coronary vessels
Many variations in the relative sizes of the right and left arteries and their branches are frequently found and there may be anomalies also in situation, distribution or origin.

Other congenital abnormalities
Numerous other variations and abnormalities exist which may be of considerable practical importance in relationship to surgical correction. However, the important common lesions are:
1 Septal defects—ASD and VSD.
2 Patent ductus arteriosus.
3 Fallot's tetralogy.
4 Coarctation of the aorta.

Dangers of congenital heart disease

Heart failure
Abnormalities of blood flow lead to increased strain on one or both ventricles with hypertrophy, but ultimately failure, of one or both chambers. Septal defects and patent ductus arteriosus cause left to right shunting of blood and pulmonary hypertension with resulting right ventricular hyptertrophy. Ultimately shunt reversal (right to left) occurs, which is of sinister significance.

Pulmonary hypertension
Particularly in septal defects and ductus arteriosus but also in the Eisenmenger complex, severe progressive pulmonary hypertension results in structural arterial

changes in the pulmonary circulation and this increases the pulmonary resistance. Sudden heart failure is common in these circumstances (see p. 94).

Endocarditis
Congenital abnormalities, particularly patent ductus and valvular lesions, predispose to the development of bacterial endocarditis (see p. 69).

Predisposition to infections
Resistance to infections is low and may be the presenting feature, e.g. frequent upper respiratory infections in patients with septal defects. The infections increase the strain on the already abnormal circulation.

Functional disabilities
These may be severe, e.g. in Fallot's tetralogy, where exercise tolerance is very poor and squatting may occur after walking a few steps. The disabilities become progressively severe with increasing age.

Cyanosis
Interference with oxygenation leads to mental and physical retardation. The cyanosis may be manifest at all times or only appear on taking exercise.

Results

Untreated
1 Minor abnormalities may cause no interference with the normal life span and are found incidentally at post-mortem examination, even in ripe old age.
2 The more serious disorders cause variable degrees of decreased life expectancy, death occurring in many during infancy, childhood or adult life.

Treated
Many of the more common conditions can be surgically corrected although not without risk, which in some cases is considerable. Complete correction of most forms of septal defect, patent ductus arteriosus and coarctation of the aorta can be carried out and should be performed before serious complications or secondary structural changes are too far advanced.

C/BLOOD VESSELS, ANEURYSMS, VEINS, LYMPHATICS, ENDOTHELIAL TUMOURS

Normal
Atheroma
Syphilis
Cystic medial degeneration
Mönckeberg's sclerosis
Buerger's disease
Arteriolar sclerosis
Vasculitis
Aneurysms
Veins
Lymphatics
Tumours of endothelium

Normal arteries
There are three groups of arteries.

Large elastic
The aorta and its major branches.

Medium muscular
Distributing arteries, e.g. renal, femoral and brachial.

Small arteries and arterioles
Mostly within the substance of tissues and organs.

Normal structure
There are three layers present in all these vessels but in differing proportions.

Intima
An endothelial cell lining with subendothelial avascular connective tissue.

Media
This is of variable thickness and is composed of muscle and elastic tissue. The latter is widely distributed in the large elastic vessels; largely condensed into internal and external elastic laminae in the medium muscular arteries; less well defined in the small vessels.

Adventitia
A poorly defined layer of connective tissue external to the media and containing nerve fibres and the vasa vasorum. These nutrient arteries are derived from branches of the same artery, pass through the adventitia into the wall and can be identified in the outer third

of the media. In the inner layers, they are poorly formed and fail to enter the intima. The amount of adventitia is relatively large in the small arteries but contains very few recognizable vasa vasorum.

Capillaries

Begin as a rather sudden transition from arterioles and consist of a layer of endothelium supported by a scanty fibrous tissue framework. The diameter varies from 5 to 20 μm. Blood flow through them is controlled by a sphincter-like action of the innervated muscle of the arterioles, so that, in health, only 2–5% of the capillary bed is open and in action at any one time.

Arterial disease

General

Arterial disease may be due to:

1 Primary vascular disease.

2 Affection of vessels by diseases of adjacent structures.

The general effects of vascular damage may be:

1 Weakening of the vessel walls with dilatation or rupture.

2 Narrowing of the lumen producing ischaemia in the tissue supplied.

3 Damage to the endothelial lining provoking intravascular thrombosis.

Incidence

Some form of vascular disease affects virtually every individual at some stage during life and, together with cardiac disease, is responsible in Western populations for 50–60% of deaths over the age of 50 years and 20–30% of deaths in the 5–50 age group.

Atherosclerosis—atheroma

Incidence

Found in Western people, in some degree in virtually every adult over the age of 40 years and in many younger individuals. The incidence has probably not significantly increased in recent years but the sevenfold increase in deaths resulting from the disease during the period 1909–49 is due to the increased frequency of the complications, particularly thrombosis.

Nature

A disease of large and medium arteries in which there is focal proliferation of smooth muscle cells and accumulation of lipid within the intima forming *plaques*.

Age

Increases with advancing age.

Sex

Up to 45 years, Male : female 2 : 1; over 45 years (postmenopausal), Male : female equal.

Sites

The arteries principally affected are:

1 Aorta: particularly the abdominal aorta.

2 Coronary arteries.

3 Cerebral arteries.

Other large and medium-sized vessels are affected less commonly and the pulmonary arteries only very rarely, unless pulmonary hypertension is also present.

The lesions are patchy along the length of a vessel and are usually most marked at the origin of branches, i.e. at the points of maximal stress. The lesions are variable in severity from one artery to another in the same individual.

Aetiological factors

Diet and fat metabolism

It is well established that accelerated atherosclerosis occurs in those with hypercholesterolaemia, particularly in diabetes, hypothyroidism and certain types of familial xanthomatosis.

Experimentally, in certain animals atheromatous-like lesions can be readily produced by feeding with prolonged lipid-rich diets, particularly with saturated fats.

Less certain is correlation between known human cases of severe atherosclerosis and identifiable abnormalities of blood lipids. In most, cholesterol levels are normal but certain lipoproteins, particularly β and very low-density lipoproteins (LDL) and triglycerides, when raised, may show better correlation between severity of atherosclerosis and its complications and blood levels.

Blood levels of HDL, *when low*, indicate a high risk factor.

It has yet to be demonstrated, however, that reduction in blood levels of such lipids by dietary or other biochemical factors decreases risks, though lowered intake of animal fats and reduction of obesity are probably desirable and helpful. This effect may, however, be more related to reduction of complicating thrombosis than of control of the atherosclerotic process.

Smoking
Epidemiological studies clearly indicate a dose-related enhanced risk in cigarette smokers.

Disturbances of blood coagulation
Encrustation may be related to enhanced deposition of fibrin and platelets by change in some parameters of blood coagulation or altered fibrinolytic activity. High blood fat content has an *in vitro* effect on decreasing clotting time. Alterations in platelet adhesiveness may also be important in this context.

Sex
Premenopausal females are 'protected' compared with men, but postmenopausally atheroma tends to develop more rapidly. Oestrogens may be the significant factor, though long-term oestrogen therapy in young women (oral contraceptives) has a significantly higher complication rate of arterial disease and thrombotic complications than controls.

Race
There are wide variations in incidence of atheroma in different countries, much of which is explicable as dietary differences, though other factors cannot be excluded. The condition is relatively uncommon in Chinese, Japanese and Africans.

Hypertension
High blood pressure, though not apparently a causative factor, appears to accelerate the progress of the disease and may also relate to accentuation of mechanical factors at certain sites.

Emotional and physical
The impact of stress and level of physical activity are well recognized as conferring a higher risk, but seem to relate more to complications of atheroma than the primary disease process.

Familial and hereditary predisposition
There is no doubt that this is a powerful factor identifiable in epidemiological studies.

Stages of development and appearances

Early pathogenesis
It seems likely that initial events are due to:
1 Endothelial cell damage allowing reaction of platelets with the intima.
2 Release of platelet mitogen factors causing smooth muscle proliferation.
3 The damaged endothelial cells allow lipid from the plasma to pass through to the intima where they accumulate—*insudation*.

Fatty streaks or dots
These are the earliest macroscopic manifestations, are barely raised and variable in size and distribution.

Simple plaque
These focal lesions are variably raised when seen in unperfused fixed tissue and also vary markedly in size and colour due to differing proportions of yellow lipid and greyish fibrous tissue—i.e. fatty or fibrous plaque. The surface is non-ulcerated. Microscopically under the intact endothelium there are lipid-rich mononuclear cells and extracellular lipid, usually with cholesterol crystals. Variable amounts of collagenous tissue and of smooth muscle are present.

Complicated plaques
Extension of the plaques may result in
1 Fissuring of the plaque with rupture into the lumen.
2 Thrombus formation at the site of rupture.
3 Pressure on the media with degeneration of the internal elastic lamina.
4 Calcification with increasing rigidity of the wall.
   Fissuring is probably the more important trigger for the development of acute occlusive episodes in coronary arteries.

Effects
1 Luminal narrowing—due to the thickening of the intima by plaques. This may be concentric or eccentric and the effect is reduction of flow and ischaemia.
2 Occlusion by superimposed thrombus.
3 Pressure destruction of muscle and elastic tissue in media leading to aneurysms.
4 Distal microembolization. From surface thrombus and atheromatous material associated particularly with fissuring.

Syphilis

Large arteries

Sites
1 *Aorta*: virtually always confined to the thoracic portion, particularly the ascending part of the aortic arch.
2 *Medium muscular arteries*: rarely affected.

Pathogenesis
Although the spirochaetes are disseminated during the primary stage of the disease, the aortitis is a manifestation of the tertiary stage (see p. 2).

Macroscopical
Pearly-grey raised plaques on the thickened intimal surface together with puckering of the intima to give stellate or longitudinal scarring, classically of 'tree bark' appearance. The plaques are maximal around the origin of vessels, e.g. coronary ostia, and the lumen is commonly dilated, with or without local aneurysm formation.

Microscopical
1 Endarteritis of the vasa vasorum with a perivascular cuffing by lymphocytes and plasma cells in the adventitia.
2 The inflammatory process and the endarteritis extend into the media with progressive ischaemia.
3 Fragmentation of the elastic tissue due to ischaemia.
4 Degeneration of the muscle due to ischaemia.
5 Replacement fibrosis.

Results
1 *Aneurysm formation*. Localized—saccular (see p. 85). More diffuse—fusiform (see p. 85).
2 *Narrowing of coronary ostia*. Coronary insufficiency (see p. 65).
3 *Aortic regurgitation*. Due to stretching of the valve ring (see p. 72).

Small arteries
At all stages of congenital or acquired syphilis, small arteries may be involved in affected organs. The resulting endarteritis is responsible for the degenerative changes in the CNS and for the necrosis and fibrosis seen in gummas.

Microscopical
The microscopical appearances of the vessels are identical in all sites—endarteritis obliterans and perivascular cuffing with plasma cells and lymphocytes.

Results
Ischaemia due to the vascular narrowing with subsequent degenerative changes and replacement fibrosis.

Cystic medial degeneration—idiopathic cystic medial necrosis

Incidence
Mild localized changes are common and are found in about 30% of autopsies, but severe and extensive medial degeneration is uncommon.

Aetiology
This is unknown, but the following factors have been suggested:
1 *Hereditary*: metabolic or biochemical abnormalities of the ground substance. The disease is sometimes associated with congenital heart disease and Marfan's syndrome (see p. 293) and other familial elastic tissue defects.
2 *Toxic*: due to bacterial toxins. There is no confirmatory evidence for this aetiological factor.
3 *Experimental*: lathyrism is a condition occurring in rats fed on extracts from sweet peas in which fundamental abnormalities occur in the chemical composition and structure of various connective tissues. One of these changes is medial degeneration and is commonly followed by a dissecting aneurysm. Similar changes also occur experimentally when aminonitriles are administered.
4 *Anoxia*: epinephrine-induced constriction of the vasa vasorum produces medial degeneration. Similarly, experimentally induced thrombosis of the vasa vasorum also causes the lesion. The suggestion is that interference with oxygenation of the media may cause the degeneration to develop.
5 *Hypertension*: dissecting aneurysms most commonly occur in hypertensive patients, but there is no evidence to suggest that the medial change results directly from hypertension.

Age
Usually 40 years of age and above, but is occasionally manifest in younger age groups.

Sex
Male : female, 2 : 1.

Site
Confined to the aorta and to the origins of its major branches.

Macroscopical
Seldom noticeable unless complicated by a dissecting aneurysm.

Microscopical
Focal degeneration of the elastic tissue and muscle of the media with poorly delineated areas of basophilic amorphous material of rather myxomatous appearance. Small cyst-like spaces are filled with this mucopolysaccharide which stains red with PAS. The distribution is variable but is usually in the outer half of the media. The intima may show unrelated atheroma but the adventitia is normal.

Results
Dissecting aneurysm, when the disease is extensive (see p. 86).

Mönckeberg's medial calcific sclerosis—Mönckeberg's medial degeneration

Incidence
A common disease. The frequency increases with advancing age and it is rare under the age of 50 years.

Sex
Male : female equal.

Sites
Medium-sized muscular arteries, particularly of the limbs; the genital arterial supply is commonly involved, e.g. uterine vessels after the menopause.

Aetiology
This is obscure. There is no relationship with atheroma, although the two diseases may coexist.

Macroscopical
Tortuous, hard, calcified vessel walls but with no diminution of the lumen—'pipe stem' arteries.

Microscopical
The media only is affected. There are deposits of calcium in the hyalinized media. Bone may form in these calcified areas which are initially patchily distributed in rings or plaques but later become more continuous.

Effects
There is no narrowing so the disorder does not, by itself, produce ischaemia. It commonly coexists with atheroma when ischaemia may follow.

Thrombo-angiitis obliterans—Buerger's disease

Nature
The disease is a segmental, thrombosing, chronic inflammation of arteries, veins and other structures in the neurovascular bundle, in the legs of young or middle-aged males. The true incidence is rare.

Age
25–40 years.

Sex
Almost exclusively males.

Sites
Muscular arteries and veins of the legs; very rare in other vessels.

Aetiology
This is obscure, but factors include an increased frequency in Jews, Japanese, heavy smokers and those in sedentary occupations. An infective agent has been postulated but not isolated, and although cold aggravates the condition, it is not primarily causative.

Macroscopical
Segmental in distribution, affecting initially the anterior and posterior tibial vessels and subsequently the popliteal and femoral arteries. Small arteries are very rarely affected. The involved segment is thickened and indurated, binding all the components of the neurovascular bundle together. The lumen is thrombosed and subsequently replaced by pale, firm, fibrous tissue. The large proximal vessels may show gross narrowing by atheroma.

Microscopical

Early
There is an inflammatory cell infiltration of the intima with endothelial and fibroblastic proliferation.

Late
The process extends to other coats of the wall but does not destroy the architecture. The lumen is thrombosed and is followed by organization and attempts at recanalization. Usually the vein is similarly involved and thrombosed. In the late fibrous stages, dense collagen binds the nerves and vessels together.

Results
There is progressive ischaemia of the limbs:
1 Intermittent claudication.
2 Trophic skin changes.
3 Gangrene.

Amputation is necessary at some stage of the disease in at least 30% of cases. Symptoms may subside in those who cease smoking.

Arteriolar sclerosis

Nature
Thickening of the walls with narrowing of the lumen of small arteries and arterioles in systemic hypertension. The hypertension precedes these structural changes (see p. 92).

Sites
Small arteries and arterioles anywhere in the body, but particularly in the kidneys, pancreas, gall bladder, small intestines, adrenals and the retina.

Macroscopical
The vessels pout from a cut surface and the lumen is narrowed.

Microscopical

Hyaline arteriolar sclerosis—benign hypertension
Hyaline and fibrous thickening of the walls with loss of muscle and narrowing of the lumen. There is also increased elastic tissue in the distributing arteries, with reduplication of the internal elastic lamina.

Hyperplastic arteriolar sclerosis—accelerated hypertension
1 Concentric, laminated, 'onion-skin' appearance, due to cellular proliferation of the endothelium, intimal fibroblasts and medial muscle cells.
2 Fibrinoid necrosis of the arterioles with an intensely eosinophilic and smudgy appearance. Haemorrhages may occur into the surrounding tissues, e.g. glomeruli.

Vasculitis including arteritis

Nature
This is now the preferred term for inflammatory conditions of blood vessels which affect variable calibre of artery and sometimes veins also. Classification is difficult; clearly one based on aetiology would be best but is often unknown. At present the size of vessel affected and the presence or not of necrosis allow useful subdivision.

Large arteries
This infers inflammation of the aorta and its main branches.

Takayasu's disease—pulseless disease
This mostly occurs in young females, many of whom are Asians, and affects the aortic arch and its main branches. Inflammatory changes occur in all coats with fibrous replacement of muscle and thickening of wall causing reduction of lumen, superimposed thrombus and loss of pulses in the arms, together with ocular and neurological symptoms due to carotid artery involvement. The aetiology is unknown.

Kawasaki's disease
In this disease of unknown cause in infants, main aortic branch arteries, and particularly the coronary arteries, are the seat of a panarteritis with marked medial fibroblastic thickening and sometimes aneurysm formation.

Rheumatoid aortitis
In rheumatoid arthritis, systemic sclerosis and ankylosing spondylitis, inflammation of the vasa vasorum of the aortic root and ascending part of the arch may occur with muscle and elastic tissue in the media replaced by collagen and subsequent dilatation. Changes microscopically are very similar to those of syphilitic aortitis (see p. 81) but occasionally rheumatoid granulomas may be seen. Clinically aortic regurgitation may result (see p. 72).

Syphilitic aortitis

This tertiary manifestation of syphilis affects the thoracic part (see p. 81).

Secondary arteritis

Vessels adjacent to inflammatory conditions in other organs may become secondarily involved. This is particularly so in the base of ulcers, e.g. endarteritis obliterans in the floor of a peptic ulcer, in tuberculous cavities and as a result of chemical injury or ionizing radiation. The usual effect is narrowing of the lumen with fibrosis of the wall and sometimes aneurysm formation (see p. 87).

Medium arteries

Giant cell arteritis—cranial arteritis

Nature

An inflammatory condition of unknown aetiology occurring in older age groups of both sexes and originally called 'temporal arteritis' because of its most frequent site. However, involvement of the occipital, carotid or cerebral arteries including the ophthalmic branch are not uncommon, and occasionally the manifestations may be systemic. There is sometimes an association with polymyalgia rheumatica (see p. 103).

Clinical

Severe headache, often unilateral, is accompanied by fever and palpable tender nodular thickening of the temporal arteries. Blood studies show a very high erythrocyte sedimentation rate and hyperglobulinaemia. Eye symptoms leading to blindness occur in 30% of inadequately treated cases.

Appearances

The segmentally affected artery is thickened nodular and indurated. Microscopically there is necrosis of the inner media with fragmentation of the internal elastic lamina and giant cells aggregated around the fragments of the degenerate elastic fibres. Inflammatory cells are present in all layers and fibrous tissue progressively replaces the muscle and necrotic material. Thrombosis with organization and recanalization is usual.

Diagnosis

Biopsy of the affected artery is usually diagnostic. The procedure often has a dramatic effect in relieving the pain.

Results

Corticosteroid therapy controls the disease but if eye symptoms were present before treatment was started, blindness in one or both eyes may ensue.

Polyarteritis nodosa

This systemic necrotizing arteritis is described on p. 102.

Wegener's granulomatosis

This granulomatous condition is accompanied by arteritis with necrosis and most commonly affects the upper respiratory tract, lung and kidney (see p.103).

Churg–Strauss granulomatosis

This angiocentric pulmonary lesion is described on p. 396.

Lymphomatoid granulomatosis

This and its related condition lymphomatoid papulosis are described on p. 419.

Small arteries and arterioles

Most vasculitides involving small vessels are necrotizing in appearance and are largely immunologically mediated. Skin vessels with production of a petechial or frankly purpuric rash, are frequently involved together with joint pain and swelling due to a concomitant polyarthritis.

Allergic vasculitis—leukocytoclastic vasculitis

Causes

The causal agents are drugs, bacteria, e.g. gonococci and meningococci and *Streptococcus viridans*, virus and mycoplasmal infections and connective tissue diseases, particularly polyarteritis nodosa and systemic lupus erythematosus (see p. 96).

Appearances

There is a necrotizing vasculitis affecting small arteries, arterioles and/or capillaries. The inflammatory cell infiltrate is perivascular and neutrophilic with eosinophils commonly present. A frequent feature is fragmentation of polymorphonuclear leucocyte nuclei—hence *leucocytoclastic*.

In some cases only skin vessels are involved; in others there is evidence of systemic involvement in which renal involvement is prognostically important (see p. 171).

Crescentic glomerulonephritis. This serious glomerular lesion is a capillary vasculitis and is described on p. 171.

Henoch–Schönlein purpura. In this remitting and relapsing disorder in children the histological features are similar to allergic vasculitis but the renal lesion is a focal proliferative glomerulonephritis. With each attack the risk of serious glomerular damage increases, progressing in some cases to end-stage renal failure (see p. 171).

Aneurysms

Definition
Abnormal localized dilatation of an artery.

Types
1 *True*: the wall is formed by one or more layers of the affected vessel.
2 *False*: the wall is formed by connective tissue which is not part of a vessel. They are usually due to traumatic or infective openings in vessels limited by the surrounding tissues.

True aneurysms

Macroscopical
1 *Fusiform*: spindle-shaped area of dilatation due to a long segment of the vessel wall being affected around the whole circumference.
2 *Saccular*: part of the circumference only is involved to produce a globular sac, usually with a narrow neck in the early stages.
3 *Dissecting*: blood tracking along a false lumen within the arterial wall.

General features
Aneurysms form as a result of weakening of the wall due to a variety of causes. Loss of elasticity and contractability due to a deficiency in the media is the most important factor.

Once the wall starts to stretch, the process is usually progressive under normal or abnormal (hypertensive) pressure forces, with increasing thinning of the wall until eventual rupture may occur. Build-up of laminated thrombus within the lumen of the aneurysmal sac is protective but only rarely is this process sufficient to repair the defect and reconstitute a normal lumen to the artery of origin.

Congenital aneurysms

'Berry' aneurysms

Incidence
This is the most common cause of subarachnoid haemorrhage and is only rarely found incidentally when death has occurred from unrelated causes.

Age and sex
The average age at presentation is 50 years. Male : female, 1 : 1.2.

Site
The vessels around the circle of Willis, particularly at the junctions of the communicating arteries. They are much more common in the anterior part of the circle (75%) than posteriorly (25%).

Pathogenesis
A congenital defect of the media in the angles formed by the junctions of vessels. The defect involves both the muscle and elastic tissue, thus, with increasing age and particularly with hypertension, this area of weak artery stretches and forms the aneurysm.

Appearances
They may be solitary or multiple or even symmetrical and form small (seldom more than 1 cm dia) sessile or pedunculated thin-walled sacs. The wall usually consists only of fibrous tissue with an endothelial lining.

Results

Before rupture
1 Pressure symptoms, which may produce localizing signs.
2 Ischaemia of adjacent brain.

Leakage. Blood staining of CSF.

Rupture
1 Subarachnoid haemorrhage.
2 Rupture into the ventricles
3 Intracerebral haemorrhage.

Prognosis
With the first bleed, untreated: 60% die; 20% disabled; 20% recover.

Treatment by direct attack or by tying the carotid

artery considerably improves this prognosis, e.g. there is about a 25% immediate mortality, but of the survivors, 75% are alive, well and at work 5 years later.

Arteriovenous malformations

Rare congenital conditions showing localized groups of poorly formed blood vessels, involving both arteries and veins. Many occur in the brain—so-called 'angioma', and at many other sites, e.g. limbs, lungs, etc. When large, they cause problems by the shunting of blood and cardiac strain. The small lesions may be symptomless or may rupture with haemorrhage.

Cirsoid aneurysms

A mass of dilated, elongated, pulsating and intercommunicating arteries and veins—'bag of worms'. About 80–90% are congenital and the remainder traumatic in origin. Most occur in the scalp connected with the frontal or temporal arteries. They increase in size gradually and may cause destruction of the surrounding tissues or rupture with haemorrhage.

Atheromatous aneurysms

Incidence
Common in the older age groups where they form the most frequent type of aneurysm.

Sites
The abdominal aorta and the common iliac arteries particularly, but any atheromatous artery, may also be affected.

Appearances
Usually fusiform dilatation of the wall due to involvement of the media by the advanced atheromatous process (see p. 80). They only occur therefore in the late stages of the disease, mostly in elderly males and are frequently multiple; they are by far the most common cause of abdominal aortic aneurysm. Most of them are situated below the origin of the renal arteries and are thus amenable to resection and replacement by a graft.

Results
There is a gradual increase in size and they may eventually rupture with a fatal outcome. The aneurysm may be surgically excised or bypassed and continuity of the vessel restored by a graft or prosthe-

sis. The prognosis is then that of the severity of atheroma present in other organs, e.g. coronary and cerebral arteries.

Syphilitic aneurysms

Incidence
Formerly common, but now rare.

Sites
The thoracic aorta, particularly the ascending and transverse portions of the arch.

Appearances
Mostly saccular in type. The wall of the adjacent vessel shows the scarring of syphilitic aortitis (see p. 81).

Results
May reach an enormous size, press on adjacent structures and eventually rupture. They are often associated with aortic incompetence due to dilatation of the valve ring.

Dissecting aneurysms

Site
Aorta

Aetiology
Due to cystic medial degeneration (see p. 81).

Pathogenesis
Entry of blood into the diseased media whence it separates the wall into an inner layer of intima and part of the media and an outer layer of part of the media and the adventitia. Blood may enter this false lumen via:
1 Intramural haemorrhage from the vasa vasorum.
2 A break in the intima at a site of particular weakness, often in the ascending portion or arch of the aorta and rarely at the site of an atheromatous plaque.

The false lumen may be long but inevitably must rupture:
1 *Internally*: to recommunicate with the true lumen or
2 *Externally*: to produce a catastrophic haemorrhage. This is more common and results in:
   (a) intrapericardial haemorrhage—haemopericardium with cardiac tamponade;
   (b) mediastinal haemorrhage;

(c) pleural cavity—haemothorax;
(d) abdominal haemorrhage.

Appearances
A double-barrelled aorta, often extending from its origin to the bifurcation, but it may not involve the whole circumference of the wall. Acute cases show little blood in the false lumen due to its escape into the para-aortic tissues; in the rarer, more chronic, forms which re-enter the true lumen, variable amounts of blood clot are present in the lumen of the sac. In other rare cases, the entire aortic blood flow may pass through the area of dissection in the wall, the original lumen of the aorta having been blocked due to the pressure of blood in the false lumen.

Effects
1 *Rupture*: with rapid death.
2 *Chronic dissecting aneurysm*: when re-entry occurs. This usually ruptures after a short period of time, e.g. months.
3 *Obliteration of branches*: as the blood extends in the wall it dissects the origins of branches resulting in their occlusion and thus causing renal or mesenteric infarction or gangrene of the lower limbs. The carotid and subclavian vessels are usually spared.

Mycotic aneurysms

Nature
Formed by weakness of the wall due to bacterial infection.

Causes
Nearly all are associated with infective endocarditis (see p. 69) and the low-grade inflammation which accompanies impaction of embolic material.

The process is also seen in vessels in the walls of tuberculous cavities, abscesses and rarely adjacent to foci of acute or chronic non-specific inflammation.

Appearances
Usually small saccular dilatations with destruction of the muscle and elastic tissue by the inflammatory process, the wall then being formed by thin, stretched, fibrous tissue in which there may be scanty residual inflammatory cells.

Sites
Aorta, coronary, cerebral and mesenteric arteries are most commonly affected.

Effects
1 *Rupture*: uncommon, except as a late manifestation.
2 *Thrombosis*: in the lumen of the aneurysms and later involving the lumen of the vessel of origin, thus resulting in ischaemic changes in the region supplied.

Loss of support
Destruction of soft tissues around blood-vessels may occasionally lead to loss of support and aneurysmal dilatation. This is stated to occur in the brain substance following cerebral softening and in the lungs as a sequel to pulmonary destruction, e.g. tuberculosis. However, other factors causing damage to the vessel wall are usually also present, e.g. inflammation.

Polyarteritis nodosa
A common sequel to the necrotizing arteritis is the dilatation of weakened arterial walls (see p. 102).

Appearances
Usually multiple and commonly numerous along the course of vessels as nodules of about twice the normal diameter. They frequently become filled with firm thrombus.

Sites
Small arteries, but the disease may affect medium-sized muscular vessels. The classical sites are the kidneys, heart, intestines and lungs.

Effects
1 *Thrombosis*: producing infarction.
2 *Rupture*: producing haemorrhage; however, this is unusual.

False aneurysms—traumatic aneurysms

Pulsating haematoma

Nature
A false aneurysm resulting from a small perforation in the wall of an artery.

Aetiology
Trauma, usually due to a sharp instrument.

Pathogenesis
The small aperture is sufficiently large to permit the

escape of blood into the surrounding tissues where it collects until the pressure within the haematoma approaches that of the blood pressure. At this point, the haematoma no longer enlarges as the blood then re-enters the artery in diastole and refills in systole resulting in a 'to-and-fro' murmur.

Appearances
The walls of the haematoma are formed by the compressed adjacent tissues, e.g. muscle and fascia of the arms and legs. The lumen is filled with laminated clot externally and fluid blood in the centre.

Results
The false aneurysm may be removed and the arterial perforation sutured. If the haematoma persists, pain due to pressure or ischaemia due to progressive pressure on the vessel, may ensue.

Arteriovenous fistulae

Nature
A false aneurysm communicating with both an artery and a vein.

Aetiology
Trauma, penetrating the walls of both an artery and a vein.

Pathogenesis
The haematoma communicates with the lumen of both the artery and the vein so that there is a fistulous communication between the two via the haematoma. A continuous murmur is produced due to the arterial blood flowing constantly into the vein.

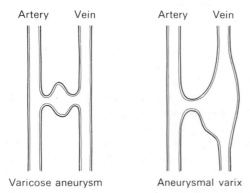

Fig. 10 Arteriovenous fistulae.

Appearances
Usually there is a false aneurysm containing blood, situated between the artery and the vein and through which blood flows—'*varicose aneurysm*' (see Fig. 10).

Sometimes there is only a small haematoma when the trauma has resulted in an immediate communication between the artery and the vein. The pressure of the arterial blood then distends the vein—'*aneurysmal varix*' (see Fig. 10).

Results
1 Increased blood flow in the artery above the fistula causes dilatation and hypertrophy of the wall with subsequent degenerative changes.
2 Decreased blood flow in the artery distal to the fistula may result in peripheral ischaemia.
3 Venous enlargement at the site of the fistula due to excessive blood flow and pressure. The vein dilates and the wall hypertrophies until it attains the histological features of an artery—venous arterialization.
4 Gross enlargement of the false aneurysm to produce pressure symptoms.
5 Cardiac hypertrophy due to the shunting effect of the arteriovenous communication which may terminate in heart failure if the fistula is not closed.

Veins

Varicose veins

Nature
Abnormally dilated tortuous veins.

Sites
1 Systemic—usually leg veins.
2 Portal—in portal venous hypertension, e.g. oesophagus, haemorrhoids, umbilicus.

Incidence
Common in legs; 10–20% of the general population develop this disorder at some age.

Age
Increasing incidence with age, most common above 50 years.

Sex
Male : female, 1 : 4

Pathogenesis

Factors involved include:

1 *Relating to support of the venous wall.*

(a) *Familial*: a relative weakening of the wall. There is a familial incidence in about 40% of all cases.

(b) *Obesity*: poor support by the adipose tissue of the leg.

(c) *Age*: loss of support by degenerative changes in the surrounding tissues and decreased activity of the muscles.

(d) *Posture*: the dependent position is a predisposition and occupations involving prolonged standing or sitting show an increased incidence.

2 *Increased pressure within the lumen.*

(a) *Pregnancy*.

(b) *Intravascular thrombosis*.

(c) *Tumour masses pressing on veins*, e.g. uterine fibroids and ovarian tumours.

(d) *Garters and other constrictions*.

Appearances

More common in the superficial veins where support is least effective, but they may occur at any site where local obstruction is present. Asymmetrical dilatation and tortuosity of the veins occurs with elongation and varying thickness of the wall. Later, there is hypertrophy of the muscle but this is ineffectual and the valves become incompetent due to the uneven stretching and deformity of the wall.

Complications

1 Oedema.

2 Trophic skin changes—varicose or gravitational ulcers.

3 Thrombosis.

4 Haemorrhage.

5 Infection—thrombophlebitis.

6 Embolism.

Venous thrombosis

Phlebothrombosis

Bland thrombosis of non-inflammatory origin but with secondary inflammatory changes in the vessel wall.

Thrombophlebitis

Thrombosis initiated by inflammation.

In most cases, the differentiation between the two types is impossible and is of little significance, although sometimes the embolic sequelae may be different due to the presence or absence of infection within the thrombus.

Incidence

Common.

Predisposing factors

Cardiac failure; pregnancy; prolonged bed rest; immobilization; varicose veins.

Although these factors which give rise to stasis are the most important, direct injury or infection may be the precipitating cause. The condition may also occur in young and otherwise healthy ambulant individuals in whom the aetiology is obscure.

Sites

Anywhere, but most common and important in:

1 Legs—95%, particularly the lower leg where the deep veins are often involved.

2 Skull and dural sinuses—this is now rare.

3 Portal venous tributaries.

4 Pelvic veins.

Appearances

Similar in both types; the veins are distended by laminated thrombus. The bland type of thrombus is only locally attached to the wall in the early stages whereas the thrombi seen in pre-existing inflammation are usually more firmly adherent. Later, organization of the thrombus and subsequent recanalization may occur.

Complications

Embolism:

1 *Phlebothrombosis*: more common, causing infarction by aseptic thrombus.

2 *Thrombophlebitis*: less common, resulting in septic infarcts or pyaemic abscesses.

In many cases of fatal pulmonary embolism, the venous thrombosis of the legs or pelvis has remained clinically 'silent'.

Thrombophlebitis migrans

An uncommon disease characterized by transient venous inflammation which migrates from one area of the body to another. The aetiology is unknown but a number of cases are associated with malignant disease, particularly carcinomas of the bronchus and pancreas.

Lymphatics

Lymphangitis

The lymphatic channels draining any focus of inflammation are inflamed, dilated and contain inflammatory cells. They may be responsible for the spread of the infection in some cases, e.g. in tuberculosis, and sometimes the inflammation is very marked clinically with tender swelling of the regional lymph nodes (see p. 266).

Appearances

Usually only seen in the subcutaneous channels as red streaks. When chronic, there may be fibrous blockage of the lymphatics resulting in lymphoedema.

Lymphoedema

Nature

Brawny induration of tissues due to blockage of the lymphatics. When severe, the thickening of the skin and the overgrowth of the dermal connective tissues results in elephantiasis.

Causes

1 Malignant tumours with mechanical blockage by tumour cells.
2 Radical surgery with resection of lymphatics.
3 Post-irradiation fibrosis.
4 Filariasis (see p. 8).
5 Post-inflammatory fibrosis—e.g. lymphogranuloma venereum (see p. 203).
6 Primary lymphatic disorders.
  (a) *Milroy's disease*: an inherited lymphoedema in which there is faulty development of the lymphatic channels, usually of the lower limbs. It is present from birth but is frequently not clinically apparent until after puberty.
  (b) *Lymphoedema praecox*: a rare condition of females aged 10–25 years, remaining localized to the feet or extending on to the trunk. The aetiology is obscure.

Effects

In addition to the swelling, which may be very gross, the oedematous part is very susceptible to attacks of lymphangitis and to ulceration. Surgical treatment may produce considerable improvement.

Tumours of vascular and lymphatic endothelium

Nature

Tumours or malformations of vascular and lymphatic endothelium.

Haemangioma

Capillary

A lesion composed of capillary blood vessels.

Cavernous

A lesion composed of cavernous, endothelial-lined spaces.

Sclerosing

Produced as a result of fibrosis or sclerosis of a capillary haemangioma; a predominantly fibrous nodule containing iron pigment remains.

Glomus tumour—glomangioma

Nature

Rare tumours arising from the cells of the glomus organ.

The glomus organ

This is a convoluted arteriovenous anastomosis with modified muscle cells—glomus cells, in the walls, which have a cuboidal epithelial-like appearance. The glomus organ is richly supplied with nerves and is believed to be responsible for temperature regulation by modifying the calibre of the vessels and thus blood flow through the area. The glomus organs are situated predominantly in the peripheral parts of the limbs, but also are widely distributed throughout many viscera.

Age

Usually present in adult life and only very rarely in children.

Sites

Periphery of the limbs, especially the fingers, but rarely elsewhere.

Macroscopical

Painful red or purple tumours on the fingers usually less than 2 cm diameter.

Microscopical
Multiple, small, vascular spaces surrounded by sheets of uniform glomus cells; special stains reveal a profuse nerve supply to the tumour, which possibly accounts for the pain.

Results
Local excision is curative and the pain disappears; the tumours are benign.

Haemangiopericytoma
This is a rare tumour occurring in relation to a blood vessel which appears to be a variant of the glomus tumour, being derived from the haemangiopericytes. These are contractile cells in close relation to capillary walls. They form well-defined tumours in the limbs, mediastinum, retroperitoneal tissues or elsewhere and are composed of multiple vascular spaces surrounded by the plump polyhedral pericytes. Though formerly regarded as benign, it is now quite clear that these can be malignant tumours though the course is variably prolonged.

Angiosarcoma
A rare but true tumour of endothelial origin composed of highly atypical vasoformative tissue. The tumour invades locally and commonly metastasizes widely (see p. 256). Breast, head and neck and the extremities are the most frequent sites.

Lymphangioma
These are almost identical to the haemangiomas in type and structure but the lumen contains lymph.

Simple or capillary
Masses of small lymphatic channels.

Cavernous
Cavernous lymph spaces, rare but most common in the spleen.

Cystic
Results in a 'cystic hygroma'.

Lymphangiosarcoma
This malignant tumour is very rare and almost exclusively arises in areas of lymphoedema, the neoplasm being derived from the endothelium of the dilated lymphatics.

D/HYPERTENSION

Systemic hypertension
   Essential
   Secondary
   Mechanisms
Pulmonary hypertension
   Passive
   Due to increased flow
   Due to vascular obstruction
   Structural changes
   Primary plexogenic arteriopathy
   Pulmonary veno-occlusive disease

Systemic hypertension

Definition
A sustained rise of the systemic blood pressure above 140 mmHg systolic and 90 mmHg diastolic.

Types

Primary or essential
1 Benign hypertension.
2 Accelerated or malignant hypertension.
Ninety per cent of hypertensives are of this type with no known cause.

Secondary
That is, follows a number of known conditions, many of which are renal.

Primary essential hypertension

Benign hypertension

Clinical
An extremely common condition in which there is a slowly progressive rise in the blood pressure over a period of many years. Five per cent of such patients enter an accelerated phase after many years of benign progression.

Age
Usually 50 years or above.

Sex
More common in males.

Effects
The hypertension precedes and produces arteriolar

sclerosis (see p. 83) and mild renal damage. In addition other organ changes result.

Organ changes

Cardiovascular
1 *Heart*: concentric left ventricular hypertrophy (see p. 73).
2 *Large arteries*: although not causative, atheroma is potentiated by hypertension, particularly in the aorta, coronary and cerebral vessels.
3 *Muscular arteries*: medial hypertrophy and intimal thickening.
4 *Small arteries*: arteriolar sclerosis (see p. 83).
  (a) Hyaline thickening of the wall.
  (b) Increased elastic tissue with reduplication of the elastic lamina.

Brain
The combination of hypertension and potentiated atheroma commonly leads to cerebral vascular accidents (see p. 322).

Kidney
Results in benign nephrosclerosis. Renal function is unimpaired in the large majority of cases (see p. 175).

Prognosis
From the age of diagnosis the average course in untreated cases is in excess of 10 years, but much longer when therapy effectively controls the pressure. The additional mortality of a blood pressure of 150/100 mmHg is 125% in males over 40 years and 85% in females of similar age. Men with blood pressure higher than 178 mmHg systolic and 108 mm Hg diastolic, have an excess mortality of 600%. Treatment of minor degrees of hypertension—diastolic pressures of 90–95 mmHg—does not decrease incidence of myocardial infarction.
  Death may be due to:
1 Congestive heart failure—45%.
2 Coronary insufficiency or infarction—35%.
3 Cerebral vascular accident—15%.
4 Renal failure—5%.

Accelerated—malignant hypertension

Nature
Most cases arise *de novo*, but some are due to a malignant termination of benign hypertension.

Clinical
A more rapidly progressive form of hypertension in which very high levels are commonly reached, e.g. 280 mmHg systolic and 180 mmHg diastolic. This is accompanied by severe headaches, papilloedema and other hypertensive retinal changes, severe renal functional impairment, albuminuria and haematuria.

Age
Mostly occurs in patients younger than 45 years of age.

Organ changes

Cardiovascular
1 *Heart*: the degree of left ventricular hypertrophy depends upon the duration of the disease. In rapidly progressive cases it may be minimal.
2 *Vessels*: usually uncomplicated by any significant degree of atheroma. The small arteries show malignant arteriolar sclerosis (see p. 83) with:
  (a) fibrinoid necrosis;
  (b) hyperplasia of the 'onion-skin' type.

Kidney
Accelerated nephrosclerosis (see p. 176).

Brain
Cerebral vascular accidents are relatively uncommon.

Prognosis
This is poor in untreated cases, but well managed and treated cases have a good survival. Untreated patients die from:
1 Renal failure—90%.
2 Heart failure.
3 Cerebral vascular episode.

Secondary hypertension

Nature
This is hypertension secondary to a pre-existing disease.

Causes

Renal disease
1 *Parenchymal*: chronic pyelonephritis; glomerulonephritis; polycystic kidneys; amyloidosis; infarction; toxaemia of pregnancy.

2 *Renal vessels*: vascular obstruction: thrombosis; atheroma; ligatures; pressure from tumours; dissecting aneurysm involving renal vessels; polyarteritis nodosa.

3 *Obstruction*: hydronephrosis.

Whilst more common in bilateral disease, unilateral renal lesions may also result in hypertension.

Blood
Polycythaemia.

Endocrine
1 Cushing's syndrome due to pituitary or adrenal hypersecretion or steroid therapy (see p. 118).
2 Phaeochromocytoma—the hypertension is commonly intermittent (see p. 119).
3 Diabetes with renal involvement—Kimmelstiel–Wilson disease (see p. 167).
4 Conn's syndrome due to hyperaldosteronism (see p. 118).

Cerebral
1 Increased intracranial pressure due to: trauma; tumours; haemorrhage; inflammations.
2 Lesions of the hypothalamic region.
3 Lesions of the brain stem.

Drugs
Adrenaline and related sympatheticomimetic drugs.

Cardiovascular
Coarctation of the aorta; arteriovenous fistulae and shunts.

Mechanism of causation of hypertension

Experimental procedures
A large number of differing procedures will cause sustained hypertension in animals.

Infusion of pressor substances
1 *Renin*: only mild elevation of pressure is possible.
2 *Angiotensin*: particularly angiotensin II, which has a marked vasoconstrictive effect.
3 *Adrenaline and noradrenaline*: potent vasoconstrictive effects which can be sustained for long periods of time.

Overdosage with salt and adrenal cortical hormones
1 *Salt*: high dietary salt intake causes sustained hypertension in some animals but not in others.
2 *Deoxycorticosterone acetate (DOCA)*: administered to rats with high dietary salt produces sustained hypertension.

Interference with kidneys
Hypertension can be produced by renal irradiation or removal of both kidneys or wrapping kidneys in silk or cellophane.

More relevant however to disease in man is the effect of interference with renal arterial flow.
1 *Unilateral renal artery constriction*: humans appear to behave like the rat in producing prolonged severe hypertension associated with rise in renin and probably maintained and potentiated by angiotensin II.
2 *Unilateral renal artery constriction after nephrectomy on other side*: this produces a persistent, usually very high level of hypertension not associated with excess renin or angiotensin II.

Secondary hypertension in humans
1 Renal diseases:
   (a) excess renin;
   (b) sodium and water retention.
2 Adrenal diseases:
   (a) aldosterone excess induces sodium retention;
   (b) glucocorticoid excess probably operates similarly;
   (c) adrenaline and noradrenaline produce vasoconstriction.

Primary or essential hypertension in humans
The mechanism in benign hypertension is not understood, but the condition may be initiated by response to emotional stress in genetically susceptible individuals via the sympathetic nervous system, with resulting renal vasoconstriction and sodium retention. If sufficiently prolonged, organic vascular narrowing of renal vessels will effect a permanent rise in the threshold for sodium excretion and further vasoconstriction.

In accelerated hypertension it is thought likely that renin and angiotensin II have a role initiated by damage to renal afferent arterioles caused by a severe and steep rise in arterial pressure. The primary initiating factors may also be related to genetic predisposition and nervous and emotional causes.

Pulmonary hypertension

Nature
Pulmonary arterial pressure in excess of 30 mmHg.

Normal pulmonary vasculature
Normal pulmonary blood flow—5–8 litres/min at rest. Normal pressure—16–17 mmHg. With exercise, the flow increases up to 16 litres/min but the pressure does not rise significantly.

The requirement of the pulmonary circulation is to transmit the total right ventricular output with the minimum of resistance through the lungs. The vessels are therefore capacious and thin-walled. Elastic arteries extend as far as the end of the cartilaginous bronchi and the muscular arteries are short, ending at the level of the respiratory bronchioles, and are thinner than their systemic counterparts. The arterioles soon lose their muscle and consist mostly of intima, external elastic tissue and adventitia. They end in the capillaries which are in close relationship to the alveoli.

Mechanisms in the production of pulmonary hypertension
1 *Precapillary*: caused by increased flow or by increased resistance. The alveolar walls are normal.
2 *Capillary*: due to destruction of alveoli or distortion of the alveolar capillary bed.
3 *Postcapillary*: from passive congestion of alveolar parenchyma.

Passive pulmonary hypertension

Causes
1 Chronic left ventricular failure.
2 Mitral stenosis or incompetence.

Effects
1 *Chronic left ventricular failure*: the degree of pulmonary hypertension is seldom marked. There is slight atheroma and increased thickening of the muscle in the muscular arteries.
2 *Mitral valve disease*: more severe changes occur:
  (a) atheroma is usually marked as superficial fatty streaking;
  (b) muscular hypertrophy of elastic and muscular arteries;

(c) arterial thrombosis may occur;
(d) embolism may also be found.

Pulmonary hypertension due to increased blood flow

Causes
1 Atrial septal defect (ASD).
2 Ventricular septal defect (VSD).
3 Other left to right shunts, e.g. ductus arteriosus, Blalock's operation, etc. (see p. 75).

Effects
1 *ASD*: left to right shunt with a massive increase in the blood flow and a marked rise of pressure. Initially, the increased pressure is reversible, but later is constant. In the late stages the resistance increases to a sufficient degree to reverse the shunt from right to left.
2 *VSD*: the pulmonary vessels are exposed to the full force of the left ventricular pressure from birth. As a result the pressure is higher and the damage is greater.

Pulmonary hypertension due to organic vascular obstruction

Causes
1 Thromboembolic disease. Particularly when small, multiple and recurrent.
2 Loss of pulmonary tissue:
  (a) *Pulmonary fibrosis*: from any cause, but particularly in fibrosing alveolitis (see p. 392).
  (b) *Emphysema*: partly due to spasm but also to compression of the alveolar blood vessels by the raised intra-alveolar tension and to loss of tissue with reduction of the capillary bed.
  (c) *Lung resection*: more than a third of the lung tissue needs to be removed before hypertension is likely to result.

Structural changes in arteries
Changes can be graded on biopsy material and, particularly in congenital heart disease, may be prognostically important. *Grade 1*—Congenital heart disease present from birth causes retention of fetal structure in lung vessels. Small arteries and arterioles show muscle thickening but no fibrosis. *Grade 2*—Intimal proliferation as well in small arteries. *Grade 3*—Involvement of medium-sized vessels by muscle hypertrophy and intimal proliferation. *Grades*

4–6—There are dilatation lesions as well—plexiform, vein-like branches, angiomatoid and cavernous. Haemosiderosis is present in grade 5 and necrotizing changes in grade 6.

Primary pulmonary hypertension—primary plexogenic pulmonary arteriopathy

This is due to increased arterial tone with a raised peripheral resistance of vascular origin and is thus analogous to essential systemic hypertension.

In this rare condition, which predominates in young females, the median age at death is 34 years. The aetiology is, by definition, unknown.

Exclusion of recurrent thromboembolic disease (particularly in those taking oral contraceptive agents) is often very difficult, but clinical features may be almost specifically diagnostic. Lung biopsy may be helpful in identifying a marked decrease in arteries less than 40 μm diameter in the primary type, together with the non-specific muscular medial thickening which, however, does not extend into normally non-muscular vessels.

Pulmonary veno-occlusive disease

A rare condition of unknown cause which often dates from an influenzal-like illness in 15–20-year-olds. Veins as well as arteries show obliterative changes and there is haemosiderosis and alveolar wall thickening. Fragmentation of elastic tissue is seen.

Chapter 5
Connective Tissue Diseases

These diseases, which include systemic lupus erythematosus, rheumatoid arthritis, scleroderma, dermatomyositis and various vasculitides, have features in common such that they are acceptable as a clinical grouping; however, they do not have a unifying pathological or immunological basis. Many are autoimmune diseases and a minority of patients demonstrate considerable overlap within the group, having features of more than one disease. Historically the term 'collagen diseases', was applied to these conditions, but this has been superseded by the title connective tissue diseases. The latter term must not be confused with hereditary defects in collagen such as Marfan's syndrome.

Their aetiology is unknown, but a combination of immunological, environmental and genetic factors are involved. Many of these diseases are characterized by the presence of autoantibodies, some of which are pathogenetic, e.g. in the haemolytic anaemia of systemic lupus erythematosus (SLE), whilst others are merely epiphenomena, reflecting a dysregulated immune system. These diseases predominantly affect women but none has a clear inheritance pattern; however, family and twin studies suggest an important role for genetic factors in their aetiopathogenesis.

Systemic lupus erythematosus

Prevalence
SLE affects all races but rates vary from country to country, and up to 1:1000 black women in North America may be affected. It is uncommon in the UK, 30 per 100 000 of the population being afflicted. Peak age of onset is 45–50 years of age.

Aetiology

Environment
SLE studies in mice implicate viruses in its aetiopathogenesis but convincing human studies have not yet corroborated this. Clusters of SLE patients have been identified and this would strongly suggest environmental factors. Sunlight is known to exacerbate SLE. Drug-induced SLE related to hydralazine and phenytoin is recognized; acetylator status is relevant, leading to rapid or slow metabolism of the drug, the slow acetylators being more at risk.

Constitutional factors
Women with SLE outnumber males 9 : 1, and a strong hormonal influence is emphasized by the detrimental effect that pregnancy and oestrogen therapy can have on some patients with SLE. The concordance rate for SLE in monozygotic twins is only 23%, emphasizing the importance of environmental influences. Individuals with inherited complement deficiencies, especially the early classical components (C2 and C4) have a marked propensity to develop SLE.

Immunological changes
Generalized B lymphocyte overactivity leads to the production of a wide variety of autoantibodies, especially to nuclear proteins, and this probably results from defective T cell control. The formation of immune complexes composed of DNA and antibody become deposited in various tissues, and are considered central to the development of many of the pathological lesions.

Sex and age
SLE affects both females and, to a lesser extent, males of all ages; however, it is unusual in children.

Organ changes
Any organ of the body can be involved, though the liver is rarely affected. In many patients, however, it is confined to skin and joints.

Kidney

Significant renal involvement is common and important. The five differing patterns are described on p. 168.

Skin

Mucocutaneous involvement occurs in 80% of cases and includes cutaneous vasculitis, alopecia, mouth ulcers, butterfly facial rash and photosensitivity. Skin biopsies of clinically uninvolved, light-exposed skin can be diagnostically useful, demonstrating granular deposition of immunoglobulin (IgG) and complement at the dermal–epidermal junction (lupus band test). Such a biopsy should be fresh-frozen in liquid nitrogen, not fixed.

Heart

The commonest cardiac lesion is fibrinous pericarditis and, less frequently, myocarditis with focal fibrinoid change in the walls of small arteries. 'Libman Sachs' endocarditis—non-bacterial verrucous endocarditis, with vegetations on the ventricular side of the mitral valve, is very uncommon and until recently was an autopsy diagnosis (see p. 70).

Lungs

Fibrinous pleural inflammation is common and can be accompanied by effusions. The pathology associated with progressive elevation of the diaphragms, the so-called 'shrinking lungs', is poorly understood.

Musculoskeletal system

Arthralgia occurs in up to 90% of patients and tendon involvement is common. The arthritis of SLE is usually polyarticular and symmetrical, most commonly affecting the small joints of the hands, wrists and knees. It is characteristically non-erosive, and in only 10% of patients do joint deformities occur resulting from laxity of the joint capsule—*Jaccoud's arthritis*. Lymphocytic vasculitis in the muscle capillaries/venules is notable in active disease.

Brain

Neuropsychiatric involvement includes epilepsy, hemiplegia, depression and psychosis. The deposition of immune complexes in the cerebral vasculature accounts for some of the neuropathology, and the effects of their deposition in the choroid plexus have received much attention and speculation. Micro-infarcts secondary to thrombosis are seen.

Spleen

The classical pathological finding is fibrous 'onion-skin' thickening of arteries in the Malpighian bodies.

Microscopical

Typically fibrinoid necrosis is seen in vessels of affected organs, especially small arteries, arterioles and capillaries (see p. 168). Fibrinoid necrosis also affects the interstitial collagen and membranes such as pleura and joint capsules, the latter contributing to the hand deformities. Inflammatory cell reaction is usually slight but the presence of haematoxyphil bodies is diagnostic.

Diagnosis

The disease commonly presents with malaise, weight loss, fever, marked musculoskeletal symptoms and a rash.

1 *Leucopenia*—especially an absolute lymphopenia—is often a clue to the diagnosis of SLE. Thrombocytopenia occurs, but is only severe in 5% of cases. The historical 'LE cell' test has been replaced by the antinuclear antibody test (ANA).

2 *ANAs* are present in the serum in 90% of cases. Antibodies to double-stranded DNA (dsDNA) are more specific for SLE than ANA, though not diagnostic. Antibodies to extractable nuclear antigens (ENAs) such as 'Sm' also have a high specificity for SLE, and antibodies to ribonuclear protein (nRNP) may help identify certain clinical subgroups such as those with severe Raynaud's disease accompanied by muscle and lung involvement, the so-called *mixed connective tissue disease* (MCTD). Such patients usually have a speckled ANA pattern whereas SLE patients have homogeneous or rim pattern. In SLE anti-Ro antibodies (another ENA) are associated with photosensitivity, may be positive in the so-called ANA-negative SLE, and help identify lupus patients who develop clinical features of Sjögren's syndrome. Drug-induced SLE typically has very high-titred ANA and absent dsDNA antibodies.

3 *Hypergammaglobulinaemia.*

4 *Elevated ESR*, interestingly often with a normal C-reactive protein (CRP). In the presence of serositis or infection, the CRP level will rise.

5 *Complement studies* are useful in monitoring SLE, particularly C4 and C3 with low levels indicating active disease.

6 *Proteinuria* indicates renal involvement and can be of nephrotic proportions (> 3 g/24 h).

7 *Anaemia*—normochromic normocytic in type.

8 *Skin and renal biopsies.*

9 *Wasserman reaction* (WR)—a false-positive result may be noted.

10 *Lupus anticoagulant and antiphospholipid antibodies* are associated with an increased risk of major arterial and venous occlusions, and spontaneous abortion.

11 *Rheumatoid factor* (RF) positive in 40% of cases.

12 *Haemolytic anaemia*—Coombs positive.

Prognosis

Lupus is characterized by exacerbations and remissions, and whilst it was once thought to lead to premature death in the majority of cases, the identification of milder cases and the judicious use of cytotoxic drugs, and often with steroids in active disease, have improved the prognosis considerably. Renal, central nervous system and cardiac lesions are the most important prognostically. Currently a 10-year survival in excess of 90% can be anticipated.

Progressive systemic sclerosis—scleroderma—PSS

Nature

A chronic progressive disease characterized by widespread and diffuse fibrosis/sclerosis affecting the skin and internal organs. Raynaud's phenomenon is a regular and frequent early accompaniment. Some patients do not get systemic involvement and others get only a very localized form of the disease, e.g. morphoea or linear localized scleroderma.

Age

Most commonly 30–50 years; rare in children.

Sex

Female : male, 4 : 1.

Aetiology

Unknown, but it may be a primary vascular phenomenon. Workers exposed to vinyl chloride, and people treated with the cytotoxic agent bleomycin, can develop scleroderma-like changes and pulmonary fibrosis. A proportion of the people who developed Spanish oil disease in 1981 after ingesting rapeseed oil, also developed an illness not dissimilar to PSS.

Organ involvement

There are no pathognomonic features.

Skin

An increase in collagen without fibroblast proliferation but with a reduction in elastic tissue is seen, and this leads to the skin thickening and immobility noted clinically. Late features include telangiectasia, loss of the pulp of fingertips, ulceration of skin over bony prominences, e.g. knuckles and medial malleoli, and subcutaneous calcification affecting terminal phalanges and extensor surfaces.

Gastrointestinal

Progressive replacement of the smooth muscle of the gut by fibrous tissue leads to hypomotility of the lower two-thirds of the oesophagus in 90% of cases, and in 50% the loss of peristalsis results in reflux oesophagitis and dysphagia. Involvement of the small intestine leads to malabsorption, abdominal fullness and cramps, and in the large intestine, wide mouthed colonic diverticula are uncommon but specific findings.

Heart and skeletal muscle

Progressive fibrosis in cardiac muscle leads to myocardial fibrosis and conduction defects, whilst in skeletal muscle extensive fibrosis with fibre degeneration is seen. Rarely inflammatory polymyositis may occur.

Lungs

Interstitial fibrosis predominantly affects the lower lobes and in the later stages a honeycomb lung with pleural thickening develops (see p. 392). Pulmonary hypertension is a frequent cause of death in PSS and there is a rare association with alveolar cell carcinoma.

Kidney

Renal involvement is predominantly vascular, producing ischaemic nephron loss (see p. 178).

Joints

In 25% of cases an inflammatory polyarthritis may occur, usually involving the small joints of the hands; however, the joint limitation and stiffness in advanced cases is related to thickening of skin and underlying tissues.

Other features
Dry eyes and dry mouth may occur from fibrosis of the lacrimal and salivary glands, but a true Sjögren's syndrome with lymphocytic infiltration may also be seen. Dryness of the mouth may compound the swallowing problems.

Blood vessels
The earliest pathological changes are intimal proliferation, adventitial fibrosis and sometimes mucoid or fibrinoid degeneration, affecting small arteries and arterioles. The severe concentric bluish-staining mucoid change is particularly notable in the arteries of the kidneys and its presence, though not pathognomonic, suggests PSS when seen in renal biopsy material (see p. 178). Subsequently the vessel lumen becomes reduced and secondary ischaemic changes follow.

Diagnosis
The skin and visceral organ involvement is the hallmark of PSS. Typical investigations might include:
1 *ESR and C-reactive protein*—normal.
2 *Anaemia*—secondary to malabsorption or renal failure.
3 *Hypergammaglobulinaemia* in 30% of cases.
4 *Antinuclear antibodies*—positive in 90% of cases, often nucleolar or speckled in pattern.
5 *Scl-70 antibodies* in 20% and not found in other connective tissue diseases.

Crest syndrome
*C*alcinosis, *R*aynaud's, *O*eophageal dysfunction, *S*clerodactyly, *T*elangiectasia denote the features of this syndrome. It is typified by the presence of anticentromere antibodies, and although systemic involvement is not prominent for many years, pulmonary hypertension can be a late complication. Primary biliary cirrhosis (see p. 244) can be associated with this syndrome.

Prognosis
Disabling deformities can profoundly affect quality of life. Death when due to PSS is related to progressive cardiac, renal or pulmonary involvement.

Polymyositis and dermatomyositis

Nature
Polymyositis is an uncommon chronic inflammatory condition involving skeletal muscle, usually symmetrically. When skin is involved it is called dermatomyositis.

Age
Any, but most commonly 40–60 years.

Sex
Female : male, 2 : 1.

Classification of these conditions
Adult polymyositis, 33%.
Adult dermatomyositis, 33%.
Myositis associated with malignancy, 8%.
Childhood poly/dermatomyositis, 6%.
Myositis with another connective tissue disease, 20%.

Aetiology
Cell-mediated immunity plays a major role in this condition and the infiltrating cells are activated T lymphocytes and macrophages. T cells from patients with polymyositis have been shown to have the capacity to damage muscle cells in culture. Virus-like particles of myxovirus and picornavirus have been demonstrated in involved muscle.

Tumour-associated poly/dermatomyositis occurs in 8% of cases, but if only men over 50 years with dermatomyositis are considered the association may be as high as 60%. As these malignancies are often occult, all patients over 50 years should initially have non-invasive investigations to detect these malignancies: the commonest ones being sited in lung, breast and ovary.

Muscle
The muscle fibres become swollen and undergo necrosis and degeneration, but at the same time there is regeneration of other muscle cells. An inflammatory cell infiltrate, predominantly lymphocytes and macrophages with occasional plasma cells, is prominent around vessels and between muscle fibres. In dermatomyositis the muscle damage is predominantly perifascicular.

Skin
Perivascular lymphocytic and plasma cell infiltrates occur in the dermis and subcutaneous tissues with

a slight mucoid or fibrinoid degeneration of the dermis.

Clinical

Commonly an insidious onset of symmetrical proximal muscle weakness which progresses over weeks/months, with variable involvement of respiratory and pharyngeal muscles. The latter may lead to dysphagia and aspiration pneumonitis. General malaise, fever and weight loss are common and symmetrical polyarthritis occurs in 20%. Symptomatic cardiac involvement resulting in dysrhythmias and heart failure is unusual, but in up to 50% of cases, non-specific ECG abnormalities may be seen—T wave/ST segment abnormalities. In dermatomyositis the dusky purple rash may affect the eyelids—heliotrope, cheeks and other light-exposed areas, whereas the scaly erythematous dermatitis is notable over extensor surfaces of knuckles, elbows and knees. Periorbital oedema may occur in the absence of other dermatological findings.

Diagnosis

1 *ESR*—usually but not invariably elevated.
2 *Serum creatine kinase and aldolase levels* are usually elevated, often to dramatic proportions.
3 *Autoantibodies*, including ANA and rheumatoid factors, are not uncommon.
4 *Anti Jo-1 antibodies*, although uncommon, are disease-specific and are directed against a soluble nuclear component.
5 *Electromyography (EMG)* can demonstrate typical changes.
6 *Muscle biopsy*, usually from the quadriceps muscle, is required to confirm the diagnosis and should not be taken from sites previously subjected to EMG studies, otherwise false-positive results may be obtained.
7 *Myoglobinuria*.
8 *Pulmonary function tests*, especially forced expiratory volume (FEV), are needed to assess respiratory muscle strength.

Prognosis

This has improved considerably with the introduction of steroids, and the value of cytotoxics is increasingly recognized. However, clinical improvement is rarely seen before 6 weeks of steroid therapy has elapsed. Those with associated malignancy, or with aspiration pneumonia, have the worst prognosis.

Rheumatoid arthritis—rheumatoid disease

Nature

A chronic inflammatory condition of joints in which systemic involvement is not uncommon.

Prevalence

This is the commonest connective tissue disease, having a worldwide distribution and being unaffected by climate. Its severity can vary, being more erosive and deforming in Europe. It appears to be a disease of modern times as no evidence for rheumatoid arthritis (RA) exists in ancient human remains, and there are indications that it is becoming less common and/or less severe.

Age

30–50 years.

Sex

Female : male, 3 : 1.

Aetiology

The precise aetiology of this autoimmune condition is unknown, but it is hypothesized that RA occurs in constitutionally susceptible individuals who encounter certain triggering factors. The association of HLA-DR4 with development of RA may be such a constitutional factor. Interestingly HLA-DR3 is associated with side-effects to drugs such as gold and penicillamine used in the treatment of RA. Possible trigger factors include infections such as herpes, rubella or Epstein–Barr viruses and mycoplasma, dietary substances and psychological factors.

Pathogenesis

The rheumatoid synovium demonstrates a marked mononuclear cell infiltrate with the development of lymphoid follicles, reminiscent of a secondary lymphoid organ. B cells predominate and some differentiate into plasma cells which produce rheumatoid factors which are antibodies to the Fc portion of the IgG molecule itself, i.e. IgM and IgG autoantibodies to IgG antibodies. Immune complex formation follows and activation of the classical complement pathway can trigger an inflammatory cascade. This B cell overactivity may be related to a defect of T cell-mediated immunity. Only indirect evidence for a T lymphocyte defect exists, namely impaired delayed hypersensitivity responses to tuberculin in active RA and the beneficial clinical response to T cell depletion by thoracic duct drainage and clinical deterioration noted if these cells are reinfused.

Organ changes

Joints

The inflammation can affect all synovial linings in the body, e.g. in joints, around tendons and bursae. The earliest change appears to be capillary damage with leakage of plasma constituents with the development of oedema. The synovial cell layer hypertrophies and lymphoid aggregates form in the deeper layers. A profuse granulation tissue consisting of proliferating fibroblasts, blood vessels and chronic inflammatory cells—*pannus* (see p. 314), spreads over the articular cartilage and leads to cartilage and bone erosion, probably mediated by release of proteases and collagenases.

Extra-articular manifestations

Nodules. Rheumatoid nodules occur, often at pressure points such as elbows, and consist of areas of fibrinoid necrosis of dermal collagen surrounded by a palisade of fibroblasts and histiocytes. Such nodules can also occur in the lung when they need differentiating from neoplasms (see p. 101).

Vasculitis. Occurs with more severe disease and affects small arteries (see p. 83). It is most commonly seen at the ends of the fingers, but when more widespread it leads to skin ulceration and neuropathy. Rarely a necrotizing vasculitis can occur with bowel and/or myocardial infarction, and this form carries a poor prognosis—'*malignant RA*'.

Eye. Scleritis and episcleritis are not uncommon, but penetration of the eye by scleromalacia perforans is an unpleasant rare complication of aggressive disease. Iritis is rare in RA, but more common in the so-called seronegative arthropathies.

Lymphoid tissue. In active disease, lymphadenopathy and splenomegaly may occur, the latter being clinically detectable in only 5% of cases. Few of these will progress to *Felty's syndrome*—RA, splenomegaly and leucopenia (often neutropenia).

Lungs. Pleurisy with or without effusion, interstitial fibrosis, pneumoconiosis—*Caplan's syndrome*—and pulmonary nodules are recognized (see p. 391).

Heart and aorta. Cardiac involvement in RA is usually subclinical and consists of granulomatous inflammation, arteritis or pericarditis. These changes are most commonly detected at post-mortem but aortic root involvement may cause aortic regurgitation (see p. 83).

Clinical

A classical case of RA is easy to recognize in a young woman with flitting pains in the small joints of the hands followed by synovitis with early-morning stiffness a few weeks or months later. Various atypical presentations are recognized and include the explosive onset and a polymyalgic onset seen in the older age group, the systemic onset seen particularly in males when the arthritis may be minimal or absent, the palindromic onset, and even a mono- or oligo-articular type when synovial biopsy may be required to exclude other causes of monoarthritis e.g. tuberculosis and pigmented villonodular synovitis (PVNS) (see p. 314).

Diagnosis

1 *Radiological*—the diagnosis is essentially clinical, but radiological examination may confirm the typical pattern of marginal erosions with joint space narrowing and periarticular osteoporosis, particularly at the metacarpophalangeal and interphalangeal joints.
2 *Anaemia*—normochromic or hypochromic.
3 *ESR and CRP levels*—the acute phase response seen in active disease leads to an elevated ESR and CRP level, often accompanied by thrombocytosis.
4 *Rheumatoid factors* (RF) are present in 85% of adult RA patients. The latex agglutination test—human IgG on latex beads—and the Rose-Waaler (RW) agglutination test—rabbit IgG on sheep red cells—are commonly used for their detection. The latex test is more sensitive but less specific, whereas the RW test is more specific yet less sensitive.
5 *Antinuclear antibodies* are present in low titre in many cases of RA.
6 *Synovial fluid analysis* has no specific diagnostic features in RA but in early cases it can help to differentiate infective synovitis.
7 *Biopsies*—there are no specific diagnostic changes

in RA synovium but it is sometimes of value to biopsy it in order to exclude infection. Nodule biopsies can be more helpful in defining RA, especially if the joint disease is minimal.

Prognosis

The course of RA is unpredictable, but joint destruction can lead to physical disability in about 30% of cases. The prognosis is dependent on the complications that may ensue:

1 *Amyloidosis*—RA is one of the commonest causes of reactive systemic amyloidosis AA amyloid and occurs in about 3% of cases. It usually presents with proteinuria or renal failure.

2 *Atlanto-axial subluxation*—resulting from rheumatoid erosion of the odontoid peg leading to direct pressure on the cervical cord.

3 *Bone marrow failure*—as consequence of treatments such as gold and penicillamine—and *gastrointestinal haemorrhage* resulting from treatment with non-steroidal anti-inflammatory agents, are unfortunate iatrogenic complications.

4 *'Malignant rheumatoid'*, see above.

Polyarteritis nodosa (PAN)

Nature

An acute/subacute disseminated vasculitis classically characterized by intense focal necrotizing inflammation confined to the walls of medium-sized arteries though overlapping considerably with other types of vascular inflammatory disease generally categorized as vasculitis (see pp. 83–85).

Incidence

Uncommon, but can occur in all age groups.

Sex

Female : male, 1 : 4.

Aetiology

The presence of *antineutrophil cytoplasmic antibodies* (ANCA) may suggest an autoimmune pathogenesis. Although these antibodies are very useful in the investigation of a suspected case of PAN, they may be only epiphenomena. Circulating hepatitis B antigenaemia has been implicated by studies from the USA, and was the first example of virus-containing immune complexes in the pathogenesis of a connective tissue disease. It occurs in up to 40% of cases in the USA, though such an association has not been prominent in the UK.

Pathology

Focal necrotizing lesions in small and medium-sized arteries involving all three layers of vessel walls, with intimal oedema and narrowing of the vessel lumen. Fibrinoid change follows but this is not universal, and then infiltration by polymorphs and occasionally eosinophils occurs. In chronic stages the infiltrate becomes mononuclear and ultimately fibrous healing occurs with disappearance of all the inflammatory cells, smooth muscle and elastic tissue in the vessel. Weakened by inflammation the vessel walls undergo aneurysm formation (nodosa) (see p. 87). All vessels are not synchronously involved and therefore vessels at different stages of evolution may be seen in an affected organ at any given time.

Organ involvement

The arteritic process may affect all organs of the body, though arteritis and/or infarcts are prominent in kidney, muscle, brain, peripheral nerves, vasa nervorum involvement, heart, lungs, liver, gall bladder and gastrointestinal tract.

Clinical

The clinical manifestations are variable, with weight loss, fever and malaise accompanied by any combination of arthritis, myalgia, abdominal pain, neuropathy, hypertension due to renal involvement, and pulmonary and cerebral changes.

Diagnosis

1 *Blood*—neutrophil leucocytosis, often with an eosinophilia and a high ESR.

2 *Antineutrophil cytoplasmic antibodies* (ANCA) are present in the serum of the majority of cases, and may be useful in monitoring the progress of the disease.

3 *Tissue biopsy*. This is the only certain way of making the diagnosis of PAN, but because of the random distribution of the vascular lesions a negative biopsy does not exclude the diagnosis. Kidney and symptomatic muscle are the best sources of biopsy material.

Prognosis

This depends on the intensity and type of vasculitis and the pattern of organ involvement. Cyclophosphamide is considered the cytotoxic of choice and, with corticosteroids, has significantly improved the outcome. Thirty per cent of patients develop renal failure and antihypertensive drugs have reduced the morbidity from hypertensive complications.

Wegener's granulomatosis

The major pathological lesion is a necrotizing vasculitis of the upper and lower respiratory tracts, associated with granuloma formation and glomerulonephritis (see p. 395 and p. 171). It is similar to PAN in that males are more frequently affected than females, and although it can affect any age, onset aged 40–60 years is common. Anaemia and a raised erythrocyte sedimentation rate (ESR) is usual, as is the presence of antineutrophil cytoplasmic antibodies. The prognosis has improved dramatically with the use of the immunosuppressive agents such as cyclophosphamide. Limited Wegener's granulomatosis, i.e. without renal involvement, does have a more favourable prognosis (see p. 396).

Sjögren's syndrome

The full triad of Sjögren's syndrome consists of keratoconjunctivitis sicca, xerostomia and a connective tissue disorder, usually rheumatoid arthritis. The term sicca syndrome is reserved for cases where only the first two features are present. Hypergammaglobulinaemia is common, as are non-organ-specific autoantibodies, especially RF and ANA. The condition is more fully described on p. 19.

Behçet's disease

This is best considered as a systemic vasculitis in which recurrent orogenital ulceration is prominent, accompanied by features such as arthritis, uveitis, retinal vasculitis and erythema nodosum. It is rare in Britain, more common in the Eastern Mediterranean, and can affect up to 1 : 1000 of the population of Japan. An association with HLA-B5 is recognized, but environmental factors such as infections—viral and bacterial—are thought to be important in its pathogenesis. There are no characteristic blood changes but an acute-phase response is often seen in active disease.

Polymyalgia rheumatica—PMR

This is a clinical syndrome of unknown aetiology, characterized by aching and stiffness in the proximal muscles especially around the shoulder girdle. The patient is usually over 60 years of age, females being affected more than males—male : female 1 : 2, and the ESR is commonly elevated to high levels. Twenty per cent of patients with PMR demonstrate giant cell arteritis in temporal artery biopsies (see p. 84). Although muscle symptoms are prominent, biopsy of symptomatic muscle is either normal or demonstrates a non-specific type II muscle fibre atrophy. The response to steroids is often described as 'magical', and the condition has a self-limiting course lasting from a few months to several years.

Ankylosing spondylitis

This is a member of the seronegative spondarthritides, therefore not strictly a connective tissue disease, and is discussed more fully on pp. 311–312. It has a male preponderance 2 male : 1 female, and can affect 1–2% of the population, with underdiagnosis being common in women. A strong disease association with HLA-B27 is recognized (> 90%) and this contrasts with a 6% frequency of HLA-B27 in the healthy British population. In addition to constitutional factors, environmental agents may play a significant role and the organism *Klebsiella aerogenes* is considered a strong candidate. Usually the sacroiliac joints are involved first, resulting in stiffness and back pain, and then the disease tends to ascend the spine. All axial joints can be affected. Progressive loss of the normal lumbar lordosis followed by an increase in the thoracic and cervical kyphoses results from fibrous and bony ankylosis. This spinal limitation makes daily living increasingly difficult, including lifting and driving, etc., and this can be further compounded by an asymmetrical large joint arthritis in 40% of cases. Ocular involvement includes acute iritis in 25%, and conjunctivitis in 20%.

A chronic mononuclear cell inflammation of the proximal aortic vasa vasorum leads to medial necrosis and subsequent fibrosis, and in some cases this results in aortic incompetence (see p. 72). Fibrotic changes also occur in the myocardium, producing conduction defects, and in the lung they lead to upper lobe fibrosis and even cavitation. Ventilation is well maintained by the diaphragm despite the rigid spine and fusion of the thoracic joints; however, chest infections including pneumonia remain a problem. Vertebral fractures can result from relatively minor trauma because of the rigidity of the spine.

Chapter 6
Soft Tissue Tumours

This group of tumours of mesenchymal origin may present in almost any anatomical site and most are therefore best described separately from specific organ systems. They are a complex mixture of benign, malignant and tumour-like but non-neoplastic lesions, which have proved easier to identify histologically, and thus classify, by more recently introduced techniques, including immunocytochemistry, enzyme histochemistry, tissue culture and electron microscopy.

Tumours and tumour-like proliferations of fibrous tissue

The fibromatoses

Congenital and juvenile

Congenital fibromatoses
Included in this group are rare multiple fibrous 'tumours' affecting the soft tissue, bones and viscera of the newborn.
1 With visceral involvement—*congenital generalized fibromatosis*. This is almost always fatal.
2 Without visceral involvement—*congenital multiple fibromatosis*. The tumours regress over the ensuing few months.

Juvenile fibromatosis

Fibromatosis colli—'sternomastoid tumour'
This tumorous, sometimes infiltrative mass affects the sternomastoid muscle of infants but normally spontaneously resolves in 3–4 months. Scarring leading to torticollis may occur.

Idiopathic gingival fibromatosis
This is a benign fibrous tumour of the gums appearing in childhood and autosomally dominant in inheritance. It is slowly growing but requires surgical removal.

Fibrous hamartoma of infancy
A benign lesion presenting before 2 years of age usually in the axilla, shoulder or upper arm. It is situated in deep dermis and subcutaneous tissue and has a characteristic mixed histological appearance of mature adipose tissue, interlacing fibrous bundles and islands of primitive mesenchyme with spindle or stellate cells.

Juvenile aponeurotic fibroma—calcifying fibroma
This lesion of the hands and feet of children consists of plump proliferating fibroblasts, dense collagen and islands of chondroid tissue with foci of calcification. It is benign.

Infantile digital fibromatosis—recurrent digital fibroma of childhood
An infiltrative cellular tumour-like lesion involving only the toes and fingers of infants and rarely young children. They may be multiple and recur after excision. The spindle cells contain round eosinophilic cytoplasmic inclusions.

Adult

Palmar and plantar fibromatosis
Palmar—*Dupuytren's contracture* and plantar—*Ledderhose's disease*, fibromatoses form slowly growing nodules and plaques which infiltrate into tissue surrounding the aponeurotic structures in hands and feet and may lead to serious contractures. The proliferating cells are *myofibroblasts*. Surgery may be required to free tendons but the lesions frequently recur.

Penile fibromatosis—Peyronie's disease
This is an almost identical myofibroblastic proliferation affecting the penis.

Musculo-aponeurotic fibromatosis— desmoid tumour—aggressive fibromatosis

Typically these occur in the rectus sheath usually in parous women but may occur in musculoaponeurotic structures in extra-abdominal sites particularly neck, shoulder and upper limbs. They may be difficult to differentiate from fibrosarcomas and have a high risk of recurrence after excision.

Keloid

This cellular fibroblastic proliferative lesion of wounds affecting the deep dermis is much more common in Negroes, particularly in adolescents and young adults. It is self-limiting but often disfiguring and its pathogenesis is obscure.

Pseudosarcomas

1 *Nodular fasciitis*: this proliferative benign lesion of myofibroblasts occurs in subcutaneous fat and deep soft tissues usually of the trunk, proximal extremities or head with ill-defined infiltrative margin and histological appearances which may be difficult to differentiate from fibrosarcoma, though there are regional varieties of pattern and uniform nuclear characteristics.

2 *Proliferative myositis*: this is a tumour-forming benign fibroblastic proliferative lesion in voluntary muscle and is thought to be initiated by trauma. Bizarre fibroblastic cells separate muscle fibres but do not destroy them, and characteristic 'ganglion' cells are usually present.

Fibromas

Many lesions previously identified as benign fibroblastic tumours are now known to be non-neoplastic fibroblastic or myofibroblastic proliferations and others recognized as fibrohistiocytic (see below). The encapsulated pure fibromas do occasionally occur, particularly in the ovary (see p. 244).

Myxoma

These encapsulated tumours have a soft, mucoid or gelatinous appearance and are composed of stellate cells in a mucoid matrix. They must be differentiated from degenerate neurofibromas (see p. 109) and are found in fascial planes, subcutaneous tissues and intermuscular septa. There is also the specific cardiac entity of the left atrium (see p. 74).

Fibrosarcoma

Formerly believed to be a relatively common tumour, exclusion of non-neoplastic fibroblastic proliferation and recategorization of fibrohistiocytic and nerve sheath tumours, has greatly reduced the incidence of true fibrosarcomas.

Most are found in superficial soft tissues retroperitoneally or in bones (see p. 305).

They are composed of fibroblasts with cellular atypical features and with a 'herring-bone' pattern. Their behaviour ranges from low to high grade of malignancy and reflects grades of fibroblastic differentiation.

Myxofibrosarcoma

This is a fibrosarcoma in which extensive myxomatous degeneration has occurred.

Fibrohistiocytic tumours

Nature

A distinct group of neoplasms with well-established clinicopathological manifestations and believed to have histiocytic features. The histogenesis is still somewhat uncertain and their admixture of differing cellular elements and growth pattern suggest that they may not all have a common ancestry.

They may arise from a primitive mesenchymal cell which gives rise to fibroblastic and histiocytic elements, or from a tissue histiocyte which acts as a facultative fibroblast.

Malignant fibrous histiocytoma

Sites

Extremities, trunk and retroperitoneally. Rare in head, neck and viscera. Peak age incidence is in the seventh decade.

Appearances

Whilst apparently circumscribed they are not encapsulated and are usually bulky, often with foci of haemorrhage and necrosis. Histologically there is a wide spectrum of cellular constituents—fibroblastic, rounded histiocytic, giant, foam and inflammatory cells, with fibroblastic cells characteristically spindle-shaped and arranged in cartwheel-like formations around slit-like vessels—storiform pattern.

Based on the relative predominance of the cell types, subtypes are described but do not appear to have significant prognostic effects.

1 Fibrous.
2 Giant cell.
3 Myxoid.
4 Inflammatory.
5 Angiomatoid—primarily in extremities of young persons.

Effects

1 Bulky painless masses.
2 Systemic effects—particularly with retroperitoneal tumours. These include pyrexia, weight loss, fatigue and gastrointestinal symptoms. Episodic hypoglycaemia sometimes occurs.
3 Associated with lymphoproliferative disease—lymphoma, leukaemia, myeloma and Langerhans cell granulomatosis (see p. 297).

Prognosis

1 Deep tumours notably retroperitoneal, are almost invariably fatal, partly from difficulty of surgical extirpation.
2 Superficial subcutaneous tumours have the best prognosis but with high local recurrence rate after excision. The deeper the tumour the higher the risk of metastases.

Dermatofibrosarcoma protruberans

This cutaneous tumour (see also p. 419) is clinically characteristic with, as its name implies, a bulky protuberant exophytic appearance and slow growth. Arising in the dermis there is usually a clear zone of upper dermis between the mass and the epidermis. There is a marked storiform pattern but there is little or no polymorphism, the cells appearing solely fibroblast-like.

Recurrence after local excision is common but metastases are exceptional.

Other probable histiocytic skin tumours

Benign fibrous histiocytoma—dermatofibroma—sclerosing haemangioma

This common upper dermal fibrohistiocytic nodule (see p. 419) has a bulging flat top and contains many vessels, variable numbers of giant cells (usually of Touton type) and iron pigment as well as fibrocytes and histiocytes.

Atypical fibroxanthoma

An ulcerated polypoid rapidly growing lesion of damaged skin—sun, X-irradiation, thermal. It is composed of pleomorphic spindle epithelioid and giant cells and its histiocytic origin is challengeable. Local excision may lead to recurrence.

Fibrous xanthoma and neuroxanthoendothelioma

These are other rare skin lesions of possible histiocytic origin.

Tumours of adipose tissue

Lipoma

Sites and incidence

Benign, lobulated, encapsulated fatty masses are very common in subcutaneous tissues but are also found in intestinal submucosa, retroperitoneal tissues, bone, kidney and intramuscularly. They may be multiple and sometimes painful—*diffuse lipomatosis*.

Microscopically

In 'pure' lipomas the mass is composed of mature regular adipocytes. Variable mixtures of other connective tissues may uncommonly occur to give variants—*fibrolipoma, angiolipoma, angiomyolipoma* (see p. 183) and *myelolipoma*—myeloid tissue component.

Other variants are *hibernomas*—brown tumours containing fat cells of fetal type, *spindle cell lipoma*, *pleomorphic lipoma* and *atypical lipoma*. In these latter conditions the presence of atypical fibroblasts and distorted lipocytes has in the past caused difficulties in differentiation (see below) but lipoblasts are not found.

Liposarcoma

Incidence

The second commonest type of soft tissue sarcoma affecting adults, and usually arising from deep tissues of the extremities, particularly the thigh and retroperitoneal tissues.

Types

1 *Myxoid*: this tumour is often enormous and usually has a good prognosis though occasionally metastasizing. Histologically lipoblasts are set in a myxoid stroma with abundant vascular capillaries.

2 *Well differentiated*: regularly arranged but nuclearly distorted lipoblasts with collagen bands and associated with a good prognosis and only slight risk of metastases.

3 *Round cell*: the lipoblasts are rounded with vacuolated fat-containing cytoplasm and vacuolar nuclei. About 50% develop metastases within 5 years.

4 *Pleomorphic*: spindle cell and bizarre lipoblasts predominate with signet ring forms and multinucleated cells. Haematogenous spread, usually to lung, is common—50% at 5 years.

Tumours of smooth muscle

Leiomyoma

Sites

Uterus (see p. 219), gastrointestinal tract (see p. 31), walls of blood vessels, skin (see p. 419).

Incidence

Very common, the uterine tumour being the most frequent benign tumour in women.

Appearances

Grossly the tumours are usually circular, pale, whorled, encapsulated and frequently multiple. Histologically they are comparatively cellular and composed of myofibrils with blunt-ended nuclei arranged in a whorled pattern. Mitoses should be virtually absent.

Variants

1 *Bizarre or atypical leiomyoma*: these are most frequently found in the uterus and show cellular pleomorphism but mitoses are absent.

2 *Intravenous leiomyomatosis*: this is growth of benign leiomyomatous tissue intravascularly which is usually seen in the uterus and may extend deep into the wall but have a benign behaviour.

3 *Leiomyoblastoma—epithelioid leiomyoma*: these have polygonal cells with clear cytoplasmic zones surrounding the nuclei, the result of artefact by formalin fixation. However, occasionally tumours of this appearance may be unpredictably locally aggressive or metastasize, so separation as an entity is justified. Most frequent sites are stomach (see p. 31), intestines and uterus.

Leiomyosarcoma

Sites

These uncommon tumours most frequently arise in deep tissues in the genital tract, gastrointestinal tract, retroperitoneal tissues and extremities. The more superficial lesions are located in the thigh, head, neck and trunk, arising usually from blood vessel walls.

Appearances

Grossly they are soft, pale and frequently bulky and poorly encapsulated or frankly infiltrative. Foci of necrosis and haemorrhage are common. Histologically they show spindle-shaped or epithelioid cell features with variable pleomorphism, giant cells and mitoses which are often bizarre.

Prognosis

Differentiation from benign-behaving smooth muscle tumours is largely dependent on mitotic counts. Less than five mitoses per 10 high-power fields—behaviour is benign; five to nine mitoses/10 HPF—uncertain malignant potential; 10–15 mitoses/10 HPF—low-grade malignancy; more than 15 mitoses/10 HPF—high-grade malignancy.

Tumours of striated muscle

Rhabdomyoma

Sites

These very rare benign tumours are almost exclusively found in the head and neck, vagina and vulva. Tumour-like hamartomas of striped muscle are found in the myocardium (see p. 74), usually associated with tuberous sclerosis.

Types

1 *Fetal*: composed of elongated spindle cells with small uniform nuclei often in a myxoid stroma or as interlacing fascicles in the cellular variant. Striations are readily seen and mitoses are infrequent.

2 *Adult*: these occur mostly in the head and neck region of adult males. Composed of large round or polygonal cells with peripheral vacuolation around centrally located granular eosinophilic cytoplasm, thin strands of which may extend to the cell membrane forming a typical 'spider cell' appearance.

Rhabdomyosarcoma

Incidence
Mostly occur under 10 years of age and are uncommon, though not as rare as rhabdomyomas.

Types
1 *Embryonal*: most common and usually arises in the orbit or other parts of the head and neck, the deep soft tissues of the limbs and in the urogenital tract where they form oedematous polypoid masses—*sarcoma botyroides*, in bladder and vagina (see p. 209). Appearances vary from one part of the tumour to another from round cells to elongated cells with central nuclei and abundant eosinophilic cytoplasm. Myxomatous areas are common. Cross-striations are usually very scanty but myofilaments on electron microscopy or positive myosin or myoglobin immunoperoxidase stains are diagnostic.

2 *Alveolar*: more common in adolescents in the extremities, and composed of round cells with scanty cytoplasm characteristically arranged in a lobular alveolar pattern due to separating strands of collagen. Multinucleated tumour cells may be present, striations are very uncommon.

3 *Pleomorphic*: the least common variant composed of spindle cells and very frequent giant cells with abundant eosinophilic cytoplasm. Cross-striations are seldom identified.

Prognosis
More than 50% of patients, irrespective of tumour type, die within 3 years of diagnosis, though results are improving with new chemotherapeutic regimes. Blood spread to lungs and lymph node metastases are common.

The alveolar type is the most aggressive—less than 10% survival at 5 years.

Tumours of peripheral nerves

Schwannoma—Neurilemmoma

Sites
A common tumour arising from intracranial nerve roots, spinal nerves and peripheral nerves of scalp, face, neck, mediastinum, intercostal nerves, pelvis and extremities.

Age and sex
Middle decades in women more than men.

Origin
From Schwann cells of nerve sheaths. The cells have elongated, serpentine, completely entangled processes lined by continuous basal laminae and do not invest axons.

Appearances
Macroscopically the tumours are fusiform or globoid, greyish or focally yellow on cut surface and with the nerve of origin compressed to one side. Microscopically there are two types:

1 *Antoni type A*: compact spindle cell tumours with interwoven sheets bearing long oval nuclei and pale eosinophilic fibrillar cytoplasm. Palisading of cells forms *Verocay bodies* characterized by rows of nuclei separated by anuclear zones.

2 *Antoni type B*: the tissue has a spongy quality and is sparsely cellular with bipolar cells similar to those in type A areas and other foci with hyperchromatic small round nuclei and xanthoma cells.

Most tumours are a mixture of these types and also contain prominent thick-walled blood vessels. Immunocytochemistry shows strong positivity to S100 antiserum.

Effects
Most are removed as benign tumours and can be dissected free of the parent nerve if the true nature is anticipated.

Space-occupying nerve compression can occur in anatomical situations with surrounding rigid structures, e.g. intracranially and in spinal nerve foramina. Malignant change rarely, if ever, occurs.

Neurofibroma

Sites
Small nerves, deep major nerves and nerves of the retroperitoneal tissues and gastrointestinal tracts. Cranial and spinal nerves are only rarely affected. The most frequent presentation is as an isolated sessile or pedunculated cutaneous lesion, often with pigmentation of overlying epidermis.

Origin
Arise from neural crest cells which form collagen and are perineurial rather than Schwann cells.

Appearances

Microscopically they produce fusiform to ovoid swellings on nerve trunks with a grey, soft, gelatinous cut surface. Nerve fibres are intimately intermingled in the tumour mass so that the lesion cannot be separated from the parent nerve without sacrifice of axons.

Microscopically there is a background of collagenous fibres in a mucinous matrix, thin-walled blood vessels and a generally wavy arrangement of the collagen bundles in which the tumour cells with oval spindle-shaped nuclei with attenuated cytoplasmic processes are set. Degenerative changes are uncommon. Staining for S100 is strongly positive.

Effects

The tumours seldom cause pain but cannot be removed except with nerve sacrifice. Malignant change may occur (see below).

Von Recklinghausen's neurofibromatosis—VRN

Nature

A protean hamartomatous disorder inherited as an autosomal dominant trait, affecting all ethnic groups and involving tissues of both ectodermal and mesodermal origin. Two syndromes occur (see p. 332).

Appearances

1 Hallmarks are a plexiform neurofibroma or numerous skin café-au-lait spots and multiple cutaneous neurofibromas.
2 Other less consistent features include:
  (a) elephantiasis—redundant folds of soft tissue,
  (b) localized soft tissue gigantism,
  (c) bilateral acoustic Schwannomas,
  (d) meningiomas—often multiple,
  (e) bilateral uveal tract naevi,
  (f) mental retardation,
  (g) gliomas,
  (h) bone and joint involvement—kyphoscoliosis, rarefaction,
  (i) phaeochromocytomas (see p. 119).
3 Minimal requirements for diagnosis are not agreed. A single café-au-lait spot is not by itself diagnostic of VRN but more than six such spots, each more than 1.5 cm diameter, presumes the diagnosis even in the absence of a positive family history.

Malignant nerve sheath tumours

Nomenclature

Doubts about the histogenesis of these tumours have created a varied terminology—*malignant Schwannoma, malignant neurilemmoma, nerve sheath fibrosarcoma.*

Origin

Much evidence, but not all, suggests a Schwann cell origin and it could be that some are derived from nerve sheath fibroblasts. They arise either (a) from nerve sheath *de novo*, or (b) from a pre-existing neurofibroma. About half arise in individuals with von Recklinghausen's neurofibromatosis.

It is probable that about 2% of cases of neurofibromatosis develop malignant nerve sheath tumours.

Age–sex

In patients with neurofibromatosis—early 30s. In *de novo* tumours—at least a decade later. Age range is from childhood to the 90s. Male : female equal.

Site

Sciatic nerve is most common for either group of patients but both intracranial and peripheral sites anywhere may be the site of origin.

Appearances

These tumours are usually large, mostly 4–15 cm diameter, and larger in cases with neurofibromatosis. They tend to extend along nerves of origin both proximally and distally.

Microscopically they are fibrosarcomas usually showing interwoven fascicles of plump and elongated or small and oval spindle cells, with pleomorphic and multinucleated foci. Mitoses are invariably present and more than 10 per high-power field is associated with necrosis.

Some tumours contain heterologous elements— *neural crest mixed tumours*, either epithelial, mesenchymal or melanotic and of either benign or malignant cytology. They are most common in von Recklinghausen's disease. Mesenchymal elements include cartilage, osteoid, rhabdomyosarcoma—*malignant Triton tumour*, osteosarcoma, liposarcoma.

Prognosis

Local recurrence even with low-grade tumours is common. With high-grade tumours recurrence and metastasis are usual; 5-year survival figures overall range from 15–35%.

Peripheral neuroectodermal tumours

Rare peripheral *medulloepitheliomas* (see p. 344) and peripheral *primitive neuroectodermal tumours* (see p. 343) occur.

Ganglioneuroma

This benign tumour of the autonomic nervous system occasionally occurs also in von Recklinghausen's neurofibromatosis. It arises from sympathetic nerves, most commonly in the posterior mediastinum (see p. 285) or adrenal medulla in young adults.

They are composed of myxomatous fibrous stroma with nerve fibres and large mature ganglion cells and are slowly growing.

Occasionally neuroblasts are present as well as ganglion cells—*ganglioneuroblastoma*, which frequently behaves in a malignant manner (see p. 121).

Tumours of blood vessels and lymphatics

These are described on pp. 90–91.

Synovial sarcoma

This tumour is described on p. 317.

Mesenchymoma

This term is reserved for rare tumours containing two or more distinct types of mesenchymal derived tissue not usually associated with each other, and occurring in parts of the body where those tissues are not normally found.

Benign tumours contain various mixtures of adipose tissue, smooth and striated muscle, blood vessels, cartilage, myxomatous and fibrous tissue and lymphoid tissue. Whether they are true tumours or hamartomas is not resolved. They most frequently occur in the kidney and limbs, often in children.

Malignant mesenchymomas are composed of two or more sarcomas.

Tumours of uncertain histogenesis

Alveolar soft part sarcoma

This rare tumour usually occurs in the thigh of young adults or head and neck region of children. Tumour cells have abundant eosinophilic cytoplasm with PAS-positive crystals, arranged in an organoid or alveolar pattern. It is of high-grade malignancy, with 50% survival at 5 years. An origin from peripheral nerve endings is presently favoured.

Epithelioid sarcoma

A rare tumour of young adult men and adolescents most frequently in fingers, palms of hands, forearms, legs, thighs and gluteal regions of limbs.

Single or multiple nodules in the dermis ulcerate mimicking an inflammatory process but also infiltrate tendons and deeper soft tissues. The cells are characteristically 'epithelioid' in appearance, grouped in nodules with central necrosis and hyalinization.

The course is protracted with local recurrences and lymph node metastases frequent.

The tumour is possibly of fibrohistiocytic origin.

Clear cell sarcoma of tendons and aponeuroses

This rare tumour, usually of the foot or knee of young adults, infiltrates fascia and tendons. The cells are rounded with clear cytoplasm arranged in fascicles and clusters.

Extraskeletal chondrosarcoma and osteosarcoma

These are very rare malignant tumours, usually in adults, occurring primarily in soft tissue.

Chapter 7
Diseases of the Ear

External ear

Inflammations—otitis externa

Inflammations are common in the skin of the ear and the meatus and, if severe, may lead to destruction of the underlying external cartilage, a feature which may occur following furunculosis. Probably the most common causes of inflammation affecting the ear are seborrhoeic dermatitis and an external otitis secondary to chronic suppurative otitis media.

Other inflammations may be caused by bacterial infections, especially streptococci and staphylococci, or due to fungi, e.g. aspergilli (otomycosis) or viruses, e.g. herpes zoster.

Trauma

Cauliflower ear

Nature
Irregular and nodular thickening of the pinna following organization of haematomas in subcutaneous or perichondrial layers. This is due to repetitive trauma (boxers).

Chondrodermatitis nodularis chronica helicis

Aetiology
The aetiology is not definitely known, but multiple minor injuries may be responsible.

Macroscopical
One or more painful and hard nodules on the upper margins of the ear. The surface is hyperkeratotic and may be ulcerated.

Microscopical
1 Hyperkeratosis.
2 Irregular acanthosis.
3 Central ulceration.
4 Chronic inflammatory cell infiltration of the dermis and of the surface of the cartilage—perichondritis, with cartilaginous degeneration.

Results
When the condition is long-standing, the overlying skin may show pseudo-epitheliomatous hyperplasia.

Other lesions

Gouty tophi
The ear is a classical site of gouty tophi (see p. 315).

Tumours
1 *Osteoma* of the bony portion of the external auditory canal.
2 *Ceruminous gland neoplasias*: adenoma and adenocarcinoma.
3 *Basal cell carcinoma* (see p. 416).
4 *Squamous cell carcinoma* (see p. 416).

Aural polyp

Nature
This is an inflammatory lesion often presenting in the auditory canal through a tympanic membrane perforation. It is composed of non-specific granulation tissue.

Tympanic membrane
The tympanic membrane divides the external auditory canal from the middle ear.

111

Myringitis

This membrane may be infected from the middle ear (see below) or from an external otitis. A special type producing haemorrhage bullae—bullous myringitis, is probably due to a virus infection and is most commonly seen during influenzal epidemics.

Middle ear

Acute otitis media

Nature
An acute non-specific infection of the middle ear.

Aetiology
The infection is usually caused by β-haemolytic streptococci, staphylococci, pneumococci or *Haemophilus influenzae*.

Pathogenesis
Any infection involving the upper respiratory tract, especially in children, associated with swelling of lymphoid tissue, e.g. adenoids, predisposes to blockage of the Eustachian tube and thus to otitis media. The condition therefore usually occurs as a complication of tonsillitis, pharyngitis, scarlet fever, influenza, measles and the common cold.

Route of infection
Almost always via the Eustachian tube.

Clinical
Earache and pyrexia, associated with hyperaemia and bulging of the drum.

Appearances
The middle ear is filled with pus or mucopus with an intense acute polymorph reaction in the Eustachian tube and in the middle ear.

Results

Resolution
The condition may resolve, especially if the purulent exudate is drained by myringotomy, by re-establishing the patency of the Eustachian tube, or by antibiotics.

Perforation
Of the tympanic membrane and drainage.

Organization
Organization of the exudate may result in fibrous tympanosclerosis producing permanent impairment of hearing.

Chronic otitis media—'glue ear'
Continuation of the infection with persistence of the inflammatory process results in a chronic 'wet' ear with aural discharge. Often the contents are of very tenacious mucoid material which drains poorly. Cholesterol granulomas may also occur.

Epidermoid cholesteatoma

Nature
This sequel is the formation of a cystic structure containing desquamated keratin and purulent and necrotic matter produced by inverted squamous epithelium, which migrates to the middle ear from adjacent areas. Some cholesterol may be present. It can also occur in the mastoid air spaces.

Results
The cholesteatoma may grow externally through the drum and present as a polyp. More frequently it extends medially from the mastoid or middle ear and progressively erodes the temporal bone to reach vital structures, e.g. the lateral sinus or cranial cavity. Infection is thereby introduced into these areas, e.g. thrombophlebitis of the sinus, meningitis, cerebral abscess.

Local spread
Mastoiditis, petrositis, labyrinthitis, thrombophlebitis of communicating petrous veins and cerebral extension as meningitis or abscess.

Mastoiditis
Due to extension of inflammation from the middle ear, with which it is in direct communication.

The mucosa of the mastoid air cells is infiltrated by polymorphs with pus formation. The condition may resolve under treatment or extend. Extension through the bone internally may lead to epidural abscess or meningitis; external spread may lead to an abscess—*Bezold's abscess*, in the upper portion of the neck, or to cellulitis of the overlying soft tissues.

Petrositis
Inflammation of the air cells in the petrous portion of

the temporal bone by infection extending from the middle ear. This may result in severe headache and oedema of the canal in which the sixth nerve lies and result in its paralysis—*Gradenigo's syndrome*.

Inner ear

Inflammation—labyrinthitis

Aetiology
Usually secondary to an acute or chronic otitis media or associated with a cholesteatoma. The condition may occasionally complicate suppurative meningitis.

Routes of infection
Usually through the oval window, following damage to the footplate of the stapes or through the round window, but it may also occur by direct extension through the bone.

Results
Impairment of both hearing and labyrinthine functions. In the acute cases, secondary to an acute otitis media, a meningitis may supervene.

Otosclerosis

Nature
A rare disease in which there is progressive bilateral deafness, starting at about puberty. The condition is more frequent in females and there is usually a family history.

Clinical
A progressive conduction deafness starting in one ear but subsequently involving the other. Speech is quiet as, due to bone conduction, the patient's perception of his own voice is not impaired.

Appearances
Irregular formation of vascular, spongy new bone around the oval window and the promontory, sometimes extending on to the cochlear side of the oval window. This new bone shows both osteoclastic and osteoblastic activity with the formation of 'cement lines' of irregular bone similar to that seen in Paget's disease (see p. 296). This results in loss of mobility and finally in fixation of the footplate of the stapes.

Results
The stapes ankylosis interferes with transmission of sound waves to the inner ear and the operations for its relief are designed to mobilize the stapes. The results are good.

Ménière's disease

Nature
A disease characterized by sudden attacks of giddiness, vomiting and tinnitus, accompanied by some degree of deafness. The attacks tend to become progressively more frequent and severe.

Appearances
The basic change is an increased pressure of unknown aetiology in the endolymph in the inner ear resulting in dilatation of the endolymphatic system. The hair cells of the organ of Corti show a progressive degeneration following the pressure increase.

Tumours

In addition to squamous cell carcinomas of the external ear and rarely in the middle ear arising from squamous metaplasia, there is also a distinct tumour entity, the non-chromaffin paraganglioma—*chemodectoma*.

Paragangliomas

Nature
Tumours arising from non-chromaffin paraganglia which are chemoreceptors, i.e. sensitive to changes in the chemical composition of the blood. These tumours may arise from the carotid body, aortic bodies and from the glomus jugulare. They should not be confused with the chromaffin tumours of adrenalin-producing cells, e.g. phaeochromocytoma of the adrenal medulla (see p. 119) or in other sites.

Glomus jugulare tumour

Origin
From the glomus jugulare, a small chemoreceptor organ, situated in the wall of the jugular bulb.

Clinical
The tumour frequently presents as a vascular polypoid tumour in the auditory meatus. It is associated with some deafness and usually occurs in middle-aged females.

Appearances

It is composed of clumps of large polyhedral cells in a fibrous stroma containing many vascular spaces. The tumour cells show no chromaffin reaction.

Results

The tumour slowly spreads from its site of origin in the jugular bulb to invade the petrous portion of the temporal bone and thus invade and destroy the ear to present as a polyp in the external auditory meatus or as destructive lesions of cranial nerves in the base of the skull. Biopsy will reveal the true nature of the tumour but its vascularity is such that biopsy, trauma, or any subsequent operative procedure, may be attended by torrential and even fatal haemorrhage. Thus, irradiation is usually employed in an endeavour to restrict further invasion.

Carotid body tumour

Incidence

A rare tumour, but this is the commonest type of paraganglioma.

Origin

From the carotid body at the bifurcation of the common carotid artery.

Age

Usually between 30 and 60 years of age.

Sex

Male : female equal.

Appearances

Presents as a firm, solid, 'potato tumour' enveloping the carotid vessels at the bifurcation. It consists of masses of polyhedral, large and often fat-containing cells in a fibrous stroma in which there are large vascular spaces. The cells are regular in formation and show no mitoses.

Results

They are slowly growing and increasingly compress the carotid arteries, but only very rarely are they malignant. Surgical removal may become necessary to relieve the arterial obstruction.

Other sites

The other examples elsewhere in the body are very rare; they have similar appearances to the carotid body tumour and behave in a benign manner.

Chapter 8
Endocrine Gland Diseases

A/ADRENAL

Cortical hypofunction
Medullary hypofunction
Cortical hyperfunction
Medullary hyperfunction
Tests of adrenal function
Tumours
   Adenoma
   Carcinoma
Medulla
   Phaeochromocytoma
   Neuroblastoma
   Ganglioneuroma
   Secondary

Each adrenal is composed of two structurally, functionally and embryologically distinct parts: cortex and medulla. The combined normal weight of the adrenals is 12–14 g.

Cortex
Of mesodermal origin from the urogenital ridge. It is composed of three zones (Fig. 11).
1 *Outer—glomerulosa*: small nests of cells.
2 *Intermediate—fasciculata*: parallel cords of cells.
3 *Inner—reticularis*: interlacing cords.

The cells are similar in appearance, having a polygonal shape with a foamy cytoplasm containing large amounts of lipid which imparts the yellow colour to the cortex.

Medulla
The brown central portion of the gland derived from neuroectoderm, which is composed of small clusters of large chromaffin cells, nerve fibres, sympathetic ganglion cells and supporting tissue.

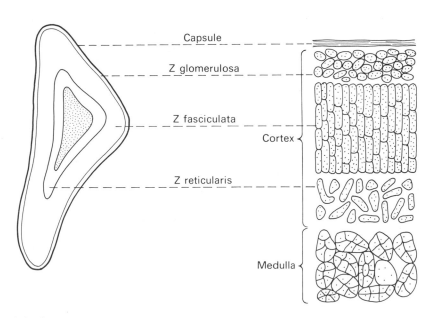

Fig. 11 Adrenal gland structure.

Hormones

Cortex

Glucocorticoids

Mostly produced in the zona fasciculata. The most important glucocorticoid is hydrocortisone which:

1 Stimulates gluconeogenesis from protein.
2 Inhibits peripheral utilization of glucose.
3 Antagonizes some actions of insulin.

In addition to these effects on carbohydrate metabolism, the glucocorticoids have some mineralocorticoid action and also cause:

4 Involution of lymphoid tissue and a fall in blood lymphocytes.
5 Reduction of the blood eosinophil count.
6 Suppression of some aspects of the inflammatory response, and of fibroblastic activity.

They also interfere with antigen–antibody reactions:

7 By suppressing protein synthesis in tissues other than the liver.
8 By suppressing ACTH secretion by the pituitary.

Mineralocorticoids

Mainly formed in the zona glomerulosa. The most potent mineralocorticoid is aldosterone which:

1 Increases sodium reabsorption by the renal tubules.
2 Increases renal potassium excretion.
3 Decreases sodium loss at other sites, e.g. sweat, bowel.

Sex hormones

Produced in the zona reticularis. They are mostly androgens with smaller amounts of oestrogen. Adrenal sex hormones are probably responsible for most of the early changes of puberty.

Medulla

Produces adrenaline and noradrenaline in the proportion of approximately 4 : 1. It may also produce neurotransmitter peptides such as enkephalins.

Adrenaline

By stimulating both α and β adrenergic receptors, it increases cardiac output but has a less marked effect than noradrenaline on peripheral arteriolar resistance. It increases glycogenesis, increases the metabolic rate and causes bronchodilatation.

Noradrenaline

Stimulates predominantly α adrenergic receptors causing vasoconstriction and increased blood pressure.

Cortical hypofunction

Primary

Nature

As a result of necrosis, replacement or atrophy of adrenal cortical tissue, inadequate amounts of adrenal cortical hormones are produced, thus limiting the ability to resist stressful stimuli.

Causes

1 Addison's disease:
   (a) atrophy—idiopathic or autoimmune—80%,
   (b) tuberculosis—now uncommon.
2 Metastatic carcinoma.
3 Previous adrenalectomy.
4 Treatment with adrenolytic drugs, e.g. ortho-para-DDD (opDDD, mitotane).
5 Haemochromatosis, and other infiltrations.
6 Infections—particularly in children with meningococcal septicaemia (Waterhouse–Friderichsen syndrome), influenza, diphtheria.
7 Haemorrhage—traumatic, haemorrhagic diatheses including anticoagulant therapy.
8 Burns.
9 Abrupt withdrawal from long-standing corticosteroid therapy.

Adrenal

Appearance depends on the cause, with glands either atrophied or replaced by other tissue. Haemorrhages commence in the medulla with little or no inflammatory reaction.

Chronic cortical hypofunction—Addison's disease

Nature

The destruction of the adrenal cortices in Addison's disease may proceed over months or years. The symptoms and signs are equally insidious and only become marked when crisis is imminent.

Effects

1 Pigmentation. Due to increased secretion of ACTH

and related peptides by the pituitary, in response to decreased negative feedback by corticosteroids.

2 Hyponatraemia with hyperkalaemia.

3 Decreased plasma volume with raised blood urea and postural hypotension.

4 Eosinophilia.

5 Hypoglycaemia.

Incidence
Rare.

Age
Any age, but usually early adult life.

Adrenal
Atrophied with variable lymphocytic infiltration. In tuberculous cases replaced by caseous and partly calcified material.

Other organs
Skin pigmentation affecting particularly exposed and pressure areas, scars, fingernails, palmar creases and buccal mucosa. Slight lymphadenopathy with enlargement of the thymus. Wasting and atrophic changes are found in many other organs.

Results
Replacement therapy with glucocorticoids (hydrocortisone or cortisone acetate) and mineralocorticoids (fludrocortisone) must be maintained indefinitely.

Acute cortical hypofunction—Addisonian crisis
May occur spontaneously or in patients with pre-existing Addison's disease. The predominant clinical feature is of hypotensive shock although any of the features of chronic cortical hypofunction (see above), and also low-grade fever may be present.

Treatment
Urgent administration of intravenous saline and commencement of corticosteroid substitution therapy is life-saving.

Secondary

Nature
Adrenal atrophy may be caused by chronically inadequate secretion of ACTH. This may result from hypothalamic or pituitary tumours, or may be iatrogenic—following destructive treatment to the pituitary, or treatment with drugs such as corticosteroids which suppress ACTH secretion.

Effects
Are those of primary adrenal atrophy, although pigmentation does not occur and the tendency to hyponatraemia and hyperkalaemia may be less.

Results
Substitution therapy with glucocorticoids alone is required since the zona glomerulosa is independent of ACTH stimulation.

Medullary hypofunction
Removal or destruction of the adrenal medulla produces no functional disturbance.

Cortical hyperfunction
Overproduction of hormones may result from excessive stimulation by the trophic hormones, ACTH and renin, or it may result from autonomously functioning adrenal tumours.

Glucocorticoid excess—Cushing's syndrome

Causes
1 Adrenal adenoma or carcinoma—commonest cause of Cushing's syndrome in children.

2 Adrenal hyperplasia secondary to excessive secretion of ACTH by the pituitary gland (Cushing's disease).

3 Adrenal hyperplasia secondary to excessive secretion of ACTH by a non-pituitary source (ectopic ACTH syndrome).

4 ACTH or corticosteroid therapy.

5 Alcohol-induced pseudo-Cushing's syndrome.

Effects
The effects of sustained elevation of glucocorticoid secretion are:

1 Central obesity and moon face.

2 Muscle wasting and weakness.

3 Osteoporosis—may cause collapse of vertebrae, rib fractures (see p. 299).

4 Atrophy of skin and dermis—paper thin skin with bruising tendency, purple striae.

5 Impaired glucose tolerance.

6 Relative polycythaemia—lowered plasma volume results in high haemoglobin concentration.

7 Hypertension.

8 Ankle swelling.

9 Hirsutism.

10 Menstrual disorders.

11 Hypokalaemia—especially in the ectopic ACTH syndrome.

12 Pigmentation—may occur, but only if plasma ACTH levels are elevated.

Adrenal

In the overactive gland there is increase in the zona fasciculata and to a lesser extent the z. reticularis. (For adrenal tumours see p. 121).

Pituitary

In Cushing's syndrome irrespective of aetiology, areas of the pituitary are replaced by pink, hyaline material (Crookes' hyaline change). In pituitary dependent Cushing's disease there may be a small adenoma (microadenoma)—large tumours are uncommon. Immunofluorescent or peroxidase techniques may show increased pituitary content of ACTH, β lipotrophin, endorphins and related peptides, sometimes with increased prolactin.

Ectopic ACTH syndrome

Benign or malignant non-pituitary tumours may secrete sufficient ACTH to cause Cushing's syndrome. Those most commonly involved are:

1 Oat cell carcinoma of the lung.

2 Carcinoid tumour of foregut origin—situated in thymus, thyroid, lung, upper intestine, pancreas (see p. 36).

3 Adrenal medullary tumours.

4 Ovarian and other tumours—rarely.

Results

The prognosis in untreated Cushing's syndrome is poor. The object of treatment is:

1 To lower elevated plasma cortisol—by bilateral adrenalectomy or with enzyme blocking drugs such as metyrapone.

2 Treatment of the cause.

Mineralocorticoid excess

Causes

1 Primary hyperaldosteronism—Conn's syndrome, due to single or multiple adenomas of the zona glomerulosa, with or without surrounding glomerulosa hyperplasia.

2 Secondary hyperaldosteronism:

(a) renin-secreting tumours—rare;

(b) conditions associated with secondary hyperreninaemia: congestive cardiac failure, cirrhosis with ascites, renal disease.

Effects

1 Hypertension—in primary type only, which is usually severe.

2 Hypokalaemia—usually marked in Conn's syndrome. Associated with alkalosis and muscle weakness.

3 Sodium at the upper limit of normal, or slightly raised.

4 Raised plasma aldosterone with, in Conn's syndrome, suppressed plasma renin.

Results

Tumours are rarely, if ever, malignant and hyperaldosteronism is cured by their removal. Hypertension may persist if arteriolar changes and renal damage have already occurred. The aldosterone antagonist, spironolactone, may be used.

Sex hormone excess

Virilization may occur as a result of excessive androgen production in women with Cushing's syndrome. Purely virilizing and feminizing (in men) tumours are exceedingly rare. Most cases of virilization and of feminization occur as part of mixed syndromes (see below).

Effects of excessive androgens

1 *Males*: boys will pass through a phase of rapid growth with well developed muscles, increasing body hair and with enlargement and maturation of the penis and scrotum (precocious pseudo-puberty). As a result of early epiphyseal fusion, growth ceases early and final adult height is stunted. Testes remain prepubertal. In adult men the effects of increased androgens would probably not be detected.

2 *Females*: girls pass through a phase of rapid growth with muscular 'tom-boy' development. Final adult height will be stunted. Body hair will be male in pattern with frontal balding, facial hair, chest, shoulder and abdominal hair, hair on the thighs and increased hair growth on forearms, lower legs and digits. Breast development may be normal, although menstruation is absent or infrequent. There may be clitoromegaly and acne. The voice may deepen.

Effects of excessive oestrogens

1 *Males*: gynaecomastia may occur in adults or children. Although this may rarely be the result of an adrenal tumour, most cases of gynaecomastia are of uncertain aetiology (*see* p. 59).

2 *Females*: the effect of increased oestrogens are usually those of menstrual irregularity, with menorrhagia and breakthrough menstrual bleeding.

Mixed syndromes

Congenital adrenal hyperplasia

A rare inborn autosomal recessive enzyme deficiency resulting in deficiency of glucocorticoids, with or without deficiency of mineralocorticoids—'salt-losing' type. The tendency to low plasma cortisol leads to raised ACTH. This in turn causes adrenal hypertrophy and excessive production of androgens.

Effects

See effects of androgens on p. 118.

1 Rapid growth in children but premature epiphyseal fusion.

2 Precocious pseudo-puberty in boys.

3 Masculinization of girls with delayed or absent menstruation.

4 Pseudo-hermaphroditism of genetically female infants (*see* p. 206).

Adrenal

Both adrenals are hyperplastic.

Results

Replacement with glucocorticoids, and mineralocorticoids if necessary, results in normal development although external genitalia may require corrective surgery in girls.

Polycystic ovary syndrome— Stein–Leventhal syndrome

Variants of this complex adrenal–ovarian disorder are common in women. Increased secretion of androgens occurs from the adrenal or ovary or both, with increased peripheral conversion of androgens to oestrogens.

Effects

1 Menstrual irregularity.

2 Infertility.

3 Mild virilization.

4 Acne.

5 Occasional galactorrhoea.

Adrenal

The adrenal is histologically normal.

Ovary

In any condition associated with increased serum levels of androgens, multiple small follicular cysts develop beneath a thickened white ovarian capsule.

Medullary hyperfunction

Phaeochromocytoma

Incidence

Rare.

Age

Any age, but commonly young adults.

Macroscopical

Usually well encapsulated, unilateral, red–brown or haemorrhagic tumours arising in the centre of the adrenal gland. They are bilateral in 10% and may very rarely arise outside the adrenal, in the carotid body, the organ of Zuckerkandl, etc., in which sites they are also hormonally active. Tumours may reach 5–6 cm in diameter. They become dark brown in colour when fixed in bichromate solutions.

Microscopical

Nests of cells resembling the normal adrenal medullary chromaffin cells.

Effects

Those of hypersecretion of catecholamines:

1 Hypertension—this is usually intermittent but is sometimes sustained (*see* p. 93).

2 Hypermetabolism.

3 Hyperglycaemia.

Results

Most of the tumours are histologically and clinically benign and the hypertension is usually relieved following their removal. Five per cent are malignant, metastasizing to the other adrenal and to lymph nodes, lungs, liver and bone. Occasionally phaeochromocytomas occur as part of multiple endocrine adenomatoses, especially associated with medullary (calcitonin-secreting) carcinoma of the thyroid (see p. 137). In von Recklinghausen's disease, phaeochromocytoma or medullary carcinoma of the thyroid may be associated with multiple cutaneous neurofibromas (see p. 109).

Tests of adrenal function
The details given below are meant only as a simple guide. In each case the need for a test, and its subsequent interpretation, are dependent on the clinical circumstances.

Cortical hypofunction—Addison's disease
1 Hyponatraemia, hyperkalaemia and raised blood urea.
2 Occasional eosinophilia.
3 Plasma cortisol may be normal but is diagnostic if less than 220 nmol/l at 9 a.m., or in the stressed patient.
4 Plasma ACTH and β-lipotrophin are grossly elevated.
5 Synacthen test—absent or diminished rise in plasma cortisol following administration of a synthetic analogue of ACTH—*Synacthen*.

Cortical hyperfunction—Cushing's syndrome

Diagnosis
1 Loss of circadian rhythm in ACTH and/or cortisol.
2 Elevated 24-hour urinary excretion of cortisol and metabolites.
3 Overnight, or low-dose dexamethasone suppression tests.
4 Hypoglycaemia stress test—insulin tolerance test—no rise in ACTH and/or cortisol.

Differential diagnosis
1 Plasma ACTH—suppressed in adrenal tumour.
2 High-dose dexamethasone test—partial suppression in pituitary-dependent disease, but not in adrenal tumour or ectopic ACTH syndrome.
3 Metyrapone test—exaggerated rise in cortisol precursors in pituitary-dependent disease.
4 Hypokalaemia—if marked, usually indicates the ectopic ACTH syndrome.

5 Procedures, such as X-rays and isotope scans, to demonstrate directly the presence or absence of adrenal, pituitary or other tumours.

Conn's syndrome
1 Hypokalaemia, with high normal or slightly elevated sodium.
2 Alkalosis.
3 Raised aldosterone levels, with suppressed renin.
4 Adrenal isotope scan.
5 Selective adrenal vein sampling for aldosterone.

Congenital adrenal hyperplasia
In the commonest form (21-hydroxylase deficiency) any of the following may be used to diagnose the condition and to monitor response to therapy:
1 Raised ACTH or β-lipotrophin.
2 Raised urinary 17 oxo- or oxogenic-steroids.
3 Raised urinary pregnanetriol.
4 Raised 17-hydroxyprogesterone in blood.
   Most agree, however, that the best way to monitor therapy in children is clinically, by documentation of growth rate.

Medullary hyperfunction— Phaeochromocytoma
1 Estimation of excretion of catecholamines or their metabolites.
2 Effect on blood pressure of sympathetic blocking agents, such as phentolamine.
3 Demonstration of adrenal tumour, e.g. radiographically by scan.
4 Selective adrenal vein sampling for catecholamines.

Tumours

Cortical adenoma

Incidence
Extremely common as an incidental finding in up to 30% of all post-mortem examinations.

Macroscopical
Small, encapsulated, yellow nodules which are unilateral or bilateral, single or multiple.

Microscopical
The adenomas resemble the normal cortex although the zonal arrangements may be disorderly.

Effects

1 Inactive—the vast majority have no clinical effects.
2 Functional—these tumours are usually larger:
 (a) Cushing's syndrome;
 (b) Conn's syndrome;
 (c) virilization or feminization.

Immunocytochemistry can identify cells which produce specific hormones. Radioimmunoassay techniques can measure their amounts.

Cortical carcinoma

Incidence
Rare.

Age
All ages, but in children functional cortical carcinoma is the commonest cause of Cushing's syndrome.

Macroscopical
Globular, large, soft, lobulated, yellow tumours with a soft, haemorrhagic and necrotic cut surface. Adjacent organs, particularly the kidney, are commonly invaded. The tumour is bilateral in 10%.

Microscopical
Very variable, from tumours showing a close resemblance to normal cortical cells to anaplastic types containing bizarre giant cells. The best guide to the malignancy of a functioning adrenal tumour is its size, not its microscopical appearance: those less than 40 g are benign, whereas those greater than 100 g are malignant in their behaviour.

Effects
1 Endocrine
 (a) Inactive—the tumours have no functional activity.
 (b) Functional—Cushing's syndrome, often with particularly marked tendency to virilization in females. Glucocorticoid production can be demonstrated by immunocytochemistry.
2 Local: there is normally a large mass with invasion of neighbouring organs.

Spread
1 *Direct*: kidney, posterior abdominal wall, diaphragm, liver, spleen, etc.
2 *Lymphatic*: invaded regional lymph nodes are commonly seen by the time of diagnosis.
3 *Blood*: spread to the other adrenal is common, as are metastases to the lungs, bone and brain.

Prognosis
Extremely poor; most are dead within 2 years and a 5-year survival is very uncommon.

Medulla

Phaeochromocytoma
See p. 119.

Neuroblastoma

Nature
A tumour of neuroectodermal origin derived from neuroblasts, cells normally found in the intermediate stages of development of the sympathetic nervous system.

Age
Children are almost exclusively affected. The tumour is rare above the age of 5 years, but adult cases do very occasionally occur.

Incidence
Rare, although neuroblastoma is one of the commoner malignant tumours in children.

Sites
1 Adrenal medulla.
2 Mediastinum—posteriorly. Usually in the posterior mediastinum in relation to the sympathetic chain (see p. 285).
3 Coeliac plexus and other sites of autonomic nerve tissue within the abdomen.

Macroscopical
Bulky, fleshy, greyish-white masses which may be bilateral when arising in the adrenals. They attain a large size and obliterate the cortical tissue. On section they are soft, and often show areas of haemorrhage, necrosis and calcification.

Microscopical
The cells are small with hyperchromatic nuclei and very little cytoplasm. They may be arranged in sheets or, more typically, in rosettes. Ganglion cells may sometimes be present—*ganglioneuroblastoma*. This tumour is thus intermediate between the differentiated ganglioneuroma and the undifferentiated neuroblastoma (see p. 110).

Evidence of differentiation and maturation may be identified and electron microscopy may show diagnostic features in the apparently undifferentiated 'small dark cell tumours' which also include Ewing's sarcoma (*see* p. 307), embryonal rhabdomyosarcoma, malignant lymphoma or anaplastic carcinoma in adult tumours.

Spread

1 *Direct*: early invasion of the adjacent organs and tissues.
2 *Lymphatic*: regional lymph nodes are commonly invaded.
3 *Blood*: occurs early and widely but with a particular predilection for bone, liver and the other adrenal.

Results

A highly malignant tumour which is usually inoperable. It is very radiosensitive but long-term results are poor, though chemotherapy has helped to improve prognosis to 3-year survival rates of 30%. Some cases spontaneously regress or mature.

Ganglioneuroma

Ten per cent of these tumours arise in the adrenal medulla (*see* p. 110).

Secondary tumours

The adrenal gland is a common site for carcinomatous metastases, especially from the bronchus and from the breast, but less commonly from other tumours. Only rarely do they cause hormonal insufficiency due to complete cortical destruction.

B/PITUITARY

Normal structure and function
Hypofunction
   Anterior lobe
   Posterior lobe
Hyperfunction
   Anterior lobe
   Posterior lobe
Tumours
   Secondary

Development

1 From the stomodeum—Rathke's pouch—to form the adenohypophysis—anterior pituitary.
2 From the brain—a downgrowth from the floor of the third ventricle to form the neurohypophysis—posterior pituitary.

Structure

This is illustrated in Fig. 12. Unlike the majority of mammals humans do not usually have a pars intermedia sandwiched between the anterior and posterior lobes. There is evidence, however, that a pars intermedia is present in the fetal pituitary, as well as in the pituitary of pregnant women.

Anterior lobe—adenohypophysis— pars anterior

Anatomically divided (a) pars distalis (PD) and (b) pars tuberalis (PT)—surrounding the infundibular stem. The blood vessels of the pituitary stalk represent an extensive portal system carrying releasing and inhibitory factors down from the hypothalamus, as well as pituitary hormones up from the pituitary.

Cell types

Formerly characterized on the basis of staining reaction (acidophil, 40%; basophil, 10%; chromophobe, 50%). Now cells are more usually characterized on the basis of immunocytochemistry and the specific hormones which they elaborate.

Posterior lobe—pars nervosa— neurohypophysis

The posterior lobe is connected to the hypothalamus by the supra-optico-hypophyseal and tuberohypophy-

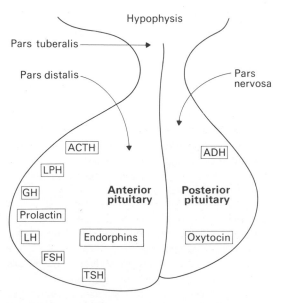

Fig. 12 Anatomical structure of pituitary gland.

seal tracts. These fibres end in perivascular arborizations in all parts of the neurohypophysis.

Hormones

Anterior lobe

Hormones are synthesized in the pituitary and their release is controlled by hypothalamic releasing or inhibiting factors carried in the hypothalamo–hypophyseal portal tract.

1 *Corticotrophin. Adrenocorticotrophic hormone— ACTH.* Probably released by hypothalamic corticotrophin releasing factor—*CRF.*

2 *β-lipotrophin—β-LPH.* Made in the same cells as ACTH, cleaved from the same precursor molecule and controlled by the same factor(s).

3 *The opioid peptides, the endorphins.* Are structurally related to β-LPH and are probably released from the anterior pituitary in man.

4 *Growth hormone—GH.* Release apparently under inhibitory control by somatostatin from the hypothalamus.

5 *Prolactin.* Phylogenetically and structurally very similar to GH. Also under dominant inhibitory control, by prolactin inhibitory factor (almost certainly dopamine).

6 *Thyrotrophin—TSH.* Released by the hypothalamic tripeptide, thyrotrophin releasing hormone— *TRH.*

7 *Follicle stimulating hormone—FSH and luteinizing hormone—LH.* Are both released by the same hypothalamic factor—*LHRH.* Like TSH, they are glycoproteins, whereas the other pituitary hormones are all peptides.

Functions

Undoubtedly our present understanding of pituitary hormones is simplistic. It is not known what role GH plays in the adult, or what role prolactin plays except in the initiation of normal lactation.

1 ACTH releases cortisol and other corticosteroids.

2 β-LPH—function unknown.

3 Endorphins have actions similar to morphine but their physiological role in plasma is not known.

4 GH. Necessary for normal growth.

5 Prolactin. Necessary for the initiation of normal lactation. Like ACTH, β-LPH, endorphins and GH, prolactin is released in response to stress.

6 TSH stimulates the thyroid gland to release thyroid hormones, thyroxine and triodothyronine. These in turn exert feedback inhibition on TSH release (see p. 128).

7 FSH.

(a) Female—stimulates ovarian follicular development in the follicular phase of the menstrual cycle.

(b) Male—together with testosterone is essential for spermatogenesis.

8 LH

(a) Female—released in a burst at mid-cycle to induce ovulation.

(b) Male—stimulates the interstitial (Leydig) cells to produce androgens.

Posterior lobe

Hormones synthesized in the supraoptic and paraventricular nuclei of the hypothalamus and conducted to the posterior lobe by nerve axons, whence they are released into the blood stream.

1 *Oxytocin.*

2 *Antidiuretic hormone—ADH,* vasopressin.

Functions

1 *Oxytocin.*

(a) Contraction of the pregnant uterus at parturition.

(b) Ejection of milk during suckling by action on the mammary myoepithelial cells.

2 *ADH.* Has a stimulatory effect on water reabsorption by the distal tubule of the kidney, resulting in the excretion of urine with increased concentration.

Hypofunction

Anterior lobe

Causes

1 Hypothalamic tumour, usually craniopharyngioma, more rarely pinealoma, teratoma or secondary from another site.

2 Pituitary tumour. Expanding to impair production or release from normal pituitary cells.

3 Idiopathic deficiency of one or more pituitary hormones, or of their releasing factors. Isolated GH deficiency is a cause of small stature in childhood. Isolated LHRH deficiency (also called isolated gonadotrophin deficiency) is a cause of hypogonadism presenting either at puberty or in adult life.

4 Spontaneous infarction. Occurs either in pre-existing pituitary tumour, or else following torrential post-partum haemorrhage—Sheehan's syndrome.

5 Iatrogenic. Previous surgery or radiotherapy to the hypothalamus or pituitary.
6 Miscellaneous. Rare causes include:
(a) Tuberculosis, sarcoidosis, syphilis.
(b) Trauma—with or without skull fracture.
(c) Giant cell granuloma of the anterior lobe—a very rare giant cell lesion of unknown aetiology.
(d) Metastatic tumour.

Effects

1 Secondary hypoadrenalism—ACTH deficiency.
2 Secondary hypothyroidism—TSH deficiency.
3 Impotence or amenorrhoea—LH and FSH deficiency.
4 Small stature—GH deficiency in childhood.
5 Failure of lactation. If post-partum haemorrhage complicates delivery, the first indication of pituitary infarction—Sheehan's syndrome, is failure of lactation. Paradoxically, in non-pregnant females, as well as in males, the first sign of pituitary tumour may be inappropriate milk production—*galactorrhoea*, due to elevation of serum prolactin.

Apart from failure of lactation, prolactin deficiency is without known effect in man, as is GH deficiency in the adult. Hypogonadism secondary to gonadotrophin deficiency is associated with the development of fine, wrinkled skin, and loss of stature secondary to osteoporotic collapse in the spine. Hypogonadism occurring before epiphyseal fusion in the long bones leads to the development of a eunuchoid habitus (span exceeds height) provided GH reserve is intact.

Tests to exclude hypofunction of anterior pituitary

This list is not comprehensive and as with all tests, the results need to be taken in clinical context.
1 ACTH reserve. Adequate if:
(a) random plasma cortisol >550 nmol/l;
(b) stress-induced cortisol rise >550 nmol/l.
2 GH reserve. Adequate if:
(a) random plasma level >20 mU/l;
(b) stress or otherwise elevated GH peak >20 mU/l.
3 TSH reserve adequate if serum thyroxine is in the normal range.
4 LH reserve adequate if:
(a) males have a normal testosterone;
(b) females are ovulating.
5 FSH reserve adequate if:

(a) males have normal spermatogenesis;
(b) females are ovulating.

Other tests of gonadotrophin reserve, e.g. LHRH test, clomiphene test, will indicate whether it is possible to elevate serum gonadotrophin levels, but will not necessarily indicate whether the reserve is adequate.

Mixed syndromes

A number of congenital syndromes are associated with various aspects of hypofunction of the anterior pituitary. This pituitary hypofunction is usually secondary to defective hypothalmic function.
1 *Kallman's syndrome*: Isolated LHRH deficiency with defective or absent sense of smell.
2 *Laurence–Moon–Biedl syndrome*: Isolated LHRH deficiency with mental subnormality, retinitis pigmentosa and syndactyly.
3 *Prader–Willi syndrome*: Isolated LHRH deficiency with hyperphagic obesity, mental subnormality and intrauterine or neonatal hypotonia.

Posterior lobe

Diabetes insipidus (cranial)

Causes

1 *Surgical trauma*: usually involving stalk section.
2 *Head injury*: with or without skull fracture. As with surgical trauma, diabetes insipidus occurring in these circumstances is often transient.
3 *Hypothalamic tumour*: either primary or secondary.
4 *Infiltrative disease of the hypothalamus*: sarcoidosis, Hand–Schüller–Christian disease (see p. 297).
5 *Idiopathic*: in approximately 30% no cause is found.
6 *DIDMOAD syndrome*: the acronym, DIDMOAD, applies to the components of this hereditary syndrome (which has complex and uncertain penetrance): cranial diabetes insipidus, diabetes mellitus, optic atrophy and dementia. Formes frustes occur.

Effects

Inability to concentrate urine leads to passing of copious dilute urine with a tendency to dehydration. The night time (11 p.m.–7 a.m) urine volume nearly always exceeds 1.5 litres. If there is associated disease of the anterior pituitary, diabetes insipidus may be masked since adequate levels of cortisol are required to excrete a water load. Polyuria may then occur when replacement therapy is commenced with corticosteroids. Diabetes insipidus may occur also as a result of renal tubular disease—the tubules being unresponsive to normal levels of ADH (nephrogenic diabetes insipidus). There are no known effects of oxytocin deficiency.

Test of posterior pituitary function
Water deprivation test. The object of the test is to demonstrate progressive haemoconcentration (with unaltered urine concentration) when access to water is restricted. It serves to differentiate diabetes insipidus from psychogenic polydipsia, but is potentially dangerous in patients with diabetes insipidus and should be undertaken only under controlled circumstances.

Hyperfunction

Anterior lobe
Hyperfunction of the anterior pituitary occurs if functioning adenomas are present. Hypersecretion of the glycoprotein hormones, TSH, LH and FSH is exceedingly uncommon.

Growth hormone

Effects
1 *Before epiphyseal union*: if a GH-secreting tumour occurs in a child there is excessive growth in a regular and initially well-proportioned manner—*gigantism*. Most giants show some features also of acromegaly, with disproportionate enlargement, e.g. of the hands and jaw.
2 *After epiphyseal union*: excessive GH in an adult results in *acromegaly*:
    (a) large hands and feet;
    (b) overgrowth of jaw, and prominence of supra-orbital ridges and malar bones;
    (c) increased soft tissue in skin and subcutaneous tissue; increased sweating;
    (d) kyphosis;
    (e) splanchnomegaly;
    (f) hypertension and cardiomyopathy;
    (g) diabetes mellitus;
    (h) hyperprolactinaemia with associated menstrual irregularity or impotence;
    (i) thyroid disorders.

Prolactin

Causes
1 Large pituitary adenoma (macroadenoma).
2 Small pituitary adenoma (microadenoma).
3 Drugs:
    (a) oestrogens;
    (b) phenothiazines;
    (c) methyldopa;
    (d) some antidepressants.

Effects
Abnormally increased prolactin secretion is associated with menstrual irregularity or infertility in women, and ejaculatory failure or impotence in men. Galactorrhoea may occur in either sex.

ACTH/β-LPH

Causes
1 Physiological: decreased plasma cortisol, e.g. Addison's disease, congenital adrenal hyperplasia.
2 Pathological: Cushing's disease.

Effects
When the adrenals are intact, the effect of increased ACTH secretion is to cause Cushing's syndrome (see p. 117). When the rise in ACTH is a physiological response to falling cortisol, as in Addison's disease, the only effect of increased ACTH/β-LPH secretion is increased skin pigmentation.

Posterior lobe

Inappropriate ADH secretion
The syndrome of inappropriate ADH (SIADH) occurs as a complication of other diseases. Primary hypersecretion of ADH, or of oxytocin, is not recognized.

Causes
1 Head injury.
2 Any intracranial pathology.
3 Any thoracic disease, especially carcinoma of the bronchus, pneumonia, pulmonary embolus.
4 Transiently following major trauma, or general anaesthesia.
5 Idiopathic. In some cases the cause is not known.

Pathogenesis
Increased ADH secretion may occur from direct

hypothalamic derangement, or alternatively from involvement of intrathoracic baroreceptors in disease processes. Some carcinomas of the lung secrete ectopic ADH.

Incidence
Common.

Effects
Water retention with haemodilution. In severe cases cerebral oedema supervenes with impaired consciousness.

Tumours

Macroadenoma of the anterior lobe

Incidence
About 15% of all primary intracranial tumours. Adenomas of the posterior lobe do not occur.

Types
1 GH-secreting. Acromegaly, gigantism.
2 Prolactin-secreting. Prolactinoma.
3 ACTH/β-LPH-secreting. Cushing's disease.
4 Mixed. Especially GH with prolactin and Cushing's disease with hyperprolactinaemia.
5 Non-functioning. True non-functioning macroadenomas are uncommon.

Effects
1 Endocrine effects.
2 Local pressure symptoms.
  (a) On the remainder of the pituitary, resulting in hypofunction.
  (b) On the optic chiasm causing visual field defects, usually bitemporal hemianopia.
  (c) On the brain. Large tumours result in distortion of the midbrain with internal hydrocephalus.
  (d) On the pituitary fossa. Causing progressive enlargement of the fossa, with erosion of the bones of the sphenoid and of the dorsum sellae.

Microadenoma of the anterior lobe

Incidence
Common. Occurs in approximately 30% of the population.

Effects
The vast majority are functionless, being incidental findings on skull X-ray or at post-mortem. A minority appear to be the source of increased prolactin secretion, presenting clinically with the same symptoms as large prolactinomas.

Craniopharyngioma

Origin
From vestigial remnants of Rathke's pouch.

Macroscopical
Solid, or more commonly part cystic and part solid, tumours anywhere along the craniopharyngeal canal. The cysts are multilocular containing granular brown debris and brown fluid with cholesterol crystals. Calcification in the wall is common.

Microscopical
Nests or cords of squamous epithelium in a loose fibrous stroma. Some have an outer layer of columnar-shaped cells which resemble the adamantinomas of the jaw (see p. 16) whilst others may be reminiscent of a basal cell tumour.

Effects
Pressure effects on adjacent structures, e.g. hypothalamus, optic nerves and the pituitary.

Behaviour
Slowly growing and only very rarely invasive. Complete removal is technically extremely difficult but decompression and radiotherapy is usually curative.

Carcinoma

Origin
Most examples arise *de novo* but a few have their origin in a pre-existing adenoma.

Microscopical
Usually of chromophobe type. Very rarely they are of mixed cell type and may have hormonal effects. The cells show nuclear irregularity and mitotic activity with evidence of local invasion of the capsule and adjacent soft tissues and bone.

Effects
1 Local invasion with destruction of surrounding tissues.

2 Only rarely hormonally active.

Chordoma

Thirty-five per cent of these tumours occur in the base of the skull and may extend to the pituitary fossa or adjacent tissues with consequential pituitary destruction (see p. 312).

Secondary tumours

The pituitary is an uncommon site for metastases although deposits from carcinomas of the lung and breast occasionally occur. The posterior lobe is mostly affected and the anterior lobe only rarely. A secondary deposit is an occasional cause of hypopituitarism.

C/THYROID

Normal
Congenital
Inflammations
  Infective
  Non-infective
Goitre
  Simple
  Colloid
  Toxic
Hypothyroidism
Tests of function
Tumours
  Benign
  Malignant

Normal thyroid

The normal adult gland weighs 20–40 g and consists of two lateral lobes connected by the isthmus, which occasionally has a pyramidal lobe attached to its superior border.

Development

A median outgrowth from the floor of the pharynx—*foramen caecum*, which descends into the neck—*thyroglossal duct*, and proliferates to form the adult gland.

Microscopical

Consists of acini lined by cuboidal epithelium containing colloid. There is a loose interacinar connective tissue containing the blood vessels and there may be a sparse lymphocytic infiltration.

    Within the follicular basement membrane are the parafollicular or *C cells*, large, rather triangular in shape and 'light' in appearance due to lack of eosinophilia. These are of neural crest, ultimobranchial origin and are part of the diffuse endocrine system (see p. 36).

Hormones

1 Thyroxine—T_4.
2 Triiodothyronine—T_3.
3 Reverse triiodothyronine—rT_3—inactive as a thyroid hormone. Within the thyroid gland these compounds are bound to thyroglobulin. In the plasma, thyroxine (99.97%) and triiodothyronine (99.5%) are bound to thyroid-binding globulin, thyroid-binding pre-albumin and other proteins. Extensive peripheral conversion of T_4 to T_3 and rT_3 occurs, predominantly in the liver.
4 Calcitonin—produced by the parafollicular, C cells, of the thyroid. Originally thought to oppose the action of parathyroid hormone by lowering serum calcium and increasing calcium deposition in bone. Physiological role is unknown, although often produced by ectopic hormone-secreting tumours (see p. 139).

Effects of thyroxine and triiodothyronine

They are qualitatively similar and probably both T_4 and T_3 are active *in vivo*. They play a regulatory role in cell metabolism: thyroid hormone deficiency leads to decreased cell metabolism; in hyperthyroidism cell metabolism is increased.

Metabolism of thyroid hormones

This is illustrated in Fig. 13. Stages which appear to be enhanced by thyroid-stimulating hormone—TSH—are indicated by double arrows.

Congenital

Lingual thyroid

Failure of descent, with development of all or part of the gland in the region of the foramen caecum.

Aberrant thyroid

1 Mid-line: anywhere along the line of the thyroglossal duct.
2 Lateral: true ectopic thyroid tissue may rarely be found medial to the sternomastoid muscle. Thyroid tissue lateral to the sternomastoid, even when of very regular appearance, always represents lymph node metastases from a carcinoma of the thyroid. The

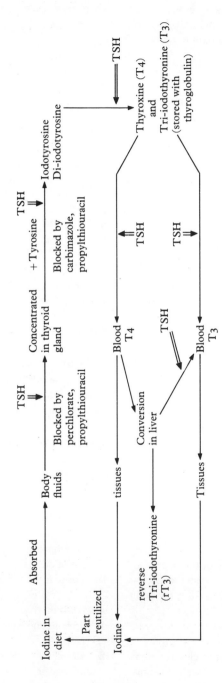

Fig. 13 Metabolism of thyroid hormones.

primary is often very small and occult which led to the use of the erroneous term 'lateral aberrant thyroid' (see p. 136).

Persistence of a thyroglossal duct
1 Thyroglossal duct.
2 Thyroglossal cyst.
3 Thyroglossal fistula. Usually following inflammation in a thyroglossal cyst.

Any of these lesions may be above, in, or below the hyoid bone and be lined by columnar or squamous epithelium.

Aplasia
This is a rare cause of cretinism (see p. 133).

Inflammations

Infective

Acute bacterial thyroiditis
This is very rare but can occur of haematogenous, lymphatic or local spread of bacteria, usually staphylococci or streptococci. Resolution usually occurs with antibiotic therapy.

Acute viral thyroiditis

Synonyms
Subacute thyroiditis, non-suppurative thyroiditis, de Quervain's disease, granulomatous or giant cell thyroiditis.

Incidence
Rare.

Age
30–50 years, but may occur in the elderly.

Sex
More common in females.

Clinical
An acute, or subacute, onset with fever, malaise, pain in the throat. The thyroid may be enlarged, but is always tender, often markedly. The pain makes swallowing and coughing difficult.

Aetiology
Coxsackie virus infection is the most common, although other viruses have also been implicated.

Macroscopical
The thyroid is enlarged to about twice the normal size. It is smooth, firm and tender; slight adhesion of the gland surface to the adjacent muscles may occur but these adhesions are readily broken down. The cut surface shows focal pale areas poor in colloid.

Microscopical
Focal granulomatous inflammation with numerous foreign body giant cells, often engulfing colloid material—*colloidophagy*, degeneration of the follicles and epithelium and an inflammatory cell infiltration by plasma cells, lymphocytes and histiocytes. Later, fibrous scarring and thyroid acinar regeneration may occur.

Results
The acute glandular destruction may result in transient elevation of thyroid hormones, with or without thyrotoxicosis. The illness is usually self-limiting and settles in 1–3 weeks. Less often there are relapses, of lessening severity, over a period of several months. Rarely, the patient may become myxoedematous. Severe thyroiditis may be fatal in the elderly and debilitated.

Non-infective

Hashimoto's disease—autoimmune thyroiditis—lymphadenoid goitre—struma lymphomatosa

Nature
A disorder characterized by variable degrees of diffuse thyroid enlargement with circulating antithyroid antibodies and showing features of an autoimmune destructive process in the gland.

Incidence
Although detectable thyroid antibodies are found in up to 2% of the population only a relatively small proportion have a clinical goitre.

Age and sex
Maximal between 35 and 55 years, but at any age though rare in children. Female : male, 12 : 1.

Macroscopical

The gland is usually diffusely enlarged and commonly 2–5 times normal size, firm and lobulated. The borders are distinct but displacement or slight tracheal compression may occur. Adjacent cervical lymph nodes are often slightly reactively enlarged and rubbery. The cut surface shows marked pale greyish lobulation with diminution of colloid components.

Microscopical

A diffuse process confined within the thyroid capsule, showing:

1 Lymphoid infiltration with lymph follicle formation.
2 A diffuse plasma cell infiltration.
3 Epithelial metaplasia with large, eosinophilic, thyroid epithelial cells—Askanazy cells.
4 Diminished colloid in the disrupted acini.
5 Increased fibrous tissue producing a lobulated pattern.
6 Elements of regeneration and increased activity induced by TSH in non-affected acini.

Biochemical changes

1 Elevated TSH level.
2 Exaggerated TSH response to the intravenous injection of thyrotrophin releasing hormone—TRH (TRH test).
3 Low T_4 level—usual.
4 Low T_3 level—becomes manifest only in later stages.

Immunology

Serum autoantibodies of three types are identified:
1 Precipitin test—detects antithyroglobulin antibodies.
2 Tanned red cell—TRC—also detects antithyroglobulin antibodies and is more sensitive.
3 Complement fixation test—CFT—microsomal antibody.

In Hashimoto's disease TRC levels of one in 25 000 or more and a CFT of even one in 64 are common and respective titres of one in 1 000 000 and one in 1000 are not uncommon.

The TRC titre is particularly high in the more fibrotic examples.

Other conditions with thyroid antibodies

1 *Hyperthyroidism*: present in high proportions (65%) usually in low titre but if CFT is one in 16 or more this indicates a high risk of myxoedema developing after thyroidectomy or radioiodine treatment.
2 *Primary atrophic thyroiditis*: low-titre antibodies are present in 80% of cases of 'primary' myxoedema with thyroid atrophy. However, even though similar pathogenetic factors may operate, it is misleading to define primary atrophic thyroiditis (see p. 134) as 'Hashimoto's disease without goitre'.
3 *Focal lymphocytic thyroiditis*: patchy histological changes of a similar type to that seen in Hashimoto's thyroiditis are seen in 5–10% of autopsy thyroids. Similar focal changes can occur in nodular colloid goitre. There is a spectrum of severity from scattered to diffuse (in 2% of autopsies) and in the more severe forms clinically occult myxodema is common retrospectively.

Association with other diseases

Other 'autoimmune diseases' are commonly associated with thyroiditis including: SLE (see p. 96), rheumatoid arthritis (see p. 100), Sjögren's syndrome (see p. 103), pernicious anaemia (see p. 27), acquired haemolytic anaemia, adrenal cortical atrophy (Addison's disease) (see p. 116), diabetes mellitus (see p. 355). Antibodies involved in this autoimmune spectrum include, in particular, organ-specific examples, e.g. pernicious anaemia (parietal cell antibodies) and Addison's disease (CFT adrenal cortical antibodies) and, additionally, a wide range of antinuclear factors, rheumatoid factors, anti-red-cell antibodies, etc.

Familial

There is a definite genetic predisposition to autoimmune disease development and relatives of Hashimoto's disease patients have a high incidence of circulating thyroid antibodies.

Results

Myxoedema usually results if the condition is not treated, but this may be delayed for many years by compensatory hyperplasia and regeneration of the thyroid epithelium, induced by TSH, which balances to some extent the progressive destruction of thyroid tissue. Thyroxine replacement therapy will reverse the clinical manifestations of myxoedema and will cause regression of any thyroid enlargement which results from TSH stimulation. Thyroid enlargement resulting from the underlying thyroiditis is unaffected by thyroxine treatment.

Riedel's thyroiditis—invasive fibrous thyroiditis—ligneous thyroiditis

Nature
A very rare thyroiditis of distinctive hardness and with involvement of adjacent tissues. There is an association with retroperitoneal and/or mediastinal fibrosis in about 30% of cases.

Aetiology
Unknown, but possibly autoimmune though antibodies are lacking.

Age
Variable, but usually in middle age.

Sex
Male : female, 1 : 4.

Macroscopical
Irregular enlargement of the thyroid gland with a densely hard and nodular surface inseparable from the surrounding tissues. On section the gland is grey, gritty and fibrous.

Microscopical
Obliteration of the thyroid architecture with replacement by mature collagen containing foci of lymphocytes, plasma cells and scanty polymorphs.

Results
1 Tracheal compression—relieved by wedge resection of the isthmus.
2 Myxoedema—25%.
3 Part of the gland only involved—rarely.
4 Frequently mistaken clinically for thyroid carcinoma.
5 Thyroid antibody studies inevitably give negative results.

Goitre

Definition
Any enlargement of part or whole of the thyroid gland.

Types
1 Simple goitre:
   (a) endemic;
   (b) sporadic;
   (c) physiological.
2 Colloid goitre:
   (a) diffuse;
   (b) nodular.
3 Toxic goitre:
   (a) Graves' disease;
   (b) toxic nodular goitre;
   (c) other.
4 Infective thyroiditis, including granulomatous.
5 Autoimmune thyroiditis.
6 Riedel's thyroiditis.
7 Adenoma.
8 Carcinoma.

Simple goitre

Nature
Diffuse enlargement of the thyroid gland due to an absolute or relative deficiency of iodine, or to goitrogenic agents.

Endemic type

Aetiology
Iodine deficiency in food and water, particularly in geographical areas remote from the sea. In most countries iodine is now added to foods, e.g. bread, salt, but iodine deficiency is still common in the Himalaya and High Andes. The addition of iodine to the diet of schoolchildren in Ohio reduced the prevalence of goitre from 20% to 0.2%.

Sporadic type
Goitre occurring in individuals where there are adequate supplies of iodine in the food and water.

Aetiology
1 Goitrogens.
   (a) Ingestion of certain of the cabbage species (Brassicas) is said to be goitrogenic in some, possibly because of their thiourea content.
   (b) Drugs and chemicals, e.g. perchlorate, resorcinol, paraminosalicylic acid, as well as drugs used in the treatment of thyrotoxicosis.
2 Familial: due to inherited autosome recessive traits which interfere with hormone synthesis at differing enzyme pathways—dyshormonogenetic goitres (see p. 134).

Appearances
A vascular, diffusely and moderately enlarged gland,

with hyperplasia, as evidenced by an increased number of acini, tall columnar epithelium and some colloid deficiency. Later, patchy involutionary changes may occur.

Results
If iodine is supplied, or the goitrogen removed, the gland returns to normal.

Physiological goitre

Nature
In girls the thyroid gland may enlarge at the time of puberty, or during pregnancy. The reason is not clear.

Colloid goitre

Incidence
A common disease in districts with endemic iodine deficiency: not uncommon elsewhere.

Aetiology
In endemic districts it represents an end-result of iodine deficiency, and follows involution of the hyperplastic gland. In non-endemic districts the cause is not known although a serum thyroid growth factor has been postulated.

Sex
Male : female, 1 : 6.

Diffuse colloid goitre

Macroscopical
Diffuse enlargement with an exaggerated vesicular pattern and a pale brown, glistening colloid appearance on the cut surface.

Microscopical
Less vascular than normal; the epithelium is low cuboidal and there is an increased amount of colloid within the distended vesicles.

Nodular colloid goitre
May follow the diffuse type, or may arise *de novo*.

Macroscopical
Nodular enlargement of part, but more usually the whole, of the gland with encapsulated appearance of the nodules. The cut surface is predominantly of a pale brown, colloid appearance with areas of haemorrhage, cyst formation, fibrosis and calcification. Some of these goitres reach an enormous size and they may show retrosternal extension.

Microscopical
The vesicles are distended with colloid and the epithelium is flattened and inactive but a few areas may show residual hyperplastic activity. There may be some areas of focal infiltration by lymphocytes and plasma cells (see p. 130).

Results
The majority of patients are symptom-free and although the gland may enlarge slowly with time, the goitre may be left provided complications do not occur. Plasma levels of T_4 and T_3 are normal.

Complications
1 *Pressure*: especially on the trachea or oesophagus, particularly where there is retrosternal extension.
2 *Haemorrhage*: into the nodules producing a rapid increase in size. This may accentuate the pressure symptoms to a dangerous degree and result in asphyxia.
3 *Toxic change*: one or more nodules may develop secondary toxic changes.
4 *Malignancy*: if this occurs, it is exceedingly rare (see p. 136).

Toxic goitre

Graves' disease—exophthalmic goitre

Incidence
Common.

Age and sex
Usually 20–40 years. Male : female, 1 : 8.

Clinical
Enlargement of the thyroid is usually diffuse or may be slightly nodular. Increased blood flow may be seen, or heard (bruit) pulsing through the enlarged gland. There are associated signs of:
1 Thyroid gland overactivity—weight loss, agitation, tremor, lid lag and stare, atrial fibrillation, etc.
2 The autoimmune process involving other tissues—exophthalmos with or without ophthalmoplegia and, rarely, pretibial myxoedema.

Aetiology

An autoimmune process characterized by the presence of circulating thyroid antibodies. Unlike the antibodies of Hashimoto's disease, these act on the TSH receptor to result in stimulation of the gland. Measurement of these antibodies (variously named thyroid stimulating immunoglobulin—TSI, human thyroid stimulator—HTS, long-acting thyroid stimulator protector—LATSP) is difficult. Thyroid stimulating immunoglobulins may cross the placenta and cause intrauterine thyrotoxicosis in the infant of a woman who has had Graves' disease.

Macroscopical

Diffuse, vascular, fleshy and moderate enlargement of the gland, with lack of colloid seen on the cut surface.

Microscopical

The epithelium is hyperplastic, tall and columnar, often with papillary processes projecting into the thyroid acini. The vesicles are deficient in colloid and show a 'scalloping' of the colloid margins. There is marked vascularity and a variable lymphocytic infiltration frequently with lymph follicle formation. In addition, the changes of focal thyroiditis are present in scattered areas in 20–30% of cases.

Results

Treatment of Graves' disease is aimed at correcting circulating levels of thyroid hormones.

1 *Surgical removal*: partial or subtotal thyroidectomy.

2 *Antithyroid drugs*:

    (a) Iodine, Lugol's iodine. The mechanism by which iodine acts is uncertain. Since its effect is only transient (1–2 weeks), it is employed mainly to decrease vascularity of the thyroid gland, prior to thyroidectomy.

    (b) Carbimazole, propylthiouracil, etc. These act on both iodine trapping and incorporation into iodotyrosine (see p. 128).

3 *Radioactive iodine*: the isotope is administered orally and is selectively taken up in the thyroid gland, causing local involution. The effects of radioiodine continue for many years, and may cause insidious hypothyroidism years after the patient has been lost to follow-up.

Toxic nodular goitre

Occasionally, toxic change occurs in a multinodular colloid goitre. Alternatively, a single autonomous nodule—'hot nodule', may develop. The aetiology is uncertain, although presumed to be autoimmune.

Incidence

Uncommon.

Age

Mostly in the older age group, e.g. middle age and upwards.

Macroscopical

Fleshy areas in one or more nodules of a nodular colloid goitre, or a single, clearly defined nodule.

Microscopical

The changes in multinodular goitre are identical to those found in primary thyrotoxicosis, but arise in a gland also showing changes of a nodular colloid goitre. Areas surrounding a single 'hot nodule' are suppressed.

Clinical

Exophthalmos and pretibial myxoedema do not usually occur. Although antithyroid drugs or radioiodine may be effective, most respond best to partial thyroidectomy.

Others

1 *Trophoblastic tumours*: tumours of placental origin may secrete large amounts of human chorionic gonadotrophin (HCG) which resembles TSH in being a glycoprotein. Either HCG itself, or closely related glycoproteins may have TSH-like activity and cause thyrotoxicosis.

2 *Pituitary*: thyrotoxicosis from excessive production of pituitary TSH occurs, but is extremely rare.

Hypothyroidism

Congenital cretinism

Nature

Hypothyroidism which is manifest at birth.

1 *Endemic*: occurs in the offspring of mothers who have iodine deficiency and who are themselves goitrous.

2 *Sporadic*: thyroid agenesis—failure of the thyroid anlage or arrested development during its descent from the floor of the fetal mouth. There is no goitre. Occurs in 1 : 4000 live births.

3 *Genetic: dyshormonogenetic goitre*—a rare autosomal recessive condition characterized by the inability to synthesize thyroid hormones. As blood T_3 and T_4 levels are low, TSH secretion rises and the gland enlarges. When treated with thyroid hormones, the gland regresses. Dyshormonogenesis may be associated with congenital neural deafness—*Pendred's syndrome*.

Appearances

1 Failure of normal mental and bodily development, particularly of the bones.
2 Dry skin.
3 Coarse facial features with puffed lips.
4 Large tongue.
5 Abdominal distension, often with an umbilical hernia.

Results

Unless treated with thyroid replacement therapy, prognosis is poor. Even when diagnosed early and treated adequately, mental deficiency may still be marked—*cretinism*, as a result of thyroid hormone deficiency *in utero*.

Myxoedema

Nature

Primary hypothyroidism (i.e. not secondary to TSH deficiency) developing after birth.

Age

Mostly occurs in older age groups, but can affect children, when it may present with slowed growth or delay in puberty.

Sex

More common in females.

Incidence

Common. If subclinical cases (i.e. diagnosed on basis of biochemistry alone) are included, may affect up to 2% of the population.

Causes

1 *Iodine deficiency*: very rare. Iodine has to be virtually absent from the diet before myxoedema develops.
2 *Hashimoto's thyroiditis* (see p. 129) and chronic atrophic thyroiditis (see p. 130).

3 *Riedel's thyroiditis* (see p. 131).
4 *Graves' disease*: approximately 5% of patients with thyrotoxicosis develop hypothyroidism in later years, unrelated to any treatment they may have received. Presumably these patients have a spectrum of antithyroid antibodies: some of which stimulate the TSH receptor and some of which are destructive (see p. 133).
5 *Treatment of Graves' disease*: possibly the commonest cause of myxoedema. The condition may be transient (caused by antithyroid drugs) or permanent (following surgery or radioactive iodine). Permanent myxoedema may occur many years after thyrotoxicosis was treated.

Effects

1 *General metabolism*: metabolism is slowed and patients feel cold and lethargic, constipated and mentally dull. Skin is puffy and facial features are coarsened. Hair is lost and the voice is gruff as a result of oedema of the vocal cords.
2 *Myxoedema*: the condition derives its name from the presence of mucinous, protein-rich extra-cellular material in many tissues. Increased albumin leakage occurs from the vessels.
3 *Cardiovascular*: bradycardia is common, as is pericardial effusion.
4 *CNS*: mental slowing, progressing to stupor or coma. Psychosis may occur in some, and may be precipitated by the start of replacement therapy.

Results

Myxoedema usually responds well to thyroxine replacement therapy. However, patients who present in coma have a high mortality.

Tests of thyroid function

In thyroid disease, as in all of endocrinology, the results of function tests must be interpreted in the light of clinical findings.

Thyroxine (T_4)

Total serum thyroxine levels vary from approximately 55 to 130 nmol/l, but the result is largely dependent on circulating levels of thyroid binding globulin (TBG). TBG levels may be low because of congenital deficiency, liver or renal impairment, and may be elevated by pregnancy and the oral contraceptive pill.

Low serum thyroxine is the best indicator of established hypothyroidism.

Tri-iodothyronine (T_3)

Measured T_3 levels are also dependent on TBG concentration, although less so. T_3 is depressed in acute ill-health, especially in the elderly, in liver disease as well as in a variety of other conditions (those in which preferential formation of the biologically inactive, reverse T_3, is formed). In myxoedema T_3 is usually maintained in the normal range until late in the illness. For these reasons low T_3 is not a good guide to hypothyroidism.

High serum T_3 is the best indicator of thyrotoxicosis.

T_3 uptake (T_3 resin uptake: thyroid hormone uptake test)

T_3 uptake tests measure the number of unsaturated thyroid hormone binding sites, and are thus used to indicate TBG concentration. TBG may be measured directly.

Free T_4 (and free T_3) index

Mathematical correction of measured total T_4 (and T_3) dependent on result of T_3 uptake test. The free indices do not, however, correct adequately for large alterations in TBG concentration.

Free T_4 (and free T_3)

Techniques are becoming available to measure only that concentration of thyroid hormone which is unbound (and hence the metabolically active fraction). It seems likely that these techniques will replace the calculated free indices in due course.

TSH

Elevated TSH levels occur in primary hypothyroidism. Because the TSH assay is relatively insensitive, it is not possible to discriminate the suppression of basal TSH which occurs in thyrotoxicosis from normal.

TRH test

The intravenous injection of hypothalamic thyrotrophin releasing hormone (TRH) releases TSH, with a peak at 20 min. Although an exaggerated response may be sought to confirm the diagnosis of myxoedema, the test is usually reserved to confirm thyrotoxicosis: there is no response to TRH in this condition.

Tumours

Benign

Thyroid adenoma

Nature

Solitary or multiple circumscribed nodules in an otherwise normal or, not uncommonly, a multinodular colloid goitre of different histological structure from that of the surrounding distorted, compressed thyroid tissue. They are found in more than 10% of thyroid glands at autopsy.

Types

1 *Follicular adenoma*: these show a varied pattern of large and small, colloid-containing, small-celled microfollicles and columns of somewhat larger cells of alveolar arrangement, mixed or composed wholly of one of these forms. The solid microfollicular nodule is sometimes inappropriately termed *fetal adenoma*.

2 *Hürthle cell adenoma*: oxyphilic cell metaplasia (resembling the Askanazy cells of Hashimoto's disease) may affect most or all of an adenoma.

3 *Atypical adenoma*: these uncommon cellular examples with foci of cells with bizarre giant nuclei have infrequent mitoses and do not invade veins. Their natural history is benign.

4 *Papillary 'adenoma'*: although occasional papillary-like foci are seen in follicular adenomas, true papillary lesions are usually regarded as malignant tumours albeit very well differentiated. This term is therefore best avoided.

5 *Toxic adenoma—'hot nodule'*: some adenomas cause hyperthyroidism unassociated with the presence of thyroid stimulating antibodies in serum (see p. 133).

Behaviour

Histological differentiation of follicular adenoma from well-differentiated follicular carcinoma (see p. 136) can be extremely difficult. Vascular invasion is the most commonly accepted criterion for a diagnosis of malignancy. Capsular penetration is also significant.

It is generally accepted that malignant change from adenoma to follicular carcinoma is rare and that most examples of follicular carcinoma arise *de novo*.

Malignant

Carcinoma of thyroid

Incidence

Geographically variable: in England and Wales 0.3% of deaths from malignant disease with three times as many females as males; about twice this frequency in the goitrous areas of Switzerland and higher still amongst the endemic goitrous zones in Colombia. However, though goitre is common, carcinoma is rare.

Predisposing factors

1 *Nodular goitre*: carries a small increased risk of follicular carcinoma.
2 *Adenomas*: probably only very rarely undergo malignant change (see p. 135).
3 *Radiation*: it is clear that external radiation to the thyroid area causes increased risk of carcinoma, largely papillary but sometimes follicular.
4 *Dyshormogenetic goitre*: adenomas are a consistent feature due to the high TSH levels and atypical hyperplastic features are often seen, though metastatic spread of such lesions is rarely recorded.

Papillary carcinoma

Age

Any age including childhood.

Macroscopical

The primary tumour in the thyroid may be single or multiple and can be quite small and occult. Cystic lesions of the gland should always be carefully examined and if they contain even small amounts of papillary tissue in the lining should be regarded as carcinomas. The papillary structure is usually grossly apparent and the lesions are frequently well circumscribed. Cervical lymph nodes are often enlarged by tumour at original presentation and in many cases this is the first symptom. The term '*lateral aberrant thyroid*' was, at one time, used for a very well-differentiated papillary thyroid carcinomatous deposit which had completely destroyed the lymphoid tissue of the node to which it had metastasized and where the thyroid primary was not clinically apparent. Aberrant thyroid tissue does not, however, occur in this anatomical site, posterior and deep to the sternomastoid muscle.

Microscopical

Papillary fronded tumours, usually exceptionally well differentiated and showing little cytological manifestation of malignancy. Calcified laminated 'psammoma bodies' are seen in about 50%. Most papillary carcinomas have cells with a characteristic large, pale, misshapen nucleus—'Orphan Annie' nuclei.

Foci of follicular pattern may be present but when any true papillary areas are identified the behaviour and terminology are those of papillary carcinoma.

Spread

1 *Direct*: this is seldom clinically significant.
2 *Lymphatic*: cervical lymph node metastases occur in about 50% of cases.
3 *Blood*: this is rare in papillary tumours.

Prognosis

Eighty-five per cent are alive and well at 10 years and 75% at 20 years. The prognosis is less good in older age groups. Most tumours grow slowly and therapy can be conservative with local removal of lymph node metastases.

Follicular carcinoma

Age

Rare under 30 years.

Macroscopical

Most are slowly growing and encapsulated varying from a few centimetres to massive tumours. Usually solid, fleshy and opaque, sometimes with foci of necrosis but uncommonly haemorrhagic.

Microscopical

1 *Slightly invasive*: resembles follicular adenoma but has evidence of sparse vascular invasion, usually after prolonged scrutiny, at the capsular margin and sometimes foci of necrosis.
2 *Overtly invasive*: this type is less common and occurs in older age groups. Direct extension outside the capsule is usually obvious histologically and sometimes grossly. Solid pleomorphic foci, numerous mitotic figures, foci of necrosis and marked venous invasion are usual features.

Spread

1 *Direct*: important in the overtly invasive type.
2 *Lymphatic*: relatively common.

3 *Blood*: metastatic deposits in bone or lungs are not infrequent but may themselves be very slowly growing.

Behaviour

Thyroidectomy is the treatment of choice. The long-term prognosis is excellent in the slightly invasive tumours but 5-year survival is only 50% in the overtly invasive and 30% at 10 years.

Radioactive iodine therapy in differentiated carcinoma

Therapy by radioiodine may be very effective in both papillary and follicular differentiated thyroid carcinomas. Uptake by the tumour, both primary and metastatic, is considerably assisted if the normal thyroid tissue is first ablated by total thyroidectomy.

Anaplastic carcinoma

This highly malignant tumour accounts for 10–15% of thyroid carcinomas. It is most frequent in the elderly and usually presents with a short history and a clinically obvious malignant local appearance. Lymphatic and blood spread is common and death is usually inevitable 6–12 months after diagnosis.

Histologically, though follicular elements may be seen, the dominant features are of either a spindle-cell tumour with or without giant cell areas or a small cell pattern which may be difficult to differentiate from lymphoma (see below) (immunocytochemistry is now usually diagnostic). Squamous cell carcinomas rarely occur.

Medullary carcinoma

Nature

A malignant tumour of C cells (see p. 127) and thus hormonally active in production of calcitonin and other substances.

Age and incidence

About 10% of thyroid carcinomas—mostly in persons over 40 years but also in the young where it is commonly familial, multiple and associated with other endocrine tumours (see p. 139)—*MEN syndromes IIA, IIB*.

Macroscopical

Grey, discrete but not encapsulated and sometimes multiple. Mostly 2–3 cm and with cervical lymph node metastases in about 50% of cases.

Microscopical

Nests and masses of closely packed eosinophilic, granular, polygonal cells with, characteristically, *amyloid* material in the stroma. The cells contain neurosecretory granules.

Spread

1 *Direct*: marked tendency to extend into superior mediastinum.
2 *Lymphatic*: common.
3 *Blood*: common in fatal cases in bones, lungs and liver.

Prognosis

If no lymph node spread at time of diagnosis normal life expectancy. If lymph node positive 42% 10-year survival.

Associated factors

About 5% of medullary carcinomas are familial with autosomal dominant inheritance. These families show high incidence of adrenal phaeochromocytomas, often bilateral, and may also have neurofibromas of skin, ganglioneuromas of intestinal plexuses, parathyroid adenoma and diarrhoea in addition to rather characteristic facies and body habitus.

Some tumours secrete not only calcitonin but also 5-hydroxytryptamine or corticotrophin.

Non-epithelial malignant tumours

Lymphomas

Primary non-Hodgkin's lymphoma of the thyroid is probably more common than originally believed, as many examples were previously included in the anaplastic carcinoma group. The patients are mainly elderly with a short history of fleshy enlargement of one or both of the lobes of the gland. Histologically, these are mostly of *MALT*-like type and B cell (see p. 37). It is likely that some cases arise in pre-existing Hashimoto's disease.

In most cases the prognosis is bad with death in a few months, but a few live for some, or many, years after X-ray or cytotoxic therapy.

Other tumours

Sarcomas occasionally occur and the thyroid gland may be involved by blood spread in disseminated carcinoma arising from many sites, e.g. breast, lung or malignant melanoma.

D/PARATHYROIDS

Normal
Primary hyperparathyroidism
Secondary hyperparathyroidism
Tertiary hyperparathyroidism
Hypoparathyroidism

Normal

There are usually two pairs of glands, each pale yellow–brown in colour and up to 0.5 cm diameter. Together they weigh about 0.1 g. The upper pair are fairly constant in position in relation to the posterior aspect of the superior poles of the thyroid gland. The lower pair are more inconsistent in position, often being found in the carotid sheath or in the mediastinum.

Microscopical

Nests or cords of epithelial cells in a vascular fibro-fatty stroma. With advancing age increasing amounts of fat appear in the glands.

Cell types

1 *Chief cells*: most numerous, with the 'water clear' cell as a vacuolated variant.
2 *Oxyphil cells*: these increase in number with age.

Functions

Parathyroid hormone (PTH) secreted by the parathyroid glands acts on bone to increase calcium resorption, and on the kidney in three ways:
1 Increase in calcium reabsorption.
2 Increase in phosphate excretion.
3 Increase in 1-hydroxylation, i.e. activation of vitamin D.

The combined effect of these actions is to raise serum calcium and to lower serum phosphate.

Congenital abnormalities

Abnormalities in number (2–5), or position, e.g. mediastinum, are relatively common and are of importance to the exploring surgeon.

Primary hyperparathyroidism

Causes

1 *Tumour*: 85%. Malignancy is rare.
2 *Hyperplasia*: 15%.

Incidence

Common, affecting approximately 0.1% of the population. In many cases the biochemical abnormality induced is very mild.

Macroscopical

1 *Adenoma*: usually solitary but multiple in 1% of cases; 75% occur in the lower glands. They are orange-brown, well encapsulated nodules of very variable size but are seldom more than 1 cm diameter. They have a homogeneous cut surface.
2 *Hyperplasia*: all the glands are enlarged with an average total weight of 19 g.
3 *Carcinoma*: these tumours usually resemble adenomas but are poorly encapsulated or sometimes frankly invasive.

Microscopical

The histological appearances vary markedly. In more than 50% the chief cell is dominant and in most of the remainder there is a mixture of cell types. Only rarely are 'pure' water-clear cell or oxyphil cell lesions found. Hyperplastic glands may be either diffuse or variably nodular in appearance.

Diagnosis of autonomous functional adenoma(s) from hyperplasia is important and may be difficult unless the appearances of all the parathyroids are known. In individual glands a helpful feature may be the presence of a rim of 'normal', though compressed, parathyroid tissue around the capsule of an adenoma. The presence of fat in enlarged glands suggests hyperplasia rather than adenoma.

Effects

Elevated secretion of PTH results in elevation of serum calcium. The elevated calcium may result in rather non-specific symptoms of polyuria, depression, constipation or it may result in calcification in blood vessels, renal substance (nephrocalcinosis) or urinary tract (stone formation) (see p. 180). Most frequently hypercalcaemia is detected as the result of routine calcium measurement. PTH results in excessive bone resorption by the osteoclasts and this may be detected as subperiosteal erosions in the phalanges. Rarely, the osteoclasts form large aggregations and the resultant swelling (brown tumour, von Recklinghausen's disease of bone) may be the presenting complaint (see p. 301).

Diagnosis
In the majority of cases the diagnosis is biochemical, and not clinical and depends on the demonstration of raised serum calcium with inappropriately elevated PTH, together with any or all of: decreased fasting serum phosphate, decreased tubular reabsorption of phosphate, increased tubular reabsorption of calcium, increased urinary hydroxyproline excretion and increased serum alkaline phosphatase.

Results
Surgical extirpation usually results in cure, although on occasion the disease recurs or it may not be possible to localize all hyperfunctioning glands. Visualization of enlarged glands by scanning techniques has enabled more accurate exploration. Carcinomas are usually slow-growing and tend to spread locally.

Associated conditions
Chief cell hyperplasia is a characteristic finding in patients with the syndrome of *multiple endocrine neoplasia type 1—pluriglandular 'adenomatosis'*, in which hyperplasia with variable nodularity of the parathyroids is associated with adenomas of the anterior lobe of pituitary, pancreatic islets and adrenal cortex, sometimes with foregut carcinoid tumours (see p. 36).

A further association occurs in *multiple endocrine neoplasia type 2*, in which nodular parathyroid hyperplasia is familialy present along with medullary carcinoma of the thyroid (see p. 137) and adrenal phaeochromocytomas (see p. 119).

Secondary hyperparathyroidism

Nature
Compensatory hyperplasia of the parathyroid glands occurs in conditions which lower blood calcium or raise the blood inorganic phosphorus level.

Causes
1 Chronic renal failure and some renal tubular disorders (see p. 300).
2 Steatorrhoea and other malabsorption syndromes (see p. 34).
3 Pregnancy and lactation.

Macroscopical
All the glands are enlarged but to a much less degree than in the hyperplastic type of primary hyperparathyroidism.

Microscopical
There is increase in the 'water clear' cells and chief cells, associated with loss of stromal fat cells.

Diagnosis
The diagnosis, which is usually presumptive and only of importance in renal failure, depends upon the demonstration of elevated PTH, alkaline phosphatase and radiological changes—'rugger-jersey spine' (see p. 301). Serum calcium is low to normal, while phosphate is elevated as a result of the underlying renal disease.

Tertiary hyperparathyroidism
Chronic overstimulation of the parathyroid glands in renal failure may result in one or more becoming autonomous, with resultant hypercalcaemia.

Hypoparathyroidism

Causes
1 *Surgery*: temporary or permanent hypoparathyroidism may result from neck surgery, including treatment of hyperparathyroidism.
2 *Autoimmune hypoparathyroidism*: the presence of circulating antiparathyroid antibodies leads to atrophy of the glands, with decreased PTH secretion and tendency to hypocalcaemia. The disease may pursue an insidious course for many years and non-specific symptoms of dizziness, gastrointestinal upset, etc., may not point to the diagnosis.

Effects
Hypoparathyroidism may result in:
1 Tetany.
2 Tendency to abdominal discomfort and diarrhoea.
3 Epilepsy.
4 Chronic monilial infection of the skin and nails.
5 Cataract.

Apart from 1 and 2, these are rare in surgically induced hypoparathyroidism, perhaps because the disease is more abrupt in onset and hence more frequently recognized early.

Diagnosis
Depends on the demonstration of hypocalcaemia (which cannot be explained by coincidental hypoalbu-

minaemia) together with tendency to high serum phosphate and inappropriately low PTH. Parathyroid antibodies may be demonstrated. In the differential diagnosis it is important to exclude hypomagnesaemia.

Results

Treatment with cholecalciferol, with or without oral calcium supplements, leads to resolution of all but cataract and, possibly, any tendency to epilepsy.

Chapter 9
Diseases of the Eye

A/EYELIDS, CONJUNCTIVA, CORNEA

Eyelids
  Inflammations
  Cysts
  Tumours
Conjunctiva
  Conjunctivitis
  Degenerations
  Cysts
  Tumours
Cornea
  Keratitis
  Dystrophies
  Degenerations
  Tumours

Eyelids

Inflammations

Stye—hordeolum
Staphylococcal infection of an eyelash follicle and its associated gland of Zeis. There is cellulitis of the lid followed by localization and pointing, usually at the lid margin.

Chalazion

Nature
A chronic granuloma developing within an obstructed Meibomian gland.

Appearances
A firm and painless lump usually in the upper lid, composed of granulation tissue rich in epithelioid and giant cells. The whole reactive area is surrounded by fibrous tissue, but multiple clear small cystic spaces are present in the main mass containing lipid material. Confusion with tuberculosis may arise but caseation and organisms are not present.

Molluscum contagiosum
This warty swelling with an umbilicated centre is caused by a virus infection of the prickle cells. This skin lesion is described on p. 416.

Cysts

Sudosiferous
The clear cyst which arises due to duct obstruction of the modified sweat gland of Moll.

Sebaceous
These cysts arise within the sebaceous Zeis's gland.

Dermoid
Inclusion dermoids, associated with the suture lines in the orbital bones, may extend into the lids. They are most commonly present at the outer angle of the orbit—*external angular dermoid*.

Meibomian
Blockage of the duct of a Meibomian gland may result in a cyst lined by flattened epithelium.

Tumours

Benign

Xanthelasma

Nature
This lesion may be a manifestation of a hypercholesterolaemic condition, e.g. diabetes, or occur as an isolated lesion, particularly in middle-aged women.

Appearances
An elevated yellowish plaque usually situated near the inner canthus—*Xanthelasma palpebrum*, containing large lipid-rich foam cells.

141

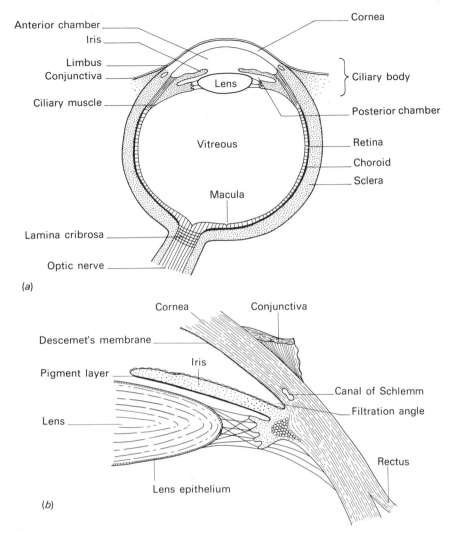

Fig. 14 (a) The eye. Diagram of the main structures. (b) Ciliary body and adjacent structures.

Neurofibroma
In von Recklinghausen's disease, the eyelid is frequently involved by extension of neurofibromas from the frontotemporal region and orbit.

Squamous cell papilloma
These are simple sessile or pedunculated papillary tumours of the squamous epithelium and are commonly seen on the lids.

Seborrhoeic keratosis
These pigmented skin lesions are very common in this site (see p. 415).

Lipoma
Adipose tissue is not normally present in the lid, thus lipomas only occur in this situation as extensions from the orbital fat.

Benign calcifying epithelioma of Malherbe
This uncommon lesion shows calcifying squamous epithelium in the dermis. The condition is entirely benign and occurs at any skin site, especially in children.

Haemangioma
All types occur in the lid, identical to similar lesions in other cutaneous sites. The cavernous variety may be

associated with haemangiomas and cysts elsewhere—von Hippel–Lindau disease (see p. 154).

Lymphangioma
Rarely found in the lids.

Naevus
These are common lesions of the lids and occur as compound, junctional and intradermal types (see p. 417).

Malignant

Primary acquired melanosis
See p. 145.

Intra-epidermal carcinoma
See p. 145.

Squamous cell carcinoma
This tumour behaves in a similar manner to squamous cell carcinoma elsewhere in the skin. There is an irregular ulcerated area which is capable of causing extensive lid destruction with invasion of surrounding structures.

Basal cell carcinoma—rodent ulcer
This is the most common malignant tumour of eyelids; indeed this is one of the commonest sites for such a tumour to develop. There is at first a small nodule, later an ulcerated centre and a rolled edge. Direct invasion of adjacent structures may result in a very considerable area of destruction involving the globe, orbit and adjacent bone (see p. 416).

Malignant melanoma
This arises in a pre-existing naevus or in an area of pre-cancerous melanosis (see p. 145).

Adenocarcinoma
This is an uncommon tumour which can arise in the sebaceous glands of Zeis, Meibomian glands, sweat glands of Moll or the accessory lacrimal gland of Krause.

Sarcoma
Very rare, but types reported include spindle cell, round cell, angiosarcoma, myxosarcoma, leiomyosarcoma and rhabdomyosarcoma.

Lymphoma
Hodgkin's and non-Hodgkin's deposits and leukaemic tissue are very occasionally seen in the lids.

Conjunctiva

Inflammations

Simple bacterial conjunctivitis

Acute
Conjunctivitis is extremely common and may be due to a large number of different organisms of variable pathogenicity. The condition usually resolves completely with local treatment.

Chronic
Usually arises as a continuation of acute conjunctivitis with only slight discharge, although the lids feel heavy and gritty. Microscopically, there is a mild chronic inflammatory cell infiltrate and epithelial hyperplasia.

Follicular conjunctivitis
A response to many irritants including viral and toxic agents. Pinhead-sized elevations, often in rows, occur on the conjunctiva of the lower lid. They are composed of aggregations of mononuclear cells in the subepithelial layer; in those cases due to chlamydial infection, inclusion bodies may be demonstrable.

Trachoma—chlamydia trachomatis

Nature
This important chlamydial infection is one of the most common cause of blindness in the world, being particularly frequent in Africa and the East.

The organism is closely related to that of virus inclusion conjunctivitis—*Chlamydia oculogenitale*, an acute viral conjunctivitis of newborn.

The sexual partners of trachoma sufferers are frequently found to harbour the infective agent in the urethra or cervix and babies born to mothers with cervicitis and/or trachoma, have been found to have the agent in their conjunctivae.

Macroscopical
In the early stages, there is an acute conjunctivitis but eventually extensive conjunctival and corneal scarring ensues. The diagnosis can be made with certainty in the early stages by the demonstration of inclusion bodies in desquamated epithelial cells. Immunocytochemistry is also diagnostic.

Microscopical

In the acute stage there is a heavy mononuclear cell infiltration, both diffuse and aggregated into follicles. This is accompanied by epithelial proliferation with invaginations and downgrowths which may become sequestrated to form pseudocysts. Later, the follicles are composed of pale-staining macrophages surrounded by lymphocytes and plasma cells. These follicles eventually rupture through the epithelium, or are absorbed and replaced by scar tissue with resulting lid deformity. Moreover, the inflammatory process extends into the cornea as a pannus starting at the limbus. Bowman's membrane is destroyed and blood vessels migrate into the substantia propria with inevitable scarring and opacity leading to blindness. Antibiotic therapy may cure the condition.

Spring catarrh—vernal conjunctivitis

Nature

Occurs in springtime, mostly in young boys, due to a reaction to exogenous allergens, e.g. pollen and moulds.

Macroscopical

The lid conjunctiva shows an hyperaemic 'cobblestone' appearance, associated with a considerable mucoid discharge rich in eosinophils.

Microscopical

There is proliferation of the goblet cells and the subepithelial tissues. The 'cobbles' and pseudo-cysts are formed from the epithelial invaginations in a similar way to those of trachoma. An infiltration of mononuclear cells and eosinophils is later replaced by fibrous tissue. Follicles are not formed.

Tuberculosis

Primary lesions are rare and secondary infections uncommon but may occur by extension of disease from the lacrimal gland, lacrimal sac and lids.

Phylctenular conjunctivitis

Nature

Although this condition can occur as an allergic reaction to any protein substance, most cases are caused by tuberculoprotein hypersensitivity.

Appearances

Pinkish-yellow spots in the conjunctival epithelium, limbus and cornea with, except in the cornea, surrounding vascular engorgement and with an exudate within the subepithelial tissues containing leucocytes and mononuclear cells. No tuberculous giant cell systems are found.

Sarcoidosis

Incidence

Ocular involvement occurs in about 25% of cases of this systemic granulomatous disease (see p. 394).

Appearances

The conjunctiva may show pinhead-sized sarcoid lesions in the fold between the bulbar and palpebral conjunctiva—lower fornix.

Degenerations

Ageing

With increasing age, the conjunctiva loses its clear whiteness and becomes slightly roughened and less transparent. The epithelium shows a tendency to keratinization and the subepithelial tissues become hyalinized and thinned.

Pinguecula

Nature

Exposure to sun, wind and dust enhances degenerative changes, especially at the interpalpebral margin of the cornea.

Macroscopical

A raised, opaque, triangular, yellow spot close to the limbus, usually on the nasal side.

Microscopical

There is patchy atrophy and thickening of the epithelium with elastosis and subsequent hyalinization and fragmentation.

Concretions

Nature

White or yellow spots within the tarsal conjunctiva of elderly or debilitated persons, due to obstructed serous glands containing inspissated epithelial cells and mucus which form concentrically laminated bodies. They may calcify and thus damage the corneal epithelium.

Cysts

Traumatic
Implanted epithelium, particularly goblet cells, may form a mucinous cyst surrounded by a fibrous capsule.

Retention
These vary greatly in size and may arise from mucous glands, from the epithelial downgrowths of trachoma and spring catarrh, or within Krause's gland.

Lymphatic
Thin-walled dilated lymphatics may rarely be seen on the bulbar conjunctiva.

Tumours

Benign

Papilloma
These sessile or pedunculated epithelial papillomas frequently arise around the caruncle and are rich in goblet cells.

Epithelial plaque
A whitish area at the limbus consisting of simple and regular proliferation of the epithelial layer, with or without keratinization.

Naevus
In addition to the usual types of naevi seen elsewhere, there is a particular form found only in the conjunctiva: *cystic naevus of conjunctiva*: a smooth, variably pigmented, mobile nodule composed of downgrowths of epithelium which form cystic structures and are surrounded by naevus cells.

Haemangioma
Capillary or cavernous types occasionally occur.

Dermolipoma
A yellow, triangular, congenital tumour which presents between the superior and external rectus muscles. The fatty element is continuous with the orbital fat and, in addition, there are hair follicles,

sebaceous and sweat glands. The mass is covered by thickened conjunctival epithelium.

Malignant

Intra-epidermal carcinoma—Bowen's disease
This carcinoma in situ is similar to that of the skin (see p. 416). Initially it remains localized as a reddish-grey plaque at the limbus or lid margin. Eventually after several years, if untreated, it becomes frankly invasive and subsequently behaves as a squamous cell carcinoma. The irregular and atypical epithelial overgrowth is confined by an intact basement membrane until invasive characteristics appear.

Squamous cell carcinoma
This may arise *de novo*, or from a papilloma, an epithelial plaque or in an area of Bowen's disease. It is seen as a warty non-pigmented tumour in the elderly and is most frequently found at the limbus from whence it may spread across the cornea and invade adjacent tissues.

Basal cell carcinoma
Primary basal cell tumours of the conjunctiva do not occur due to the absence of basal type cells. However, extension from a lid rodent ulcer may cause a secondary tumour.

Primary acquired melanosis—precancerous melanosis

Macroscopical
This may occur in both the skin of the lid and conjunctiva, and first appears in middle age. The lesions are flat, irregular and variably pigmented, commonly of a widespread and bespattered 'gunshot' distribution.

Microscopical
There is intra-epithelial proliferation of pigmented basal epithelial cells over a wide area resulting in a multilayered structure. Bud-like clusters of cells may extend into the dermis but the lesion remains precancerous for a variable period of time and is analogous to a junctional naevus except for its widespread distribution (see p. 417). Malignant melanoma develops within 5–10 years in 15–20% of cases.

Malignant melanoma

Arises most frequently from precancerous melanosis but may also develop in a previously simple naevus present from birth—*congenital ocular melanocytosis*. Compared with skin melanomas prognosis is markedly better.

Benign lymphoma

This sharply demarcated, pinkish fleshy nodular lesion is reactive with benign behaviour. The lymphoid cells are polymorphous with prominent follicle formation.

Malignant lymphoma

Leukaemic deposits, non-Hodgkin's and Hodgkin's lymphoma, are occasionally found in the conjunctiva as a manifestation of generalization of these diseases.

Cornea

Inflammations—keratitis

Ulcers

Marginal

Simple catarrhal

Commonly associated with acute conjunctivitis due to staphylococci or the Koch–Weeks bacillus. A small ulcer develops in the marginal corneal epithelium and is accompanied by an inflammatory cell infiltration. Healing rapidly occurs when the infection is eliminated, and corneal perforation is rare.

Mooren's ulcer

This occurs in the elderly and is usually bilateral. A shallow ulcer with an overhanging edge forms at the corneal margin and there is a chronic inflammatory cell infiltration with some necrosis of the superficial substantia propria. The ulcer may extend across the entire corneal surface but perforation is uncommon.

Central

Central ulcers usually commence as primary pyogenic infections of the cornea. An example is the hypopyon ulcer.

Hypopyon ulcer

Macroscopical. A corneal ulcer associated with cloudy exudate within the anterior chamber.

Microscopical. Acute and chronic inflammatory cells are present in the region of the ulcer and also infiltrate the iris, ciliary body and anterior chamber forming a sterile but cloudy exudate—hypopyon. There is necrosis of the substantia propria, the filtration angles are occluded by exudate and the iris margin frequently adheres to the lens. Thus, anterior and posterior synechiae are formed.

Results. The ulcer either penetrates all layers with resulting perforation or heals with the formation of dense scar tissue.

Herpes simplex ulceration

This virus infection is a relatively common condition and a significant cause of corneal scarring due to repeated attacks.

Sequelae of corneal ulceration

Opacities
Due to scarring.

Facet
A shallow surface depression resulting from loss of tissue.

Ectatic cicatrix
An outward bulging of scar tissue.

Descemetocoele
Ulceration may leave only Descemet's membrane—the innermost layer, which, as a result of intra-ocular pressure, may bulge outwards.

Perforation
Rupture of the cornea, which may be followed by prolapse of the lens and iris through the perforation.

Anterior staphyloma
If a corneal perforation becomes sealed by the iris and the anterior surface is later epithelialized, intra-ocular pressure may cause bulging of the 'plug' producing the staphylomatous deformity.

Interstitial keratitis

Nature
Inflammation of the deeper layers of the cornea.

Origin

Although sometimes the result of extension from superficial inflammatory lesions, this is more usually syphilitic in origin or due to tuberculosis, leprosy, onchocerciasis or sarcoidosis.

Appearances

The fibres of the substantia propria become swollen and later necrotic. Vessels and lymphocytes infiltrate from the limbus and there is degeneration of Descemet's membrane. The superficial layers are not involved.

Results

Dense opacity of the cornea follows.

Corneal dystrophies

Hereditary bilateral degenerations of the cornea, usually appearing at the time of puberty. There are three main types.

Granular

Hyaline nodules in all layers with clear intervening zones.

Macular

Central hyaline nodules with opacity of the intervening stroma.

Lattice

Superficial, doubly contoured, bifurcating lines of granular and hyaline material crossing one another.

Degenerations

Arcus senilis

This presents in middle age, is caused by fatty infiltration and appears as a pale ring at the periphery. The outer border is sharply defined but the inner margin indefinite.

Pannus degenerativus

This occurs in eyes which are either senile or in which there has been longstanding inflammation. There is vascularization and round cell infiltration in the superficial layers at the margin with overlying epithelial thickening. The central cornea remains unaffected.

Pterygium

A sun damage induced wing-shaped ingrowth of conjunctival epithelium appearing on the nasal or lateral sides of the cornea and progressing towards its centre. Dysplastic atypicality are common, associated with the underlying solar elastosis.

Keratoconus—conical cornea

Probably has both a congenital and a degenerative aetiology and appears at puberty as apical bulging, rendering the patient grossly myopic. There is thinning of the central cornea.

Tumours

The majority of corneal tumours have their origin in the conjunctiva or limbus but primary lesions which have occasionally been described include the following.

Epithelial plaques

Benign overgrowth of squamous cells.

Squamous cell carcinoma

Usually arising within an epithelial plaque or pterygium.

Fibroma

Following corneal trauma.

Dermoid

A fibro-fatty mass with projecting hairs.

B/LENS, UVEAL TRACT, RETINA

Lens
   Structure
   Cataract
   Pseudo-exfoliation
Uveal tract
   Uveitis
Retina
   Vascular
   Retrolental fibroplasia
   Degenerations
   Cysts
   Congenital
   Glaucoma

Lens

Structure

The lens is a unique avascular structure formed entirely by epithelium. It is enclosed by a hyaline capsule; beneath this is the epithelium which produces the keratinized lens fibres. These, as they mature, become backed into the centre to form the 'nucleus' of the lens which inevitably becomes both larger and denser with advancing age.

Cataract

Nature
Any opacity of the lens.

Lens changes
There are two main senile types.

Nuclear cataract—hard
This is an extension and intensification of the physiological sclerosis which occurs with ageing. The fibres of the nucleus are progressively compressed at the centre into laminated layers which coalesce to form a homogeneous opaque mass.

Cortical cataract—soft
In this type the changes occur in the cortical fibres that surround the central nucleus. These fibres become oedematous with the deposition of albuminous material which coalesces to form Morgagnian globules; it is this denatured protein material which forms the opacity. Finally the entire lens cortex becomes a pultaceous mass of globules and granular debris enclosed within the capsule.

Clinical types

Congenital cataract
This is usually of the nuclear type and the condition may be familial as an autosomal dominant. In other cases it is associated with multiple intra-ocular congenital abnormalities, but some cases presenting at birth are due to maternal rubella infection during pregnancy.

Senile cataract
This is the common form of lenticular opacity which becomes increasingly frequent with advancing age. The lens may show either the nuclear or cortical form of cataract. If the latter form occurs, the altered and liquefied lens material may remain within the lens capsule but frequently this ruptures and releases material into the globe resulting in absorption without reaction or *phagolytic glaucoma* or lens-induced uveitis—*phacoanaphylactic endophthalmitis*, due to an immunologically mediated granulomatous reaction to lens antigens (see p. 150).

Other types of cataract

Traumatic
Following penetration of the lens, the capsule retracts away from the area of injury. The defect is frequently filled by optically dense reparative fibres.

Complicated cataract
A cataract following other intra-ocular diseases, e.g. iridocyclitis, retinitis pigmentosa, choroidoretinitis, detached retina, etc.

Diabetic cataract
In severe cases of diabetes in young individuals, a bilateral and rapidly progressive form of cataract frequently occurs. Elderly diabetics are also prone to cataract but it is then indistinguishable from the senile type.

Cataract due to physical causes
Lens opacities may follow exposure to ionizing radiations, lightning or electric shocks; glassworker's cataract occurs due to damage by heat whilst intra-ocular metallic objects, especially iron and copper, may also induce a lens opacity.

After or secondary cataract
This is the development of an opacity in the intra-capsular lens residue after nuclear extraction. This is largely due to epithelial proliferation which grows through the capsule incision on to its outer surface and is followed by adhesions to other intra-ocular structures.

Pseudo-exfoliation of the lens capsule
A collection of fluffy white material of unknown composition which forms within the anterior chamber, on the surface of the iris, ciliary body, zonules and lens capsule. The material shows eosinophilic staining, and is of a feathery shrub-like appearance. It may peel off the lens surface and be carried to the filtration angles resulting in glaucoma.

Uveal tract
The uveal tract consists of the iris, the ciliary body and the choroid.

Inflammations—uveitis

Non-specific

Acute uveitis

Origin
Arising from perforating wounds, corneal ulcers or septicaemic conditions.

Macroscopical
Purulent infection of the uveal tract—*purulent endophthalmitis*. Localization and abscess formation usually occur with subsequent fibrosis, intra-ocular disorganization, contraction of the entire globe, calcification and ossification—*phthisis bulbi*.

An even more widespread infection of the eye involving the retina and vitreous in addition—*panophthalmitis*—may result in abscess formation within the vitreous with danger of global rupture.

Microscopical
The predominant picture is a widespread polymorph infiltration of the affected tissues. When localization takes place fibrosis occurs, its extent varying with the size of the inflammatory mass. If confined to the anterior segment, dense scar tissue may form on the anterior surface of the iris covering the pupil—*occlusio pupillae*, and the filtration angles may become occluded—*peripheral anterior synechiae*. In the posterior segment, localization leads to abscess formation within the vitreous where the organisms are free from inhibiting structures. Regression is followed by fibrosis in the form of a transverse membrane—*cyclitic membrane*, which, by contraction, may detach the retina, if this has not already occurred due to a subretinal purulent exudate.

Chronic uveitis
The distinction between acute and chronic uveitis is not always clearly defined, but in the usual non-specific infections by organisms of low pathogenicity, the appearances in the uveal tract are as follows.

Iris
There is a focal chronic inflammatory infiltration, heavy in the region of the sphincter muscles. Adhesions in the filtration angles—*peripheral anterior synechiae*, commonly develop and eversion of the pupillary margin—*ectropion uveae*, may occur due to

fibrosis. Posterior synechiae, adhesions between the iris and lens, usually form and thus the entire pupillary margin becomes adherent to the lens—*seclusio pupillae*. Rising intra-ocular tension is then inevitable and causes the anchored iris to balloon forwards—'*iris bombé*', narrowing even further the anterior chamber. The pigmented epithelium shows patchy degeneration and proliferation, whilst chronic inflammatory cells wander from the iris into the anterior chamber and aggregate in small clumps on the corneal endothelium—'*keratitis punctata*'.

Ciliary body
There is fibrosis and a chronic inflammatory cell infiltration, usually focal and maximal posteriorly.

Choroid
Dense focal aggregations of lymphocytes and scattered plasma cells which may extend into the retina destroying the pigmented epithelium and outer layers—*choroidoretinitis*. Healing causes dense sclerotic patches within the choroid and overlying retina and the formation of small round hyaline nodules—*colloid bodies*, which may distort the retinal surface.

Granulomatous

Tuberculosis
This is almost always secondary.

Iris and ciliary body
An exudate is unusual but pale 'mutton-fat' precipitates of endothelial cells may be deposited on the posterior surface of the cornea.

Choroid
This layer may be involved as part of a generalized miliary tuberculosis but more commonly appears as chronic tuberculous choroiditis. Both eyes commonly show typical caseating tuberculous granulation tissue, often involving the retina. Healing is prolonged, with frequent relapses.

Syphilis
Manifestations are common in congenital syphilis. In the acquired disease iridocyclitis is common in the secondary stage and gummatous choroiditis extending frequently to the retina and sclera is seen in tertiary syphilis.

Sarcoidosis

Sarcoid granulomas are found in the iris, ciliary body and choroid. The eye is affected at some stage in about 40% of cases of the systemic disease.

Toxoplasmosis

In both congenital and adult types, the disease is mostly confined to the choroid but with infrequent retinal and scleral involvement. Focal granulomatous lesions may be mistaken for those of tuberculosis. Diagnosis is made by the finding of the protozoon— *Toxoplasma gondii*, either in pseudo-cysts or extracellularly (see p. 6).

Toxocara canis

The migrating larvae of the dog nematode, *Toxocara canis*, are capable of lodging in the uveal tract of children forming a granulomatous lesion. On ophthalmoscopy this can closely resemble a neoplasm.

Lens-induced uveitis— phagoanaphylactic endophthalmitis

Nature

Following the release of lens protein in the opposite eye at an earlier date, release of protein in the second eye may precipitate an anaphylactic anterior uveitis (see below).

Appearances

The eye is acutely inflamed. The iris, ciliary body, anterior choroid and cortex of the ruptured lens are infiltrated by eosinophils, polymorphs, plasma cells, lymphocytes, giant cells, macrophages and endothelial cells. Glaucoma is a common sequel.

Sympathetic ophthalmitis

Nature

This is a bilateral cellular reaction of the entire uveal tract following a penetrative injury to one eye—the 'exciting' eye, 2 weeks to 1 year previously. The response in the non-injured, 'sympathizing' eye, can be avoided if the injured 'exciting' eye is urgently enucleated within 1 week of the injury. If sympathetic ophthalmitis is allowed to proceed, blindness in both eyes is inevitable.

Pathogenesis

It is believed that this is an autoimmune reaction in both eyes to uveal pigment released on injury of the 'exciting' eye.

Macroscopical

Clinically, both eyes resemble any of the other granulomatous conditions previously described. Evidence of previous injury to the 'exciting' eye is present but it is the only feature distinguishing the two eyes.

Microscopical

The cellular reaction is contained almost entirely within the uveal tract and consists of:
1 A massive infiltration of lymphocytes.
2 Collections of endothelial cells with scattered giant cells.
3 Eosinophils.
4 Dalen–Fuch's nodules—aggregations of the above cells between the retina and the choroid.
5 Perivascular collections in the sclera and tumour-like cellular aggregations on its outer surface.

The retina remains intact except for slight thinning over the Dalen–Fuch's nodules.

Retina

Vascular diseases

General features

The central artery of the optic nerve, although structurally similar to other arteries of similar size, loses its elastic tissue after the first and second divisions and the muscle separates into isolated fibres leaving a wall composed of endothelium and adventitia only. Thus vascular disease in the retina varies somewhat from arterial lesions elsewhere. Moreover the vessels are readily visible through an ophthalmoscope so that changes seen in this way may provide important information regarding the state of the vascular system in general.

Involutionary sclerosis

An ageing process not associated with hypertension but in which arterioles are narrowed, pale and variable in calibre. Histologically, there is fibrosis and patchy endothelial proliferation.

Arteriolar sclerotic retinopathy

Nature

Retinal changes associated with hypertension (see p. 83).

Appearance—benign hypertension

Early. Narrowing due to endothelial proliferation and deposition of hyaline material. This produces the characteristic 'copper and silver wire' ophthalmoscopic appearance.

Later. Segmental dilatation due to hypertension results in tortuosity and compression at the arteriovenous crossings.

Late. Eventually thin, white, parallel lines of fatty material surround the vessels—'pipe-stem sheathing'. Retinal haemorrhages occur but are small and are usually rapidly absorbed.

Accelerated hypertension

Papilloedema, exudates and small haemorrhages are present. The vessels show irregular narrowing and areas of fibrinoid necrosis with surrounding extravasated blood.

Atheroma

Although the retinal artery is not a common site of atheroma, when present it may cause vascular occlusion and serious atrophy of the inner retinal layers. The outer layers are supplied by choroidal vessels and are thus unaffected.

Cytoid bodies

These are fluffy white patches in the retina which are found in cases of accelerated hypertension, systemic lupus erythematosus and dermatomyositis. The cytoid body is actually a nodular swelling on the injured axon—Cajal node, and consists of an eosinophilic pseudo-nucleus lying within a 'cytoplasm' of swollen axon material.

Central retinal vein thrombosis— thrombotic glaucoma

Thrombosis of retinal veins at points of arteriovenous crossing. This occurs in hypertensives and frequently at the site of global entry of the optic nerve—*lamina cribrosa*. Retinal haemorrhagic infarction follows and new vessels grow on the surface of the iris and into the filtration angles, thus leading to glaucoma. In the area of the retina drained by the thrombosed vein, haemorrhages occur in great numbers and the veins are engorged. At a later stage the retinal haemorrhages are absorbed, leaving cystic spaces and the thrombus may partially recanalize. Cupping of the optic nerve head follows the glaucomatous rise of intra-ocular pressure.

Diabetic retinopathy

Both retinae are affected, the first abnormality being the appearance of 'dot' haemorrhages due to capillary microaneurysms. Later, the aneurysms rupture, producing 'blot' haemorrhages, accompanied by small yellow–white exudates which may become confluent. Haemorrhages spread into the vitreous, provoking development of new blood vessels and fibrous tissue— 'retinitis proliferans'. This condition frequently leads to retinal detachment degeneration and ultimately *phthisis bulbi*.

Eales's disease

Recurrent vitreous and retinal haemorrhages occurring in young adults; the aetiology is unknown. Absorption of the haemorrhage is followed by vascularization, fibrosis of the vitreous and eventual retinal detachment.

Coat's disease

A disease due to multiple intraretinal vascular anomalies also occurring in young adults in which haemorrhagic lipid-rich exudation into the subretinal space occurs, causing retinal detachment.

Retrolental fibroplasia

Detachment and fibrosis of the retina, usually bilateral and occurring in premature babies after removal from an incubator in which the oxygen concentration has been greater than 40%. There is angioblastic activity in the inner retinal layer with haemorrhages and formation of new vessels in the vitreous. This leads to retinal detachment and conversion into the retrolental fibrous membrane.

Senile macular degeneration (HAAB)

The blood supply of the macula is dependent upon choroidal vessels. Sclerosis of these vessels will result in retinal damage and loss of central vision—*central scotoma*.

Disciform degeneration of the macula (Junnis and Kuhnt)

A degenerative process of the macula of unknown aetiology and characterized by irregular white–yellow swellings. These consist of organized exudates between the choroid and retina, the outer layers of which are atrophic and replaced by glial tissue.

Degenerations

Retinitis pigmentosa

Nature
Premature degeneration of the retinal neuroepithelium which commences in early adult life and is manifest by progressive night blindness and loss of visual fields, with total blindness by 50–60 years of age. Inheritance is variable and the result of multiple gene abnormalities.

Macroscopical
Pigmentary migration and clumping at the fundus, usually more advanced on one side. The arteries are attenuated and the discs pale and waxy.

Microscopical
The rods and cones are almost entirely missing, the outer nuclear and plexiform layers atrophic and the pigmented epithelium disorganized. Cells of this layer migrate haphazardly into the retina and also form proliferating masses. Phagocytes, engorged with pigment granules, are carried towards the retinal perivascular spaces. In many cases the optic disc shows atrophy.

Cysts

Nature
Cystic change in the peripheral part of the retina occurring in middle age. Rupture of one of these cysts may result in retinal detachment.

Microscopical
Small spaces develop within the outer and inner nuclear layers which fuse forming interlacing channels. At a later stage, all surrounding retinal tissue is destroyed, the channels lying between the internal limiting membrane and a compressed layer of rods and cones.

Congenital

Coloboma of the choroid and retina

Nature
A congenital fissure of the eye.

Appearances
May be associated with a similar lesion of the optic nerve, ciliary body and iris. The defect, if complete, extends from the optic disc downwards and inwards to the pupillary margin of the iris. It is due to an anomalous closure of the fetal cleft with ectodermal hyperplasia at the margins. The sclera and choroid are thin, Bruch's membrane is absent and the fault is covered by atypical retinal tissue.

Persistence of the hyaloid artery—persistent hyperplastic vitreous

Appearances
The remains of the hyaloid artery may be found as a cord stretching from the optic disc to the posterior surface of the lens. Often other congenital abnormalities are also found—microphthalmia, ectopic lens or ectopic pupil. Posteriorly, the artery may be patent and contain blood. Anteriorly, the fibrotic remnants are adherent to a retrolental membrane which incorporates the posterior lens capsule and stretches across the globe from one retinal surface to the other, frequently detaching it from the choroid.

Glaucoma

Nature
Increased intra-ocular tension. The condition may be acute, subacute or chronic and of the following types:

Primary

Nature
Glaucoma presenting without other detectable intraocular disease.

Pathology
This is due to failure of the normal drainage mechanisms of the aqueous humour although the exact cause or the site of this failure remains uncertain.

Congenital
This type is due to a congenital anatomical defect in which either Schlemm's canal is absent or in eyes

which have an abnormally shallow anterior chamber so that the root of the iris is very close to the corneo-scleral trabeculae of the filtration angle—*closed angle glaucoma*. Any swelling of the ciliary body, e.g. by congestion or oedema, will then block the channels leading to the canal of Schlemm and thus produce glaucoma.

Secondary

Nature
Glaucoma occurring secondarily to previous intra-ocular disease which obstructs the drainage of intra-ocular fluid.

Aetiology
1 *Iridocyclitis*: the presence of inflammatory cells, exudate or adhesions—*anterior synechiae*, obstructs the tissues at the filtration angles. A ring adhesion of the pupillary border of the iris with the lens—*iris bombé*, also prevents drainage.
2 *Trauma*: perforation of the cornea may lead to a diminution of size of the anterior chamber or result in anterior synechiae, with narrowing of the filtration angle. In addition, blood clot may block the drainage channels. Penetration or dislocation of the lens may displace the iris anteriorly, block the pupil or obstruct the drainage channels with disintegrating lens matter.
3 *Intra-ocular tumours*: space-occupying lesions may push the lens and iris forwards to block the filtration angles. Tumours also predispose to glaucoma by thrombosis of the retinal vein or by producing inflammatory synechiae.
4 *Retinal vein thrombosis—thrombotic glaucoma.* (see p. 151).

Results
Any of these types, if unrelieved, may result in an absolute glaucoma in which the following changes are usually present.
1 Obliteration of the filtration angles by anterior synechiae.
2 Oedema of the cornea.
3 Atrophy of the iris, ciliary body and retina, due to the raised tension and ischaemia.
4 Cupping of the disc with optic atrophy.
5 Cataract.

C/INTRA-OCULAR TUMOURS, LACRIMAL ORGANS, ORBIT, OPTIC NERVE

Intra-ocular tumours

Benign

Benign epithelioma of the iris
A rare condition which is merely hyperplasia of pigmented epithelium and appears as a pigmented mass, often at the pupillary margin, consisting of overgrown and invaginated pigment epithelium.

Benign epithelioma of the ciliary body—adenoma
A more frequent but otherwise similar lesion to that of the iris described above. Symptomless and usually found as a round lesion about 1 mm in diameter in an eye removed for some other condition.

Naevus
Benign melanomas are seen as elevated, variably pigmented masses on the anterior surface of the iris, in the ciliary body and on the choroid in relation to the ciliary nerves.

Haemangiomas

Iris and ciliary body
These are rare tumours and are of the capillary type.

Choroid
Usually found posteriorly as flat tumorous masses.

They are of cavernous type and ill-defined, tapering off into the surrounding choroid. Calcification and ossification commonly occur.

Retina

Vascular masses in the retina are often associated with haemangioblastoma in the brain and there may be associated tumours or cysts of the kidney, pancreas, liver and epididymis—von Hippel–Lindau's disease. The tumour is spherical and consists of capillary plexuses in the retina with solid areas of angioblastic cells. Scattered amongst the vessels are swollen endothelial cells containing phagocytosed fat. Haemorrhages are numerous and may extend into the retina, vitreous or subretinal space.

Leiomyoma

These are rare tumours, usually of the iris where they arise from the sphincter and dilator muscles. Occasionally they occur in the ciliary body.

Malignant

Medulloepithelioma of ciliary epithelium

This includes diktyoma and malignant ciliary epithelial tumour.

Diktyoma

Origin

Arises in young persons from the non-pigmented epithelium of the ciliary body and is a counterpart of the retinal retinoblastoma.

Appearances

A white non-metastasizing but locally malignant tumour which may fill the entire globe. Non-pigmented epithelial cells are arranged in tubules or rosettes. Mitotic activity is marked and the lesion resembles the early embryonic retina.

Malignant ciliary epithelial tumour

Origin

Occurs in adults, often in chronically inflamed eyes and arises from both layers of the ciliary epithelium.

Appearances

Pigmentation may be heavy. The lesion does not usually grow to a large size, in contrast to the diktyoma,

and metastases have not been reported. Microscopy shows proliferating epithelium in the form of strands and tubules, resembling a diktyoma but better differentiated.

Retinoblastoma

Origin

A congenital tumour arising from primitive cells in the retina.

Incidence

Presents in early childhood, 90% before 3 years of age; 20–30% of cases are bilateral, the other eye always being the site of an independent focus, i.e. a separate primary tumour.

Aetiology

Most cases develop sporadically, but the influence of heredity is well proven, 6% being inherited in an autosomal dominant fashion but with incomplete penetrance (50–85%); 25% of sporadic cases are from transmissible genetic mutations.

Macroscopical

A pink–white lobulated mass extending in several directions:
1 Endophytum—into the vitreous.
2 Exophytum—into the subretinal space.
3 Planum—within the retina.
4 Diffuse infiltrating—within the retina, ciliary body and iris.

All eventually cause glaucoma and fill the entire globe. Extra-ocular spread takes place along the optic nerve into the brain and blood-borne metastases are frequent with a predilection for bone.

Microscopical

Masses of round or carrot-shaped cells with hyperchromatic nuclei and little cytoplasm, arranged in dense sheets, around blood vessels as pseudo-rosettes and as true rosettes of 16–30 cells around a central lumen—*Flexner–Wintersteiner rosettes*. Mitoses are numerous and necrosis or calcification is frequent; rarely this leads to retrogression of the tumour. Seedling deposits on other intra-ocular structures are common. Pigmentation does not occur.

Results

Five-year survival is 87%. In treated cases death

usually occurs in the first year after enucleation, recurrence being exceedingly rare after a 4-year survival period. Extent of invasion of the optic nerve is an important prognostic indicator.

Malignant melanoma

Site
Eighty-four per cent in the choroid; 10% in the ciliary body; 6% in the iris.

Incidence
This is by far the most frequent intra-ocular tumour.

Macroscopical

Choroid
An elliptical mass, initially confined by the sclera and Bruch's membrane. Eventually, the tumour mushrooms into the subretinal space, lifting the retina and causing its destruction. In time the entire globe may be filled and finally the tumour may burst out of the globe into the orbit. Extra-ocular spread may occur sooner via the channels of the perforating retinal vessels and rarely along the optic nerve. The degree of pigmentation is variable and this feature may be almost absent. Haemorrhages and areas of necrosis are common. Glaucoma may occur due to blockage of the filtration angles by the growing mass or by cellular debris from the neoplasm.

Ciliary body and iris
Glaucoma commonly appears early and the lens may be dislocated and become cataractous. Rarely the lesions spread around the entire iris—'ring melanoma'.

Microscopical
Two types are recognized although mixtures are common.

Spindle cells
Elongated cells with oval nuclei which are arranged in groups and bundles. Mitotic figures are scanty. They are subdivided into types A and B.

Epithelioid cell
Large, polygonal and pleomorphic cells with pale nuclei. Mitoses are numerous and giant cells are often present. Tumours predominantly of this type are the most malignant.

The pigment content varies in different areas of the tumour but can be so heavy that bleached sections are necessary for cellular recognition. Granules of melanin, although produced within the cells, may be phagocytosed to other parts of the globe. Heavy pigmentation is considered to carry a poor prognosis.

Variable amounts of reticulin are formed, the amount being of prognostic significance, i.e. the more reticulin present the more favourable the prognosis.

Spread
1 *Local*: extension outside the globe to the orbit.
2 *Blood*: as with malignant melanomas elsewhere, blood spread is frequent with metastases to any site, but particularly the liver. This may occur at variable lengths of time after removal of the primary tumour—'the big liver and glass eye' syndrome.

Results
Spindle A tumours—92% 15-year survival.
Spindle B tumours—75% 15-year survival.
Pure epithelioid tumours—28% 15-year survival.
Mixed tumours (most common)—41% 15-year survival.

Secondary tumours
Many forms of carcinoma have been found within the eye. The usual site is the posterior segment of the choroid.

Rarely, deposits of malignant lymphomas are found in the uveal tract.

Lacrimal organs

Lacrimal gland

Acute dacryoadenitis
May follow virus infections, e.g. mumps and influenza, but 50% are due to *Staphylococcus pyogenes*.

Sjögren's syndrome—benign lymphoepithelial lesion
In this condition there is immunological destruction of glandular tissue resulting in dry conjunctivae, atrophic rhinitis and pharyngitis. It may be primary—*sicca complex*, or secondary (see p. 19).

Tumours

Pleomorphic adenoma
The appearances of this tumour in the lacrimal gland are similar to those occurring in the parotid and other salivary glands (p. 19).

Adenoid cystic carcinoma
This is the most common malignant tumour of the lacrimal gland, locally destructive and with a median survival of 4.5 years: only 14% survive 15 years (see p. 20).

Adenocarcinoma
Malignant change occurring in a pleomorphic adenoma or *de novo*.

Lymphomas
All types have been reported in the lacrimal glands.

Lacrimal passages

Chronic dacryocystitis

Nature
A non-specific inflammation of the tear sac due to stasis in the nasolacrimal duct.

Microscopical
In addition to the non-specific inflammatory cell infiltration, the epithelium shows some areas of hyperplasia with increase of the goblet cells and desquamation.

Tumours of the lacrimal sac

Papilloma
A benign but potentially malignant papillary overgrowth of columnar epithelium.

Carcinoma
Most are squamous cell carcinomas arising in metaplastic epithelium.

Others
Sarcomas, secondary carcinoma and deposits of malignant lymphomas occur, but they are all extremely rare.

Orbit

Congenital

Cysts

Dermoid cysts
These inclusion dermoid cysts are relatively common and may occur at any site along the cranial suture lines. Peri-orbital dermoids are most frequent at the outer and upper angle—the frontomalar or the frontotemporal suture. Intra-orbital dermoids are outside the muscle cone but secondary inflammation may cause adhesion to muscle, optic nerve or other orbital contents.

Meningoceles and encephaloceles
Protrusion of meninges—meningocele, or brain—encephalocele, into the orbit through a bony defect. They are soft elastic swellings which are sometimes pulsatile but are compressible (see p. 330).

Vascular lesions

Vasculitis
Orbital tissues are commonly involved by cranial (temporal) arteritis. Systemic vasculitides, including Wegener's granulomatosis, not uncommonly have orbital involvement (see p. 84).

Aneurysms

Saccular
Arising from the ophthalmic artery—rare.

Cirsoid or arteriovenous
May be traumatic or congenital (see p. 86).

Infections
Orbital cellulitis may be caused by pathogenic bacteria—e.g. extension from air sinuses, or by fungi. The latter may occur in healthy persons—usually *Aspergillus* or by opportunistic infection by *phycomycosis*.

Tumours

Haemangioma
Cavernous, capillary and sclerosing types are seen.

Lymphangioma
Rare and of the cavernous type.

Teratoma
These tumours usually contain representatives of all three germinal layers and thus may contain skin, teeth, bone, muscle, internal organs or almost a complete fetus. They are occasionally found in the orbit where malignant change frequently supervenes.

Benign connective tissue tumours
These are all rare and are identical to similar tumours occurring at other sites. They include fibroma, lipoma, myxoma, chondroma, osteoma and neurofibroma.

Malignant tumours

Rhabdomyosarcoma
This is the most common malignant mesenchymal orbital tumour presenting in childhood. Alveolar and pleomorphic types occur in the orbit but most are embryonal. Long-term cures are now achievable in 75% of cases (see p. 108).

Sarcoma
Most arise from the periosteum or fascia and are fibrosarcomas.

Lymphoma
Deposits of leukaemia, Hodgkin's disease and other malignant lymphomas are sometimes found in the orbit.

Meningioma and glioma
Meningiomas may extend through the optic foramen from the cranial cavity or arise from the optic nerve sheath. Intra-orbital optic gliomas occur, including the juvenile pilocytic astrocytoma.

Secondary tumours
1 *Malignant melanoma*: direct extension from the globe (see p. 155) or by metastasis.
2 *Carcinoma*: rare, but may occur from many primary sites.
3 *Neuroblastoma*: a relatively common site for metastases from an adrenal neuroblastoma—Hutchison's syndrome (see p. 121).

Pseudotumour of the orbit

Nature
A non-specific chronic granuloma of the orbit of unknown aetiology. Some are thought to follow infection of the adjacent sinuses, lacrimal glands or teeth; others may be immunologically induced.

Macroscopical
A unilateral rapidly developing lesion, clinically closely simulating a tumour.

Microscopical
The appearances are very variable:
1 Lymph follicles enclosed by fibrous tissue.
2 Focal and perivascular collections of lymphocytes involving the muscles.
3 Diffuse acute or chronic inflammatory cell infiltration of the orbital tissues, frequently with an excess of fibrous tissue and giant cells. Fat necrosis may be found in this type.
4 Dense fibroblastic proliferation with minimal inflammatory cell infiltration.

Results
The great majority regress spontaneously, but occasionally the lesion may persist for a considerable period of time and create painful proptosis, with diagnostic difficulty in differentiation from true tumours.

Optic nerve

Inflammations

Perineuritis

Nature
Inflammation of the nerve sheath.

Causes
Usually secondary to inflammation of the meninges or orbit by pyogenic organisms, tuberculosis or syphilis.

Optic neuritis

Nature
Inflammation of the nerve tissue.

Causes
1 *Pyogenic infections*: secondary to perineuritis, purulent endophthalmitis, orbital infection or metastatic abscess.
2 *Tuberculosis*: by spread from the choroid or meninges.
3 *Syphilis*: may occur early or in the tabetic stage.
4 *Multiple sclerosis*: usually retrobulbar in situation (see p. 334).

Results
Destruction of nerve fibres with optic atrophy is common. With multiple sclerosis, which is the commonest cause, pallor of the temporal parts of the disc usually remains, although vision commonly returns to normal.

Optic atrophy

Causes
The more common causes of optic atrophy include the following.

Optic neuritis
Any of its causes as above.

Trauma

Pressure
From glaucoma, aneurysm, etc.

Vascular
Central retinal artery thrombosis.

Papilloedema
Of longstanding.

Poisons
Especially methyl alcohol and tobacco.

Papilloedema

Nature
Oedema of the optic disc (papilla).

Causes
1 *Raised intracranial tension*: due to space-occupying lesions in the skull, e.g. tumour, abscess, haemorrhages, meningitis.
2 *Optic neuritis.*
3 *Accelerated hypertension.*
4 *Venous drainage obstruction*: by thrombosis, e.g. cavernous sinus thrombosis, or by pressure, e.g. from a tumour.

Appearances
Stages:
1 Congestion of retinal veins.
2 Blurring of disc margins.
3 Filling of the physiological cup.
4 Protrusion of the optic disc.
5 Haemorrhages in and around the disc.
6 Optic atrophy with pallor of the disc subsequently.

Results
In addition to deterioration in visual acuity, optic atrophy results when the papilloedema is of long standing.

Primary tumours
The optic nerve should be regarded as part of the brain tissue and most of its tumours are therefore similar to those of cerebral tissue.

The most frequent are meningiomas, gliomas and neurofibromas.

Secondary tumours

Direct spread
1 *Retinoblastoma*: the most frequent (see p. 154).
2 *Malignant melanoma*: rarely spreads into the optic nerve (see p. 155).

Metastases
Very rare but metastases have been reported from the breast, lung, kidney and stomach.

Chapter 10
Diseases of the Genito-Urinary System—Kidney

A/CONGENITAL, INFECTIONS

Normal kidney
  Renal function
  Examination of kidneys
Congenital
  Agenesis, hypoplasia, dysplasia
  Horseshoe kidney
  Others
  Cystic diseases
Infections
  Pyogenic
  Granulomatous
  Interstitial nephritis

Development
The kidneys are of mesodermal origin but arise in two parts:

1 From the ureteric bud of the Wolffian duct—this forms the ureter, pelvis, calyces and collecting tubules.

2 From the urogenital ridge:

(a) pronephros ⎱
(b) mesonephros ⎰ both transient structures;

(c) metanephros—develops at the pelvic brim and forms the nephrons.

After the two parts have united, the organs migrate along the posterior abdominal wall to the loins, obtaining their blood supply successively from the iliac arteries, lower abdominal aorta and finally the upper abdominal aorta.

Normal structure
Each kidney weighs about 150 g.

Nephron
There are about 2 million of these basic units, each formed by a glomerulus and a tubule (see Fig. 15).

Glomerulus
Consists of a mass of capillaries fed by an afferent arteriole, which rejoin to form the efferent arteriole. The capillaries perforate the capsule at the hilum and are lined by endothelial cells lying on a basement membrane. Externally situated are the epithelial cells of the visceral layer which have numerous slender foot processes investing the surface of the capillary tuft. The glomerular epithelium is continuous at the hilum

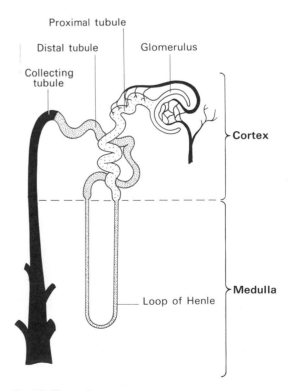

Fig. 15 The nephron.

with the parietal layer of epithelial cells which forms the lining of Bowman's capsule. The space between this capsule and the tuft is the capsular space. Between the capillary loops in the stalk of the lobules are *mesangial cells* and the *mesangial substance (matrix)* which they produce. The glomeruli all lie within the renal cortex.

Tubules

1 *Proximal convoluted tubule*: this forms the bulk of the nephron and is composed of cuboidal cells with a brush border; it lies in the cortex.
2 *Descending loop of Henle*: flattened cuboidal cells; in the medulla.
3 *Ascending loop of Henle*: low cuboidal cells with a rather dense cytoplasm; also in the medulla.
4 *Distal convoluted tubule*: cuboidal cells with no brush border; it is found in the cortex.
5 *Collecting tubule*: low cuboidal epithelium; confined to the medulla.

Cortex

There is an outer fibrous capsule which strips easily to reveal a smooth surface. It measures about 1.2 cm in depth and is sharply demarcated from the medulla. The pattern is formed by vasa recta, straight lines perpendicular to the capsular surface. In addition to the glomeruli, the cortex contains the convoluted tubules, interlobular arteries and small amounts of loose connective tissue.

Medulla

The pyramids end in blunt tips—papillae, which protrude into the calyces. Separating the pyramids are the broad bands of renal substance containing the loops of Henle—columns of Bertini. The medulla also contains collecting tubules, interstitial tissue and the main blood vessels with their arcuate branches at the cortico-medullary junction.

Calyces and pelvis

Lined by transitional epithelium—urothelium.

Some aspects of renal function

Blood flow

The renal blood flow accounts for 25% of the cardiac output. It passes to the glomeruli where the difference between the hydrostatic and osmotic pressures produces the glomerular filtrate. Blood in the efferent arterioles passes into a second capillary bed which then supplies the remaining parts of the nephrons in the cortex at a somewhat lower pressure (see Fig. 16).

Glomerular filtrate

About 170 litres/day. The filtrate passes from the capsular space to the tubules where it is altered by:
1 Selective reabsorption—99% of its bulk.
2 Tubular secretion, e.g. ammonia.

The altered filtrate then passes to the collecting tubules in which it is carried to the calyces and pelvis as urine—approximately 1700 ml/day.

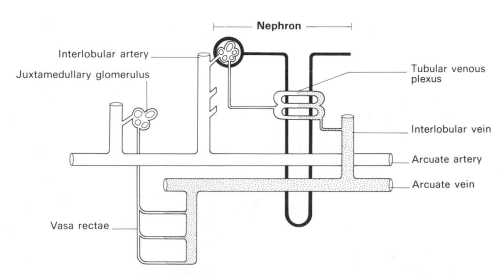

Fig. 16 Diagram of blood supply to the nephron.

Renal functions

The chief functions of the kidney are:

1 Elimination of water.
2 Excretion of certain substances normally present in plasma when their concentration rises above a certain level—renal threshold.
3 Selective reabsorption of substances necessary for the body, e.g. sugar, electrolytes, etc.
4 Excretion of waste products, e.g. urea.
5 Plays an important role in the regulation of acid–base balance.

Factors necessary for normal renal function

1 Adequate blood flow and pressure to allow the formation of a normal glomerular filtrate and to maintain tubular function.
2 Normal glomerular structure to allow the filtrate to form in normal quantities and of normal composition.
3 Normal tubules to alter the composition of the filtrate according to the requirements of the body.
4 Unhindered passage of the urine thus formed into the calyces and thence outside the body via a normal lower urinary tract.

Disordered function

This may therefore follow disease processes affecting:

1 Renal blood flow and blood vessels.
2 Glomeruli.
3 Tubules.
4 Obstruction to the urinary flow at any level.

Tests of renal function

1 Blood urea (or non-protein nitrogen). Rises above the normal upper limits of 6 mmol/l may be from prerenal causes, e.g. dehydration, haemorrhage, congestive heart failure, in addition to renal and postrenal obstructive lesions.
2 Blood creatinine. If this is raised along with the urea, the failure is likely to be of renal origin.
3 Electrolyte and acid–base blood levels.
4 Clearance rates. Rates of blood clearance of urea, creatinine or inulin are only rarely used in clinical practice.
5 Urine. The volume and relative density of urine are important, as is the appearance of the centrifuged deposit.
6 Plasma osmolality.

Examination of the kidney

A systematic method of examination of both the macroscopic and microscopic appearances is necessary, not only in respect of local lesions but, more particularly, for diffuse parenchymal disease.

Macroscopical appearances

1 *Size, weight, shape, colour.*
2 *Capsule:* ease of stripping and appearance of the capsular surface.
3 *Cortex:* width, demarcation from the medulla, pattern, colour.
4 *Medulla:* size, pattern, colour.
5 *Pelvis and calyces:* mucosal appearance, contents, size.
6 *Blood vessels:* prominence, thickening, occlusion.

Microscopical appearances

1 *Glomeruli:* tuft and capsule.
2 *Tubules:* including contents.
3 *Interstitial tissue.*
4 *Blood vessels.*
5 *Calyces and pelvis.*

Congenital

Agenesis

Failure of development of the kidney.

1 Bilateral—incompatible with life.
2 Unilateral—compensatory hypertrophy of the other kidney occurs.

The ureteric remnants may be present or they too may be aplastic.

Renal hypoplasia and dysplasia

Most congenitally small kidneys show evidence of anomalous metanephric differentiation and are termed dysplastic. The renal tissue is disorganized and shows fetal type of structures usually including primitive ducts and cartilage often together with cysts. Other congenital abnormalities of the urinary tract are often present.

True hypoplasia shows reduction in number of calyces and papillae and is uncommon.

Fusion—'horseshoe kidney'

This is quite common—1 in 500 births, affecting the lower pole in 90% of cases and the upper pole in 10%. The function of the fused organ is unaffected.

Abnormal sites

Development in ectopic foci or, more commonly,

failure of migration, results in normal kidneys within the pelvis or at the pelvic brim. Kinking of the ureters may occur, predisposing to pyelonephritis.

Ureteric anomalies

1 Double ureter with double pelvis.
2 Stricture.
3 Megaureter—commonly associated with megacolon.

Vascular

Anomalous arteries from the iliacs or lower aorta may occur and an additional vessel to the lower pole may cross the pelvi-ureteric junction and be associated with hydronephrosis (see p. 179).

Cystic diseases of kidney

Simple cysts

These are common and occur as solitary, or occasionally multiple, cystic spaces in otherwise normal kidneys. They are usually 1–5 cm in diameter, although they may be 10 cm or more, are filled with clear fluid and lined by a smooth glistening membrane of flattened cuboidal epithelium surrounded by a thin fibrous capsule. They are non-uriniferous and have no communication with the pelvis, usually being cortical in situation. They may cause renal enlargement and distortion and thus require clinical differentiation from tumours.

Polycystic disease

Nature

An hereditary disease occurring uncommonly and equally between the sexes, in which both kidneys are progressively replaced by numerous cysts lined by flattened cuboidal epithelium. The cysts communicate with the calyces and with each other and the contents indicate traces of renal function.

Types

Adult polycystic disease
Inherited as autosomal dominant, but 50% of cases are new mutants. Present in fourth decade or later usually with very large lobulated loin masses containing cysts up to 5 cm or so in diameter. Associated features are:
1 Berry cerebral aneurysms in 10%.
2 Cysts of liver, pancreas and lung.

Infantile polycystic disease
Less common than the adult type, this is autosomal recessive inherited. Usually presents in stillborn or neonates with enlarged kidneys which preserve their reniform outline but on section show radiating, finely cystic pattern in medulla and cortex. The cysts are composed of dilated tubules and collecting ducts.

In the liver there are abnormal and sometimes dilated bile ducts with cysts also occasionally present in lungs and/or pancreas.

Polycystic disease of kidneys and liver
This spectrum of variable degrees of renal and liver involvement is also of autosomally recessive inheritance but can present in infants, children or adults. The liver changes may be severe—as in *congenital hepatic fibrosis*, with minor renal abnormalities or the converse or variable mixtures.

Effects

Adult type
1 Hypertension—in 50%.
2 Abdominal swelling—often massive.
3 Renal failure—life may be preserved by dialysis or transplantation.
4 Infection of cysts.
5 Haemorrhage into cysts.

Infantile type
1 Most cases die as neonates or are stillborn.
2 A small minority present later in childhood with renal failure or hypertension.

Polycystic disease of liver and kidneys
1 Portal hypertension when liver changes dominate.
2 As for infantile polycystic disease.

Medullary cystic disease

Medullary sponge kidney
This is a predominantly radiological diagnosis of dilated medullary collecting ducts usually associated with urinary tract infections and calculus formation. It is not a familial condition.

Juvenile nephronophthisis—medullary cystic disease
An hereditary nephropathy causing polyuria and renal

failure in children. Salt loss, growth retardation and renal osteodystrophy are prominent and a disproportionately severe normochromic anaemia is usual. There is extensive glomerulosclerosis and a variable degree of cystic change at the corticomedullary junctional area.

Renal dysplasia
Multiple cysts are usually present (see p. 161).

Acquired cystic disease
1 Numerous small cortical cysts are consistently associated with renal scarring from pyelonephritis, vascular disease or in end-stage glomerular disease.
2 In long-term dialysis patients, multiple cysts are usually present and may be large and numerous resulting in mechanical problems—*acquired polycystic kidneys*.

Infections

Pyogenic

Blood-borne

Pyaemia
In pyaemia, lodgement of infected emboli leads to the formation of multiple abscesses throughout the renal substance. Small, rounded, numerous, yellow areas with a surrounding zone of hyperaemia are visible, maximally in the cortex. The usual organisms are staphylococci.

Carbuncle of the kidney
Blood-borne spread of organisms, usually staphylococci, to the kidney may result in a solitary large abscess in the cortex, sometimes multiloculated. Extensive destruction of renal tissue may occur.

Perinephric abscess
Abscess formation in the perinephric tissue may result from:
1 Spread from intrarenal inflammation, e.g. carbuncle of the kidney, pyelonephritis.
2 Primary focus in the perinephric fat without renal involvement.

Pyelonephritis

Definition
Inflammation of the renal pelvis and renal parenchyma. Pyelitis, inflammation of the pelvis alone, is so exceedingly uncommon that the name should be abandoned, as some degree of parenchymal involvement is inevitable.

Acute pyelonephritis

Incidence
Common.

Age
There are three peaks of incidence—childhood, pregnancy and the elderly.

Sex
Females rather more commonly than males.

Organisms
Fifty per cent are due to *Escherichia coli*, others to *Aerobacter aerogenes*, *Proteus vulgaris*, *Streptococcus faecalis*, *Staphylococcus pyogenes* or *Pseudomonas aeruginosa*, in descending order of frequency.

Pathogenesis
Urinary stasis or urinary tract obstruction is an important and almost invariably predisposing factor, hence the peaks of incidence at the following ages.
1 *Childhood*: major or minor degrees of congenital urinary tract abnormalities and ureteric reflux of urine during micturition.
2 *Pregnancy*: pressure of the gravid uterus on the ureters at the pelvic brim.
3 *Elderly*: women—prolapse of the uterus and cystitis; men—prostatic enlargement.
　　Two pathways by which the organisms may reach the kidneys are propounded:
1 Haematogenous.
2 Ascending via the ureters or peri-ureteric lymphatics.
　　The latter is much the more likely usual mechanism.

Macroscopical
The condition may be unilateral or bilateral and the involved organs are enlarged with a tense capsule; small abscesses may be seen beneath the stripped capsule. On section, there are numerous small

abscesses in the cortex with linear streaks of yellowish colour in the medulla—'surgical kidney'. The pelvis is usually hyperaemic and granular with purulent urinary contents. Earlier cases show less abscess formation and focal areas of hyperaemia.

Microscopical

Acute inflammation with infiltration by polymorphs in the renal tubules and in the interstitial tissue, later causing necrosis and abscess formation. The inflammatory process is focal and a bacterial inflammation is present also in the calyceal and pelvic mucosae.

Results

1 *Resolution*: before there is frank suppuration; however, some scarring usually occurs.
2 *Healing*: with scarring.
3 *Chronic*: chronic pyelonephritis.
4 *Suppuration*: if associated with total urinary obstruction will produce a pyonephrosis.
5 *Death*: in uraemia.

Healed pyelonephritis

Nature

The end stage of scarring due to a previous acute pyelonephritis or in childhood without demonstrable obstruction, as a result of vesico-ureteric reflux—*reflux nephropathy*.

Macroscopical

The kidneys are small, unequal, and irregularly scarred and contracted. The capsule is thickened and adherent revealing a variably scarred surface with minute and focal or more generalized depressed areas according to the severity of the previous acute inflammation. These scars are irregularly distributed, flat, broad or 'U-shaped' depressions, usually 0.5–2 cm in diameter, which extend into the cortex but do not involve the medulla.

Microscopical

Focal areas of parenchymal replacement by fibrous tissue with occasional lymphocytes. In adjacent areas there are dilated atrophic tubules filled with albuminous material of 'colloid' appearance.

Effects

Although renal function may be unimpaired and the patient remains normotensive in this condition, there is loss of some renal parenchyma which may become significant should further episodes of pyelonephritis occur. Reflux nephropathy of childhood often presents as renal failure.

Chronic pyelonephritis

Incidence

Formerly identified as the most common form of fatal primary renal disease, this is now no longer true.

Origin

In only a relatively small proportion of cases is there good evidence of either:
1 long-continued low grade infection, or
2 recurrent attacks of acute pyelonephritis with scarring.

Although usually bilateral, unilateral local abnormalities may give rise to involvement of only one kidney.

Macroscopical

The kidneys are small, sometimes very small—50 g or less. The capsule is firmly adherent and thickened with numerous irregular, wedge-shaped, flat scars on the surface. Occasionally, when the changes are very diffuse, a fine granularity may be seen. On section, the cortex is thinned, particularly at the sites of scarring and the pattern and corticomedullary differentiation are indistinct. The organs are pale and the medulla is contracted. The pelvic mucosa is usually thickened, pale, fibrotic and granular whilst dilatation of the pelvis and calyces may be present due to a concomitant obstructive lesion. The blood vessels are prominent.

Microscopical

Fibrous replacement in the scarred areas with hyalinized glomeruli and increased interstitial fibrous tissue in which there are dilated atrophic tubules containing albuminous material which mimics colloid—'thyroid kidney', accompanied by a variable lymphocytic infiltration. There is usually also evidence of inflammatory activity with a focal infiltrate of polymorphs and lymphocytes. The calyces show increased submucosal fibrosis with a lymphocytic infiltration and sometimes cyst-like invaginations of the epithelium—*pyelitis cystica*. The blood vessels are often markedly thickened due to widespread endarteritic or hypertensive changes. A variant is *xanthogranulomatous* pyelonephritis.

Results

Clinically, some cases give a clear history of past episodes of urinary tract infection or have identifiable predisposing structural abnormalities; in many, however, the disease may remain latent for many years and then present as:

1 Hypertension.
2 Renal failure with uraemia.

Death results from either or both of these sequelae.

In unilateral pyelonephritis associated with hypertension, nephrectomy of the affected kidney may occasionally lead to reversal of the hypertension. More commonly, however, irreversible structural changes have already occurred (see p. 92) and, after a temporary remission following operation, the hypertension returns and progresses.

Papillary necrosis and analgesic abuse nephropathy

Nature

Necrosis of medullary pyramids may occur as a variant of acute suppurative pyelonephritis, particularly in the elderly or in diabetics. The condition is also increasingly recognized in those taking grossly excessive amounts of analgesic substances, particularly those containing phenacetin, over a long period of time. In this situation of analgesic abuse, corticomedullary interstitial fibrosis is usually also marked.

Macroscopical

The distal portion of the pyramids are brownish or grey or necrotic, separated from the upper medullary tissues by a sharp hyperaemic demarcated zone. Some or all of the papillae may have been shed leaving an ulcer at the apices of the calyces. Scarring of cortex may be considerable in analgesic nephropathy.

Microscopical

The dominant feature is ischaemic necrosis with marginal inflammatory reaction only prominent at the demarcation zone.

Results

Renal failure is inevitable whatever the cause but the time scale is very variable.

Transitional cell carcinomas of the pelvis and calyces, and less commonly of ureter and bladder are increasingly recognized as late complications (see p. 185).

Granulomatous

Tuberculosis

Miliary

Diffuse involvement of both kidneys as part of generalized haematogenous spread. The organs are usually normal in size and on section show numerous greyish-white pinhead-sized tubercles.

Focal

Pathogenesis

Haematogenous; it is probable that all cases are due to blood-borne infection from a distant site. Twenty-five per cent show evidence of active pulmonary tuberculosis, other possible sources being the intestines, tonsils and bone.

Sites

Although clinically unilateral, before antibiotic treatment changed the course of the disease 50% of the cases would eventually show active bilateral disease. It seems probable that most cases are bilaterally infected but most commonly the lesion heals in one kidney and progresses in the other. The lesion frequently starts in the cortex and spreads locally to involve the apices of the pyramids and the walls of the calyces.

Macroscopical

1 *Early*: an irregular, pale, yellow, necrotic, caseating lesion is seen near the corticomedullary junction.
2 *Later*: the apices are irregularly ulcerated with the formation of a cavity lined by caseous material and communicating with the pelvis.
3 *Late*: the pelvis becomes filled with caseous material and lined by tuberculous granulation tissue. The cavities extend to destroy large areas of renal substance.

Involvement of the pelvi-ureteric junction by tuberculous granulation tissue leads to obstruction and tuberculous pyonephrosis, whilst extension of the tuberculous process down the ureter is common.

Microscopical

Caseating tuberculous giant cell systems.

Fate

Untreated:

1 Healing with fibrosis and calcification; this only occurs at very early stages.

2 Tuberculous pyonephrosis due to ureteric occlusion.

3 Auto-nephrectomy—the pyonephrosis becomes spontaneously sterile with fibrosis and calcification producing a completely enclosed caseous mass which may partially absorb—*'putty kidney'*.

4 Spread of infection to the lower urinary tract, particularly the bladder, epididymis and seminal vesicles.

Treated (antibiotics):

1 Early lesions heal by fibrosis.

2 If involvement of a calyceal or pelvi-ureteric junction has already occurred before treatment is instituted, healing by fibrosis may still lead to stricture formation, obstruction and subsequent loss of function.

Diagnosis

Urine. Deposit—red cells, pus cells, debris; acid–alcohol fast organisms are commonly seen on ZN staining.

Culture—sterile on ordinary media.

TB cultures on early morning specimens—positive.

Results

Prognosis is good unless diagnosis is delayed and bilateral obstructive complications develop.

Actinomycosis

The kidneys are very rarely involved in the disseminated type of actinomycosis.

Interstitial nephritis

Nature

True examples of primary interstitial inflammation of the kidney are very uncommon but do occur in:

1 Adverse drug reactions, e.g. phenindione and hypersensitivity to some antibiotics (methicillin, etc.)

2 Brucellosis, leptospirosis—Weil's disease (see p. 235) and some cases of glandular fever.

3 Non-infective causes, e.g. irradiation, analgesic abuse nephropathy, hypercalcaemia, etc.

4 Reflux nephropathy.

Appearances

Glomeruli are normal or show only mild ischaemic changes. In true interstitial inflammation, interstitial tissue and tubular epithelial cells shows patchy infiltration by polymorphonuclear leucocytes often eosinophils with variable admixture of plasma cells and lymphocytes in the more chronic cases. Also related to chronicity is an increasing fibrosis and tubular atrophy.

B/GLOMERULAR LESIONS

Steps in diagnosis
Patterns of reaction
   Minimal change
   Obvious glomerular lesions
   Proliferative
   Glomerulosclerosis
   Membranous
   Hereditary
Associated diseases

Since Richard Bright's original, and in some ways still classical, description of acute nephritis in 1827, there had been a bewildering succession of classifications of glomerular diseases, particularly of glomerulonephritis. The advances in knowledge of renal pathology which have stemmed from needle biopsy and immunological techniques have led to an awareness that a simplistic approach has considerable advantages, at least until more information is available regarding aetiological factors. The classification given on p. 169 has the marked advantage that it enables decisions about patient management to be taken without the necessity of exact pigeon-holing, and that it can absorb additional knowledge without needing fundamental alteration.

Steps in diagnosis

Diagnosis based on this classification is made in several steps:

1 Identification of clinical presentation and type of urinary abnormality.

2 Identification of pattern of glomerular response to injury, i.e. histological classification—including electron microscopy where relevant.

3 Immunological abnormalities—deposition of immunoglobulins, complement, fibrin and serological changes.

4 Addition of:
   (a) aetiological mechanism, if known;
   (b) associated disease process, if present;
   (c) specific clinical syndromes.
5 Time scale, i.e. acute or chronic (if known).

Clinical presentation and urinary abnormalities

1 *Nephritic*—haematuria, proteinuria, often with urinary casts.
2 *Nephrotic*—proteinuria (usually >3.5 g/24 h) with hypoproteinaemia and oedema.
3 *Asymptomatic proteinuria* (>0.3 g/24h) without haematuria:
   (a) continuous;
   (b) orthostatic;
   (c) transient.
4 *Haematuria*—without significant proteinuria:
   (a) continuous;
   (b) intermittent.
5 Renal failure.
6 Hypertension.

Histology of patterns of glomerular reaction

Methods
Techniques used in the study of renal histology include:
1 Standard paraffin-wax-embedded needle biopsy material for thin (3 μm) sections. Useful stains, in addition to haematoxylin and eosin are; PAS—for mesangium and basement membrane in particular; silver impregnation, particularly methenamine silver-PAS, for basement membrane detail; connective tissue stain, e.g. Mallory trichrome, for collagen, hyaline material, fibrin.
2 Very thin (1 μm) resin-embedded, glutaraldehyde-fixed biopsy material stained with toluidine blue—for deposits.
3 Electron microscopy—for ultrastructural abnormalities and identification of position of immune deposits.
4 Immunoperoxidase techniques—for composition and distribution of immune substances.

Definitions
1 *Diffuse*—lesions involving all glomeruli.
2 *Focal*—lesions of some glomeruli but not others.
3 *Global*—involvement of the whole of the glomerular tuft.

4 *Segmental*—segment of glomerular tuft only involved.

Minimal glomerular lesion—lipoid nephrosis

Appearances
As the name suggests, the essential feature is that glomeruli are normal on light microscopy. On electron microscopy glomerular epithelial cells are swollen by protein droplets and their foot processes are fused—these changes are believed secondary to the escape of protein.

Incidence
This lesion accounts for less than 20% of cases of the nephrotic syndrome in adults but about 50% in children.

Immunology
Appearances on immunofluorescent techniques are non-specific and usually negative for immunoglobulins and complement.

Clinical
Most patients with the disease present with the nephrotic syndrome in which the proteinuria is highly selective. Response to corticosteroid therapy is usually good with occasional relapses requiring a further course of therapy. Lack of remission suggests that the diagnosis was incorrect, particularly in relationship to focal glomerulosclerosis (see p. 172) or early membranous nephropathy (see p. 172). The long-term prognosis is very good.

Aetiology
Virus infection has, along with other factors, been postulated but there is no substantial evidence in favour. There is likewise no evidence of an immune complex origin for the minimal lesion.

Obvious glomerular lesions

Specific
In this group the glomerular abnormalities are commonly (or usually) sufficiently characteristic to be able to make a definitive diagnosis of a clinical entity.
1 *Diabetic nephropathy*. The characteristic glomerular abnormalities are of diffuse or nodular—

Kimmelstiel–Wilson nodules—deposition of eosinophilic, PAS-positive material in basement membranes and endothelial cells (see p. 355). These tend to be maximal towards the central parts of the lobules. Occasionally, quite marked diabetic changes are seen in the absence of overt glycosuria or other manifestations of diabetes. Also specific when present, are the *fibrinoid caps* seen at the periphery of the affected glomerulus and *capsular drops*.

Vascular lesions are also usually present as hyaline arteriolar sclerosis or microaneurysms of afferent arterioles. Accelerated atherosclerosis, pyelonephritis and papillary necrosis often complicate the renal diabetic picture (see p. 165).

2 *Amyloid*. The nephrotic syndrome or renal failure are common presenting features of amyloidosis and renal involvement is frequently dominant. Eosinophilic amyloid material of homogeneous appearance is seen variably diffusely or in a more nodular distribution in the intercapillary areas, in blood vessels and in tubular basement membranes. Specific staining by Congo red, Sirius red or thioflavine-T-fluorescence is diagnostic.

3 *Disseminated intravascular coagulopathy* (DIC). Renal involvement in this systemic disorder is usual and oliguria or anuria common, often being responsible for death.

Glomeruli show intracapillary fibrin and platelet plugs with similar changes in arterioles. A variable number of glomeruli may be involved.

4 *Malarial nephropathy*. In endemic areas, particularly for *Plasmodium malariae* infection, the nephrotic syndrome is common. When associated with parasitic infection many cases show a proliferative glomerulonephritis with segmental thickening of capillary walls leading to progressive sclerosis of the tufts. Electron-dense subendothelial deposits are seen and immunofluorescence shows granular deposits of IgM on the epithelial side of the basement membrane. Malarial antigen can be demonstrated in these deposits.

5 *Systemic lupus erythematosus—lupus nephritis*. Renal involvement in SLE is commonly the most important manifestation in respect of therapy and prognosis. Estimates of the frequency of renal involvement vary from 55% to 80% with renal failure in 15% or more. The only specific and pathognomonic abnormality is the presence of *haematoxyphil bodies*. Five patterns of involvement are described:

(a) *Glomeruli normal*—on light, immunological and electron microscopy. Very infrequent—good prognosis.

(b) *Mesangial lupus nephropathy*—mesangial deposits only with variable mesangial proliferation—good prognosis.

(c) *Focal and segmental proliferative GN*—up to 50% of glomeruli involved in focal or segmental areas of cellular proliferation and small occasional subendothelial deposits as well as abundant mesangial—intermediate prognosis.

(d) *Diffuse proliferative GN*—more than 50% of glomeruli have endocapillary cellular proliferation, sometimes with crescents. Necrosis is usual and large subendothelial deposits—*wire loops*, are seen, as well as in the mesangium. Appearances may mimic mesangiocapillary glomerulonephritis—grave prognosis.

(e) *Membranous*—diffuse uniformly thickened basement membranes due to subepithelial deposits sometimes with 'spikes' seen on silver stains. Deposits present in the mesangium as well, differentiate from idiopathic membranous glomerulonephropathy—slowly progressive decline in renal function.

Immunology of lupus nephritis

Immune substances are consistently found in the glomeruli except in type (a), although there is a wide range of appearances. Granular, or occasionally linear, deposits of IgG are almost always present, usually with IgM, IgA, fractions of complement and fibrin.

Levels of complement and anti-DNA antibodies in serum are useful parameters for monitoring activity of the disease.

Prognosis of renal lesion in lupus

Treatment by corticosteroids and/or other immunosuppressive drugs has led to much improvement in prognosis but requires careful monitoring to avoid deaths from complications of therapy rather than disease processes.

6 *Infective endocarditis and shunt nephritis*. A range of proliferative glomerular abnormalities can be seen in endocarditis particularly when of *Streptococcus viridans* origin. Similar lesions are found as infective complications of ventriculocaval and dialysis shunts—usually from coagulase-negative staphylococci. Most common is a focal segmental proliferative lesion with fibrin and immune deposits present but no

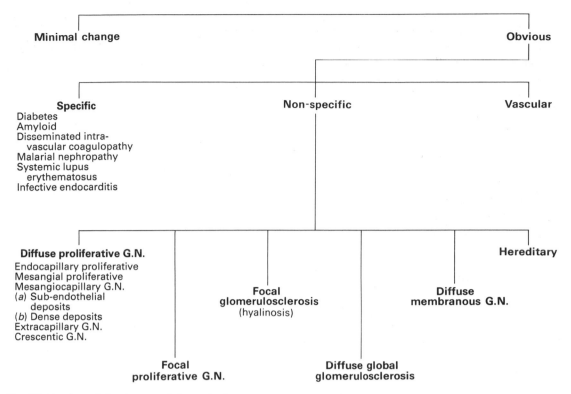

Fig. 17 Histological classification of glomerular lesions.

organisms—previously called focal embolic nephritis but *not* embolic. Crescents are quite common and diffuse global abnormalities may occasionally occur.

Non-specific

Nature

Most or all of these glomerulonephritic lesions are the result of immunological disturbances and two types of mechanisms are involved:

1 *Anti-GBM disease.* Specific antiglomerular basement antibodies become fixed to the membrane. Immunological staining techniques show the deposition to be linear.

2 *Soluble immune complex disease.* Antigen–antibody complexes in the circulation are incidentally cleared by the kidney and become trapped in glomeruli where they can be demonstrated as *granular* deposits. Their size and position and immunoglobulin composition are very variable in the different subgroups of glomerulonephritis.

Relatively little is known about the nature of the

antigen in most cases in this group.

Proliferative glomerulonephritis

Diffuse

Nature

Hypercellularity of virtually all glomeruli and all parts of the glomerular tuft.

There are a number of subdivisions depending on:
1 The presence or absence of polymorphs.
2 Increase in mesangial cells and/or matrix.
3 Presence of adhesions to the capsule.
4 Presence or absence of crescents from epithelial cell proliferation and, when present, the percentage of glomeruli thus involved.

Endocapillary proliferative glomerulonephritis

Microscopical

In this pattern there is a predominance of endothelial

cell proliferation which may be very uniform in appearance in *post-streptococcal glomerulonephritis* and rather more irregular in distribution in bacterial endocarditis, systemic lupus erythematosus and in some other cases where the aetiology is unknown.

In the acute stage there is often an increase in polymorphs—*exudative change*, together with endothelial cell proliferation predominantly axial and loss of capillary lumen with resulting 'bloodless' appearance. Capsular adhesions and some epithelial proliferation may also occur.

Electron microscopy demonstrates subendothelial immune complex deposits in infected children but in adults these deposits of IgG and complement are usually subepithelial—'lumpy-bumpy' appearance.

Clinical
This condition is commonly preceded by pharyngitis or tonsillitis due to type 12 group A β-haemolytic streptococci and serum anti-streptolysin titres may be raised. Presentation may be as an acute nephritic illness as described originally by Richard Bright with oliguria and hypertension. This is followed in the majority of cases by resolution, which may be complete in 85% of children and 60% of adults, or incomplete with persistent urinary abnormalities and a progressive proliferation and subsequent hyalinization in glomeruli leading to renal failure in a time span varying from a few to more than 30 years. A very small number of patients may die in the acute phase and the clinical pattern may be nephrotic at almost any stage during the progressive illness. In many adult patients the onset is often clinically more insidious.

Mesangial proliferative glomerulonephritis

Microscopical
Diffuse expansion of the mesangial regions of the glomerular tufts by mesangial cell proliferation and variable increase in mesangial matrix. The capillary loops appear normal at the periphery.

Clinical
Sometimes associated with systemic diseases, e.g. SLE and Henoch–Schönlein syndrome, this pattern also occurs in the resolving stage of diffuse endocapillary post-streptococcal glomerulonephritis.

May be associated with nephrotic syndrome or the recurrent haematuria syndrome. In the latter case

large deposits of mesangial IgA are usually seen, sometimes with C_3 and IgG also (see p. 171).

In most cases of diffuse mesangial proliferative GN, the course is benign with spontaneous resolution.

Immunology
Many cases are entirely negative but some show mesangial C_3 and IgG in addition to the clear-cut cases of *IgA disease* described above.

Mesangiocapillary glomerulonephritis— membranoproliferative glomerulonephritis

Microscopical
There are two types:

Type I: subendothelial deposits
The characteristic appearances in this condition is of '*double-contour*' basement membranes due to interposition of PAS-positive mesangial matrix. The change is usually diffuse though not necessarily uniform in distribution and is best demonstrated by the PASM (PAS methenamine silver) method. In addition to this feature there is increased cellularity of the tufts due to endothelial cell proliferation. There are considerable variations in appearance and this mesangiocapillary pattern is seen in more than one disease entity, e.g. also in some cases of SLE, bacterial endocarditis; more usually aetiological factors are not identifiable. Sometimes when the mesangial increase is more nodular the term *lobular glomerulonephritis* was previously used.

Immunology. Marked hypocomplementaemia is noted at some stage in nearly all patients. The glomeruli consistently show deposits of complement (C_3) and granular IgG and some have considerable IgA.

Type II: dense deposits
A further group of patients have very dense intramembranous deposits—these have a worse prognosis. Adhesions and/or epithelial crescents are also frequently seen in this group. Low serum complement levels are associated with C_3 glomerular deposition but other immunoglobulins are usually absent. Some cases are associated with a partial lipodystrophy.

Clinical
Most patients present with insidious renal failure or

hypertension. The nephrotic syndrome is a less common feature and appears to confer a worse prognosis. Present methods of treatment appear to influence the course very little. The natural history is not identified with certainty but the prognosis is, on the whole, poor and certainly worse than diffuse membranous glomerulonephritis (see p. 172). There is a rather high recurrence rate in transplants particularly in type II.

Extracapillary proliferative glomerulonephritis—crescentic GN— rapidly progressive GN

Microscopical

The dominant feature is of proliferation of epithelial cells into the capsular space together with varying degrees of endothelial and/or mesangial proliferation which is usually overshadowed. The capsular space is commonly completely obliterated by these extensive crescents involving 80% or more of glomeruli. Fibrin is often present.

Immunology

Granular deposits of IgG and complement are present in most cases but about one quarter show no significant immunoglobulins and in a minority there is linear deposition of IgG, complement and other immunoglobulins.

Pathogenesis

In many cases aetiological factors cannot be identified but some are due to bacterial endocarditis, SLE, vasculitis, Henoch–Schönlein syndrome, Wegener's granulomatosis (see p. 103) and, particularly with linear deposits, in *Goodpasture's syndrome* (see p. 386). In this last condition, the deposits are antiglomerular basement membrane—anti-GBM, a common antigen shared with lung basement membrane hence the haemorrhagic pulmonary lesions. Many cases are, however, focal rather than diffuse (see below).

Clinical

The onset is acute with severe oliguria, rapidly progressive uraemia and a very high and speedy mortality. Immediate prognosis is related to the percentage of glomeruli with crescents, being particularly grave in those with more than 80%. If trans-

planted, anti-GBM cases have a high risk of recurrent disease in the graft.

Focal and segmental proliferative glomerulonephritis

Definition

Whilst some cases of diffuse proliferative glomerulonephritis undoubtedly start as focal or segmental lesions, a group of conditions exists where only some glomeruli (focal) or parts of the tufts (segmental) are involved by a proliferative process.

Microscopical

Affected segments show increased cellularity in which endothelial, epithelial and mesangial cells may all take part. One or more lobules may be affected and adhesions and crescents may occur. Fibrinoid areas may be seen and there may be increase in polymorphonuclear leucocytes.

Pathogenetic factors

Focal proliferative lesions may be associated with a wide range of disorders including post-streptococcal glomerulonephritis, bacterial endocarditis, Henoch–Schönlein syndrome, systemic lupus erythematosus, polyarteritis nodosa and other vasculitic conditions. Some are 'idiopathic'. Many cases of Goodpasture's syndrome show focal glomerular disease rather than diffuse, although the linear IgG deposition is diffuse (see above). The focal glomerulosclerosis of children (hyalinosis) needs separation from this proliferative group.

Clinical

The picture is very variable reflecting the range of factors above. Microscopic haematuria is common, particularly so with IgA disease.

Immunology

The syndrome of recurrent haematuria commonly shows deposition of considerable quantities of IgA in the mesangium—*IgA disease*. Whilst this is often associated with focal proliferation, minimal or no proliferation may be seen in patients with marked IgA deposition or they may show diffuse mesangial proliferation (see p. 170). In other cases of focal proliferative GN, immunoglobulin deposition is usually present and focal but not specific in pattern, usually comprising complement and IgG.

Focal glomerulosclerosis—focal and segmental hyalinosis

Nature
This is an important cause of the nephrotic syndrome, most commonly occurring in childhood. The pathogenesis is possibly related to fibrin deposition but aetiological factors are not identified.

Microscopical
Segmental adhesions of glomerular tufts to capsule are associated with hyaline eosinophilic subendothelial nodules in the earlier stages. Later, one or more segments show sclerosis and this extends to an increasing number of glomeruli and parts of the tuft. Even in the presence of a grossly nephrotic clinical picture there may be only occasional foci of glomerular involvement and, as a result, some cases are initially misdiagnosed as 'minimal change'.

Immunology
Characteristically, IgM and C_3 are present in glomeruli, often segmentally, and only in the sclerotic areas.

Clinical
The presentation is typically in childhood with the nephrotic syndrome. Progression of the lesion may be rapid and there is steroid-resistance. The overall prognosis is poor and the disease commonly recurs in those initially successfully transplanted.

Diffuse global glomerulosclerosis

Nature
Diffuse glomerular scarring associated with widespread tubular atrophy and compensatory increase in interstitial tissue.

This occurs with the later stages of any type of glomerulonephritis with masking of differentiating features so that more specific histological identification is not possible.

The term is synonymous with *end-stage nephritis*.

Membranous glomerulonephritis— membranous nephropathy

Microscopical
All glomeruli are uniformly involved and show basement membrane thickening by PAS-positive material which commonly shows 'spikes' of silver-positive material on the epithelial aspect of capillary loops and on electron microscopy shows deposition of proteinaceous material on the outer side of the membrane— *epimembranous*. Progression of the lesion leads to capillary luminal obliteration, hyalinization and renal failure.

Immunology
Capillary loop beaded deposits of granular IgG and C_3, sometimes also with IgM and IgA, are the most typical.

Pathogenetic factors
Most cases are 'idiopathic' but, in adults, a few are associated with malignant disease, particularly in the lung, in which case the deposits are of tumour-associated products. The lesion may also occur in systemic lupus erythematosus, with some drugs—gold and penicillamine, and as a result of HB_sAg.

Clinical
The majority of cases present with the nephrotic syndrome and progress to renal failure, often in a 5-year period. About one-third of the cases of the 'idiopathic' type progress more slowly and some patients have a prolonged course into renal failure up to 25 years later.

Hereditary nephritis

Nature
Glomerular lesions with a familial incidence are relatively common and include most patterns of disease in which more than one member of a family is affected. The pathogenesis of many such cases is obscure and will probably remain so until more is known about glomerular disease antigens. Some are likely to prove to be the result of an infective agent to which sibs are exposed.

Additionally, there are clear-cut inherited conditions.
1 Alport's syndrome.
2 Congenital nephrotic syndrome.

Alport's syndrome

Clinical
The fully developed syndrome consists of deafness and progression to renal failure with variably associ-

ated features including giant platelets, ocular lesions, neuropathy and bony abnormalities. The renal lesion usually presents as microscopic haematuria and proteinuria appearing in childhood, progressing through a phase of nephrotic syndrome to end-stage failure.

Microscopical
In the early stages, light microscopical appearances are near normal with slight mesangial increase. Electron microscopy is necessary to make the definitive diagnosis by identifying splitting and lamellation of the lamina densa of the basement membrane. Glomerulosclerosis follows.

Inheritance
This is very complex but is basically autosomal dominant with incomplete penetrance in females.

Congenital nephrotic syndrome
Classically, this relates to nephrotic syndrome occurring at or shortly after birth often associated with bulky placenta, congenital heart disease and raised α-fetoprotein level in maternal amniotic fluid.

The *Finnish type* shows slight glomerular mesangial proliferation and progressive glomerulosclerosis.

In *non-Finnish type* there is focal and segmental glomerulosclerosis.

Both types progress inexorably to renal failure.

Aetiological mechanisms, clinical syndromes and associated disease processes
In only a relatively small proportion of the patients with glomerular lesions can the exact aetiological mechanism be identified but, in a rather higher percentage, a defined clinical syndrome may be apparent or the renal involvement is part of a more systematized disease. This is true of the group of 'specific' abnormalities identified earlier in this chapter.

Other clinical syndromes include:
1 Henoch–Schönlein—purpura and proliferative glomerulonephritis largely focal (see p. 171).
2 Infective endocarditis—in *Streptococcus viridans* endocarditis in particular (see p. 70).
3 Goodpasture's syndrome—lung haemorrhages and a rapidly progressive type of glomerulonephritis associated with linear deposition of anti-GBM immunoglobulins on the basement membrane (see p. 386).

4 Wegener's granulomatosis—necrotic vasculitic granulomatous lesions affecting upper and lower respiratory tract particularly (see p. 395) and with an associated severe focal proliferative glomerulonephritis with abundant fibrin, crescent formation and no other immune deposition.
5 Poststreptococcal—raised anti-streptolysin and other antibody titres are found in a proportion of cases of focal and diffuse proliferative glomerulonephritis. There may be typical clinical manifestations of infection by particular strains (e.g. type 12) of β-haemolytic streptococci.

C/TUBULAR, VASCULAR

Tubular disorders
   Morphological
   Cell changes
   Substances in tubules
Vascular
   Hypertensive
   Atherosclerotic
   Renal artery stenosis
   Infarction
   Renal vein thrombosis
   Cortical necrosis
   Haemolytic uraemic syndrome
   Vasculitis
   Systemic sclerosis
   Toxaemia of pregnancy

Disorders of tubules

Alterations in basic tubular morphology

Atrophy
Tubular loss usually follows glomerular diseases in which there is progressive hyalinization of the tufts. Thus it may follow the various types of glomerulonephritis, the specific glomerular lesions identified in Section B and ischaemic conditions including hypertension and renal artery atherosclerosis. Shrinkage of tubular lumina is accompanied by reduction in height of the epithelium and loss of specialized features. There is a concomitant increase in interstitial tissue by fibrosis and a lymphocytic infiltrate which is quite non-specific in origin.

Atrophy is also a feature of *obstructive uropathy* (see p. 179).

Hypertrophy

A compensatory mechanism involving surviving nephrons where there is progressive chronic renal damage, particularly in hypertension and glomerulonephritis. The enlarged tubules contrast with adjacent patchy areas of atrophy and fibrosis and are responsible for subcapsular granularity.

Tubular dilatation

Distended thin-walled tubules with epithelium of collecting duct type are frequently seen in obstructive uropathy and in many other chronic renal diseases at a relatively late stage.

Tubular necrosis

Acute necrosis of renal tubules usually occurs in the absence of glomerular abnormalities.

There are two types:
1 Nephrotoxic.
2 Ischaemic.

Aetiological factors

1 *Nephrotoxic*: circulating toxins of chemical or bacterial origin producing a direct effect on tubular epithelial cells, particularly in the proximal convoluted segment. Substances include heavy metal salts particularly mercury and uranium, ethylene glycol and carbon tetrachloride.
2 *Ischaemic*: usually associated with hypotension or hypoperfusion of glomeruli from other causes. Particularly important predisposing factors are burns, blood loss particularly uterine, traumatic injuries particularly crush injuries—*crush syndrome*, incompatible blood transfusion and the hepatorenal syndrome, seen in cases of severe jaundice or other forms of liver disease.

Pathogenetic factors

Direct toxic effect of poisons are easy to understand but the exact mechanism in the ischaemic group of cases is more obscure. Reduction of blood flow and of pressure in the tubular vascular plexus appears to be dominant with resulting anoxia and damage particularly to the more sensitive specialized convoluted epithelium.

Macroscopical

Swelling and pallor of the cortex with loss of cortical pattern.

Microscopical

There is considerable variability in morphology of involved tubular segments partly dependent on the cause. A wide range of degenerative changes from swelling, granularity and vacuolation of cytoplasm, to complete necrosis of lining cells and filling of lumina with debris.

Interstitial oedema often with some lymphocytic cellular infiltrate may be prominent but glomeruli are usually structurally intact.

Additional features in specific situations include presence of myoglobin casts in crush syndrome, haematin casts in incompatible blood transfusion kidney and bile staining in hepato-renal syndrome when jaundice is severe.

Secondary calcium deposition is common at an early stage as is the presence of oxalate crystals.

Clinical

Correlation of morphological changes and clinical severity is unrewarding. Severe acute renal failure can be present with little histological evidence of necrosis or cell damage although biopsy evidence of necrotic tubules is also invariably associated with acute renal failure.

Results

1 Acute renal failure with death if untreated.
2 A period of oliguria or anuria is followed by clinical and pathological recovery often heralded by a diuretic phase.
3 Correction of the cause and treatment of the renal failure by attention to fluid and electrolyte balance with or without supportive dialysis usually leads to complete recovery of structure and function.

Alterations in tubular cells hydropic or vacuolar change—osmotic nephrosis

Nature

Cytoplasmic swelling with granularity or vacuole formation occurring in tubular epithelial cells, usually in the proximal convoluted tubule. It is believed that this results from disturbance of the normal osmotic relationships within the cells.

Aetiology

Most commonly seen after treatment with sucrose, dextrose and mannitol.

Similar changes are found in some cases of severe or prolonged potassium deficiency.

Substances present in tubular cells or lumina

Hyaline (protein) droplets
Protein aggregates forming droplets of hyaline eosinophilic, PAS-positive material in tubular cell cytoplasm. These may be found in a wide range of renal diseases in which there is proteinuria.

Calcium—nephrocalcinosis
Deposition of calcium salts can occur in damaged tissues as dystrophic calcification or due to abnormal serum calcium levels—*metastatic calcification* (see p. 138). The most marked examples of nephrocalcinosis are seen in hypercalcaemia due to hyperparathyroidism, malignant disease, sarcoidosis, milk-alkali syndrome and hypervitaminosis D.

Myelomatosis
Renal failure associated with characteristic 'hard' tubular casts and cellular reaction is common in myelomatosis which may also be complicated by secondary renal amyloidosis. The casts are densely eosinophilic usually with multinucleated cells at their periphery which appear to be derived from tubular epithelium.

Gout
In both primary and secondary gout (see p. 315) renal involvement is common but seldom clinically important. Deposits of urate crystals and surrounding inflammatory reaction including foreign body giant cells may be quite marked. These are usually in the medulla and, whilst starting in the tubules, later appear to be interstitial.

Vascular disorders

Hypertensive nephrosclerosis— arteriolar sclerosis

Benign nephrosclerosis

Nature
The renal disease associated with benign hypertension (see p. 92) though some similar changes may just be due to ageing.

Incidence
This is the most common form of nephropathy and is found in approximately 75% of autopsies over the age of 60 years.

Aetiology
Most commonly seen in the essential type but it may also be found in cases of hypertension secondary to renal disease and this, therefore, may then complicate the appearances of the kidneys. The hypertension antedates and produces the renal changes in uncomplicated cases.

Kidneys
Diffuse, symmetrical, ischaemic atrophy and scarring in uncomplicated cases of long-standing hypertension.

Macroscopical
1 *Size*: small and pale.
2 *Capsule*: moderately adherent.
3 *Cortex*: fine, even granularity of the surface, the cortex being pale grey and narrow, with some loss of pattern.
4 *Medulla*: demarcation from the cortex is usually preserved but there is a decrease in size with some pallor.
5 *Blood vessels*: the arcuate arteries are particularly affected and are prominent on the cut surface with thickening of their walls.
6 *Calyces and pelvis*: normal.

Microscopical
1 *Glomeruli*: progressive wrinkling of basement membrane and fibrosis which is maximal in the periglomerular and capsular interstitial tissues—extracapsular glomerulofibrosis, cf. the intracapsular fibrosis of glomerulonephritis.
2 *Tubules*: atrophic.
3 *Interstitial tissue*: increased fibrosis with a very scanty lymphocytic infiltration.
4 *Blood vessels*: thick-walled arterioles and small arteries which have a markedly decreased lumen. The thickening is due to hyaline material which at first is subendothelial but later replaces the muscle of the media.

These arteriolosclerotic changes are present in other organs and may also be superimposed on other forms of renal disease which cause hypertension, e.g. chronic pyelonephritis and glomerulonephritis.

Results

Not more than 5% of patients with well-developed benign nephrosclerosis die from renal failure. Death in the great majority of cases of benign hypertension occurs from congestive heart failure, coronary insufficiency and cerebral vascular accidents (see p. 321).

Accelerated nephrosclerosis

Nature

Renal disease produced by accelerated malignant hypertension (see p. 92).

Origin

1 In previously normotensive individuals.
2 Superimposed on pre-existing renal disease or benign hypertension.

Age

In the pure form, the disease usually presents under 40 years of age, but as a complication of benign hypertension is most frequently seen between 60 and 70 years of age.

Kidney in the pure type

Macroscopical

1 *Size*: normal or slightly enlarged and congested.
2 *Capsule*: strips easily.
3 *Cortex*: normal pattern and size with small pinpoint haemorrhages on the surface.
4 *Medulla*: demarcation from the cortex is preserved and the medullary pattern is normal.
5 *Blood vessels*: normal or slight vascular prominence.
6 *Pelvis and calyces*: normal.

Microscopical

1 *Glomeruli*: sometimes focal necrosis may be seen in the capillaries, but more often they appear normal.
2 *Tubules*: minor degenerative changes in the proximal convoluted tubules.

Blood vessels

1 Fibroblastic proliferation and muscular hypertrophic thickening of the arterioles and small arteries. There is the appearance of concentric fibrous lamination—'onion-skin'; the lumen is narrowed.
2 Fibrinoid necrosis of the afferent arterioles often with rupture producing haemorrhages or thrombosis; this is the pathognomonic lesion.

Kidney in the secondary type

The appearances are those of a pre-existing renal disease, e.g. chronic pyelonephritis, or of benign hypertension with superimposed fibrinoid necrosis of the blood vessels.

Results

Untreated accelerated hypertension causes death from renal failure in 90%, usually with marked rapidity. If the hypertension is treated adequately before there is evidence of impairment of renal function by a raised blood urea, prognosis is good and subsequent renal failure unusual.

Senile arteriosclerotic kidney—atherosclerotic nephrosclerosis

Aetiology

Atheromatous narrowing of the main renal arteries and branches leading to ischaemic atrophy of the renal substance. Although the renal arteries are not a very common site for atheroma, the mouths of the vessels are frequently involved by aortic atheromatous plaques.

Appearances

1 *Main arteries involved*: diffuse symmetrical contraction producing a pale, granular, small kidney similar to that of benign nephrosclerosis except that the blood vessels within the renal substance do not show hypertensive changes.
2 *Branch arteries involved*: asymmetrical, patchy, focal, depressed scars of the cortical surface. These are pale, granular, wedge-shaped areas of fibrosis extending into the medulla and showing ischaemic atrophy with fibrous replacement of the glomeruli and tubules.

Results

1 Usually there is no interference with renal function.
2 When there is unilateral renal artery obstruction, hypertension may ensue which may occasionally be relieved by removal of the ischaemic organ.
3 Occasionally, severe bilateral main artery involvement may lead to renal failure.

Renal artery stenosis

Whilst atheroma is by far the most common cause there are uncommon cases of luminal narrowing due to segments of *fibromuscular hyperplasia* or *fibro-elastosis*, usually in younger persons and causing hypertension.

Infarction

Incidence

A common site of infarction.

Causes

1 *Arterial*: 98%.
  (a) *Embolic*, e.g. mural thrombus from a cardiac infarct, left atrial thrombus in mitral stenosis. Atheromatous material rich in cholesterol crystals is an increasingly recognized cause of multiple small or fewer large emboli to the kidney, particularly as complications of invasive intra-arterial or aortic investigative procedures.
  (b) *Thrombotic*: due to advanced atheroma, occlusion of renal artery orifices by aortic thrombus, polyarteritis nodosa.
2 *Venous*: 2%—renal thrombophlebitis with sudden occlusion is usually associated with perinephric abscess or other intra-abdominal infections.
  Gradual venous occlusion does not cause infarction but may cause the nephrotic syndrome (see below).

Appearances

Infarcts in the kidneys are anaemic in type and within 24 hours there is a wedge-shaped, sharply demarcated, pale, yellow–white area with a hyperaemic border, usually confined to the cortex. Later, a V-shaped scar develops.

Renal vein thrombosis

Nature

This uncommon condition is an occasional cause of the nephrotic syndrome, usually in adults over 50 years of age. Rapid occlusion of renal veins, e.g. by extension of inferior vena caval thrombus, is likely to produce renal infarction, but the mechanism of a presumed more insidious venous thrombosis is obscure. Some cases are associated with renal amyloidosis, accelerated hypertension, acute pyelonephritis or glomerulonephritis. Extrinsic pressure from metastatic tumour in adjacent lymph nodes is also a frequent cause. Many cases, however, have to be classified as 'idiopathic'.

Appearances

The diagnosis can often be suspected on renal biopsy material when:
1 Tubular damage, atrophy and interstitial oedema and fibrosis are disproportionately greater than glomerular abnormalities.
2 Mild to moderate diffuse basement membrane thickening of glomeruli is present but lacks 'spikes' and other features of membranous glomerulonephritis (see p. 172).

Results

If infarction occurs then renal failure is inevitable. When the presentation is by the nephrotic syndrome, this may be progressive with developing renal failure, or spontaneously improve, or improve following anticoagulant therapy.

Acute cortical necrosis

Nature

Acute massive usually bilateral symmetrical necrosis of the cortical tissues.

Aetiology

This very rare condition occurs most frequently with placental abruption during pregnancy, but may also follow severe infections, burns and shock.

Mechanisms

1 There is a close association with disseminated intravascular coagulopathy (DIC) and the haemolytic—uraemic syndrome of children (see p. 178).
2 Appearances are very similar to the experimentally produced Schwartzmann reaction.

Macroscopical

1 *Size*: enlarged.
2 *Cortex*: the surface shows areas of congestion and haemorrhage alternating with pale yellow areas of massive necrosis. Double contour (tramline) calcification commonly develops in the subcapsular tissue and at the sharp zone of demarcation between necrotic and normal cortex.
3 *Medulla*: usually completely normal.
4 *Blood vessels*: thrombosed vessels may be seen within the necrotic zones.

Results

When cortical necrosis is bilateral, there is complete anuria and acute renal failure.

Haemolytic uraemic syndrome

Nature

The combination of haemolytic anaemia, thrombocytopenia and renal failure mostly in children, usually under 4 years of age. There is often a preceding infective episode.

Clinical

Acute onset of jaundice, thrombocytopenia and haemolytic anaemia with *schistocytes*—fragmented erythrocytes, in the peripheral blood and acute renal failure, sometimes with hypertension.

Kidney

There is widespread fibrin and platelet deposition in vessels and glomerular tufts with endocapillary proliferation of global or segmental distribution. Apart from fibrin deposition, immunohistological studies are negative.

Arterioles and branch arteries may show intimal fibrous thickening with luminal narrowing, changes which are also notable in *postpartum renal failure*, a rare complication of parturition and probably initiated through fibrin deposition.

In severe cases of the haemolytic uraemic syndrome cortical necrosis occurs (see p. 177).

Pathogenesis

Many of the features are similar to those of disseminated intravascular coagulation (DIC).

Results

The prognosis depends largely on the severity of the acute attack and mortality may be as high as 40%.

Polyarteritis nodosa and vasculitis

Incidence

Renal involvement is common and is often the determining prognostic factor in this multisystem disease (see p. 102). Necrotizing lesions of arteries of varying size and age are seen in renal vessels and also sometimes in glomerular capillaries. A focal and segmental proliferative glomerulonephritis may occur, sometimes with crescent formation (see p. 171).

Progressive systemic sclerosis

The renal arteries are frequently involved in this systemic type of scleroderma (see p. 98) with resulting luminal narrowing by intimal fibroelastic thickening, ischaemia and renal failure.

Toxaemia of pregnancy—eclampsia

The lesions in the kidneys in this disease consist of diffuse glomerular swelling primarily involving the endothelial cells, deposition of protein material related to fibrin adjacent to the basement membrane and swelling of mesangial cell cytoplasm reducing intercapillary spaces.

The condition usually resolves following evacuation of the uterus but if essential hypertension preceded the pregnancy, its progression may be accelerated.

D/MECHANICAL, RENAL FAILURE, RENAL TRANSPLANTATION

Granular contracted kidneys
Hydronephrosis
Calculi
Proteinuria
Uraemia
Renal transplantation

Granular contracted kidneys

Many serious renal diseases lead to renal failure and are associated with small granular contracted kidneys. Characteristic and diagnostic features may be present but often the changes, grossly and histologically, are non-specific.

Chronic glomerulonephritis

Diffuse fine granularity with a uniform loss of pattern and prominent blood vessels. The pelvis and calyces are normal.

Chronic pyelonephritis

Irregular granularity with large, flat areas of cortical scarring, the intervening zones often appearing normal. The pelvis and calyces are thickened, pale and granular (see p. 164).

Analgesic abuse nephropathy

Cortical scarring pallor and interstitial fibrosis are marked but non-specific. Necrotic papillae, when present, are obvious but identifying the absence of shed papillae is more difficult (see p. 165).

Vascular diseases

1 *Benign nephrosclerosis*. Fine, even granularity of the cortex with slight loss of the cortical pattern but preservation of corticomedullary differentiation. The vessels pout from the cut surface and the calyces and pelvis are normal (see p. 175).

2 *Atherosclerotic nephrosclerosis*. Asymmetrical, focal, wedge-shaped cortical scars extending deeply into the medulla with severe atheroma of the large vessels. When the main arteries are involved, however, the kidneys are symmetrically contracted with a fine granularity (see p. 176).

3 *Vasculitis*. Petechial haemorrhages and infarcts of varying age are usually seen in addition to a fine cortical granularity. The blood vessels are commonly aneurysmally dilated and may be thrombosed.

Diabetes

Usually a mixed picture due to the common concurrence of pyelonephritis and nephrosclerosis with the rather more streaky and mottled appearance of the Kimmelstiel–Wilson lesion (see p. 167).

Hydronephrosis—hydrocalycosis

Nature

Dilation of the renal pelvis and calyces.

Mechanism

Due to slowly progressive obstruction at any level of the urinary tract. Ureteric ligation may cause renal atrophy without significant hydronephrosis. However, intermittent, partial, or progressive obstruction leads to distension of the renal pelvis with a rise of pressure, atrophy of the renal parenchyma and subsequent loss of function.

Age and incidence

Common in differing age groups according to the cause.

Causes

These are many and include:
1 *Lumen*: calculi, blood clot.
2 *Wall*.
  (a) *Congenital*: valves, strictures, abnormalities of peristalsis at the pelvi-ureteric junction.

  (b) *Acquired*: post-traumatic and post-inflammatory stricture, prostatic enlargement, tumours of the renal pelvis, ureter, bladder and urethra.
3 *External*: gravid uterus; pressure from ovarian or uterine masses; retroperitoneal fibrosis; invasion by tumour from adjacent organs or by enlarged lymph nodes.

An aberrant renal artery crossing the pelvi-ureteric junction probably perpetuates hydronephrosis arising from other causes.

Macroscopical

Hydronephrosis may be unilateral or bilateral. The most severe examples are seen in unilateral lesions due to obstruction proximal to the bladder, especially the pelvi-ureteric type. There is gross enlargement of the kidney with saccular distension of the pelvis, much of which becomes extrarenal in position. The calyces are flattened and the renal parenchyma is thinned and atrophied, in severe cases leaving only a thin rim of recognizable renal tissue. The external surface may be lobulated.

Microscopical

Marked atrophy of the tubules, the glomeruli at first being spared but subsequently becoming hyalinized.

Results

1 *Bilateral*: prolonged bilateral hydronephrosis leads to hypertension and/or renal failure.
2 *Unilateral*: the opposite kidney may become hypertrophied and maintain normal function but hypertension may result from the unilateral renal ischaemia (see p. 93).

In both forms, infection is a common complication causing *pyonephrosis*, i.e. pus in the distended pelvis and calyces. Pyelonephritic changes, spreading from the pelvis, speed the progression of the renal atrophy.

Calculi

Nature

Urinary calculi may form in the kidney and bladder but are also seen in passage down the ureter and urethra. These stones are composed of urinary salts in amorphous form bound by a colloid matrix and consist of a nucleus, usually organic, around which are deposited concentric layers of one or more of the salts.

Constituents

Principally
1 Uric acid.
2 Calcium oxalate.
3 Triple phosphates.

Others
4 Amino acids, e.g. xanthine, cystine.
5 Calcium carbonate.

They may occur in pure form, but are more frequently mixtures.

Types of stone

1 *Primary stone*: no antecedent inflammation. They are usually composed of uric acid, urates or calcium oxalate and the urine is acid.
2 *Secondary stone*: associated with inflammation. They are mostly triple phosphates or occasionally ammonium urate; the urine is alkaline.

Appearances

1 *Uric acid stones*: may occur alone or more usually combined with urates and oxalates. They are of moderate hardness, light or dark brown in colour with wavy concentric markings.
2 *Oxalate stones*: these are often in pure form and are extremely hard with a dark colour due to blood staining resulting from the production of local injury. They are laminated and show a spiny or prickly exterior—'mulberry calculus'.
3 *Phosphatic stones*: occur in a pure form or as a surface covering of primary stones. They are white, smooth and friable.

Pathogenesis

Renal stone formation is of frequent occurrence and the pathogenesis in most cases remains unknown. However, the following factors may be contributory:
1 *Hypercalciuria*: this occurs in hyperparathyroidism due to parathyroid adenoma or secondary hyperplasia (see p. 138).
2 *Urinary infection*: some urea-splitting organisms cause alkalinity of the urine.
3 *Urinary stasis*: favours the development of infection and the retention of organic substances.
4 *Microliths*: small foci of calcification are commonly seen in the medullary interstitial tissue and within macrophages in lymphatics. They have, however, no constant relationship to the presence or absence of calculi.
5 *pH of urine*: alkalinity of the urine renders calcium phosphate and triple phosphates less soluble.

Sites

Renal pelvis
Solitary or multiple, unilateral or bilateral and usually composed of oxalates or urates. Small stones are the commonest but large branched 'stag-horn' calculi may occur and completely fill the pelvis and calyces.

Bladder
1 Originate in the kidney with subsequent enlargement in the bladder due to phosphatic encrustation.
2 Formed primarily in the bladder usually of phosphates.

Effects

Obstruction
1 At the pelvi-ureteric junction.
2 Ureter.
3 Bladder neck.

Ulceration
Of calyces and pelvic mucosa.

Chronic infection
Predisposed to by the stones and by the stasis they cause, thus, pyelonephritis or pyonephrosis are induced if obstruction is present.

Proteinuria

Nature
Although albumin is the most important constituent of urinary protein loss, normal and abnormal globulins may be present and, indeed, normal persons pass up to 50 mg of total protein daily comprising twenty or more different types, ten closely related to serum proteins. Proteinuria may be selective or not.

Normal glomerular filtrate contains protein but at a concentration of less than 50 mg/100 ml and nearly all is reabsorbed by the tubule.

Origin
1 Escape of normal plasma proteins through a defective glomerular membrane.

2 Failure of normal tubular reabsorption.

3 Abnormally increased concentration in the plasma of normal plasma proteins.

4 Abnormal plasma proteins passed in the urine due to small size or failure of tubular reabsorption due to qualitative abnormality.

5 Abnormal secretions of proteins by the cells of the kidney, ureter, lower urinary tract and accessory glands.

In massive proteinuria leading to the nephrotic syndrome (see p. 167) factor 1 is largely responsible because of the glomerular abnormality. Factors 1 and 2 are effective in 'nephrosis' and factor 3 may operate in patients given protein infusion and in certain diseases causing high plasma proteins. Factor 4 is operative in conditions such as haemolytic states with haemoglobinuria and in myeloma and factor 5 comes into play with local abnormalities such as calculi and infections in the urinary tract.

Causes
The main causes are:

Postural (orthostatic) and exercise proteinuria
The physiological mechanisms are poorly understood but the protein content qualitatively is a reflection of plasma protein levels. If protein is detected in an ambulant or erect person then it should not be detectable after a period of rest or after a time in the supine position for a diagnosis of orthostatic or exercise proteinuria to be acceptable.

The urinary deposit should likewise be normal.

Renal diseases
1 Nephrotic syndrome (see p. 167).
2 Renal vascular disease (see p. 175) and congestive cardiac failure.
3 Glomerulonephritis of all types and stages (see p. 169).
4 As a constituent of escaped blood in any renal cause of haematuria—red cells identified in urinary deposit.
5 In renal infections (see p. 163)—pus cells and organisms usually identified in urinary deposit together with cultural isolation.

Post-renal diseases
Disorders of the ureters, bladder and lower urinary tract may cause proteinuria associated with infections, bleeding from these structures, calculi, etc.

Uraemia

Nature
A clinical state associated with a raised blood urea.

Causes

'Pre-renal'
1 Acute circulatory failure, e.g. shock.
2 Dehydration and severe electrolyte imbalance; due to excessive loss, e.g. vomiting, diarrhoea and sweating, or to inadequate fluid intake.
3 Bleeding into the gastrointestinal tract with absorption of breakdown products.
4 Massive tissue necrosis, e.g. gangrene of the leg, large infarcts, etc.

Renal
The most common causes are:
1 Vascular disease—accelerated nephrosclerosis, polyarteritis nodosa and vasculitis.
2 Glomerulonephritis—acute and chronic.
3 Diabetes mellitus.
4 Chronic pyelonephritis and analgesic nephropathy.
Less common renal causes include:
5 Acute tubular necrosis.
6 Polycystic kidneys.
7 Renal tuberculosis.
8 Myeloma kidney.

'Post-renal'
Any severe long-standing obstruction in the urinary tract may produce a bilateral back pressure effect on the kidneys. This is most commonly due to:
1 Hydronephrosis.
2 Calculi.
3 Carcinoma of the bladder.
4 Prostatic enlargement.
5 Carcinoma of the cervix.

Metabolic changes
The most important changes are:
1 *Blood urea and non-protein nitrogen*: raised.
2 *Metabolic acidosis*: there is a low bicarbonate due to failure of ammonia production and to electrolyte disturbances aggravated by vomiting, diarrhoea, etc.
3 *Electrolytes*: the changes are variable:
(a) When the decrease in glomerular filtration rate is dominant, there is sodium and potassium retention with raised blood levels.

(b) When failure of tubular reabsorption is dominant, there is sodium and potassium depletion with lowered blood levels. The urinary volume remains large, causing excess water loss.

This is particularly well seen in analgesic nephropathy. chloride levels are very variable.

4 *Phosphate and calcium*: phosphates are retained with increased blood levels. As a result the ionized serum calcium level falls and secondary hyperparathyroidism may ensue (*see* p. 139).

Organ changes

These are very variable but some or all of the following may be seen at post-mortem examination:

1 *Heart*: fibrinous pericarditis.

2 *Gastrointestinal tract*: mucosal or serosal petechial haemorrhages due to damaged capillaries are common. Stomatitis, oesophagitis, gastritis and enterocolitis are frequent, the last named often being associated with a patchy haemorrhagic and necrotizing appearance—'uraemic colitis'.

3 *Lungs*: pulmonary oedema, often associated with a fibrinous alveolar lining—'uraemic pneumonitis'.

4 *Skin*: sallow colour with a purpuric rash and frequently a 'uraemic frost'.

5 *Blood*: anaemia, which is commonly severe and of the normochromic normocytic type due to marrow depression in the presence of a raised blood urea; however, iron deficiency and macrocytic types may be found. The purpuric manifestations are non-thrombocytopenic and are due to 'toxic' capillary damage.

Renal transplantation

Functional allograft survival in excess of 5 years is now commonplace in 60–70% of patients in many centres. The best results occur when kidneys from a twin or live related donor are used, but most transplants are of fresh cadaver kidneys from unrelated persons. These are usually removed speedily at the time of death or when life support equipment is disconnected. Good HLA matching improves prognosis.

Complications

1 Technical.
2 Effects of immunosuppression.
3 Graft rejection.
4 Transmission of renal disease to graft.

Technical

1 Ureteric anastomosis—leakage or pyelonephritis.
2 Venous—venous thrombosis.
3 Arterial—kinking of supply, thrombosis or renal artery stenosis at the anastomosis.

Immunosuppression

Immunosuppressive drugs may be required in high dosage to control or prevent rejection of the graft. Cyclosporin with or without low-dosage corticosteroids and immunosuppressive agents are usually given in as low a dosage as safely possible. Complications due to this therapy include:

1 Metabolic.

2 Suppression of resistance to infection, particularly normally non-pathogenic *opportunistic* organisms, e.g. *Aspergillus* species, cytomegalovirus, *Pneumocystis carinii*. Septicaemic episodes by a wide range of microorganisms are common.

3 Induction of neoplasia—particularly lymphomas but many epithelial tumour associations are now also described.

Graft rejection

1 *Hyperacute*: this occurs within a few minutes of re-establishing blood flow to the graft. Flow quickly falls and within a few hours urine production ceases. Progressive cortical necrosis appears. Factors responsible include:

(a) Blood group incompatibility.

(b) Presensitization of recipient—from blood transfusions, pregnancy, a previous failed transplant, etc.

This type of rejection is mediated humorally by circulating cytotoxins.

2 *Acute*: episodes of acute rejection are common in recipients of grafts in the first few weeks even when immunosuppressed. There is, however, marked variability in severity and the ability to control the episode by treatment. There are two types of appearance:

(a) *Cellular (parenchymal) rejection*: marked oedema and dense focal or more generalized infiltration of the cortex by pyroninophilic lymphoid cells. Tubular degeneration and/or necrosis are usual and there may be endothelial cell swelling in capillaries. IgG and complement are not seen in capillaries or glomeruli. This type is cell mediated.

(b) *Vascular rejection*: lymphocytic infiltration is slight but platelet aggregates are found in capillaries and small venules later with fibrin and polymorphs. Fibrinoid necrosis is seen in the walls of small arteries and veins with superimposed thrombus deposition. Rupture of the internal elastic lamina of arteries may be seen. The thrombi will show progressive organization if the recipient survives. IgG, IgM, C_{1q}, C_3, fibrinogen can usually be demonstrated in vessel walls and glomerular capillaries. This type is predominantly humoral.

3 *Chronic*: rejection may occur months or years later presenting as insidious loss of graft function.

(a) *Arterial narrowing*: thickening of intima by collagen, myofibrils and fatty material often with rupture of internal elastic lamina. IgM and complement are usually present and the lesions are the result of fibrin and platelet deposits. Ischaemic glomerular changes result.

(b) *Glomerular changes*: basement membrane thickening segmental or diffuse and usually focal. Capsular adhesions sometimes with crescent formation may occur. Immunofluorescence usually shows granular IgM deposition with some C_{1q} and C_3 on capillary basement membranes: occasionally this is linear. The differential diagnosis of '*transplant glomerulopathy*' from recurrent disease in the graft may be very difficult.

4 *Cyclosporin toxicity*: blood levels need monitoring to avoid excess dosage. Toxic changes may closely mimic histological features of rejection and require very expert evaluation.

Transmission of renal disease to graft

Changes similar to those seen in the host renal disease may appear after a variable period of time in the graft. In not all such cases, however, is it possible to be dogmatic that disease transmission has occurred. A risk of transmission is, however, identifiable, particularly in focal glomerulosclerosis (see p. 172), crescentic glomerulonephritis and in type II mesangiocapillary lesions (see p. 170).

E/TUMOURS

Benign
  Adenoma
  Angiomyolipoma
  Juxtaglomerular cell tumour
  Others
Malignant
  Wilm's
  Adenocarcinoma
  Sarcoma
  Renal pelvis and ureter

Benign

Adenoma

An area of controversy. Although small yellow 'adenomas' are a not infrequent incidental finding in scarred kidneys in the elderly, it is considered by many that these are all small adenocarcinomas (see below). Well-differentiated nodules under 1 cm diameter can, for practical purposes, be called adenomas.

Angiomyolipoma

A hamartoma, and thus not a true tumour. Composed of an admixture of smooth muscle, blood vessels and fat in cortex or medulla. Many are seen in patients with tuberose sclerosis (see p. 332) either in its overt form or as a *forme fruste*.

Rarely produce symptomatology and present as an undiagnosed abdominal lump but may occasionally bleed extensively into retroperitoneum.

Never become malignant.

Juxtaglomerular cell tumour

A rare benign renin-secreting tumour causing subsequent hypertension, hypokalaemia and secondary hyperaldosteronism. Small (3–5 mm) white spherical nodule in cortex.

Other connective tissue tumours

Rarely a lipoma, fibroma and leiomyoma may be seen subcapsularly; ectopic adrenal tissue occasionally seen at this site also.

Malignant

Wilm's tumour—nephroblastoma

Nature

Thought to arise from residual embryonic mesodermal nephrogenic, metanephric blastemal subcapsular rests—*nephroblastomatosis*. This is commonly seen in kidneys of patients with nephroblastoma and in patients with genetic or teratological disorders with which this tumour is strongly related.

Age

Average presentation at 3 years, rarely after 7 years.

Incidence

Comprises 20% of malignant tumours in childhood, 5% are bilateral.

Sex
Male : female equal.

Macroscopical
Solitary, rapidly growing, demarcated spherical mass which is firm and grey–white on cut surface. Larger tumours may have areas of haemorrhage and necrosis and compression of renal parenchyma forms a pseudo-capsule. Invasion of pelvicalyceal system is uncommon such that haematuria is a late symptom and the tumours usually present as an abdominal mass.

Microscopical
Three histological elements:

1 *Blastema* which, if rosettes are formed, may be confused with neuroblastoma.

2 *Stromal cells* which may differentiate into striated muscle.

3 *Epithelial elements* forming tubules and occasionally glomeruloid bodies.

An anaplastic variety with cells containing giant nuclei also occurs.

Spread
1 *Direct*: into renal parenchyma and perinephric tissues.

2 *Lymphatic*: to regional lymph nodes—commonly invaded at time of presentation.

3 *Blood*: common to lung, less frequently liver and peritoneum and only rarely to bone.

Results
Survival rates of over 90% now achieved with modern chemotherapy regardless of metastatic spread for all except the anaplastic variety in which good results only occur when the tumour is confined to the kidney.

Adenocarcinoma—Grawitz tumour—hypernephroma—renal cell carcinoma

Incidence
Two per cent of malignant tumours in the adult.

Age
Rare below 40 years, commonly 55—70 years.

Sex
Male : female, 2 : 1.

Origin
Arise from renal tubular cells and may be subdivided into origin from the different tubular segments but this is of limited diagnostic or prognostic value. There is an increased risk of malignancy complicating the renal cysts of von-Hippel Lindau syndrome (see p. 154) and the cysts occurring in acquired cystic disease following renal dialysis (see p. 162).

Grawitz's theory of origin from adrenal nests, hence the term hypernephroma, is no longer acceptable.

Presentation
Classical triad of haematuria, flank pain and flank mass. Many present with paraneoplastic syndromes, especially pyrexia of unknown origin, and polycythaemia from erythropoietin production.

Increasingly being diagnosed at medical examination for non-associated symptomatology either by abdominal palpation or at ultrasound or computerized tomography scan.

Macroscopical
Large spherical, apparently encapsulated, masses with variegated cut surface comprising golden-yellow areas, fibrous trabeculae, cysts and areas of necrosis, haemorrhage and sometimes calcification. Ulceration of renal pelvis produces haematuria and invasion of renal vein is seen macroscopically in up to 20% of cases—on the left side obstruction of testicular vein may give a unilateral varicocele. Invasion through capsule common with large tumours.

Microscopical
1 *Clear cell carcinoma*: large cells containing much lipid to give yellow colour macroscopically. Lipid dissolved by histological processing to give clear appearance—'plant cells'. Cells arranged in alveoli, tubules or papillae.

2 *Granular cell carcinoma*: cytoplasm of cells more granular and eosinophilic.

3 *Sarcomatoid carcinoma*: undifferentiated cells resembling sarcoma but often will have areas of carcinoma if extensively sampled.

4 *Oncocytoma*: cells have eosinophilic cytoplasm and small nuclei. Macroscopically brown with central scar. Good prognosis but probably because most are grade I tumours. Grade II and III oncocytomas may metastasize.

Many tumours are composed of an admixture of two or more of the above patterns.

Spread

1 *Direct*: into renal parenchyma, renal pelvis and perinephric tissues.

2 *Lymphatic*—30% of cases have tumour in para-aortic lymph nodes at presentation.

3 *Blood*: early haematogenous spread is classically to lung and bones but metastases may occur in such unusual sites as nasopharynx where the typical histology permits accurate diagnosis.

Results

Fifty per cent or more 5-year survival with stage I or II tumours—tumours confined to renal substance or invading immediate perinephric tissue only. If renal vein is invaded prognosis is reduced to 30% or less at 5 years.

Tumour grade is an important prognostic indicator for low-stage tumours, Grade I (well differentiated) tumours having a 75% or more 5-year survival.

Sarcoma

Occasional fibrosarcomas and leiomyosarcomas occur, they must be distinguished from retroperitoneal tumours *invading* the kidney.

Secondary tumours

Metastatic carcinoma is seen in the kidney of 8% of cases of carcinomatosis at autopsy—bronchus and malignant melanoma are common primary sites. It is very uncommon for metastatic carcinoma in the kidney to produce clinical symptoms. Similarly, although malignant lymphoma is seen in renal parenchyma of 50% of autopsied cases, lymphomatous infiltration rarely produces renal problems in life.

Tumours of the renal pelvis and ureter

Incidence

These form approximately 15% of all malignant renal tumours.

Age

At 50–70 years.

Sex

Male : female, 3 : 1.

Site

Left and right sides involved equally, but 75% occur in renal pelvis and 25% in ureter—mostly in lower ureter.

As with all urothelial carcinomas they are frequently (50%) multiple but rarely bilateral.

Predisposing factors

1 Generally as for urothelial carcinoma of bladder (see p. 192).

2 Renal calculi are found with many squamous cell carcinomas.

3 *Balkan nephropathy*—most patients with this condition develop this tumour.

4 Analgesic abuse—patients with renal papillary necrosis from phenacetin overdosage have an increased incidence of carcinoma of renal pelvis (see p. 165).

Macroscopical

Identical to urothelial tumours of bladder.

1 *Papillary*: delicate fronds of tumour with no infiltration of underlying tissues.

2 *Papillary and solid*: fronded tumour but solid areas of invasion of adjacent underlying wall or kidney substance.

3 *Solid*: firm mass of pale tumour invading wall and, if in pelvis, invading renal parenchyma.

Microscopical

1 *Urothelial or transitional cell—95%*: they are identical to those seen in bladder and may be graded I—III accordingly (see p. 192).

2 *Squamous cell carcinoma*: one-third or more are associated with renal calculi and squamous metaplasia of urothelium. Highly invasive tumours with poor prognosis.

Spread

Non-invasive papillary tumours of low grade rarely ever spread or metastasize.

1 *Direct*: into pelvic or ureteric muscular wall and into renal parenchyma and adjacent connective tissue

2 *Lymphatic*: commonly to para-aortic lymph nodes.

3 *Blood*: may metastasize to lungs or other sites but death commonly from local spread.

Effects

1 Obstruction leads to hydronephrosis.

2 Ulceration of urothelium gives haematuria.

3 Renal infection.

Results

Following nephro-ureterectomy:

1 Non-invasive papillary tumours have excellent results and rarely recur.

2 Invasive tumours have a much poorer prognosis which is dependent upon tumour grade—nearly all grade III tumours are dead at 5 years but with grade II tumours only approximately 50%.

3 Squamous cell carcinoma is invariably fatal.

Chapter 11
Diseases of the Genito-Urinary System—Genito-Urinary Tract

A/BLADDER

Development
Structure and function
Congenital
Diverticula
Neurogenic
Calculi
Inflammations
  Non-specific
  Specific
Metaplasia
Carcinoma

Development
The primitive cloaca, which is the terminal segment of the endodermal tube, is connected to the allantois by the elongated urachus. A septum divides the cloaca into the posterior portion—the rectum, and an anterior chamber which connects with the ureters and forms the bladder and urethra. A downgrowth of mesoderm invests the endodermal mucosa with a musculature. At birth, the urachus becomes obliterated.

Structure and function
The bladder is lined by transitional epithelium—*urothelium*—and rests upon the connective tissue of the tunica propria. The muscularis—*the detrusor muscle*—is composed of large bundles of smooth muscle which run in all directions and condense around the ureteric orifices and internal urethral meatus to form functioning, but anatomically poorly defined, sphincters. The bladder is extraperitoneal except for the dome which has a covering of peritoneal serosa.

The bladder stores urine between the acts of voluntary voiding and has a capacity of 200–300 ml in the adult.

Congenital

Ectopia vesicae—exstrophy

Incidence
One in 40 000 births.

Sex
Male : female, 7 : 1.

Aetiology
Failure of mesoderm to migrate to the midline anteriorly.

Appearances
Absence of the infraumbilical anterior abdominal wall and of the anterior wall of the bladder results in exteriorization of the everted posterior bladder wall. There are accompanying abnormalities of the genitalia—*epispadias* is invariably present and there may be absence of the symphysis pubis. Urine is discharged from the ureters onto the exposed mucosa of the trigone.

Effects
1 *Infection*: repeated attacks of infection lead to ulceration of mucosa and replacement by granulation tissue with areas of glandular and squamous metaplasia.
2 *Pyelonephritis*: ascending infection leads to infection of the kidney (see p. 163).
3 *Hydronephrosis*: postinflammatory fibrosis of ureteric orifices leads to obstruction.
4 *Malignancy*: carcinoma—often adenocarcinoma—occurs in some long-term survivors.

Results

Many died in childhood from renal failure due to infection and hydronephrosis in the past, but with modern surgical corrective techniques more are surviving into adult life.

Persistent urachus

Types

1 Persistence as closed fibrous cord.
2 Urachus remains patent in part or whole:
   (a) fully patent—*umbilicovesical fistula*;
   (b) lower portion obliterated—*urachal cyst*;
   (c) lower portion remains patent—*urachal diverticulum*.

Effects

1 Fistulae.
2 Infection.
3 Malignancy—site of one variety of vesical adenocarcinoma (*see* p. 193).

Diverticula

Definition

Pouch-like eversion or evagination of the bladder wall.

Types

1 *Congenital*—focal failure of muscle development—usually single and uncommon.
2 *Acquired*—following obstruction to urine outflow—herniations between muscle bundles of trabeculated bladder wall and often multiple.

Incidence

Acquired type more common in males and often secondary to benign prostatic hypertrophy (*see* p. 194).

Effects

1 *Infection*—stasis of urine which is not expelled at micturition.
2 *Stone formation*—due to stasis.
3 *Malignancy*—tumours may arise in diverticula and be difficult to diagnose.

Neurogenic bladder

Nature

Disturbance of normal micturition due to interference or interruption of controlling nerve pathways. Normally two pathways operate:
1 Voluntary micturition controlled by the brain.
2 Automatic conditioned emptying reflex—an autonomic reflex activated through a spinal reflex arc.

Causes

1 Severance of brain connections above the reflex arc by trauma, tumour, inflammation or degenerative lesions.
2 Interruption of reflex arc by injuries or lesions of cauda equina, sacral plexus or peripheral nerves leads to evacuation by overflow—*autonomic neurogenic bladder*.

Results

Neurogenic bladder is extremely susceptible to infection with resulting renal failure.

Calculi

Origin

1 From the kidney—the most common site (*see* p. 179).
2 Formed primarily in the bladder—primary bladder stones.

Age

Adults over 40 years.

Sex

Male : female, 20 : 1.

Aetiology

Similar for renal calculi (*see* p. 180). Retention of urine due to incomplete emptying and subsequent infection is an important cause of 'infection' stones.

Types

1 *Non-infection*: most of renal origin—urate, oxalate, xanthine or cystine. If there is secondary infection of bladder they may have a covering of phosphate.
2 *Infection*: composed predominantly of calcium or magnesium phosphate.

Effects

1 May be asymptomatic.
2 Persistent infection—may lead to squamous metaplasia of urothelium.
3 Haematuria.
4 Obstruction at bladder neck.
5 Spontaneous passage *per urethra*.

Foreign bodies

A vast variety of foreign bodies may be found in the bladder—mostly self-introduced but some iatrogenic, e.g. catheters. Effects are similar to calculi.

Inflammations

Acute cystitis

The normal bladder remains sterile due to frequent flushing away of urine; this prevents organisms from establishing an infection. Cystitis is commonly infective in origin but may be caused by physical agents.

Infective cystitis

Incidence
Very common.

Sex
More common in females—traditionally attributed to the shorter urethra.

Routes of infection
1 *Urethral*: either ascent from urethral infection or secondary to introduction of foreign body—most commonly at catheterization.
2 *Renal*: descending infection—e.g. renal tuberculosis.
3 *Haematogenous*: rare.
4 *Lymphatic*: rare.
5 *Direct spread*: from adjacent organs, e.g. diverticulitis coli (see p. 47).

Predisposing factors
1 *Urinary retention or stasis*: obstruction, bladder paralysis, diverticula, calculi, foreign bodies, tumours, uterine prolapse.
2 *Infection of adjacent structures*: prostatitis, pyelonephritis, urethritis and diverticular disease of the colon.
3 *Diabetes mellitus*.
4 *Pregnancy*.
5 *Trauma*: especially catheterization.

Agents
1 *Viral*: adenovirus may cause haemorrhagic cystitis in children.
2 *Bacteria*: most infective cystitis cases are bacterial in origin—coliforms are the commonest but *Streptococcus faecalis*, *Pseudomonas aeruginosa* and staphylococci are also frequent and tuberculosis is not uncommon.
3 *Parasites*: *Schistosoma haematobium*—bilharzia (see p. 190).
4 *Fungi*: *Candida*.

Macroscopical
Acute inflammation causes oedema, reddening due to capillary dilatation and later friability and ulceration of the mucosa.

A number of appearances are described:
1 *Haemorrhagic*.
2 *Ulcerative*: large areas of ulceration.
3 *Bullous*: formation of vesicles containing oedema fluid.
4 *Emphysematous*: gas-forming organisms produce gas cysts in wall of bladder.
5 *Gangrenous*: necrosis of mucosa produces a membrane or pseudo-membrane of necrotic material, hence alternative name of *diphtheritic cystitis*—uncommon.
6 *Encrusted*: infection with urea-splitting organisms may result in deposition of phosphates on areas of necrosis or ulceration.

Microscopical
Histology is that of acute inflammation except for some specific infective agents (see below). Changes are usually limited to the mucosa. Ulceration may occur with a fibrin slough containing polymorphs.

Results
1 *Resolution*: usually occurs if predisposing cause is removed.
2 *Chronic cystitis*: if underlying cause untreatable.
3 *Necrosis gangrene and extension to surrounding structures*: is rare.

Specific types of cystitis

Abacterial cystitis—urethral syndrome
A condition of women with symptoms of cystitis but sterile urine. Some cases may be viral in origin but many are probably related to sexual intercourse—'honeymoon cystitis'.

Chemical cystitis
May result from:
1 Direct effect of agents instilled into the bladder for the treatment of tumours—formalin, thiotepa and mitomycin C.

2 Complication of systemic therapy—cyclophosphamide may cause severe haemorrhagic cystitis.

Radiation cystitis
A complication of excess irradiation to bladder, cervix or uterus.

Initially hyperaemia is followed by a haemorrhagic cystitis, vascular thrombosis and ulceration with marked oedema. Later the entire thickness of the bladder wall becomes fibrotic or even necrotic with sloughing of the mucosal surface, perforation, secondary infection and fistula formation. Frequently telangiectatic vessels develop and cause severe haematuria.

Mechanical irritants
Calculi and foreign bodies may produce infection. Catheters may irritate and ulcerate the mucosa, the resulting proliferative granulation tissue can simulate tumour at cystoscopy—'catheter tumour'.

Interstitial cystitis—Hunner's ulcer
Occurs almost exclusively in middle-aged women and is characterized clinically by suprapubic pain and frequency but the urine is sterile. Pathologically there is a fibrotic bladder of small capacity which when distended with fluid at cystoscopy shows linear ulceration and erythema. Histologically there is fibrosis and lymphocytic infiltration through the full thickness of the bladder wall. Many cases have a significant increase in mast cells in the wall. The aetiology is unknown.

Tuberculous cystitis

Origin
Almost always secondary to renal tuberculosis (see p. 165).

Macroscopical
Affects the trigone, especially around ureteric orifices:
1 *Early*: tubercles can be seen as small pinhead mucosal elevations.
2 *Later*: tubercles coalesce to form caseous nodules which ulcerate to reveal yellow tuberculous granulation tissue.
3 *Late*: fibrotic contraction of bladder wall may produce wide dilatation of ureteric orifices—'golf-hole' ureter.

Microscopical
Typical tuberculous giant cell granulomata but in the early lesions there may be no caseation. Identical granulomas are seen in patients with urothelial cancer treated by local instillation of BCG.

Results
1 Marked irritation and fibrotic contraction gives severe urinary symptoms.
2 Healing with fibrosis—follows appropriate antibiotic treatment.
3 Fistula formation.
4 Extension to other organs—prostate, epididymis and testis.

Schistosomiasis—bilharziasis

Organism
Schistosoma haematobium.

Source and life cycle
See p. 9.

Geographical distribution
Mainly in Africa with minor foci in the Middle East, Portugal, Greece, Cyprus and the West Indies. In some of these countries the disease is extremely common, e.g. Nile delta.

Pathogenesis
The worms attain maturity in the liver and thence travel against the venous blood flow to tributaries of the portal vein. *S. haematobium* has a trophism for pelvic plexuses, particularly vesical. The eggs, 20–30 for each pair or worms, are deposited in the small vessels of the bladder submucosa and into the lumen where they appear in the urine 1–3 months after infestation. Many eggs are retained within the wall where they instigate a dense inflammatory reaction.

Macroscopical
The trigone is first affected but later the whole organ is involved. The mucosa is initially congested and shows yellow nodules up to 2 mm in diameter, which later become elevated brown–yellow areas. These coalesce and extend. Two or more years later there is extensive fibrosis and muscular hypertrophy with mucosal thickening and bladder contraction. Similar changes are seen in the lower portions of the ureters.

Microscopical

1 *Early*: intense eosinophilia around the eggs in the submucosa.

2 *Later*: pseudo tubercles form around the eggs which subsequently calcify, and there is marked surrounding fibrosis which ultimately extends to all coats. Epithelial overgrowth and areas of squamous metaplasia develop at the trigone and may extend over the whole mucosa.

Effects

1 Contraction of the bladder.
2 Calculus formation around the eggs.
3 Ureteric obstruction leading to hydronephrosis.
4 Fistula formation.
5 Carcinoma may occur and in endemic areas bladder carcinoma is extremely common, e.g. Egypt.

Metaplastic conditions

The urothelium may undergo metaplasia into a variety of appearances some of which can cause diagnostic problems and confusion. Many have the prefix cystitis, but they are not necessarily always found in inflammatory situations.

Brunn's nest

These are small rounded collections of urothelial cells found just below the urothelial surface. They are extremely common and frequently seen in the normal bladder.

Cystitis glandularis

The term for Brunn's nests which have developed a central lumen surrounded by cuboidal or columnar cells. This is the common variety but occasionally there is metaplasia to a colonic mucin-secreting epithelium—the intestinal variant of cystitis glandularis.

Cystitis cystica

Eosinophilic fluid may accumulate within Brunn's nests to produce cystic structures beneath the urothelium; these may be microscopical or sufficiently large to be seen with the naked eye.

Squamous metaplasia

Occurs in two forms:

1 *Non-keratinizing squamous metaplasia—vaginal metaplasia*: produces white plaques seen at endoscopy, often on trigone, only occurs in women and has no pathological significance.

2 *Keratinizing squamous metaplasia—leukoplakia*: also produces white plaques. Often secondary to chronic irritation such as calculi. Occurs in both sexes and in a significant proportion of cases precedes squamous carcinoma of bladder.

Adenomatous metaplasia—nephrogenic adenoma

Metaplasia of urothelium to low cuboidal epithelium resembling collecting tubules of kidney. Commonly occurs in chronic infections like tuberculosis. A benign condition but may be misdiagnosed as adenocarcinoma.

Follicular cystitis

Not really a metaplasia. Numerous lymphoid follicles in lamina propria producing many tiny grey elevated nodules on bladder mucosa. A benign condition which may complicate carcinoma or chronic urinary infection. Must not be confused with the rare malignant lymphoma of bladder.

Miscellaneous

Amyloid

Isolated deposits of amyloid in the lamina propria not associated with systemic amyloidosis are a rare cause of haematuria.

Endometriosis

Deposits of endometrial tissue may produce cyclical haematuria. Fibrosis secondary to haemorrhage into the lamina propria or the endometrial tissue itself may block ureters to give hydronephrosis.

Malakoplakia

Soft yellow plaques of tissue in lamina propria composed of large histiocytes—von Hansemann cells—and plasma cells. Due to defective lysosomal function, coliforms ingested by histiocytes cannot be broken down and lysosomes become calcified to produce diagnostic targetoid *Michaelis–Gutmann bodies*.

Tumours

Virtually all bladder tumours are epithelial in origin.

Carcinoma of the bladder

Nature
It is important to realize that the term carcinoma is used in an imprecise way when applied to urothelial tumours. Many of the bladder tumours that are called carcinomas show no evidence of invasion and should perhaps be called papillomas. However, historically they have been called carcinoma since they are frequently multiple and/or recur and because in a significant proportion there is evolution to an invasive and metastasizing carcinoma.

Incidence
Three per cent of deaths from malignant disease but the incidence is higher than this (see above).

Age
A wide range but usually between 60 and 70 years.

Sex
Male : female, 3 : 1.

Predisposing factors
1 *Chemical substances*. Bladder cancer was the first tumour to be accepted as an occupational disease and thus to warrant compensation. It is seen particularly in aniline dye and synthetic rubber workers; chemical substances implicated include β-naphthylamine and benzidine. There is much clinical, experimental and biochemical evidence to suggest that bladder cancer may be induced by chemical substances in the urine which bathes the urothelium of the entire urinary tract. Stasis from any urinary tract obstruction renders these substances more effective so tumours are commonest in the bladder (where the urine is stored) and many bladder tumours are near the trigone.
2 *Smoking*
3 *Schistosomiasis* (see p. 190).
4 *Leukoplakia*: associated with squamous cell carcinoma.
5 *Bladder diverticula*: tumour complicates about 3% of diverticula.
6 *Ectopic vesicae*: adenocarcinoma has been reported to complicate this condition (see p. 187).

Sites
Most tumours are at the base on the trigone and around the ureteric orifices.

Macroscopical
About 20–30% of tumours are multiple, and these may be situated anywhere in the urothelium from renal pelvis down to tip of urethra. This multiplicity is considered to be a field effect of carcinogens on the urothelium rather than implantation of tumour cells from higher up the urinary tract.

The tumours may be:
1 *Papillary*: fronded masses growing into the lumen with little or no invasion of the wall. This is the more common form.
2 *Solid*: tumour growing directly into the bladder wall with little or no projection into the lumen. These are often ulcerated or encrusted.
3 *Papillary and solid*: variable mixture of 1 and 2.
4 *Flat in-situ carcinoma*: a distinct form of surface malignancy causing reddening of the bladder mucosa due to underlying telangiectatic blood vessels.

Most solid tumours are invasive from the outset and only a small percentage of papillary tumours evolve into invasive carcinoma. A significant proportion of flat in-situ carcinomas become invasive and patients with this condition need very careful follow-up such that cystectomy, if required, is performed before the tumour has spread widely.

Microscopical
Urothelial tumours are graded I to III according to the degree of differentiation.
1 *Papilloma*: many authorities do not accept this as an entity regarding tumours so-called as variants of 2 below. Can be defined as a papillary growth with no significant stroma, the urothelium of which is indistinguishable from normal.
2 *Well-differentiated (grade I) transitional cell carcinoma*: the vast majority of these (some would say all) are papillary growths with no evidence of invasion; only a very small proportion of these develop into invasive tumour. The fronds of the tumour have more cell layers than normal urothelium and cells have slightly larger nuclei than the normal.
3 *Moderately well-differentiated (grade II) transitional cell carcinoma*. These are usually papillary tumours in which a significant number are either invasive at presentation or become so. The cells of the fronds show significant atypicality and an increase in mitotic figures.
4 *Poorly differentiated (grade III) transitional cell carcinoma*: almost all of these are solid, extensively invasive tumours. The cells are pleomorphic with

numerous mitoses and may be difficult to recognize as being urothelial in origin.

5 *Squamous cell carcinoma*: bulky, widely invasive tumour of keratinizing squamous cell type arising in metaplastic epithelium—leukoplakia (see above). Commonly complicates bilharzia.

6 *Adenocarcinoma*: may arise from the urachus at the dome of the bladder or at the base where a proportion are a complication of intestinal metaplasia of the urothelium.

Spread

1 *Direct*: the TNM classification has wide international acceptance, in this p stands for pathology, T for tumour and the letter or number the degree of spread as assessed by the pathologist.

    pTa No invasion.

    pT1 Invasion confined to lamina propria.

    pT2 Extension into inner half of muscle.

    pT3 Extension into outer half of muscle.

    pT4 Extension beyond muscle.

In order to distinguish between papillary non-invasive tumours with their excellent prognosis and the *flat in-situ carcinoma* which frequently becomes invasive the term *pTis* has been introduced for the latter category.

2 *Lymphatic*: common in fatal cases to iliac and para-aortic lymph nodes.

3 *Blood*: a late phenomenon with metastases to liver and lungs most frequently.

4 *Implantation*: may occur at cystectomy with implantation recurrences in prostatic bed, urethra and scars in bladder or abdominal wall.

Effects

1 *Haematuria*.

2 *Infection*: cystitis and pyelonephritis.

3 *Ureteric obstruction*: hydronephrosis and pyonephrosis.

4 *Urethral obstruction*: retention of urine.

5 *Extension to other organs*: fistula formation; vesicocolic fistula with pneumaturia and vesicovaginal fistula giving incontinence.

Results

Very dependent upon type of tumour. Most patients with non-invasive papillary tumours will die from some other cause. Solid invasive urothelial tumours have only a 35% 5-year survival. Squamous cell and adenocarcinomas have a similarly poor prognosis.

Other tumours

Sarcoma

Rare, accounting for less than 0.5% of bladder tumours. The bladder is one of the sites where embryonal rhabdomyosarcoma occurs (see p. 108) and at this site is often a polypoid, grape-like tumour macroscopically—*sarcoma botryoides*. Leiomyosarcoma and malignant lymphoma are the relatively commoner tumours in adults.

Benign connective tissue tumours

Uncommon; leiomyomas and angiomas are reported.

Secondary tumours

Direct spread

Bladder often invaded by carcinomas of prostate, colon, rectum and cervix.

Metastatic

Uncommon but occasionally from breast, stomach and malignant melanoma.

B/PROSTATE

Structure and function
Inflammations
Benign hyperplasia
Carcinoma

Structure and function

The adult prostate gland weighs some 20 g and is roughly the shape of an inverted Spanish chestnut. It is situated at the base of the bladder and encircles the prostatic urethra. There has been a confusing variety of anatomical descriptions of the lobular structure of the gland. The essential subdivision is of a central superior portion delineated by the urethra anteriorly, and the two ejaculatory ducts posteriorly, this is the region which enlarges in benign prostatic hypertrophy—*medial lobe*, and a more inferior and peripheral area in which carcinoma develops—*posterior lobes*.

Microscopically it is a compound tubulo-alveolar gland with columnar epithelial cells set in a fibromuscular stroma. Growth of the gland is hormone-dependent but the mechanisms controlling this remain unknown.

The prostatic secretions are a constituent of seminal fluid and contain an acid phosphatase amongst other substances.

Inflammations

Small numbers of chronic inflammatory cells are commonly seen in surgically resected prostates and are probably of little significance. The presence of polymorphs usually indicates that there is a urinary tract infection rather than symptomatic prostatitis.

Acute prostatitis

This is a more ill-defined condition. Inflammatory cells are present in the prostate of many older men and to confidently make this diagnosis pus should be demonstrated in urine or urethral secretions after prostatic massage. Bacteria may not be cultured even in the presence of frank pus and many of these cases are thought to be due to *Chlamydia*. A significant number of men with perineal discomfort have no abnormal physical findings—*prostatodynia*; some of these patients will have psychosexual problems.

Granulomatous prostatitis

In this condition the prostate contains foci of granulomatous inflammation, often with foreign-body giant cells and usually arranged around a ruptured prostatic duct or acinus. It is thought that the reaction is a response to prostatic secretions which have ruptured into the stroma following obstruction to the ducts by nodules of prostatic hyperplasia. The ensuing fibrosis renders the gland very firm such that it may feel malignant on digital examination.

Tuberculous prostatitis

This is usually secondary to tuberculosis higher up the urinary tract, especially the kidney. The histological appearance is very similar to granulomatous prostatitis except that caseation may be present and acid-fast bacilli demonstrable by ZN stain. The use of BCG in the treatment of superficial bladder cancer (see p. 192) may produce an identical picture to true tuberculosis in both bladder and prostate.

Post-transurethral resection granuloma

Palisading granulomas almost identical to those of rheumatoid arthritis may be seen in prostates of men who had transurethral resection of prostate a few months previously.

Benign nodular hyperplasia

Nature

This is extremely common over the age of 50 years and indeed may almost be said to be a normal ageing process. Its aetiology is unclear, although it is certainly in some way hormonal since it does not appear in men castrated before puberty. It also responds to anti-androgen therapy although transurethral resection is almost invariably preferred for treatment.

The size of the gland at presentation is very variable, presumably reflecting the tolerance to symptoms of the patient concerned. Most resected glands are between 60 and 100 g but glands up to 200 g occur. Most patients are now treated by transurethral resection which may thus contain peripheral gland tissue. The prostate removed digitally at transvesical or retropubic resection is composed of the central portion only: carcinoma of prostate may thus present post-prostatectomy in residual peripheral gland tissue.

Appearances

Hyperplasia affects the stroma and glands of the central and superior portions—median and lateral lobes, and if extensive may protrude upwards into the base of the bladder.

On section the gland is obviously nodular, the stromal, fibromuscular nodules being solid and grey whilst the glandular nodules will have a yellow honeycomb appearance containing milky fluid. Histologically, variable degrees of hyperplasia of epithelium, muscle and fibrous tissue are seen with compression of adjacent tissue. The glandular tissue may be cystically dilated due to obstruction of ducts.

Effects

Distortion of the prostatic urethra by the hyperplastic nodules leads to difficulty with micturition with a slow stream, hesitancy, dribbling and ultimately, if untreated, to acute retention. Incomplete emptying of the bladder, accentuated by the enlarged gland protruding into the base of the bladder, results in urinary infection and dysuria. The bladder wall thus hypertrophies and becomes trabeculated, and diverticulae may develop. The raised pressure ultimately produces hydroureter, hydronephrosis and may progress to renal failure—*obstructive uropathy* (see p. 179).

Carcinoma

Incidence

Prostatic carcinoma is a disease of older men and is

distinctly uncommon below 50 years. It is increasing in importance in the Western world and is exceeded only by bronchus and colon as the cause of male cancer-related deaths.

Types

1 *Clinical* prostatic carcinoma describes patients with symptoms related to the prostate and with evidence of malignancy of the organ, either a firm irregular gland or signs or symptoms of metastatic disease.

2 *Occult* carcinoma identifies patients who present with metastatic disease.

3 *Incidental* carcinoma is used for the many cases which are discovered only after histological examination of prostatic tissue resected for benign hyperplasia. Most older patients with incidental carcinoma will die of other disease processes and thus the incidence of prostatic cancer is much higher than the number of deaths from this condition.

4 *Latent* carcinoma. Examination of the prostate at post mortem reveals an increasing incidence of prostatic cancer with increasing age, many of which have not produced problems in life. After 80 years some 80–90% of the male population will harbour a histological prostatic malignancy.

Aetiology

As with benign hyperplasia sex hormones are considered to be of considerable aetiological significance. Prostatic cancer does not occur in castrates and many tumours regress after reduction of androgens, either by castration or by administration of oestrogens such that male hormones are considered to be one contributory agent. The tumour has also been associated with the taking of anabolic steroids.

There are considerable variations in incidence between different races; it is high in Scandinavia and the USA and low in Japan and Mexico. Blacks have a higher incidence than whites in the USA and Protestants are more susceptible than Jews—this suggests a genetic component to the aetiology.

Macroscopical

Carcinoma of prostate arises in the peripheral portions of the gland and early tumours may not be sampled in limited resections. The typical tumour is firm in consistency and yellow–white on cut surface. The tumour extends locally both centrally to involve the urethra giving symptoms of prostatic obstruction and laterally into seminal vesicle, bladder base and adjacent fat. Extension into the rectum is unusual due to the dense Denonvillier's fascia between these two organs.

Microscopical

The vast majority of tumours are *adenocarcinomas*; these are of varying degree of differentiation and this variability may be seen in the one tumour. A number of grading systems have been developed using both cytological appearances and degree of glandular differentiation. The most widely used is the Gleason system, which evaluates the degree of glandular differentiation only. Grading is of value in the assessment of small incidental carcinomas in younger men since many believe that small, low-grade carcinomas do not develop into widely invasive tumour and require no further treatment. This view has recently been challenged.

Some tumours are so poorly differentiated that they may be difficult to distinguish from urothelial tumours invading the prostate from the bladder base (see p. 192) or, more rarely, arising within the prostate or prostatic urethra. Almost all prostatic tumours produce *prostatic acid phosphatase* (PSAP) and *prostatic specific antigen* (PSA), and immunocytochemical demonstration of one or both of these substances allows recognition of the primary nature of such tumours which, unlike urothelial tumours, may respond to hormone manipulation.

Other tumours, primary or metastatic are distinctly uncommon.

Spread

1 *Direct*: extensive local spread into bladder base, seminal vesicles and periprostatic tissue is common at presentation.

2 *Lymphatic*: permeation of perineural lymphatic spaces is a common histological finding and the iliac and paraortic lymph nodes are commonly grossly invaded at autopsy.

3 *Blood spread*: this is also common, frequently to bone, which may be the presenting clinical feature in occult carcinoma. Spinal vertebrae, particularly lumbar, are often affected, possibly by direct extension into Batson's paravertebral venous plexus. Bony secondaries of prostatic origin are very frequently osteosclerotic and must be distinguished radiologically from Paget's disease of bone. Liver and lung are also frequent sites of blood-borne spread.

Clinical diagnosis

When prostatic carcinoma is suspected but resection of prostate is not indicated the diagnosis may be effected in a number of ways. In men with osteosclerotic bone metastases an elevated serum acid phosphatase—above 6 IU/litre—is almost pathognomonic. Confirmation by tissue diagnosis can be effected by needle biopsy of firm suspicious nodules in the prostate via the rectum to produce either a core of tissue for histological assessment or an aspirate for cytological evaluation. Serum levels of *prostate-specific antigen* are also valuable in the diagnosis of prostatic cancer and the monitoring of its progression and response to treatment.

Results

Prostatic carcinoma was the first tumour in which hormone administration was shown to be effective. With its very variable natural history many urologists will treat older men with this disease only if they are symptomatic. Orchidectomy is often the preferred treatment since it does not have the cardiovascular and thrombotic complications associated with oestrogen therapy. Hormone manipulation is not always effective and in other patients the treatment may fail to control progression after an early response—chemotherapy may help some of these patients.

Radical prostatectomy is now available for tumour restricted to the gland in certain centres, especially in the USA. Younger men with small, well-differentiated tumours are now being treated by this method since recent studies have shown that a small but significant percentage of incidental carcinoma progress to metastatic disease if followed up for long periods.

C/URETHRA

Inflammations
Stricture
Caruncle
Carcinoma

Inflammations

Gonococcal urethritis

Aetiology and incidence

A purulent infection due to *Neisseria gonorrhoea*, a Gram-negative coccus which is invariably acquired venereally. Bacteria multiply on the intact urethral mucosa and subsequently invade peri-urethral glands in the male and endocervix, and Bartholin's glands in the female (see p. 208).

A common condition throughout the world which reflects sexual activity, particularly promiscuity.

Diagnosis

Yellow purulent discharge occurs 3–8 days after initial infection. Organisms may be visible as Gram-negative cocci inside pus cells on smears but many cases will require culture.

Course and complications

1 May resolve in 2–4 weeks either spontaneously or following treatment.
2 Chronic infection with abscesses and fibrosis of peri-urethral glands leads to stricture in the male. In the female it is an important cause of pelvic inflammatory disease (see p. 220).
3 Systemic spread is rare but produces suppurative arthritis, tenosynovitis, skin rashes and endocarditis.

Non-gonococcal urethritis

Nature

By definition urethritis in which gonococci are not cultured.

Aetiology

Most cases are venereal in origin. A variety of organisms may be cultured but in some no organism is identified—*non-specific urethritis* (NSU). Organisms implicated are *Chlamydia trachomatis*, *Ureaplasma urealyticum*, *Trichomonas vaginalis*, *Candida albicans* and Herpes simplex virus type II.

Course and complications

1 *Urethral discharge*: which is either eliminated spontaneously or becomes chronic with recurrent acute exacerbations.
2 *Reiter's disease*: chlamydial urethritis associated with conjunctivitis and arthritis: occasionally ulcerative lesions of mucous membranes and skin of feet.

Urethral stricture

Aetiology

1 Most are postinflammatory—especially from gonorrhoea.

2 Trauma—(a) instrumentation, (b) obstetric complications.

Site
Usually in bulbous or membranous urethra.

Effects
1 Urinary obstruction leads to retention.
2 Repeated instrumentation may lead to false passage formation and eventually fistula formation.

Urethral caruncle

Nature
Circumscribed prolapse of urethral mucosa in female of uncertain aetiology.

Macroscopical
Red, painful protuberance (1–2 cm diameter) at or just within urethral meatus. Commonly ulcerated and bleeds.

Microscopical
A mass of vascular granulation tissue with a variable quantity of hyperplastic but benign squamous or transitional epithelium on the surface.

Urethral carcinoma

Incidence
A rare tumour, commoner in females and occurring after the age of 65 years. Must be distinguished from urothelial carcinoma of the urethra complicating carcinoma of bladder.

Appearances
Papillary tumours which ulcerate and invade adjacent tissues at an early stage. Most are squamous cell carcinomas but adenocarcinomas may arise from peri-urethral glands.

Spread and results
1 Directly into adjacent tissues.
2 Lymphatic to inguinal nodes in the male and inguinal and iliac nodes of the female.

Progress
This is generally very poor.

D/TESTIS, EPIDIDYMIS

Congenital
Inflammations
Torsion
Tumours
Male infertility
Testicular biopsy
Seminal vesicles diseases

Congenital

Retractile testis
Testis undescended at birth but subsequently descends into the scrotal position.

Ectopic testis
Testis situated away from the normal pathway of descent of the testis.

Cryptorchidism—maldescended or undescended testis
Failure of the testes to descend into the scrotal sac from their embryonic intra-abdominal position. May be unilateral or bilateral and situated anywhere from the lumbar region of the posterior wall to the scrotal sac but most commonly in the inguinal canal.

Occurs in up to 1% of male infants.

Effects
1 Spermatogenesis requires the lower temperature found in the scrotum and the cryptorchid testis undergoes progressive atrophy of tubules with interstitial fibrosis and relative prominence of the interstitial (Leydig) cells.
2 Sterility occurs if the condition is bilateral and not treated. The endocrine function of the organ is retained.
3 Malignancy is the most important complication, the incidence of testicular malignancy being increased by up to 35 times. Seminoma is the commonest tumour but malignant teratomas occur and there is also an increased incidence of malignancy in the contralateral testis.

Miscellaneous
Absent or multiple testes—*anorchia and polyorchia*—are rare abnormalities.

Patency of the processus vaginalis leads to infantile inguinal hernia and congenital hydrocele.

Lesions of tunica vaginalis

Hydrocele
Accumulation of serous fluid in the tunica vaginalis—a common condition.

Causes
1 *Congenital*: due to patent processus vaginalis.
2 *Infantile*: when processus vaginalis is obliterated late.
3 *Secondary*: as a complication of heart failure, renal failure, trauma, infection. Most commonly idiopathic. The underlying testis should always be assessed for the possibility of an underlying tumour, although this is an uncommon cause of hydrocele and an uncommon mode of presentation.

Effects
1 Infection may occur primarily if the underlying cause is infective or as a complication of aspiration.
2 Testicular atrophy follows long-term untreated hydrocele.

Haematocele
Blood in the tunica vaginalis resulting from trauma, torsion of the testis, haemorrhage into a pre-existing hydrocele, generalized bleeding disorders or, rarely due to extension of testicular tumour through the tunica vaginalis.

Other cystic lesions of scrotum

Spermatocele
Accumulation of spermatic fluid in dilated portions of the epididymis due to obstruction of draining ducts.

Varicocele
Variceal dilatation of the veins of the pampiniform plexus of the spermatic cord. It is a treatable cause of subfertility and when localized to the left side may be a sign of renal tubular carcinoma extending into the left renal vein (into which the left testicular vein drains).

Inflammations

Non-specific epididymo-orchitis

Nature
Retrograde infection via the vas of epididymis and testis. Most cases are a complication of infections elsewhere in the urinary tract—cystitis, prostatitis, urethritis.

Organisms
Those found in urinary tract infections—coliforms, streptococci and staphyloccoci.

Macroscopical
Swelling and congestion of epididymis and the testis. Differentiation from testicular tumours is usually simple due to signs of inflammation and presence of pain.

Microscopical
Acute inflammation with pus cells in epididymis and later, if not treated, abscess formation.

Results
1 Resolution with scarring.
2 Suppuration with abscess formation and sinus tracks on to scrotal skin.
3 Chronic infection which leads to fibrosis and testicular atrophy.
4 Sterility due to:
   (a) pressure atrophy of testicular tubules,
   (b) fibrotic obstruction of ducts of epididymis.

Gonococcal epididymo-orchitis
A not uncommon complication of gonococcal urethritis (see p. 196).

Tuberculous epididymo-orchitis

Origin
Vast majority, if not all, are secondary to renal tuberculosis (see p. 165).

   As with non-specific epididymo-orchitis the epididymis is initially infected with later spread to the testis.

Macroscopical
Painless swelling of epididymis—sinus formation on to scrotal skin is common.

Microscopical
Typical epithelioid and giant cell granulomas with much caseous necrosis.

Results
1 May heal with fibrosis and calcification.

2 Secondary hydrocele.
3 Extension into testis or on to scrotal skin.

Mumps orchitis

Incidence
About one-quarter of adults with mumps develop orchitis about 7 days following the swelling of the salivary glands (see p. 19).

Appearances
Intense interstitial oedema with a patchy infiltrate of lymphocytes and plasma cells. Tubular atrophy of variable degree is a common sequel which, if bilateral, may result in sterility.

Syphilitic orchitis

Site
Unlike tuberculosis the epididymis is rarely involved.

Appearances
1 *Gumma*: nodular painless enlargement with dense fibrosis surrounding foci of yellow–white structured necrosis.
2 *Diffuse*: interstitial inflammation with endarteritis obliterans and perivascular cuffing by lymphocytes and plasma cells.

Results
Progressive fibrosis leads to atrophy and sterility.

Torsion of testis

Nature
Twisting of testis such that venous drainage is impaired and testis becomes engorged with resulting venous infarction if not treated.

Predisposing factors
1 Violent movement or trauma.
2 Abnormality of attachment of testis to cord such that it is unduly mobile.

Results
Unless the twist is reduced almost immediately, the testis will be destroyed with complete loss of function. Underlying abnormality is often bilateral, and contralateral testis should be anchored to prevent a similar fate.

Tumours
Testicular tumours are a difficult group due to their very diverse histological appearances and the multiplicity of classifications in use.

Incidence
Uncommon—some 1–2% of cases of malignancy in the male, but increasing in incidence in many Western countries, especially Denmark. Also commoner in whites than blacks. An important tumour in young adult males in whom other tumours are uncommon at this age.

Pathogenesis
Majority arise from the primordial germ cells which have their origin in the yolk sac. These cells migrate along the dorsal portion of the developing embryo to the genital ridge where the testis develops.

Germ cell tumours are subdivided into tumours showing spermatogenic differentiation—seminomas, and those retaining their totipotentiality for differentiation. The latter are called teratomas in the British nomenclature but by the name of the tissue into which the cells have differentiated in the American classifications. About one-third of germ cell tumours show both seminomatous and teratomatous differentiation—*combined tumours*.

Presentation
1 Majority present as enlargement of the testis—often painless.
2 A small number present with symptoms of metastases—this is common in malignant teratoma, especially malignant teratoma trophoblastic.
3 Endocrine effects—gynaecomastia, precocious puberty usually indicate Leydig or Sertoli cell tumours.

Seminoma
Comprises about 40% of testicular tumours and usually occur in the fourth and fifth decades.

Macroscopical
Testis is enlarged by a tumour with relatively homogeneous white cut surface, there may be yellow areas of necrosis but haemorrhagic areas are rare.

Microscopical
Rounded and polygonal cells with clear cytoplasm and vesicular nuclei arranged in sheets and columns with a

distinctive lymphocytic infiltrate which more rarely has a histiocytic component.

Spread

1 *Direct*: spread into adjacent epididymis and spermatic cord is common with large tumours.
2 *Lymphatic*: spread to para-aortic lymph nodes is common at presentation with more widespread dissemination later.
3 *Blood*: spread to liver and lungs is a later complication.

Prognosis

The tumour is very radiosensitive. Orchidectomy and adequate radiotherapy has given good results for this tumour for many years. Tumours restricted to the testis—Stage 1, have a virtual 100% survival and more advanced tumours had an 85–90% 5-year survival with radiotherapy which has been further improved by the use of platinum-based chemotherapeutic regimes to give survival rates nearing 100%.

Teratoma

Definition

The classical definition is 'a tumour showing differentiation into tissues foreign to the normal organ and derived from all three germ layers'. This is true of benign tumours but in many malignant tumours only malignant undifferentiated tissue is present. These are considered to be teratomas, as identical undifferentiated tumour is seen in other tumours which fulfil the diagnostic criteria.

Incidence

Thirty two per cent of all testicular tumours. Incidence has increased markedly, nearly doubling over the last 50 years.

Age

A tumour of young men in second and third decades.

Macroscopical

Testis is enlarged and cut surface variable with areas of haemorrhage and necrosis. Tumours with areas of differentiation into mature tissues commonly have cystic foci.

Microscopical

The British classification is based on the degree of differentiation that is present.

1 *Teratoma differentiated—TD*: contains only fully differentiated cells and organoid structures.
2 *Malignant teratoma intermediate—MTI*: both fully differentiated and obviously malignant tissues are present—the latter commonly having the appearance of a poorly differentiated carcinoma.
3 *Malignant teratoma undifferentiated—MTU*: undifferentiated tumour of carcinomatous appearance only present. No differentiated tissue present. Some tumours have tissue which has the appearance of yolk sac tissue and others may have syncytiotrophoblast cells. These are the elements which produce α-fetoprotein—(AFP) and the β unit of human chorionic gonadotrophin (βHCG) respectively. These proteins can be demonstrated in the cells by immunocytochemistry.
4 *Malignant teratoma trophoblastic—MTT*: tumour composed entirely of syncytio- and cytotrophoblast.

American and WHO classifications

These list all elements recognizable in histological sections and therefore have many more subdivisions. Certain tumours may be equated to their British counterparts (Table 11.1).

Spread

Commonly by blood to lung and liver, less frequently to para-aortic lymph nodes along the lymphatics.

Prognosis

The advent of platinum-based chemotherapeutic regimes has vastly improved the prognosis of malignant teratomas. Before their introduction 50% of patients died within 2 years; now the vast majority, even those with extensive metastases, can be cured.

Combined tumour

Nature

Tumours with both teratomatous and seminomatous components—these may be separate or intermingled.

Table 11.1 WHO and American classifications of teratoma.

British	American
Teratoma differentiated	Teratoma mature
Malignant teratoma intermediate	Teratocarcinoma
Malignant teratoma undifferentiated	Embryonal carcinoma
Malignant teratoma trophoblastic	Choriocarcinoma

Tumour markers

Malignant teratomas often produce α-fetoprotein and/or βHCG, the former from yolk-sac tissue, the latter from syncytiotrophoblast. These substances can be demonstrated in the tumour by immunocytochemical techniques and are also measurable in peripheral blood.

Applications

1 *Tissue sections*: identification of primary testicular tumours as a teratoma but more importantly identifies a non-testicular tumour as being teratomatous and most probably metastatic in nature.

2 *Serum levels*:

(a) Elevated levels indicate a diagnosis of teratoma for an enlarged testis before orchidectomy.

(b) Continually elevated levels after orchidectomy indicate presence of metastatic tumour.

(c) Rising levels during postoperative follow-up is evidence of growth of previously undetected metastases.

Other tumours

Interstitial—Leydig cell tumour

Circumscribed yellow–brown tumours forming about 2% of testicular tumours. Occur at all ages, and in childhood often present as precocious puberty, in adults as gynaecomastia. Less that 10% behave in a malignant fashion (see also p. 225).

Sertoli-cell tumour

Tubules formed of Sertoli cells in a variable quantity of stromal mesenchyme. They constitute less than 1% of testicular tumours—approximately 20% are malignant (see also p. 225).

Malignant lymphoma

The commonest tumour in the elderly with peak incidence between 60 and 80 years.

Malignant lymphoma at any site not uncommonly affects the testes in its later stages but some 7% of malignant testicular tumours are lymphomas presenting as a testicular mass, of which 20% are bilateral.

The tumours have a typical creamy-white cut surface and are non-Hodgkin's lymphomas: most are B cell in type. Prognosis is that of malignant lymphomas in general.

Adenomatoid tumour

A tumour of probable mesothelial origin composed of irregular clefts and spaces lined by flattened cuboidal cells with a superficial resemblance to carcinoma. They are always benign and found most commonly in the epididymis and fallopian tubes.

Secondary tumours

Apart from lymphoma and acute leukaemia the testis is an uncommon site for metastatic tumour, although prostatic carcinoma is occasionally seen in testes removed therapeutically for this condition.

Male infertility

Abnormalities in the male are responsible for infertility in about half of couples seeking medical advice.

In many cases there may be obvious testicular atrophy (or absence) from numerous causes.

1 Cryptorchidism (see p. 197).

2 Congenital syndromes—Klinefelter's syndrome.

3 Secondary to gonadotrophin deficiency:

(a) diseases of hypothalamus or pituitary (see p. 123);

(b) drugs—e.g. oestrogens, cypoterone acetate.

4 Irradiation.

5 Chemotherapeutic drugs.

6 Previous orchitis—especially mumps.

7 Malnutrition and cachexia.

8 Cirrhosis of the liver.

9 Alcoholism.

Testicular biopsy

This investigation is only occasionally indicated with the hormonal assays now available. It is not indicated in patients with clinically obvious testicular atrophy from the causes listed above.

A raised FSH level indicates defective spermatogenesis due to failure of the regulatory feedback mechanism and, as there are no proven drugs which can stimulate spermatogenesis, biopsy is not really indicated in this group of infertile males.

Biopsy can be recommended for those patients with presumed obstruction of the epididymis or vas in order to ascertain that the testis has normal spermatogenesis.

Diseases of the seminal vesicles

Apart from infections of non-specific, gonococcal or tuberculous nature reaching the organ from the prostatic urethra, significant conditions are extremely rare.

E/PENIS, SCROTUM

Penis
   Congenital
   Inflammations
   Premalignant conditions
   Carcinoma
Scrotum
   Inflammations
   Carcinoma

Penis

Congenital

Malformations of the urethral groove and canal

Hypospadias
The urethra opens on to the ventral surface of the penis.

Epispadias
The urethra opens on to the dorsal surface of the penis.

Both of these are commonly associated with maldescent of the testes or other more severe congenital anomalies.

Effects
1 *Infection*: particularly near the base of the penis.
2 *Sterility.*
3 *Obstruction*: when the orifice becomes stenosed.

Phimosis

Nature
The orifice of the prepuce is too small to permit its retraction.

Origin
May be congenital, or acquired following inflammatory scarring.

Effects
1 Prevents the cleansing of the glans with accumulation of secretions in the prepuce; this predisposes to infection.
2 Forcible retraction of a phimotic prepuce over the glans penis may result in constriction and swelling so

that it cannot be replaced—*paraphimosis*. This may cause urethral obstruction and urinary retention.

Other congenital lesions
Rare lesions include absence, hypoplasia, hyperplasia and duplication.

Inflammations

Balanoposthitis

Nature
Non-specific inflammation of the glans—*balanitis*—and of the prepuce—*posthitis*.

Organisms
Staphylococci, streptococci, coliforms, gonococci, *Candida* and *Chlamydia*.

Aetiology
Usually associated with phimosis or a large redundant prepuce, venereal infection and coital trauma.

Appearances
Marked congestion and oedema with exudate on the surface of the glans. If neglected, ulceration occurs and if persistent and chronic, scarring occurs with aggravation of the underlying condition—usually phimosis.

Diagnosis
Gonococci can be readily distinguished by examination of smears; other organisms can be identified by culture.

Syphilis—primary chancre
This is by far the commonest site for a chancre in the male, particularly the glans and the inner side of the prepuce, but occasionally on the shaft.

Appearances
Begins as a solitary, slightly elevated, firm papule. Later there is superficial ulceration to form a shallow, clean-based depression, with extensive surrounding induration and inguinal lymphadenopathy. Typically painless.

Course
Healing with re-epithelialization in about 2 months occurs spontaneously, or more rapidly with treatment; slight scarring usually remains.

Chancroid—soft sore—soft chancre

Organism
Haemophilus ducreyi—Gram-negative rod.

Geographical distribution
Particularly common in the Orient, West Indies and North Africa. Uncommon in Europe and North America.

Transmission
By sexual intercourse, inoculation occurring through abrasions of the surface.

Site
Usually the glans.

Appearances
A macule becomes a papule and thence a pustule which ulcerates. The ulcer is at first shallow and up to 1 cm diameter, but later deepens with necrotic purulent slough in the base and enlarges to 2–3 cm diameter. It is soft with little or no surrounding induration. Inguinal lymphadenopathy usually follows in 1–2 weeks, is markedly painful and suppurates with discharge on the skin surface—'bubo'.

Course
Spontaneous or therapeutic healing with residual scarring, usually within 1 month.

Granuloma inguinale

Organism
Calymmatobacterium granulomatis, an encapsulated coccobacillary organism found in the lesions within mononuclear cells—*Donovan bodies* (see p. 201).

Geographical distribution
Worldwide but uncommon.

Transmission
Believed to be venereal, but infectivity and invasiveness of the organism are low. The incubation period varies from 3 days to several months.

Appearances
A papule may appear anywhere in the perineal or peri-anal regions or on the penis. The papule ulcerates and spreads, with a necrotic centre and raised red and exuberant inflammatory margins. Satellite lesions may occur along involved lymphatics. It is usually relatively painless but inguinal lymphadenopathy with suppurative necrosis occurs, leading to sinus formation. Extensive fibrosis occurs in this very chronic condition.

Diagnosis
Smears or tissue biopsies show the large vacuolated macrophages containing the Gram-negative Donovan bodies.

Course
Very chronic, with extensive local destruction and distortion of the affected site.

Lymphogranuloma venereum— lymphogranuloma inguinale— lymphopathia venereum

Nature
A venereal disease caused by *Chlamydia trachomatis* (see p. 143).

Site
Glans, prepuce, urethra or perineal skin.

Geographical distribution
Worldwide but uncommon.

Stages
1 Invasive. Usually a few days after inoculation.
2 Genital or anorectal lesion. The primary lesion at the site of inoculation is usually small, transient and inapparent.
3 Lymphadenopathy: 1–2 weeks later.
4 Late complications. Elephantiasis, or rectal stricture in females, may develop at a later date due to lymphatic obstruction (see p. 207).

Appearances
1 Genital lesion. A small vesicle ruptures to form a shallow ulcer which rapidly heals.
2 Lymph nodes. Progressive painful swelling. These nodes are at first discrete, but later coalesce, with necrosis and sinus formation on to the skin surface.

Microscopical
Characteristic granulomatous lesions of central,

irregular, stellate abscesses containing polymorphs and ringed by radially arranged fibroblasts, epithelioid cells and histiocytes. Occasional giant cells of Langhans' type may be present. There is a surrounding zone of plasma cells and lymphocytes.

Course
Chronic, varying from weeks to months. Healing with fibrosis occurs, producing distortion and lymphatic blockage which may lead to elephantiasis of the external genitalia or, when the pararectal lymph nodes are involved, rectal stricture.

In females the primary lesion is frequently in the cervix and escapes notice. It is followed by pelvic lymph node inflammation and, when healing occurs, the scarring commonly produces rectal stricture or esthiomene (see p. 207).

Diagnosis
1 Frei test. Intradermal inoculation of material from an infected case. This test is not entirely specific.
2 Complement fixation test. Specific for the disease.
3 Culture of organism—special media required.

Genital warts—condylomata acuminata

Nature
Venereally acquired and caused by human papilloma viruses—HPV, 6 and 11 (see p. 210).

Site
Usually on glans but may occur in urethra, penile shaft, perineum and around anus.

Microscopical
A proliferation of squamous cells—acanthosis, with many cells having a halo around the irregular nucleus—*koilocytes*.

Balanitis xerotica obliterans

Macroscopical
Firm white areas located on the external surface of the prepuce and on the glans of circumcised individuals.

Microscopical
Histology is that of *lichen sclerosus et atrophicus* (see p. 208) Thinned hyperkeratotic epidermis with oedema of upper dermis and dense layer of lymphocytes and plasma cells in deep dermis.

Effects
1 Phimosis if on glans and situated near urethral meatus.
2 Carcinoma. This is reported but balanitis xerotica obliterans (BXO) is common and the association almost certainly coincidental.

Premalignant conditions

Erythroplasia of Queyrat
Carcinoma *in situ* restricted to the glans. Single or multiple flat red glistening patches. Histologically nuclei are enlarged with numerous mitoses, many of which are atypical.

Bowen's disease
This is similar to Bowen's disease elsewhere (see p. 416) and is found on prepuce and penile shaft as a single plaque of white tissue with identical histology to erythroplasia.

Bowenoid papulosis
Numerous small velvety papules on shaft of penis of young men. Histologically indistinguishable from Bowen's disease and erythroplasia but unlike them is not premalignant and is probably due to HPV (see p. 210).

Carcinoma of penis

Incidence
Uncommon in Western communities but causing up to 10% of male cancer deaths in some Third World countries.

Age
Fifty to 70 years.

Aetiological factors:
1 Circumcision. The condition is virtually unknown in Jews and Moslems who are both ritually circumcised. Presumed carcinogenic agent in retained smegma has not been identified.
2 Premalignant conditions described above commonly evolve into invasive carcinoma.

Macroscopical.
A papillary and ulcerating tumour often hidden by the prepuce but producing swelling and an offensive purulent discharge.

Microscopical.
Squamous cell carcinoma which is usually well differentiated.

Spread:
1 Direct. Through prepuce and proximally along shaft of penis.
2 Lymphatic. Thirty per cent have metatases in inguinal lymph nodes at presentation. Lymph nodes are almost invariably enlarged as a reaction to secondary infection of the tumour.
3 Blood spread is uncommon.

Results.
If lymph nodes are free of tumour, 80–90% 5-year survival occurs following amputation, but with node involvement prognosis is poor.

Scrotum

Inflammations
Tuberculous epididymitis not infrequently erodes through scrotal skin to form a skin sinus.

Fournier's gangrene is a rapidly extensive idiopathic process which destroys the scrotum and reveals the testis. It is assumed to be infective in nature but no organism is yet identified.

Carcinoma

Incidence
A rare tumour—less than 0.25% of male cancer deaths, and occurring only in industrial communities in elderly patients.

Aetiology
Known to be related to exposure to petroleum and coal tar derivatives. 'Chimney sweep's cancer' was scrotal carcinoma of chimney sweeps whose clothes were impregnated with soot. More recently 'mule-spinner's cancer' is scrotal cancer in lathe workers whose overalls became drenched in machine oil.

Appearances
Squamous cell carcinoma with raised ulcerated plaques.

Spread and results
A slow-growing tumour. Lymph nodes are affected in only 20% and overall prognosis is good.

F/HERMAPHRODITISM, INTER-SEX

Definitions
Hermaphroditism
Normal sex development
Abnormal sex development
   Genetic
   Phenotypic

Definitions

Sex of the individual
The sex of the individual is dependent upon the context in which the term is applied.
1 *Genetic sex:* presence of Y chromosome normally implies masculinity.
2 *Phenotypic sex:* dependent upon appearance of external genitalia.
3 *Gonadal sex:* dependent upon nature of the gonads, either testis or ovary.
4 *Sex of upbringing:* this is usually according to phenotypic sex.
5 *Behavioural sex:* usually determined by sex of upbringing. There is no evidence that homosexuality or transvestism have an organic origin.

Hermaphroditism

True hermaphroditism
The occurrence of both testicular and ovarian tissue in the same individual. Most cases are due to mosaicism.

Male pseudo-hermaphroditism
Genotypic male, with testes, who has ambiguous or female external genitalia and body habitus.

Female pseudo-hermaphroditism
Genotypic female, with ovaries, fallopian tubes and uterus but with varying degrees of masculinisation of external genitalia and body habitus.

Normal sexual development
Genetic sex is determined at the time of fertilization when the ovum containing one X chromosome fuses with a spermatozoon containing either one X or one Y chromosome. In the absence of a Y chromosome the primitive gonad and ductular system develops into a phenotypic female. The presence of the Y chromosome results in the development of the primitive testis.

Sertoli cells produce a protein—*Mullerian inhibiting factor*—MIF, which causes regression of the Mullerian system. Androgens from the testis stimulate development of the Wolffian system and the male phenotype.

Abnormalities of sexual development

Abnormalities of genetic sex

These arise either at fertilization or subsequent aberrant meiosis.

Turner's syndrome—XO—gonadal dysgenesis

Absence of the second X chromosome leads to failure of gonadal development which are represented by a small quantity of gonadal blastema—'*streak ovary*'. With lack of gonadal MIF and androgens the phenotype is female. There are other associated abnormalities: small stature, shield-shaped chest, web neck, cubitus valgus and cardiac abnormalities, in particular coarctation of the aorta.

Klinefelter's syndrome—XXY

Presence of the Y chromosome leads to the normal male phenotype but the additional X chromosome prevents maturation of the testes which remain small and the subject is infertile as the seminiferous tubules fail to develop normally. A variable degree of failure of interstitial cells may lead to under-androgenization—eunuchoid habitus, failure of epiphyseal fusion, obesity, gynaecomastia and female distribution of the body hair.

True hermaphroditism—XX/XY and variants

Most are due to mosaicism but others are more complicated. Presence of both ovarian and testicular tissue—sometimes in the same organ—*ovo-testis*—produces a spectrum of ambiguous appearances of both internal and external genitalia.

XYY Syndrome

These subjects are normal phenotypic males but are characterized by a tendency to tall stature, reduced intelligence combined with antisocial behaviour.

Abnormalities of phenotypic sex

Male pseudo-hermaphroditism

Genotypic males with female phenotype result from unresponsiveness of target organs to circulating androgens during embryological development—*androgen resistance* or *testicular feminization syndrome*.

The typical case has a normal female phenotype externally but with a short vagina and absent uterus. Testes are present and are either inguinal or intra-abdominal. Many of these patients are not diagnosed until they are investigated for amenorrhoea at puberty.

Female pseudo-hermaphroditism

These genotypic females with female internal genitalia have masculinization of their external genitalia due to circulating virilizing agents. These may result from underlying metabolic defects such as *congenital adrenal hyperplasia* (see p. 119) or follow administration of compounds to the mother during pregnancy.

A number of ovarian abnormalities and tumours in the adult may produce virilization and a degree of clitoromegaly, but never sufficient to produce ambiguous external genitalia (see p. 119).

Chapter 12
Diseases of the Genito-Urinary System—Female Genital Tract

A/VULVA, VAGINA

Vulva
    Congenital
    Inflammations
    Bartholin's cyst
    Non-neoplastic epithelial disorders
    Tumours
Vagina
    Congenital
    Inflammations
    Tumours

Vulva

Congenital

The vulva may be absent or hypoplastic, usually associated with a hypoplastic uterus and a deficiency of secondary sexual characteristics. There may be duplication of the vulva associated with a double vagina or a septate uterus. The most common congenital abnormality is an imperforate hymen, which may escape notice until the onset of menstruation occurs to produce *haematocolpos* (vagina), *haematometra* (uterus), or even *haematosalpinx* (tubes) due to the progressive accumulation of menstrual blood.

Inflammations

Human papilloma virus—HPV
This is probably the most common infection of the lower female genital tract. *Condylomata accuminata* are usually sexually transmitted; they may be verrucous, papillary or sessile. Skin involvement may be difficult to see without the application of dilute acetic acid, which turns such areas white. Associated pruritis vulvae is common.

Herpes virus
Vesicles, pustules and shallow ulcers are caused by the herpes simplex virus type II. This is a relapsing condition.

Syphilis
This venereal disease is caused by *Treponema pallidum* (see p. 2). The vulva and cervix are the commonest female sites of the primary chancre of syphilis—a painless shallow ulcer with raised edges. Secondary syphilis may include the plaque-like *condylomata lata*.

Granuloma inguinale—Calymmatobacterium granulomatis
Primary lesions are painless papules, or ulcers with rolled edges. The disease spreads by local infiltration causing gross deformity. The intracellular organisms can be seen in Giemsa or silver-stained preparations as *Donovan bodies* (see p. 203).

Lymphogranuloma venereum—Chlamydia trachomatis
The main feature of this disease is the production of painful superficial groin nodes which may rupture through the skin. The primary painless vulval ulceration is usually overlooked. Later, chronic lymphatic obstruction leads to non-pitting oedema of the external genitalia (see p. 203).

Miscellaneous infective diseases
Non-specific infections of the vulva are frequent, especially when associated with a vaginal discharge, often caused by a fungal infection. *Candida albicans* is frequently the pathogen.

Bartholin's cyst

A mucus-containing retention cyst of Bartholin's gland in the labia minora. Frequently there is superimposed infection—*Bartholin's abscess*.

The cyst is lined by cuboidal or columnar epithelium with mucous glands in the fibromuscular wall. The epithelial lining is destroyed by infection so that the cyst commonly contains inflammatory material and is lined by granulation tissue. However, some mucous glands remain in the fibrous wall which enable recognition of the tissue of origin.

Non-neoplastic epithelial disorders

Classification

1 Lichen sclerosus—lichen sclerosus et atrophicus.
2 Squamous cell hyperplasia—formerly hyperplastic dystrophy.
3 Other dermatoses.

Lichen sclerosus

There is blunting and loss of rete ridges with a concomitant homogeneous eosinophilic subepithelial layer in the dermis. There is a decrease in the number of layers of epithelial cells and the basal layer is hydropic. An autoimmune aetiology has been postulated.

Squamous cell hyperplasia

This is a diagnosis derived by exclusion. Specific cutaneous lesions or dermatoses involving the vulva may include squamous cell hyperplasia, but should be diagnosed specifically. Squamous cell hyperplasia with associated vulval intraepithelial neoplasia (VIN), should be diagnosed as VIN (see below).

Mixed epithelial disorders may occur, in which case the components of the mix should be reported.

Other dermatoses

Being covered with skin the vulva may be involved by specific skin disorders, most commonly *lichen simplex chronicus*, *lichen planus* and *psoriasis* (see p. 413). The features usually seen in skin on exposed sites may be modified in vulval lesions.

Tumours

Vulval intraepithelial neoplasia—VIN

This is graded as VIN I, II and III. Conservative therapy is recommended with wide local excision.

Laser ablation under anaesthetic is also used: 90% of VIN has evidence of associated HPV infection (see p. 210).

Paget's disease

In this disease large Paget cells occur in nests and singly within the epidermis. Their cytoplasm frequently contains mucopolysaccharides which can be identified by the diastase-PAS reaction. More reliably they stain positively with the CAM 5.2 immunoperoxidase method. Vulval Paget's disease may occur alone, but associated underlying intraductal or invasive adenocarcinomas in adnexal structures and squamous cell carcinomas have been reported. Curiously, in one study, 14% of vulval Paget's disease cases were associated with a breast carcinoma.

Squamous cell carcinoma

This tumour is responsible for approximately 1% of malignant disease. The incidence increases with age, but it is being diagnosed with increased frequency in younger women. There is a recognized association between vulval, vaginal and cervical carcinomas and 'field-changes' may occur, especially in immunocompromised women. Ninety per cent of vulval squamous cell carcinomas are well differentiated and the tumours are usually solitary. Lymph node metastasis has been shown to be related to depth of invasion at time of excision—5 mm: 15.2%; 3 mm: 12.1%. In large series collected over decades, just over 50% of cases have been recorded as having metastatic disease at presentation, but with earlier diagnosis this may well decrease.

Other tumours

The vulva is a relatively common site for malignant melanoma, basal cell carcinoma and sweat gland tumours, particularly the benign *hidradenoma*.

Vagina

Congenital

The vagina may be involved, with the uterus, in a failure of fusion of the Mullerian ducts and thus be septate, whilst atresia or even absence of the whole vagina occurs rarely. Vestigial remnants of the Wolffian ducts—*Gartner's ducts*, lie in the lateral walls of the vagina and are occasionally the site of cyst formation. They are small fluid-filled cysts with a cuboidal epithelial lining.

Inflammations

The vagina is relatively resistant to infection in women of reproductive age. Superficial squamous cells become glycogenated and the epithelium thickens as a maturation effect of oestrogen. Lactobacilli metabolize the glycogen of desquamated cells into lactic acid reducing the vaginal pH to 3–4, a deterrent to the growth of pathogens. Physiological oestrogen-deficient postmenopausal atrophy of the vaginal epithelium predisposes to low-grade infection and inflammation—the so-called *senile vaginitis*.

Gonococcal vulvovaginitis of children

Mature squamous epithelium of adult women is resistant to infection by *Neisseria gonorrhoeae*, but the thinner mucosa of children can be penetrated and the submucosa invaded giving a purulent vaginitis.

Gardnerella

This organism probably accounts for 90% of non-specific vaginal infections.

Candidiasis

Candida albicans is a yeast-like fungus which produces an infection of the superficial squamous epithelium of the vagina. Thick white plaques and a vaginal discharge result.

Trichomoniasis

Trichomonas vaginalis is a unicellular protozoan with prominent flagella. It is readily identifiable in wet preparations and in smears stained for cervical cytology. It produces a frothy and offensive discharge.

Human papillomavirus—HPV

Vaginal infection with HPV is not uncommon. Frank warts may be seen, but flat condylomata visible only after the application of dilute acetic acid may also be present.

Tumours

Benign connective tissue tumours, e.g. fibromyoma, haemangioma, etc., occur but are rare and show no special features in this site. *Fibroepithelial polyps* occur and in 50% may include large atypical-looking stromal cells. Mitotic figures are, however, uncommon. These lesions are benign and they do not recur after simple excision.

Vaginal intraepithelial neoplasia—VAIN

Intraepithelial neoplasia occurs much less frequently in the vagina than on the cervix (CIN): 80% of cases of VAIN are found in women previously treated for CIN or invasive cervical cancer.

Malignant tumours

Primary malignant tumours of the vagina are rare, secondary deposits from elsewhere occurring more frequently.

Squamous cell carcinoma

This must be distinguished from vaginal involvement by a primary carcinoma of the cervix and from metastatic carcinoma. Approximately 50% of primary tumours arise in the upper third of the vagina and 60% from the posterior wall.

Sarcoma botryoides—embryonal rhabdomyosarcoma

This is the most common neoplasm of the lower female genital tract in girls: approximately two-thirds occur under 2 years of age. It infiltrates the vaginal wall producing polypoid masses resembling a bunch of grapes (see p. 108). Extensive pelvic clearance with chemotherapy in early disease has been successful.

B/UTERINE CERVIX

Congenital
Development of transformation zone
DES exposure
Inflammations
Pseudo-tumours
Tumours

Congenital

The cervix is frequently involved by congenital abnormalities arising from faulty fusion of the Mullerian ducts. There may also be atresia of the cervical canal resulting in retention of secretions and of menstrual blood—*haematometra*.

Development of the transformation zone

The position of the junction between the ectocervical squamous epithelium and the endocervical columnar epithelium, the *squamocolumnar junction*, is hormone-dependent (see Fig. 18). In more than 95%

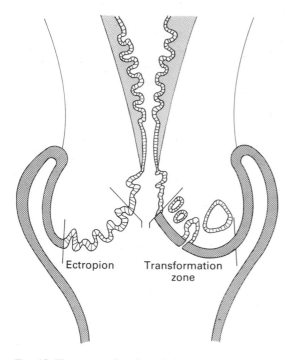

Fig. 18 The cervix: physiological changes.

of female infants it is on the cervix and approximates to the external os. In a small percentage it can be in the vaginal fornices or on the vaginal wall. At puberty, as oestrogen levels rise, the pH of the vagina decreases and exposed columnar epithelium changes into squamous epithelium. This is partly by *squamous epithelialization* from the original squamous epithelium and partly by *squamous metaplasia* from differentiation of reserve cells to squamous rather than columnar cells in the acid-exposed area. The new area of squamous epithelium which is produced is called the *congenital transformation zone*.

Eversion of columnar epithelium can occur at other times and is known clinically as an 'erosion' as it looks red and granular and bleeds easily. The area is more properly termed an *ectropion*. This too will undergo epithelialization and squamous metaplasia.

The endocervical epithelium is usually thrown into folds with villi and crypts. It is mainly the tips of the villi that undergo the squamous change and the underlying crypts may remain, to some degree, still lined by columnar epithelium surviving in its own alkaline mucus. If the openings to these crypts are blocked by squamous epithelium then mucus retention cysts

result. These are commonly known as *Nabothian follicles* (see Fig. 18).

Changes related to diethylstilboestrol (DES) exposure
Anatomical abnormalities of the upper vagina and cervix, especially the presence of a hood (cockscomb) or collar around the cervix, have been related to exposure to DES *in utero*. Also, the squamocolumnar junction is often in the vagina. The cervix and upper vagina are covered with columnar epithelium—so-called *vaginal adenosis*. Squamous metaplasia proceeds slowly, and the glandular epithelium may undergo neoplastic transformation into *clear cell adenocarcinoma*.

Inflammations

Acute cervicitis
Bacterial infection is most common. Many cases of acute cervicitis result from opportunistic infections by 'commensal' organisms when epithelial atrophy, trauma, ulceration, or some other factor renders the cervix susceptible. Additionally, sexually transmitted infections with more virulent organisms such as *Neisseria gonorrhoeae*, or *Chlamydia* occur. Clinically, acute cervicitis is important because of its association with ascending infection and transmission of infection to the placenta, fetus and neonate.

Viral cervicitis

Herpes virus (HSV)
Cervical infection with this virus can be asymptomatic. In the Papanicolaou smear, large multinucleated cells with ground-glass intranuclear inclusions are seen.

Human papilloma virus (HPV)
Frank warts can be seen on the cervix as well as on the vulva and in the vagina. Again, flat condylomata may not be visible without the aid of dilute acetic acid. In cervical smears multinucleation, *dyskeratosis* (cells with orange cytoplasm and distorted nuclear remnants) and *koilocytes* (cells with a perinuclear clear zone due to cytoplasmic necrosis) are characteristic.

Both HSV and HPV have been implicated in the formation of cervical intra-epithelial neoplasia (CIN) and cervical carcinoma (see p. 212).

Pseudo-tumours

Endocervical polyps

These result from hyperplastic endocervical folds, or from protruding mucus retention cysts—*Nabothian follicles*. In pregnancy, decidualization of endocervical stroma may produce a *decidual polyp*.

Microglandular hyperplasia

Endocervical mucus glands undergo proliferation to produce small polyp-like lesions under progestogenic stimulation. The lesions are seen in pregnancy and the puerperium and in women taking oral contraception. The microtubular pattern may be florid with areas of hyperchromatic and pleomorphic nuclei—*atypical microglandular hyperplasia*. Such lesions have been mistaken for adenocarcinoma, but are benign.

Tumours

Cervical intra-epithelial neoplasia—CIN

Site on the cervix

CIN arises in the transformation zone of the cervix. The rapidly dividing squamous cells of metaplasia seem to be particularly open to carcinogenic attack. It is the area at and around the external cervical os which must, therefore, be thoroughly sampled when cytology screening scrapes are taken.

Risk groups

1 The only well-established fact concerning cervical squamous carcinogenesis is that there is a strong sexually transmitted component. The women at highest risk are those who begin to have sexual intercourse at an early age and who have multiple partners, so combining active metaplasia with a sexually transmitted agent. It must be remembered, however, that metaplasia can occur at any age and a sexually transmitted disease can be contracted from one partner. The at-risk group, therefore, includes all women who have ever had intercourse, if only once.
2 It is possible that normal cervical mucus acts as a protector against surface acting agents and it has been suggested that cervical mucus changes at puberty, during menstruation and in women taking oral contraceptive therapy might increase cervical epithelial vulnerability.
3 Polyamines normally present in seminal fluid have been shown to be capable of producing abnormalities in the DNA of cervical squamous cells.

4 Certain types of sexually transmitted virus, especially HPV types 6, 11, 16, 18 and 33, are associated with CIN but are also frequently found in normal epithelium. Types 16, 18 and 33 have been detected integrated into the DNA of invasive cervical squamous carcinoma cells.
5 Women who smoke tobacco have been shown to be at higher risk than those who do not. Nicotine and other known carcinogenic agents in tobacco smoke are absorbed through the lungs, circulated throughout the body and have been isolated from cervical mucus. The presence of these substances is associated with the appearance of 'adducts' in cervical squamous DNA. The interplay of these factors is ill-understood and the detail of the carcinogenic process is yet to be determined.

Natural history

The natural history of the disease appears to be extremely variable. The time between the first admitted sexual contact and detection of CIN may be months in some cases, whereas in some women, despite a high risk history, CIN does not appear until 40–50 years of age. Also, CIN seems to be able to progress rapidly to invasive malignancy, or to have an apparently endless intra-epithelial phase. This almost certainly reflects the fact that cervical epithelial malignancy comprises several disease processes. Despite this, the most effective cytology screening interval has been determined to be 3 years, regardless of age or parity. Attempts have been made to identify high-risk groups for more frequent screening, but without success in further reducing mortality, perhaps because the highest risk group is still the unscreened population.

Histology and cytology

On histology CIN is graded I, II and III, by eye, based on the depth of epithelial thickness replaced by undifferentiated malignant cells (see Fig. 19). All grades of CIN are asymptomatic, but can be detected by scraping cells from the surface of the cervix. The surface cells reflect the relative immaturity of the epithelium beneath and so have an increased nuclear/cytoplasmic ratio. The abnormal cells are also seen to have irregular nuclei with an irregular chromatin distribution and are therefore termed *dyskaryotic*. Mild, moderate and severe dyskaryosis on cytology roughly equates with the finding of CIN I, II and III respectively on histological examination of cervical biopsies.

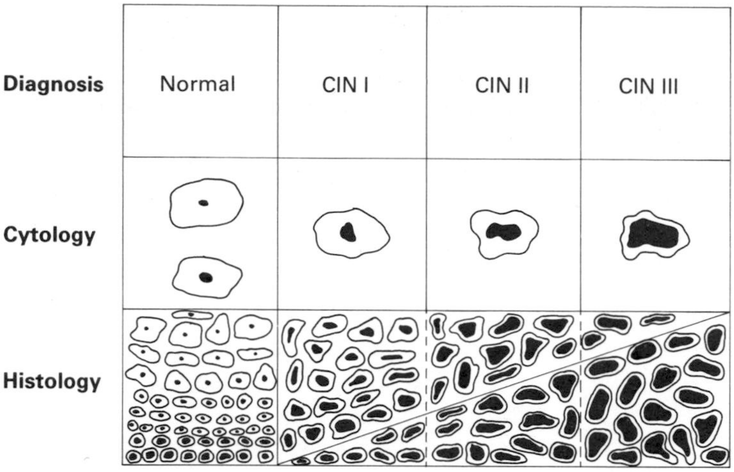

Fig. 19 Histology: Cytology correlation.

Management

Initial diagnosis from the presence of abnormal cells in cervical cytology preparations is followed by colposcopy. The cervix is painted with a dilute solution of acetic acid and viewed under magnification to determine the site of the lesion. If the whole of the squamocolumnar junction can be seen, it is less than 1 cm into the endocervical canal and there are no features to suggest the presence of an invasive focus (e.g. atypical vessels) then the lesion is suitable for treatment by local destruction, following histological confirmation of its nature. Lesions extending into the endocervical canal for more than 1 cm, where the whole of the squamocolumnar junction cannot be seen, or where there is a suspicion of invasion, must be diagnosed by an excision biopsy—cold knife cone biopsy, or diathermy loop excision.

Cervical glandular intra-epithelial neoplasia—CGIN

The endocervical epithelium may show multilayering, tufting, hyperchromatic nuclei, nuclear pleomorphism and mitotic activity. Minor degrees of abnormality may be seen in association with marked inflammation and have been termed regenerative, but true CGIN is recognized and divided into high- and low-grade lesions. CGIN has been reported in 16% of cone biopsies in which there is CIN. It is more rarely seen when CIN is not present.

Carcinoma of the cervix

In England and Wales 3800 new cases of cervical cancer are registered each year with approximately 1800 deaths. In countries where there are screening programmes reduction in mortality appears to be directly proportional to the population coverage. It can occur at any age from late teens onwards, the average age being 50 years. In the past 20 years there has been an increasing incidence in those women aged less than 35 years.

Clinical stage

The internationally accepted FIGO (International Federation of Gynaecologists and Obstetricians) staging is:

Stage 0   Carcinoma *in situ*.

Stage I   Confined to the cervix (extension to corpus disregarded).

Stage Ia   Preclinical carcinomas diagnosed by microscopy. *Microinvasive carcinoma.*

Stage Ia1   Minimal microscopically evident stromal invasion. *Early stromal invasion.* Less than 1 mm in maximum dimension.

Stage Ia2   Lesions detected microscopically that can be measured. *Microcarcinomas*—maximum depth from base of epithelium of origin 5 mm. Horizontal spread no more than 7 mm. Vascular space involvement should not alter staging, but should be specifically recorded. Larger lesions are staged Ib.

Stage Ib   Lesions larger than Stage Ia2, whether seen clinically or not.

Stage IIa   Invasive carcinoma extending to involve the upper two-thirds of the vagina without parametrial infiltration.

Stage IIb   Carcinoma involving upper two-thirds of vagina with parametrial infiltration not involving pelvic side wall.

Stage III   Spread to either lateral pelvic wall and/or lower third of vagina and/or hydronephros due to tumour.

Stage IV   Involvement of mucosa of bladder and/or rectum or extending beyond true pelvis.

Microscopy

More than 95% of malignant epithelial neoplasms of the cervix used to be classified as squamous cell carcinomas. With the routine use of mucin stains, however, and stricter criteria carcinomas can now be more accurately designated (see Table 12.1). The incidence of adenocarcinoma has been reported as increasing, particularly in women less than 45 years of age.

Management

The treatment of preinvasive disease has been described above. Microinvasive carcinomas are usually treated by local excision.

Invasive carcinoma is usually managed by radical surgery and/or radiotherapy and/or chemotherapy depending on the stage of the disease and local custom.

Results

The 5-year survival rate for adequately treated patients of all stages together is given as 60%. The 5-year survival after treatment of recurrent disease is 20–35%.

Table 12.1 Types of cervical carcinoma.

	Non-mucin secreting (%)	Mucin secreting (%)
Large cell keratinizing	26	8
Large cell non-keratinizing	26	18
Small cell	10	0
Mixed	0	2
Adenocarcinoma	0	10

Five-year survival according to stage:

Stage I   85–90%
Stage II   70–75%
Stage III   30–35%
Stage IV   10%

Survival rates are reduced to 30–50% even at stage Ib if those with lymph node metastases are analysed separately.

C/BODY OF UTERUS

Normal development
Congenital
Endometrium
   Normal cycle
   Gestational
   Trophoblastic disease
   Inflammations
   Abnormalities of cycle
   Hormone therapy
   Metaplasia
   Hyperplasia
   Tumours
Myometrium
   Adenomyosis
   Leiomyoma
   Leiomyosarcoma
Endometriosis

Normal development

The uterus, cervix and vagina are formed by fusion of the paired Müllerian ducts. The fallopian tubes arise from the unfused portions of these ducts.

Müllerian duct epithelium is of three basic types with a potential to interchange by metaplasia:

1 Endometrial.
2 Endocervical.
3 Tubal (ciliated).

Congenital

The common congenital abnormalities result from anomalies of fusion of the Müllerian ducts (Fig. 20).

If one Müllerian duct fails to develop the uterus is *unicornis*.

The uterus can be totally absent. This abnormality, referred to as the *Rokitansky–Kuster–Hauser syndrome*, is one of the more common causes of primary amenorrhoea. The aetiology of degrees of atresia may sometimes be genetic as siblings can be affected.

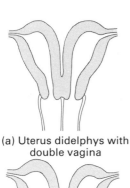

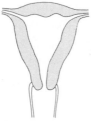

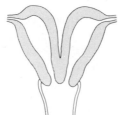

(a) Uterus didelphys with
    double vagina

(b) Uterus arcuatus

(c) Uterus bicornis

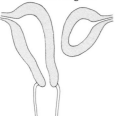

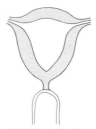

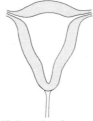

(d) Uterus bicornis unicollis.
    with rudimentary horn

(e) Atresia of cervix

(f) Atresia of vagina

Fig. 20 Schematic representation of the main congenital abnormalities of the uterus and vagina caused by persistence of the uterine septum or obliteration of the lumen of the uterine canal.

Endometrium

Normal menstrual cycle

A menstrual cycle is timed from the commencement of one period of menstrual loss to the commencement of the next, and averages 28 days. Individual variations from 24 to 30 days are not uncommon, but if outside this range are usually regarded as abnormal.

In a 28-day cycle the changes, illustrated in Fig. 21, are as follows.

Menstruation

Lasts for 3–6 days.

Follicular phase

The follicle is maturing within the ovary and this phase is associated with oestrogen production.

1 *Resting phase*: following menstruation only the basal endometrial layers remain.

2 *Proliferative phase*: this lasts until ovulation at the 14th day. Proliferative activity occurs in both endometrial tubules and stroma resulting in progressive thickening of the endometrium by simple, straight, regular, endometrial tubular glands in a cellular stroma.

Ovulation

The follicle ruptures on the 14th day.

Luteal phase

Immediately following ovulation, the ruptured follicle develops into a corpus luteum and there is associated production of progesterone.

1 *Early secretory phase*: this lasts for 2–3 days (14th to 17th day) immediately following ovulation. There is subnuclear vacuolation of the epithelial cell cytoplasm with progressive displacement of nuclei towards the lumen. The glands become less straight.

2 *Mid-secretory phase*: in the next 7–9 days (17th to 26th day)the endometrium continues to increase in depth with increasing tortuosity of the glands. The nuclei resume their basal position and the luminal border becomes less well defined with intraluminal secretion. The stromal cells become plumper and less active.

3 *Premenstrual phase*: in the 2–3 days preceding menstruation (26th to 28th day) characteristic changes occur in the stromal cells which become plump—*decidual cells*. The glands are complex and very tortuous with a 'saw-tooth' appearance, and are filled with secreted material. As menstruation approaches, there is a polymorph infiltration and haemorrhages into the stroma of the superficial layers.

4 *Menstruation*: 28th day. All but the basal layers of the endometrium are shed.

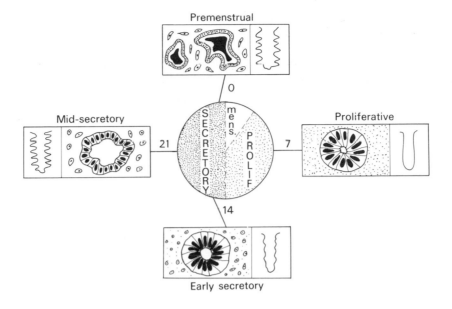

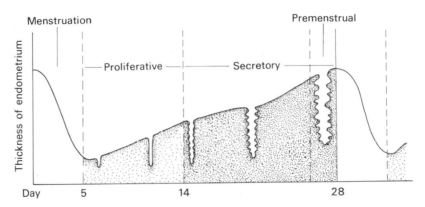

Fig. 21 Endometrial changes in the menstrual cycle.

Gestational endometrium

If the ovum is fertilized, the corpus luteum persists and secretes progesterone. The secretory changes are therefore continued in the tubules and the decidual cells of the stroma persist, becoming the decidua of pregnancy.

Gestational trophoblastic disease—GTD

Classification

1 Hydatidiform mole.
  (a) complete.
  (b) partial.

2 Invasive mole.
3 Choriocarcinoma.
4 Placental site trophoblastic tumour.

Hydatidiform mole

In the Western hemisphere hydatidiform mole occurs in 1 : 1500 pregnancies. In Japan the frequency is approximately 1 : 500 pregnancies. The reason for this difference is unexplained.

In a *complete mole* the majority of the villi are hydropic, producing the typical 'bunch of grapes' appearance. Histologically there is always trophoblastic proliferation but variable in degree, and fetal tissue is not usually present. Within the hydropic villi there is loss of vessels and central degeneration producing *cisternae*. The karyotype is usually 46 XX, all paternally derived. Clinically the uterus is large-for-dates and the human chorionic gonadotrophin (hCG) level is above normal for dates. Approximately 10% lead to persistent gestational trophoblastic disease.

A *partial mole* is a mixture of enlarged hydropic villi of irregular 'geographic' outline and normal villi. Fetal tissue is often present. The karyotype is most frequently triploid with a maternal component. Partial moles comprise 25–45% of reported molar pregnancies. The uterus is generally small-for-dates and there is a low or normal hCG, but an increase in human placental alkaline phosphatase (PLAP); 4–10% lead to persistent GTD.

Invasive mole

This is a hydatidiform mole in which hydropic villi invade myometrium, or blood vessels causing local problems. As hysterectomy is now rarely performed for persistent GTD, the diagnosis is only occasionally confirmed histologically.

Choriocarcinoma

A highly malignant tumour of both syncitio- and cytotrophoblast which occurs once in 30 000–40 000 pregnancies in the West, but more frequently in the East. Chorionic villi are not present. Most appear to follow a gestational event, with abnormal uterine bleeding being the most common presentation. Fifty per cent have a preceding hydatidiform mole, 25% follow an abortion, 22% a normal pregnancy and 3% an ectopic pregnancy. Early metastasis via the blood stream is common, but there is a good response to chemotherapy with an overall survival in persistent and metastatic GTD of 90%. If there is a histologically confirmed diagnosis of choriocarcinoma, however, this falls to 81% and in histologically confirmed choriocarcinoma with proven metastasis it is only 71%: hCG levels are raised and can be used to monitor response to treatment.

Placental site trophoblastic tumour

This is the rarest GTD and is composed of intermediate trophoblast, resembling an exaggerated placental site reaction. The biphasic pattern of choriocarcinoma is absent, as are villi. The patient presents with amenorrhoea, or abnormal bleeding, and is frequently thought to be pregnant although the serum hCG is low. The disease is generally benign in its course, but is occasionally highly malignant with a poor response to chemotherapy. The treatment of choice for early-stage disease is hysterectomy.

Inflammations

Acute endometritis

A polymorphonuclear leucocyte infiltrate, necrosis and haemorrhage occur in the endometrium in the menstrual and premenstrual phases, but micro-abscesses and gland lumina, filled or disrupted by polymorphs, form the basis of the histological diagnosis of acute endometritis. Clinically significant acute endometritis usually presents in association with pregnancy, or abortion as is most often caused by haemolytic and anaerobic streptococci, staphylococci and *Clostridium welchii*. Gonococcal endometritis rarely occurs. If the cervical canal is obstructed by tumour, or stenosis, proximal infection may give rise to distension of the endometrial cavity by frank pus; a *pyometra*.

Chronic non-specific endometritis

Chronic endometritis has been associated with a recent pregnancy or abortion in 53%, salpingitis in 25% and an intrauterine contraceptive device in 14%. The histological diagnosis rests on the presence of plasma cells, and when made in asymptomatic patients without associated factors, should prompt endocervical cultures for *Chlamydia* and gonococci (see p. 210).

Tuberculous endometritis

The endometrium in genital tuberculosis is affected by seeding directly from disease in the fallopian tubes and is involved in up to three-quarters of such cases (see p. 220). The disease may be discovered during the investigation of infertility, as the patient is usually sterile. After treatment, if fertility returns, tubal implantation frequently occurs. 'Tubercles' are most often seen if curettage is performed in the late secretory, or premenstrual phase. Caseation is rarely seen and tubercle bacilli are hardly ever seen with ZN staining, even if cultures are positive.

Abnormalities of the menstrual cycle

Anovulatory cycles

Such cycles occur typically at menarche and menopause. Bleeding is usually irregular and variable in amount. On histology the glands are typically proliferative and there may be ectatic venules containing fibrin thrombi. Prolonged unopposed oestrogen stimulation may give rise to metaplasia and/or hyperplasia (see below).

Luteal phase defect
This may be due to inadequate production of progesterone by the corpus luteum or to endometrial progesterone receptor defect. The endometrium shows a delayed secretory phase response. Luteal phase defect is thought to occur sporadically in otherwise normal women, and so should be demonstrated in at least two consecutive cycles by endometrial biopsy before it is considered to be significant.

Reduced, or absent, proliferation
Endocrinological and other abnormalities may result in insufficient oestrogen production and the proliferative changes are reduced in degree or are absent—*oligomenorrhoea* or *amenorrhoea*.

Effects of hormone therapy
The commonest histological appearance is that associated with combined oral contraceptive therapy. The endometrium is scanty and the tubules are hypoplastic and inactive. The stroma may show a pseudo-decidualized appearance. Stromal pseudo-decidualization is more marked due to progesterone-only contraceptive pill administration, and most prominent in women given progestogens in an attempt to control menorrhagia.

Unopposed oestrogen administration to women with an intact uterus is unwise, as prolonged endometrial stimulation, just as with endogenous oestrogen, may give rise to metaplasias, but more importantly hyperplasias and eventually carcinoma.

Metaplasia
These usually occur in association with hyperplasia, but *squamous metaplasia* may be seen in normal cycling endometrium. Occasionally, especially in older, postmenopausal women, the whole cavity may be lined by keratinizing squamous epithelium which grossly looks like fish scales, and is therefore known as *ichthyosis uteri*. *Tubal metaplasia*, or ciliated cell metaplasia, *mucinous metaplasia*—endocervical type epithelium—and *eosinophilic metaplasia* also occur. Eosinophilic metaplasia is more common in atypical hyperplasia. Mixtures of metaplasias are common.

Hyperplasia

Simple or cystic hyperplasia
This is the most common form of hyperplasia formed of cystically dilated glands lined by stratified columnar cells showing mitotic activity. It is distinguished from postmenopausal cystic degeneration by the fact that the cysts in this latter condition are usually lined by a single layer of low-cuboidal epithelium without proliferative features.

Complex hyperplasia, or hyperplasia with architectural atypia
Such endometria exhibit complex, crowded glands with reduced stroma. Mitotic figures may be sparse and are normal and nuclear irregularity is absent.

Atypical hyperplasia, or hyperplasia with cytological atypia
The cells lining the glands show hyperchromatic nuclei with prominent nucleoli, an increased nuclear/cytoplasmic ratio, pleomorphism and lack of basal polarity. Atypical mitotic figures may be seen.

Progression to carcinoma
Simple hyperplasia, approx. 1%
Complex hyperplasia (architectural atypia), 3%
Atypical hyperplasia:
    cytological atypia, 8%
    cytological and architectural atypia, 28%

Tumours

Endometrial polyps
These may be single, or multiple. They are overgrowths of endometrium, most frequently at the fundus and often out of phase with the remainder of the endometrium. They are usually benign, but occasionally include foci of hyperplasia, or even carcinoma.

Endometrial carcinoma

Types
There appear to be two distinct types of endometrial adenocarcinoma.

1 Occurs in pre- and perimenopausal women and is associated with endometrial hyperplasia and prolonged unopposed oestrogen stimulation of the endometrium. Such lesions tend to be well differentiated,

may show foci of benign squamous metaplasia—
adenoacanthoma—have only superficial myometrial
invasion at diagnosis and have a good prognosis.

2 Does not appear to be oestrogen related. It
occurs in older postmenopausal women, is usually
poorly differentiated with deep myometrial invasion—
adenosquamous, *serous papillary* and *clear cell* subtypes with a poor prognosis occur in this group. There
are approximately 3300 new cases of endometrial
carcinoma registered in England and Wales each year,
with 1450 recorded deaths.

Predisposing factors

An increased incidence of endometrial carcinoma is
seen in association with obesity, hypertension, diabetes mellitus and nulliparity. There is also a recognized association between breast cancer and endometrial cancer and an increased risk of either of these
two diseases in first-degree relatives of women with
either disease. By contrast cigarette smoking does not
seem to be a factor in endometrial carcinogenesis.

Stage and prognosis

The FIGO classification:

Stage I   Confined to corpus—80% of cases: 5-year
           survival 81%; 10-year 65%.
Stage II   Corpus and cervix: 5-year 41%; 10-year
           33%
Stage III Outside uterus, confined to pelvis: 5-year
           42%; 10-year 25%.
Stage IV   Outside true pelvis or involving rectal or
           bladder mucosa: 5-year 9%; 10-year 0%.

Metastases usually occur only in the poorly differentiated tumours.

Endometrial stromal sarcoma

These tumours are composed of cells resembling the
stromal cells of proliferative phase endometrium.
Low-grade lesions are slow-growing, but local recurrences have been reported in up to 50% of patients.
High-grade lesions—more than 10 mitoses/10 high-
power fields, behave badly but a 50–60% 5-year
survival is claimed for patients with disease confined to
the uterus at time of primary excision.

Mixed Müllerian tumours

Nature

Mixed tumours contain both epithelial and stromal

components and are found arising from endometrium
(usually fundal), cervix and ovary.

Classification

The classification is given in Table 12.2. The sarcomatous elements may be homologous or heterologous, i.e. connective tissues not normally found at
this site of origin including chondrosarcoma, osteosarcoma and rhabdomyosarcoma.

Results

Forty per cent of adenosarcomas recur, or metastasize, but there is a 75% survival from the disease,
whereas up to 50% of cases of MMMT have extended
beyond the uterus at time of diagnosis, such cases
having zero 5-year survival.

Myometrium

Adenomyosis

This condition, reported in up to 20% of uteri, consists
of down-growths of endometrial glands and stroma
into the myometrium. The uterus is enlarged and on
the cut surface there are haemorrhagic foci with
surrounding whorled myometrium most frequently in
the posterior wall. The usual junction between the
base of normal endometrium and myometrium is
irregular and so the diagnosis can be made with
certainty only if the adenomyotic foci are more than
2.5 mm below the lower border of the endometrium.
Serial sectioning reveals that the adenomyotic foci are
in continuity with the endometrium lining the endometrial cavity. As there is no barrier between the
endometrium and myometrium, the reason why this
endometrial downgrowth should occur in some but
not others is obscure.

Adenomyoma

In the localized form a circumscribed, but poorly
demarcated, nodule of smooth muscle and endo-

Table 12.2 Classification of mixed Müllerian tumours.

	Epithelium	Stroma
Adenofibroma	Benign	Benign
Adenosarcoma	Benign	Sarcoma
Malignant mixed Müllerian tumour (MMMT)	Carcinoma	Sarcoma

metrium is found either within the uterine wall, or presenting as an endometrial polyp.

Leiomyoma—fibroid

These extremely common uterine tumours appear to be formed by the proliferation of a single clone of smooth muscle cells. In most cases fibroids are multiple. They are hard, white, whorled, well-circumscribed nodules which may be submucosal, intramural or subserosal. The submucosal variety may present as *fibroid polyps*.

Degenerations

Degenerative changes are extremely common and may be:
1 Simple atrophy.
2 Hyaline fibrosis.
3 Cystic degeneration.
4 Mucoid degeneration.
5 Red degeneration—necrobiosis.
6 Fatty change.
7 Calcification—'womb stones'.
8 Ossification.
9 Sarcomatous change—less than 0.1%.

Leiomyosarcoma

Sarcomas may rarely arise from previously benign fibroids. The level of mitotic activity is the most important criterion in making the diagnosis of sarcomatous change. In many of the degenerative conditions above, marked cellular atypia, sometimes with *'symplasmic'* giant cells, frequently occurs and over-diagnosis of malignancy must be avoided. Cellular fibroids with more than 10 mitoses per 10 high-power fields are designated as leiomyosarcomas regardless of cellular atypia. If there are less than five mitoses per 10 high-power fields then they only very rarely behave as leiomyosarcomas. Leiomyosarcomas may also arise *de novo* from myometrium. An overall survival rate of 20% is reported, but this rises to 40–50% when the disease is confined to the uterus.

Endometriosis

Definition

Ectopic endometrial tissue in an extramyometrial site.

Sites

Ovaries (80%), round ligaments, fallopian tubes, rectovaginal septum, pelvic peritoneum, intestinal wall, abdominal wall, umbilicus, laparotomy scars, lymph nodes, lung, pleura.

Findings

At any of these sites endometriosis appears macroscopically as haemorrhagic and/or cystic foci or cysts filled with altered blood—*'chocolate cysts'*. On histology there are foci of benign endometrial glands and stroma, or if the lesion is a cyst it is lined by endometrial epithelium with an endometrial stromal layer beneath it. If there has been repeated bleeding into the cyst, the lining may be largely replaced by haemosiderin-laden macrophages. Occasionally cysts are found with no residual recognizable endometrial lining, and then the diagnosis cannot be made with certainty as similar appearances can be found in other cystic lesions into which there has been haemorrhage. In areas containing smooth muscle, e.g. intestine, adjacent muscle is hypertrophied.

Pathogenesis

No single hypothesis can explain the presence of endometrium in all of its extra-uterine sites. Pelvic endometriosis has been postulated to be due to a combination of *retrograde menstruation* with induced *metaplasia of pelvic peritoneum* and *altered cellular immunity to endometrium*.

1 Retrograde menstruation has been shown to occur in more than 90% of women with patent fallopian tubes and so can be regarded as a normal physiological phenomenon. This menstrual debris is, at least partially, viable and is capable of survival if implanted.
2 It has been demonstrated that menstrual debris may act in another way to produce endometriosis. An elegant experiment involving placing the material in millipore filters produced metaplasia of adjacent peritoneal mesothelium to endometrium. Peritoneal mesothelium is capable of metaplasia into other types of Müllerian epithelium and has been called the *extra Müllerian system*. Apparently spontaneous, tubal metaplasia—*endosalpingiosis*—and endocervical metaplasia—*endocervicosis*—are also seen. Endosalpingiosis in particular may be misdiagnosed as endometriosis.
3 It has been suggested that the reason why all women with patent fallopian tubes do not develop endometriosis is that there is a peritoneal cell-mediated cytotoxicity to autologous endometrium. Indeed a reduced cell-mediated cytotoxicity to endometrium and a decreased lymphocyte stimulation

response to endometrial antigens have been demonstrated in patients with endometriosis. The degree of deficiency in the immune response appears to be directly proportional to the severity of the disease. Women with blockage to the normal antegrade flow, however, often develop endometriosis and do not show the same altered cellular immunity.

It is possible, therefore, that pelvic endometriosis is a consequence of an imbalance between the amount of retrograde menstruation and the ability of the cell-mediated immune system to destroy the material before it either implants, or induces mesothelial metaplasia.

4 Foci of benign endometrium can be seen in lymph nodes and at the umbilicus where it is suggested that the spread is via the lymphatic system. Endometriosis at distant sites, such as in bone or in the lung, are postulated to be due to blood-borne spread, vascular intrusion being occasionally demonstrable.

D/FALLOPIAN TUBES

Congenital
Inflammations
Ectopic gestation
Cysts
Tumours

Congenital

Abnormalities of the Müllerian ducts may result in absence, reduplication or atresia of one or both fallopian tubes. Partial reduplication occurs quite frequently, producing paratubal cysts which are usually quite small. The other anomalies are rare.

Inflammations

Acute salpingitis

This is usually due to ascending infection from the uterine cavity. The infection is usually polymicrobial with *Chlamydia*, *Bacterioides* species, *Escherischia coli* and peptostreptococci commonly isolated. Gonococcal salpingitis is also common. The gonococcus most readily infects the tube at the time of menstruation with the acute symptoms occurring a few days afterwards. Whatever the organism the tube may distend with pus, especially if the fimbrial end becomes closed—*pyosalpinx*.

Chronic salpingitis

Acute salpingitis may resolve without sequelae, but residual disease may be found. There may be adhesions between the plicae of the tubal lining with blind ending multiple lumina—*salpingitis follicularis*. The wall may be thickened with fibrous tissue and diverticula-like outpouches of tubal epithelium may develop leading to a nodularity of the tube—*salpingitis isthmica nodosa*. Adhesions can develop between the serosa and adjacent structures, most particularly the ovary. The ovary may be directly involved in the inflammatory process with the production of a *tubo-ovarian abscess*. *Hydrosalpinx* may be the end-result of a pyosalpinx with a retort-shaped dilated tube filled with watery fluid.

Granulomatous salpingitis

Tuberculous salpingitis

This is usually due to secondary haematogenous infection from a primary focus elsewhere. The granulomatous reaction is firstly in the mucosa, spreading later into the muscularis and serosa. Sterility is almost inevitable. The diagnosis can be made indirectly by culture of endometrium obtained at curettage.

Other causes

Worldwide one of the commonest causes of granulomatous salpingitis is *schistosomiasis* (see p. 9). This rarely causes sterility; however, the granulomata produce nodules on the tubal serosa. Although the pinworm, *Enterobius vermicularis*, is only an unpleasant infestation in children, in adult females it may migrate into the genital tract where a granulomatous reaction is produced to portions of worm and ova. *Actinomycosis* may occur in the tube, usually in association with intrauterine contraceptive devices. *Foreign-body* reactions occur to talc, starch, mineral oil and lubricant jelly.

Ectopic gestation

The fallopian tube is the site of ectopic gestation in 95% of cases. Any delay to the passage of a fertilized ovum into the endometrial cavity may result in tubal implantation. The incidence throughout the world varies markedly, but closely follows the rate of diagnosis of salpingitis.

The tube is distended by a haemorrhagic mass—a *haematosalpinx*. On microscopy fetal parts, chorionic villi and/or trophoblast must be seen to make the diagnosis.

Cysts

Small cysts at the fimbrial end of the tube—*fimbrial cysts*—are extremely common. They are small, unilocular and benign with clear fluid contents.

Cysts of Morgagni occur adjacent to the tube near the fimbrial end and are presumed to be derived from remnants of the Wolffian duct.

Primary tumours

Intra-epithelial neoplasia

Reactive changes in tubal epithelium in association with salpingitis are frequently misdiagnosed as intra-epithelial neoplasia. True neoplasia is diagnosed when marked nuclear atypia and abnormal mitoses are present in tufted epithelium.

Invasive adenocarcinoma

This is a rare primary tumour which presents classically with a watery vaginal discharge. The tube resembles a sausage, the lumen being filled and dilated by tumour which may be solid, or papillary. There is frequently transcoelomic spread and the prognosis is poor.

Secondary tumours

These are far more common than primary tumours and usually result from direct spread from the body of the uterus, or the ovary.

E/OVARY

Development
  Developmental abnormalities
Inflammations
Follicular cysts
Endometriosis
Torsion
Tumours
  Common epithelial
  Sex cord—stromal
  Germ cell
  Gonadoblastoma
  Soft tissue tumours
  Secondary

Development of ovary

The early development is characterized by four main phases.

1 Primordial germ cells, probably of yolk-sac origin, migrate to the genital ridges which are bilateral coelomic epithelial thickenings ventral to the mesonephros.

2 Proliferation of coelomic epithelium and underlying mesenchyme.

3 Gonadal division into cortex and medulla.

4 Cortical development and medullary involution in the female and the reverse in the male.

Subsequent to this the primitive germ cells—*oogonia*—proliferate by mitosis and then subsequently by meiosis forming *oocytes*.

Developmental abnormalities

Streak gonads—ovarian dysgenesis

The uterus and tubes are small and the gonads form small streaks of tissue, normally situated. Surface epithelium covers the largely fibrous tissue centre resembling ovarian stroma. Hilar cells can often be found but germ cells are absent by the time the individual reaches puberty. Most of these patients have identifiable chromosomal abnormalities usually 45 XO—*Turner's syndrome* (see p. 206).

Hermaphroditism

True hermaphrodites with recognizable ovarian and testicular tissue, either as ovotestes or differing types of gonads on different sides, are very rare (see p. 206).

Heterotopia

Misplaced nodules of adrenal tissue may be juxta-ovarian but not within the ovarian tissue.

Inflammations

Ovarian involvement in pelvic inflammatory disease is almost always secondary to salpingitis. Mumps oophoritis is much less common than mumps orchitis, only being clinically apparent in 5% of cases. Viral oophoritis may lead to germ cell depletion with resultant premature menopause.

Cysts of follicular origin

Both the normal follicle and corpus luteum are cystic structures. Quite frequently retention cysts develop which, by definition, must be more than 2 cm diameter. *Follicular* cysts are lined by an inner layer of benign granulosa cells and an outer layer of theca cells. Luteal cysts have an inner layer of large luteinized granulosa cells and an outer layer of smaller luteinized theca cells. Rarely a fibrous-walled *corpus albicans* cyst may occur. Haemorrhage into any of these cysts may produce a 'chocolate cyst' which is indistinguishable from endometriosis macroscopically.

Endometriosis

The ovary is the commonest site of endometriosis, being recorded in 80% of cases (see p. 219).

Torsion of the ovary

Torsion of a previously normal ovary is rare in adults, but may occur in children. In adults it is most frequently associated with a pre-existing retention cyst or tumour. A swollen, haemorrhagic, plum-coloured, and occasionally infarcted tubo-ovarian mass results.

Tumours of the ovary

Primary ovarian neoplasia arise from one of the three constituent cell lines of the ovary, the surface *epithelial* cells, the *stromal* cells and the *germ* cells. The World Health Organization Classification and more recent modifications divide primary ovarian neoplasia into these three main categories of lesions. Ovarian tumours cause almost 4000 deaths in England and Wales each year; 4250 ovarian malignancies are registered annually.

Common surface epithelial tumours

These tumours are certainly not as common as retention cysts in the ovary (see p. 221), but constitute approximately 70% of primary ovarian neoplasms. Mixtures of epithelia within these lesions are frequently seen. The tumour is classified according to the predominant epithelial type.

Types

1 Serous.
2 Mucinous.
3 Endometrioid.
   (a) typical,
   (b) clear cell tumours,
   (c) mixed Müllerian tumour.
4 Brenner—transitional cell tumours.
5 Carcinoma unclassifiable.

Serous tumours

Benign serous tumours

Serous cystadenomas
These are usually thin-walled unilocular cysts containing clear watery fluid. They form approximately 20% of all benign ovarian neoplasms. They are bilateral in 7–12% of cases. The inner lining of the cysts or serosal surface may be smooth or have a variable number of papillary projections. The lining cells are predominantly cuboidal and ciliated and arranged in a single regular layer. In larger cysts the cells may be flattened and their true nature unascertainable. In such cases the name *indeterminate cyst* is used.

Cystadenofibroma
The *cystadenofibroma* includes solid, pale, whorled areas within the wall of the serous cyst or, less commonly, there may be only a minor cystic component; the lesion is then termed an *adenofibroma*.

Malignant serous tumours

Borderline serous tumours
Serous tumours are 50–70% benign, 10–15% borderline and 25–35% invasive carcinomas. Borderline tumours are bilateral in 25–35% of cases, if only at a microscopical level. The lining cells show malignant features, with multilayering, tufting, cellular hyperchromasia and pleomorphism and mitotic activity, but there is no evidence of stromal invasion. There may be serosal papillary projections and similar, non-invasive, or even benign serous foci may be seen in the omentum, or on the pelvic peritoneum of the *secondary Müllerian system—tumour implants—*but this does not alter the diagnosis, or indeed the prognosis, of the primary ovarian lesion as a borderline tumour. Ten-year survival of patients with borderline serous tumours is 75% compared with 13% with serous carcinomas.

Serous carcinoma
This is the most common malignant ovarian tumour, occurring most frequently in women aged between 40 and 60 years. They are bilateral in approximately 50% of cases. They may be largely cystic—25%, semi-solid—65% or entirely solid—10%. In well-differentiated tumours the appearances resemble those seen in borderline lesions, but the distinguishing feature is that there is stromal invasion. In poorly differentiated lesions the papillary pattern is largely obliterated and there may be just solid sheets of cells. More than 75% are at an advanced stage at primary laparotomy and there is a less than 20% 5-year survival.

Mucinous tumours

Benign mucinous tumours

Mucinous cystadenomas are thin-walled, often multi-loculated cysts predominantly lined by a single layer of tall, mucus-secreting columnar cells. The cyst contents are usually mucoid and may be gelatinous. They are bilateral in only 5%. The mucin, rather than endocervical in type, is often intestinal and Paneth cells may be seen.

Malignant mucinous tumours

Borderline mucinous tumours
Mucinous tumours are 75–85% benign, 10–15% borderline and 5–10% invasive carcinomas. They are bilateral in 5–10% and in 15% there is *pseudomyxoma peritonei*. There may also be associated mucoceles of the appendix. The mucins may be 'endocervical' or intestinal. There are malignant features in the lining epithelium, but no evidence of stromal invasion. Stromal invasion is rather more difficult to assess in mucinous lesions owing to their usual multilocular nature. Dissection of mucin through the stroma—*pseudomyxoma ovarii*, which occurs in 25% of borderline mucinous tumours, is not thought to represent invasion and does not alter the diagnosis. Excluding those with pseudomyxoma peritonei the 10-year survival in patients with borderline mucinous tumours is 90% compared with 34% for mucinous carcinomas. When pseudomyxoma peritonei is present the 10-year survival is only 20%.

Mucinous carcinoma
This tumour constitutes 6–10% of malignant ovarian primary neoplasms. Patients have a median age of 35 years. Approximately 25% are bilateral. The appearances are similar to the borderline tumours in well-differentiated carcinomas, but invasion is present. A primary *signet-ring cell* variant has been reported, although this appearance is more commonly seen in ovarian metastases from the intestinal tract. The overall 10-year survival is 34%.

Endometrioid tumours

Benign endometrioid tumours

Endometrioid cystadenomas are indistinguishable from the cysts of ovarian endometriosis. *Endo-*metrioid *cystadenofibromas* and *endometrioid adenofibromas* occur, differing from the serous tumours only in their epithelial component which frequently shows focal squamous metaplasia.

Malignant endometrioid tumours

Borderline endometrioid tumours. These are less well documented than their serous and mucinous counterparts. Borderline endometrioid cystadenofibromas appear to occur more commonly than tumours without a fibrous component. There is a recognized association with concurrent, or later development of endometrial hyperplasia, or carcinoma.

Endometrioid carcinomas. These form approximately 20% of primary ovarian adenocarcinomas and are associated with endometriosis in the same ovary in 17%. Transition from endometriosis to *in situ* and invasive carcinoma can be infrequently observed. Approximately 30–50% of the tumours are bilateral. Squamous elements occur, when benign the lesion may be termed an *adenoacanthoma*, when malignant the lesion is *adenosquamous carcinoma*. A true squamous endometrioid carcinoma is extremely rare. Coexisting endometrial carcinoma of the corpus has been reported in one series as occurring in more than 50% of cases.

Clear cell tumours

Benign, borderline and malignant clear cell glycogen-rich tumours of the ovary are now regarded by many to be variants of endometrioid tumour due to the high associated presence of pelvic endometriosis, the fact that clear cell carcinoma has been observed arising from the epithelium of endometriosis and the undoubted occurrence of a clear cell variant of endometrial adenocarcinoma of the corpus. Indeed clear cell and typical endometrioid carcinomas have a similar prognosis—5-year survival 40%, 10-year survival 30%; carcinomas confined to the ovary have a 5-year survival of 80%.

Mixed Müllerian tumours

All variants of mixed Müllerian tumour can be seen in the ovary and are regarded as endometrioid (see p. 218). The malignant mixed Müllerian tumour of the ovary has a median survival of only 6–12 months.

Brenner—transitional cell tumours

These lesions comprise approximately 1.5% of all ovarian neoplasms and are bilateral in 6.5%. The majority are firm with a grey–white whorled cut surface rather than cystic, and consist of nests of epithelial cells within a stroma of tightly packed bundles of spindle cells. The 'transitional' epithelial cell nuclei typically have a grooved 'coffee-bean' appearance. Brenner tumours frequently form a nodule in the wall of a benign cystic neoplasm, most often a mucinous cystadenoma.

The newly revised World Health Organization Tumor Classification uses the term 'transitional cell tumours' with subdivisions into: (a) Benign Brenner, (b) Borderline Brenner, (c) Malignant Brenner, (d) Transitional cell carcinoma.

Sex-cord stromal tumours

Sex-cord stromal tumours form approximately 8% of all ovarian tumours with the inert fibromas comprising about half of the cases. Most are of ovarian cell types, but some are of testicular cells. Rarely cells of both gonads are present—*gynandroblastomas*: such usually benign lesions are small and unilateral and may be associated with bizarre endocrinological clinical effects.

Fibroma

Such hard lesions with a white, whorled cut surface occur at all ages, but fewer than 10% occur under 30 years of age. They are not associated with steroid hormone production, but do occur in association with *Meig's syndrome* and *Gorlin's syndrome* (see p. 416).

Meig's syndrome is present in approximately 1% of patients with an ovarian fibroma and comprises ascites and a pleural effusion which disappears following the removal of the fibroma. In 10–15% of cases of fibromas more than 10 cm diameter, ascites alone is present.

Gorlin's syndrome includes ovarian fibromas (see p. 416).

Thecoma

Oestrogen-secreting thecomas are rare before puberty, approximately 85% occur in postmenopausal women of whom 60% have postmenopausal bleeding and 20% an endometrial carcinoma. They are typically less than 10 cm, firm, with a yellow cut surface. There may be a variable amount of admixed fibroma and when this component predominates—*fibrothecoma*—the lesion may be only very pale yellow and have a whorled cut surface. Thecoma cells contain lipid, and where there is doubt whether a lesion is a pure fibroma or has a thecal component, a frozen section stained for lipid serves to demonstrate the oestrogen-producing cells. Ninety-seven per cent are unilateral and malignant examples are extremely rare.

Granulosa cell tumour—adult type

These tumours, which also produce oestrogen, occur more often in postmenopausal women. They form 1–2% of ovarian tumours and 95% of granulosa cell tumours; only 5% are bilateral. In contrast with thecomas, the usual finding in the endometrium is benign cystic hyperplasia, with endometrial carcinoma, usually well differentiated, in less than 5%; but nevertheless more frequently than would be expected by chance. Rarely they may be androgenic. They may be solid or partly cystic with areas of haemorrhage. The nuclei are small and often grooved with scanty cytoplasm. They may be arranged in nests, or cords, or in a diffuse pattern. Microfollicles, resembling the developing Graafian follicle—*Call–Exner bodies*—are commonly found.

Prognosis

Granulosa cell tumours of all patterns are potentially malignant, but in patients with tumours confined to the ovary there is a reported 10-year survival rate of up to 96%. Tumour size as well as stage has shown to be of prognostic significance. Ten-year survival is given as 73% if the tumour is less than 5 cm diameter, 63% between 5 and 15 cm and 34% if over 15 cm. Nuclear characteristics have not been shown to be reliable prognostic indicators. Recurrences are often not evident until more than 5 years after initial diagnosis and there are many instances of recurrent disease appearing 20, or 30 years later.

Granulosa cell tumour—juvenile type

Less than 5% of granulosa cell tumours are diagnosed before the normal age of puberty; most of these are of the juvenile type. They are only bilateral in 2% of cases and spread beyond the ovary is unusual, although the average size is 12.5 cm. The macroscopical appearance differs little from the adult type, but the nuclei are generally hyperchromatic and rounded and are rarely grooved; they frequently have abundant eosinophilic cytoplasm and show microcysts.

Prognosis

Stage is the most important prognostic indicator with only 2 of 80 cases which were confined to the ovary in one series having a malignant course. This is despite a marked degree of nuclear atypicality and a high mitotic rate being commonly present.

Androblastoma—Sertoli–Leydig cell tumour

These tumours form less than 0.5% of ovarian tumours and contain Sertoli cells, Leydig cells, or both in varying proportions. Virilization occurs in about one-third of cases. Pure Sertoli cell tumours may produce oestrogen and progesterone. Most tumours are small and confined to the ovary and, if well differentiated, have virtually 100% survival. The much less common lesions which are poorly differentiated behave badly, however, even if initially confined to the ovary.

Sex-cord stromal tumour with annular tubules—SCTAT

This tumour is characterized by the presence of simple and complex tubules with central hyaline bodies. The growth pattern has features of granulosa cell and Sertoli cell tumours. These tumours vary in their behaviour depending on whether the patient has the *Peutz–Jeghers syndrome* (see p. 44). In women with the syndrome, when the ovaries are examined, two-thirds have multifocal, bilateral tumourlets with annular tubules, all benign. In those without the syndrome, tumours are almost all unilateral and of significant size. Clinical evidence of oestrogen secretion is present in 40%, and 20% are malignant.

Steroid—lipid cell tumours

Ovarian neoplasia composed of typical steroid-hormone producing cells of lutein, Leydig or adrenal cortical type are all rare.

Germ cell tumours

In adults germ cell tumours form 20% of ovarian neoplasms, being second only to common epithelial lesions. Most of these germ cell tumours are benign, mature cystic teratomas. In children and adolescent girls 60% of ovarian tumours are of germ cell type. Germ cell tumours may be of the undifferentiated germ cells themselves—*dysgerminomas*, or of mixtures of cells which have differentiated, via *embryonal carcinoma*, towards fetal—*teratomata*—or extra-fetal tissues—*endodermal sinus tumour, choriocarcinoma*.

Dysgerminoma

This tumour, which is the ovarian equivalent of the seminoma of the testis (see p. 199) provides 1–2% of primary ovarian tumours and occurs in adolescents and young adults, and has been known as *carcinoma puellarum*. It is seen more frequently in India and Japan. It is bilateral in approximately 15% of cases, but affects the right ovary alone in about 50% of patients. Bilaterality is seen more frequently when the dysgerminoma is arising in a dysgenetic gonad (see p. 221).

Macroscopical

Pure dysgerminomata are solid and may be pink or yellow. Areas of haemorrhage or necrosis can be seen, but cystic areas should arouse suspicion of additional germ cell elements. As these may affect prognosis, any atypical looking areas must be carefully sampled.

Microscopical

Dysgerminomata are composed of large uniform cells with sharply defined cell boundaries. The nuclei are vesicular and usually contain a prominent eosinophilic nucleolus. The cytoplasm is rich in glycogen, which can be used to aid diagnosis. There is a variable amount of stroma which typically contains lymphocytes, or may resemble granulation tissue with giant cells. The stromal element may predominate, leading to misdiagnoses of inflammatory or lymphomatous conditions. Stromal giant cells must also be distinguished from syncytiotrophoblastic giant cells which occur in 6–8% of dysgerminomas and produce hCG, apparently without an effect on the prognosis.

Prognosis

With pure dysgerminomas prognosis is good, the 5-year survival with unilateral encapsulated tumours is more than 90%. Patients treated with unilateral salpingo-oophorectomy have 20–50% recurrence rates, but these can be treated successfully with radiotherapy as dysgerminomas are highly radiosensitive. Poor prognostic indicators are metastatic disease, local spread, bilaterality and a large tumour at initial diagnosis. More than 75% of recurrences are said to occur in the first year.

Embryonal carcinoma

This is considered to be the least differentiated form of germ cell tumour with differentiating potential. The tumour pattern, while not uncommon in the testis (see

p. 200), is very rare in the ovary, both as a component of a mixed germ cell tumour and particularly as a pure tumour. They are seen in children and young adults, are formed of solid aggregates of medium to large cells with eosinophilic granular cytoplasm and a large hyperchromatic nucleus which frequently contains multiple nucleoli. High mitotic activity, nuclear pleomorphism and tumour giant cells are the rule. Such tumours are highly malignant, although some progress is being made with combination chemotherapy regimes.

Endodermal sinus tumour—yolk-sac tumour

These tumours resemble the endodermal sinus, or yolk-sac tumours seen in the testis (see p. 200) and occasionally elsewhere (see p. 345). They are rare, and occur in children and young women; most patients are less than 30 years of age at diagnosis. They usually present as an abdominal mass, often of considerable size and raised levels of α *fetoprotein* (AFP) can be detected in the serum. The tumours are usually bilateral, mainly solid with cystic spaces.

Microscopical

Several histological patterns may be seen including a network of microcysts, which may contain PAS-positive hyaline globules, glomerulus-like perivascular formations—*Schiller–Duval bodies*—gland-like formations, myxomatous, papillary and hepatoid patterns. Some of the PAS-positive material has been demonstrated to be AFP on immunoperoxidase staining.

Prognosis

Until recently this was appalling. Endodermal sinus tumours are not radiosensitive and they were often beyond complete surgical excision at primary diagnosis. More success had been achieved with conservative surgery and adjuvant multi-agent combination chemotherapy. The progress of the disease and the therapy can be monitored using serial serum AFP estimations. Some 5-year disease-free intervals are now being reported.

Choriocarcinoma

Pure choriocarcinoma of germ cell origin is very rare; even as an element in a mixed germ cell tumour it is rare in the ovary. The presence of other germ cell elements enables the diagnosis to be made in women

of reproductive years in whom a gestational choriocarcinoma would be a differential diagnosis. The tumour produces hCG, which can be useful in monitoring the disease and the therapeutic response. Tumours tend to be unilateral, solid and haemorrhagic. They are composed of syncytio- and cytotrophoblast with considerable variation of the proportions of each within and throughout the tumour. Both types of trophoblast must be present to make the diagnosis. They are highly malignant but, unlike gestational choriocarcinoma, they do not respond to methotrexate. They are also not radiosensitive, but some success is being achieved with combination chemotherapy.

Teratomas

These may be:

1 Immature.
2 Mature:
  (a) solid;
  (b) cystic: (i) mature cystic teratoma—dermoid cyst; (ii) mature cystic teratoma—dermoid cyst with malignant transformations.
3 Monodermal and highly specialized:
  (a) struma ovarii;
  (b) carcinoid;
  (c) strumal carcinoid;
  (d) others.

Immature teratoma

These lesions are rare and tend to occur in the first two decades. Composed of ectoderm, mesoderm and endoderm, they are usually unilateral solid tumours having a variegated cut surface. They may be composed mainly of mature elements and so careful sampling is required. They are malignant and grow rapidly. Before the advent of combination chemotherapy there was a less than 20% 5-year survival. Recurrences tend to occur early and those alive after 18 months tend to survive long term.

Mature solid teratoma

A very rare unilateral benign neoplasm occurring mainly in children and young adults. Most solid teratomata are composed partly of immature tissues and are malignant. Extensive sampling of the tumours, to exclude immature areas, must therefore be carried out before making the diagnosis. Unilateral salpingo-oophorectomy results in a complete cure.

Mature cystic teratoma—dermoid cyst

This benign tumour is the most common of the ovarian teratomata, comprising more than 10% of ovarian neoplasms. There is a wide age range, but most occur in women of reproductive age. They are usually incidental findings on pelvic examination, or at Caesarian section, but more than 10% are bilateral. The most common element is ectoderm, forming a cyst lined by skin and skin appendages and containing sebaceous material and hair. There is a protuberance in the wall and bone, or teeth when present are usually adjacent to this structure which is formed of a variety of tissues and which should always be sampled. Neuroectodermal tissues are frequently found.

Complications

1 *Torsion*: this is common.

2 *Rupture*: uncommon but may further complicate torsion or infection. Shed glial tissue may implant and form tumours on peritoneum—*peritoneal gliomatosis*.

3 *Infection*: rare but dangerous.

4 *Haemolytic anaemia* of autoimmune type occurs occasionally and disappears following tumour excision.

5 *Malignant change*: this is seen in approximately 2% of cases with an age range of 20–90 years. Most are squamous cell carcinomas. The presence of many different malignant elements indicates an immature teratoma rather than a mature cystic teratoma with malignant transformation.

Monodermal and highly specialized teratomata

1 *Struma ovarii*: most or all of the tissue is of thyroid gland, usually normal but occasionally hyperplastic and thyrotoxic. Occasional thyroid carcinomas develop.

2 *Carcinoid tumour*: similar to the intestinal tumours and occasionally hormonally active producing the carcinoid syndrome (see p. 36).

3 *Strumal carcinoid*: a mixture of thyroid and carcinoid tumour, often with other teratomatous elements. Like hindgut carcinoids (see p. 46) it is not associated with the carcinoid syndrome.

4 *Others*: malignant melanoma, some mucinous tumours, sebaceous gland tumours and epidermoid cysts without appendages are amongst other lesions in this category.

Gonadoblastoma

A very rare tumour composed of germ cells mixed with epithelial cells of granulosa cell or Sertoli cell type and, usually, stromal elements of luteal or Leydig cell appearance. They are small or microscopic and calcification is almost always present. The course is benign unless true dysgerminoma develops.

Associated features

Gonadoblastoma nearly always develops in a previously abnormal gonad. Most of the patients have a Y chromosome, many are mosaics. They have either pure gonadal dysgenesis with bilateral streak gonads (see p. 221) or mixed gonadal dysgenesis with one streak gonad and a contralateral dysgenetic testis. A few have occurred in male pseudo-hermaphrodites but very rarely in patients with somatic features of Turner's syndrome.

Soft tissue tumours not specific for ovary

These include haemangioma, lymphangioma, neurofibroma, leiomyoma, oesteoma and their malignant counterparts. Adenomatoid tumours are also sometimes ovarian in position (see p. 201).

Secondary tumours

Secondary deposits of carcinoma in the ovary are common, particularly from breast and gastrointestinal tract. A particular type is the *Krukenberg tumour* of characteristic histological appearance with signet-ring, mucus-secreting, adenocarcinoma cells in a cellular fibrous stroma. These arise from primary tumours in large intestine and stomach.

The ovaries may also be involved by malignant lymphoma either as part of disseminated disease, occasionally as an apparent primary site of origin and, in Burkitt's lymphoma, as a common presenting and clinically prominent feature (see p. 272).

Chapter 13
Diseases of the Liver and Biliary Tract—Liver

A/NORMAL, VASCULAR

Normal
Vascular
   Hepatic arteries
   Portal venous system
   Hepatic veins
   Systemic disturbances

Normal liver
A complete discussion of normal liver anatomy and physiology is beyond the scope of this book. However, many disease processes affecting the liver have a zonal distribution, which can be explained on the basis of functional differences occurring within the anatomical units of the liver.

Two anatomical units have been proposed—the hepatic *lobule* and *acinus*. The acinar concept is now preferred but the terminology used to describe different zones within these units is, to some extent, interchangeable.

Liver lobule
The lobule was, for a long time, considered to be the basic functional unit of the liver. In its classical form (Fig. 22) this is roughly hexagonal in shape with blood from portal tracts at the periphery draining into terminal hepatic venules at the centre. Three main zones are recognized:
1 *Centrilobular/perivenular*—around hepatic venules.
2 *Periportal*—around portal tracts.
3 *Mid-zonal*—between the other two.

Liver acinus
On the basis of detailed microcirculatory studies, the liver acinus is now considered to be the functional unit of the liver.

The *simple acinus* is defined as the area of paren-

chyma supplied by a single terminal hepatic arteriole with its accompanying portal venule and bile duct. (Fig. 22). It can be divided into three main zones which are increasingly distant from the axial blood supply. Zones 1, 2 and 3 correspond approximately to the periportal, mid-zonal and perivenular regions of the classical lobule.

Each portal branch gives rise to an average of three simple acini and together these form a *complex acinus* (Fig. 22). There is an overlap between adjacent simple acini, in particular between zone 3 hepatocytes.

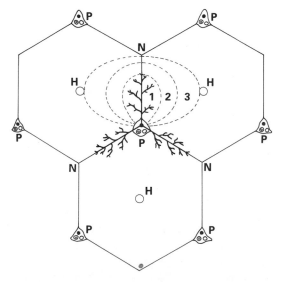

Fig. 22 Diagram illustrating the structure of hepatic acini and lobules. The portal triad in the centre gives rise to three simple acini, the afferent blood supply radiating outwards towards 'nodal' points of Mall. Each acinus is subdivided into zones 1, 2 and 3 which are increasingly distant from the afferent blood supply. The hexagonal shape of the classical liver lobule can be appreciated.
(P = portal tract, H = hepatic venule, N = 'nodal' point of Mall)

Some examples of diseases with a zonal distribution

Ischaemic lesions tend to be located towards the microcirculatory periphery, i.e. perivenular areas or acinar zones 3. Many of the enzymes responsible for producing toxic drug metabolites are also located in these areas—thus accounting for the characteristic zonal necrosis seen with some drugs, e.g. paracetamol. The acinar concept is more useful than the lobular one for explaining the lesions of bridging necrosis which occur in acute and chronic hepatitis. These represent areas of confluent hepatocyte necrosis involving acinar zones 3 forming curved bridges between portal tracts and hepatic venules (see p. 233).

Vascular disorders

The liver has a dual blood supply, approximately 75% by the portal vein, 25% by the hepatic artery.

Effects of vascular occlusion are, therefore, unpredictable.

Diseases of hepatic arteries

Congenital

Aberrant arteries

'Abnormal' branches are present in up to 45% of people but are insignificant apart from problems with surgery, e.g. accidental ligation, anastomotic problems during liver transplantation.

Acquired

1 *Polyarteritis nodosa*: hepatic arteries are involved in 60–70% of cases (see p. 102) and thrombotic occlusion may lead to infarcts. Aneurysm formation produces diagnostic lesions on angiography.
2 *Arteriolar sclerosis*: occurs in systemic hypertension, with predisposition to thrombosis.

Occlusion of hepatic arteries

Causes

1 Thrombosis: secondary to intrinsic disease of hepatic arteries (see above).
2 Embolism: infective endocarditis.
3 Accidental ligation.

Effects

Unpredictable, due to dual blood supply.

Hepatic infarction

Causes

Hepatic artery occlusion as above together with circulatory failure, e.g. eclampsia, septicaemia.

Appearances

Peripheral irregular, yellow areas of variable size. Microscopically there is coagulative necrosis of liver parenchyma and a variable infiltration by polymorphonuclear leucocytes. Portal tracts are relatively resistant to ischaemia but are also involved in more severe cases.

Diseases of the portal venous system

Congenital/neonatal

1 *Aplasia*.
2 *Neonatal obliteration*: along with the umbilical vein and ductus venosus.
3 *Cavernomatous transformation*.

Portal vein obstruction—Thrombosis

Causes

1 *Inflammatory—pyelophlebitis*: umbilical sepsis in neonates and intra-abdominal sepsis (e.g. appendicitis, cholecystitis, pancreatitis).
2 *Neoplastic*: hepatocellular carcinoma (see p. 254), spread from other intra-abdominal tumours and myeloproliferative disorders.
3 *Cirrhosis*.
4 *Splenic vein thrombosis*: by propagation.

Non-thrombotic

1 External compression (e.g. by enlarged nodes or tumour masses).
2 Cirrhosis.

Venous 'infarction' of liver—Zahn's infarct

Cause

Occlusion of medium-sized intrahepatic portal vein branches.

Appearances

Peripheral, well circumscribed, haemorrhagic areas which are not true infarcts but show intense sinusoidal congestion with atrophy of intervening liver cell plates.

Portal hypertension

Causes

1 *Diseases of hepatic veins*:
   (a) *Congestive cardiac failure*: causing venous outflow obstruction.
   (b) *Budd–Chiari syndrome* (see below).
   (c) *Veno-occlusive disease* (see p. 231).
2 *Diseases of liver parenchyma*:
   (a) *Cirrhosis*.
   (b) *Non-cirrhotic portal hypertenson*: (i) Infective—schistosomiasis; (ii) drugs—alcohol, hypervitaminosis A, vinyl chloride, arsenic; (iii) congenital—congenital hepatic fibrosis and infantile polycystic disease; (iv) nodular regenerative hyperplasia (NRH)—diffuse nodularity of liver without fibrosis; (v) 'idiopathic' portal hypertension—cause unknown but common in India, where it is responsible for up to one-third of cases.
NB: Most of the non-cirrhotic causes of portal hypertension are associated with fibrotic damage to the liver, not amounting to a true cirrhosis. Fibrosis has a variable pattern: portal in congenital hepatic fibrosis, vinyl chloride, arsenic, schistosomiasis, possibly compressing portal venules; perisinusoidal in hypervitaminosis A resulting in reduced sinusoidal blood flow; perivenular in some cases of alcoholic liver disease preventing drainage of blood into hepatic venules

In cases with no significant fibrosis (NRH, idiopathic) obliterative lesions have been described in portal veins. These are often subtle and require special techniques, including morphometry, for detection.
3 *Portal venous obstruction*:
   (a) *Non-thrombotic* (see p. 229).
   (b) *Thrombosis* (see p. 229).

Effects

1 *Portal–systemic anastomoses*:
   (a) Lower oesophagus—oesophageal varices.
   (b) Lower rectum—haemorrhoids.
   (c) Periumbilical—'caput medusae'.
   (d) Retroperitoneum.
2 *Ascites*.
3 *Splenomegaly*. Principally due to passive congestion, but progressive fibrosis occurs with time. Focal haemorrhages heal by scarring to produce siderotic nodules—*Gamna–Gandy bodies*. Hypersplenism occurs in some cases.

Diseases of hepatic veins
The Budd–Chiari syndrome and veno-occlusive disease are both associated with obstruction to hepatic venous outflow.

Budd–Chiari syndrome

Site of lesion
Usually in large hepatic veins, less commonly the intrahepatic vena cava.

Causes
1 *Myeloproliferative diseases*, e.g. polycythaemia rubra vera.
2 *Intra-abdominal neoplasia*, especially hepatocellular carcinoma.
3 *Membranous webs*, congenital or acquired.
4 *Oral contraceptive pill*.
5 *Idiopathic*.
6 *Traumatic*.

Appearances

Hepatic vein lesions
1 *Acute phase*: occlusion of hepatic veins is usually by thrombus, less commonly by tumour or membranous webs. Although the primary lesions are found in large hepatic veins, propagation of thrombi may occur into smaller vessels.
2 *Chronic stages*: in chronic cases thrombi may organize to produce fibrous cords or membranous defects. Some membranous 'webs' may therefore represent organized thrombi rather than congenital lesions as previously suspected. Small vessels often show fibrous obliteration, probably as a consequence of ischaemia. Distinction from veno-occlusive disease may be difficult in such cases.

Liver parenchymal changes
1 *Acute phase*: intense congestion involving acinar zones 2 and 3 with atrophy and/or necrosis of liver cells in affected areas.
2 *Chronic stages*: fibrous scarring in areas of hepatocyte necrosis. True cirrhosis supervenes in a minority of cases.

Veno-occlusive disease

Site of lesion
Small hepatic venules.

Causes
1 *Irradiation of liver*.
2 *Drugs*: particularly chemotherapeutic agents, e.g. cytosine arabinoside, 6-thioguanine and immunosuppressive drugs, e.g. azathioprine.
3 *Bone marrow transplantation*: probably due to a combination of irradiation and chemotherapy prior to transplantation.
4 *Secondary to other liver disease*: alcoholic liver disease and cirrhosis from many causes.

Pathogenesis
In 1–3, veno-occlusive disease is thought to be a toxic injury initially affecting perivenular hepatocytes and/or sinusoidal lining cells with secondary changes probably causing obliteration of hepatic venules.

In 4, veno-occlusive lesions are possibly related to disturbances in blood flow and in most cases have little clinical significance.

Appearances
1 *Hepatic vein lesions*: deposition of loose fibrous tissue in the intima of hepatic venules.
2 *Liver parenchyma*: as for Budd–Chiari syndrome. A similar pattern of damage is also observed in cases of severe right-sided heart failure, e.g. constrictive pericarditis (see below). Distinction between the various causes of hepatic venous outflow obstruction is often not possible on liver biopsy specimens.

Systemic circulatory disturbances

Shock
From any cause.

Effects
Severe hypoperfusion results in *zonal necrosis*, which predominantly affects acinar zone 3, though zones 2 or 1 may be involved in *severe* cases.

Ischaemic necrosis characteristically has a coagulative pattern and is associated with variable infiltration by neutrophil polymorphs—'*ischaemic hepatitis*'.

Venous congestion

Cause
Right-sided heart failure.

Effects
1 *Acute congestion—'nutmeg' liver*: there is engorgement of hepatic venules and surrounding sinusoids with compression of intervening liver cell plates. Variable fatty change, probably due to hypoxia, is seen in periportal and midzonal hepatocytes. Necrosis of hepatocytes is uncommon except in severe cases, e.g. constrictive pericarditis (see p. 61).
2 *Chronic congestion—cardiac fibrosis or 'cirrhosis'*: fibrosis and hepatocyte loss involve the peripheral acinar zones with nodular regeneration of surviving hepatocytes in acinar zones 1–2.

Fibrous septa may link to produce a picture of '*reversed lobulation*', but lobular relationships are usually still retained and true cirrhosis is uncommon.

B/INFECTIONS

Viral
Bacterial
Parasitic
Helminthic

Viral infections of the liver
Many viruses may infect the liver as part of a systemic illness but the term 'viral hepatitis' is reserved for viral infections which specifically involve the liver.

Viral hepatitis
Three main types of viral hepatitis are recognized: hepatitis A, hepatitis B, hepatitis non-A–non-B.

Hepatitis A

Epidemiology
Worldwide distribution with faecal—oral transmission. Can be sporadic or epidemic. e.g. sewage contamination of food or water.

Causative agent
RNA virus 27 nm diameter.

Incubation period
Short: 15–40 days.

Hepatitis B

Epidemiology
Mainly parenteral transmission. Screening of blood donors has greatly reduced the incidence of post-transfusion hepatitis B infection but blood spread is still an important route for intravenous drug addicts, dialysis patients and hospital workers exposed to needle-stick accidents.

Sometimes other close personal contact may be responsible as viral particles have been found in various body fluids including saliva, semen and vaginal fluid.

Causative agent
DNA virus 42 nm diameter. This is the complete infective virion—*Dane particle*. Dane particles have the following antigens:
1 *Hepatitis B core antigen*—HBcAg
   (a) Contains hepatitis B virus DNA (HBV–DNA) and HBV–DNA polymerase
   (b) Forms the central core of the Dane particle within a 27 nm nucleocapsid.
   (c) Synthesis of HBV–DNA occurs mainly in the *nucleus* of infected hepatocytes.
2 *Hepatitis B surface antigen*—HBsAg.
   (a) The outer lipoprotein envelope of Dane particle.
   (b) Antigenically heterogeneous and several subtypes are recognized.
   (c) Synthesized within endoplasmic reticulum in *cytoplasm* of infected hepatocytes.
3 *Hepatitis B 'e' antigen*—HBeAg.
   (a) Closely related to HBcAg
   (b) Involved in replication of HBV–DNA and its presence correlates with infectivity.

Incubation period
Long: 50–180 days.

Hepatitis non-A–non-B

This term has been used to describe cases of hepatitis in which a viral aetiology is suspected, but in which specific markers of viral infection are absent.

Epidemiology
At least three viruses are thought to be involved:
1 Post-transfusional—non-A–non-B hepatitis responsible for up to 90% of cases.
2 Faecal–oral.

3 Sporadic—no obvious route of transmission identified.

Causative agents
Until recently the causative agents of non-A–non-B hepatitis were unknown and the diagnosis was one of exclusion. Serological and ultrastructural studies now suggest two new agents:

Hepatitis C. A serum marker for post-transfusional non-A–non-B hepatitis has been developed and this is now known as hepatitis C.

The causative agent has not been fully elucidated but studies in chimpanzees suggest a viral particle, less than 80 nm, with the properties of an RNA togavirus.

Hepatitis E. The virus responsible for enterically transmitted non-A–non-B virus has been identified as a small RNA virus (32–34 nm) with calcivirus-like properties. This virus is now called hepatitis E.

Incubation period
Variable, 10–100 days.

Hepatitis delta—hepatitis D

Epidemiology
Always occurs in association with hepatitis B infection. Coinfection is relatively uncommon in the UK, but occurs in up to 50% of HBsAg carriers in parts of Africa, southern Italy and the Middle East.

Causative agent
A small, defective RNA virus. Can replicate only when encapsulated by hepatitis B surface antigen.

Consequences of hepatitis D infection
It modulates the effects of hepatitis B infection with two main consequences:
1 Increased risk of fulminant hepatitis in the acute phase—3–5% versus 1% in 'pure' HBV infection.
2 Higher risk of progression to chronicity—10–40% versus 5–10% in 'pure' HBV infection.

Consequences of infection with the hepatitis viruses
(See also Table 13.1 on p. 234)

Asymptomatic carriage
Viral infection in people with no symptoms and normal biochemistry.

Hepatitis A: No.
Hepatitis B: Yes—< 1% in UK, but up to 10–20% in high-incidence areas.
Hepatitis C: Yes—prevalence not properly assessed yet, but probably < 1% in UK.

Classical acute hepatitis—acute hepatitis with spotty necrosis
This is the typical presentation of the hepatitis viruses.

Appearances
In the fully developed stage inflammatory changes are present in portal tracts and the liver parenchyma. These changes probably take several weeks to evolve.

Portal tracts:
1 Diffuse infiltration by inflammatory cells, mainly mononuclear.
2 Spillover into periportal zones which may be confused with piecemeal necrosis of chronic hepatitis (see p. 238).
3 Varying degrees of bile ductular proliferation which can mimic biliary obstruction when severe.

Parenchyma:
1 *Spotty inflammation*—with mainly mononuclear cells—lymphocytes, plasma cells, histiocytes.
2 *Hepatocellular degeneration, necrosis and regeneration*—hepatocyte degeneration is seen in the form of ballooning, leading to lytic necrosis and *acidophil bodies*—eosinophilic cells with pyknotic or absent nuclei, produced by apoptosis. Regenerative changes include mitotic activity, nuclear pleomorphism with bi- or multinucleate cells and widening of cell plates.
   These lesions are diffusely distributed throughout hepatic acini but are usually most prominent in perivenular regions—acinar zone 3.
3 *Lobular disarray*—Loss of the normal regular arrangement of liver cell plates occurs as a result of the above changes.
4 *Cholestasis*—a mild degree is very common in all types of viral hepatitis. In a small proportion of cases cholestasis is severe and becomes the predominant histological and biochemical feature—*cholestatic viral hepatitis*. Distinction from other causes of cholestasis may then be difficult.
   As the disease progresses, hepatocellular damage and inflammatory changes subside. Enlarged Kupffer cells laden with ceroid and/or iron pigments may persist, providing evidence of recent liver cell damage. Minor abnormalities of the reticulin framework may also persist after other changes have subsided.
   Although some differences are described, it is not possible to make a reliable distinction between the various causes of viral hepatitis on histological appearances.

Acute hepatitis with bridging necrosis
Differs from classical acute hepatitis in having more extensive necrosis involving confluent groups of hepatocytes—*confluent necrosis*.
   Confluent necrosis mainly affects acinar zones 3 causing reticulin collapse and bridges linking hepatic venules to portal tracts—*bridging necrosis*.
   Bridging necrosis is an indicator of severity and is associated with a higher risk of mortality.

Acute hepatitis with panacinar necrosis
This represents the most severe form of hepatocyte necrosis in which there is confluent necrosis extending throughout entire acini—*panacinar necrosis*. Extensive proliferation of bile ductular structures is seen around surviving portal tracts.
   In very severe cases almost all of the liver parenchyma is destroyed, resulting in a small, shrunken organ with a wrinkled capsular surface—*massive hepatic necrosis*.
   Clinically, massive hepatic necrosis is associated with very severe hepatitis—*fulminant hepatitis*, and a high risk of mortality.
   Surviving cases have irregular nodules of regenerating liver cells separated by broad zones of fibrous scarring—*postnecrotic scarring/cirrhosis*.

Chronic hepatitis
Chronic infection, with inflammation persisting for more than 6 months, is seen in association with hepatitis B and non-A–non-B.
   The histological features of chronic hepatitis are described in detail later on p. 237.

Cirrhosis
A small proportion of patients with chronic viral hepatitis progress to develop cirrhosis (see p. 241).

Hepatocellular carcinoma—HCC
Hepatitis B is increasingly implicated as a major cause of hepatocellular carcinoma (see p. 254).
   Many patients with HCC have antibodies to

hepatitis C but the significance of this observation is uncertain.

Other viral infections involving the liver

Hepatitis may complicate infections with several other viruses. Examples include:

Epstein–Barr virus—infectious mononucleosis

The hepatitis is usually mild. Massive hepatic necrosis may occur as rare complication.

Appearances

Atypical lymphocytes are seen infiltrating portal tracts and sinusoids (can be mistaken for leukaemia).

Cytomegalovirus—CMV

A cause of neonatal hepatitis due to infection *in utero*. May also cause a mild acute hepatitis in older children and adults. CMV is an important opportunistic infection in immunocompromised patients.

Appearances

Characteristic 'amphophilic' inclusions are seen in nuclei of infected cells with a surrounding halo—'owl's-eye' appearance.

Herpes simplex

Occurs as a neonatal hepatitis or as an opportunistic infection in adults. Rare in immunocompetent people.

Appearances

Small yellow foci of coagulative necrosis surrounded by zones of congestion.

Rubella

Can cause a neonatal hepatitis which is usually mild.

Yellow fever

This group B arborvirus infection causes viral haemorrhagic fever.

Appearances

Hepatocyte necrosis, mainly involving mid-zonal regions.

Bacterial infections of the liver

Pyogenic bacteria

Infection with pyogenic bacteria is associated with formation of hepatic abscesses which are frequently multiple.

Origins

1 *Bile duct—Ascending cholangitis*: associated with biliary obstruction and showing multiple abscesses centred on portal tracts.
2 *Portal vein—portal pyelophlebitis*: from infection in organs drained by portal venous system, e.g. colon, appendix, pancreas.
3 *Hepatic artery*: involvement of the liver in septicaemia.
4 *Direct spread*: from subphrenic abscess, retroperitoneal abscess, gallbladder in acute cholecystitis.
5 *Unknown—cryptogenic*: in up to one-third of cases no primary focus of infection is found.

Table 13.1 Summary of the main patterns of damage seen with the hepatitis viruses.

	Hepatitis A	Hepatitis B	Hepatitis C
1 *Asymptomatic carrier* Incidence	No —	Yes < 1% in UK; 10–20% in high-incidence areas	Yes Not known; probably < 1% in UK
2 *Acute hepatitis*	Generally mild; mortality 0.1%	More severe; mortality 1%	Intermediate; mortality unknown
3 *Chronic hepatitis* Incidence	No —	Yes 5–10% (10–40% with superadded HDV infection)	Yes 40–60%
4 *Cirrhosis*	No	Yes	Yes
5 *Hepatocellular carcinoma*	No	Yes	?

Organisms

These vary according to the portals of entry but include:

1 In ascending cholangitis—*Escherichia coli*.

2 In portal pyelophlebitis—*E. coli, Klebsiella, Pseudomonas, Enterobacter, Bacteroides* (plus other anaerobes).

3 Particularly in cryptogenic cases—*Streptococcus milleri*.

4 In 'toxic shock' syndrome—*Staphylococcus aureus*.

Other bacteria, spirochaetes

Actinomycosis—*Actinomyces israelii*

The liver is affected by direct or blood spread from abdominal actinomyces. Multiple abscesses containing 'sulphur granule' colonies are seen.

Leptospirosis—Weil's disease—*Leptospira interrogans* complex

Pathogenesis

The spirochaetes are excreted in urine of infected animals; chiefly rats but also dogs and pigs. They can penetrate skin, conjunctiva and mucous membranes of humans.

Clinical

There is fever, meningitis, mucosal haemorrhages, jaundice, renal failure and splenomegaly. Mortality is 15–20%.

Appearances

The liver shows focal hepatocyte degeneration and necrosis with prominent mitoses and a mild infiltration by mononuclear cells together with cholestasis. Haemorrhagic foci are common.

The histological abnormalities may be mild and belie the clinical severity. The kidney is affected by an interstitial nephritis with tubular necrosis and glomerular and interstitial haemorrhages (see p. 166).

Typhoid fever—*Salmonella typhi*

Hepatomegaly due to a mild hepatitis is common in the second–third week (see p. 32). Jaundice is infrequent. The liver shows microvesicular fatty change with small foci of necrosis and mononuclear cell infiltration.

Syphilis—*Treponema pallidum*

Congenital

There is a diffuse fine pericellular fibrosis and mononuclear cell infiltration. Abundant organisms are present.

Acquired

In secondary syphilis there is a diffuse hepatitis with focal necrosis and formation of small granulomas.

Organisms are identified in less than 50% of cases.

In tertiary disease gummata form with central necrosis and progressive surrounding fibrosis which causes deep scars—*hepar lobatum*.

Organisms are rarely demonstrable.

Tuberculosis—*Mycobacterium tuberculosis*

Blood-borne spread causes irregularly distributed caseating granulomas but there is little effect on liver function. Occasionally tuberculomas may develop. Very rarely there is infection of bile ducts—*tuberculous cholangitis*. Organisms can be identified in tissue sections in less than 20% of cases.

Q fever—*Coxiella burnetti*

This produces hepatic granulomas of characteristic fibrin-ring appearance—central fat vacuoles surrounded by rings of fibrinous material. Clinical effects of hepatic involvement are usually mild in this predominantly respiratory disease (see p. 372)

Parasitic infestations

Protozoa

Malaria—*Plasmodium vivax, ovale, malariae* and *falciparum*

The liver is important in the exo-erythrocytic phase of acute malaria in man (see p. 5). There is hepatomegaly with congested sinusoids containing parasitized erythrocytes.

In chronic malaria, malaria pigment—haemozoin—formed by the breakdown of haemoglobin from ingested red cells, is deposited in Kupffer cells and, less markedly, in hepatocytes.

In the abnormal immune response to parasites of the 'tropical splenomegaly syndrome' there is marked sinusoidal infiltration by mature lymphocytes—hepatic sinusoidal lymphocytosis.

Dormant forms of parasites—*hypnozoites*, may

persist in the cytoplasm of hepatocytes for several months or years and are responsible for relapses in *P. vivax* and *P. ovale* infections.

Visceral leishmaniasis—kala azar—*Leishmania donovani*

This diffuse disease of the lymphoreticular system is described on p. 279. Hepatomegaly may be marked with distension of sinusoids by parasite-containing Kupffer cells. More rarely there is an inflammatory reaction with granuloma formation and hepatocyte necrosis. There may be some fibrosis but not cirrhosis.

Amoebiasis—*Entamoeba histolytica*

The liver is involved by spread via the portal vein from the large intestine (*see* p. 41). Presentation is usually in the form of solitary or occasionally multiple 'abscesses'. These measure up to 10 cm in diameter and are caused by cytolytic enzyme action on liver tissue by the organisms. They usually occur in the right lobe and contain reddish-brown necrotic material—'*anchovy sauce*'. There is a surrounding mononuclear cellular infiltrate and granulation tissue in which organisms can be identified as trophozoites. 'Abscesses' may rupture into the peritoneum or through the diaphragm to the pleural cavity and lung. Blood spread via the systemic circulation may cause 'abscess' formation in the brain and other organs.

Helminthic

Hydatid disease—*Echinococcus granulosus*

Life cycle

1 The adult worm, 5–9 mm long, lives in the intestine of the dog—definitive host.
2 Ova are ingested by sheep, cows or pigs eating grass contaminated with dog faeces—intermediate host. Humans are occasionally infected as an intermediate host.
3 Embryos develop in the intestine of the intermediate host and migrate by portal veins to reach liver and, in some cases, lungs and by systemic veins to reach other sites.
4 Formation of hydatid cysts containing larval forms. These have characteristic heads—*scolices*, containing several suckers and two rows of hooklets.
5 Ingestion of infected offal from sheep, cows or pigs by dogs completes the cycle.

Sites

Liver 70%, lungs 10–20%, systemic—brain, bone, kidney, 10–20%.

Appearances

At all sites progressively enlarging cystic masses develop—*hydatid cysts*. These have an outermost host fibrous capsule, inside which there is a cyst wall composed of laminated chitinous material and an innermost layer formed by a germinal membrane from which scolices develop.

Smaller '*daughter cysts*' develop from the main cyst which may enlarge gradually to a size in excess of 20 cm.

Effects

1 *Hepatomegaly*: due to space occupying lesion.
2 *Secondary infection*: results in death of the parasite, but an abscess cavity may persist.
3 *Rupture*: into peritoneum, biliary tree—causing cholangitis or pancreatitis, or pleural cavity.

Cyst fluid is highly allergenic and spillage results in a type 1 anaphylactic hypersensitivity reaction.

Schistosomiasis

Schistosoma mansoni, S. Japonicum, S. mekongi, S. intercalatum. S. haematobium does not affect the liver.

Infections with these worms are described more fully on p. 9.

Life cycle

Ova are laid by adult worms in the intestine and pass via portal venous system to enter the liver (see p. 9).

Appearances

Inflammation

Ova deposited in portal venules produce an initial eosinophilic reaction followed by formation of epithelioid granulomas.

Fibrosis

Granulomas heal with progressive fibrous enlargement of portal tracts. In some cases broad fibrous septa are formed which have been likened to a clay pipe stem—'*pipestem fibrosis*'.

In spite of considerable fibrosis, the underlying architecture remains intact and the picture is not that of a true cirrhosis.

Effects

Portal hypertension is the main feature due to portal fibrosis and obstruction of portal venules (see p. 230). Hepatocellular function remains good.

Opisthorciasis—clonorchiasis—liver fluke

Organisms

Opisthorcis (clonorchis) sinensis—Far East; *Opisthorcis felineus*—Poland, Ukraine, Siberia; *Opisthorcis viverrini*—Thailand.

O. sinensis is the most important of these three species of liver fluke, being present in up to 15% of residents in focal endemic zones.

Life cycle

1 Adult fluke, 1–2 cm long, inhabits major intrahepatic bile ducts in humans (also dogs, cats).
2 Ova are released in faeces and ingested by snails.
3 Cercariae released from snails form metacercariae beneath the scales of freshwater fish.
4 Humans are reinfected by eating raw or undercooked fish. The cysts hatch in the duodenum and flukes migrate up the bile duct.

Appearances

There is inflammation, including eosinophils, in the walls of bile ducts causing hyperplasia and infolding of biliary epithelium—adenomatous hyperplasia. Malignant transformation to *cholangiocarcinoma* frequently supervenes.

Effects

Secondary infection with ascending cholangitis. Portal hypertension. Cholangiocarcinoma.

Fascioliasis—*Fasciola hepatica*

Life cycle

1 Adult flukes (4 cm) live in the biliary tree of sheep and cattle. Humans are only occasionally infected.
2 Ova are ingested by snails, which excrete metacercariae.
3 The definitive host is reinfected by eating watercress contaminated with metacercariae. Metacerariae exist in the duodenum, larvae penetrate the gut wall, migrate into peritoneum and burrow into the liver—migrating phase. Eventually they reach bile ducts, developing into the adult forms which release ova into bile.

Appearances

Subcapsular tracts of necrosis and later fibrosis are seen at points(s) of entry. Bile duct obstruction and ascending cholangitis follow.

Ascariasis—*Ascaris lumbricoides*

This roundworm infestation of the intestine is described on p. 7. The liver is involved during two phases of the life cycle.
1 *Larval migration phase*: larvae penetrate the intestinal wall to reach lungs via the portal venous system. During this process they may cause focal parenchymal necrosis, granuloma formation and an eosinophilic infiltrate.
2 *Adult worm phase*: worms in the intestine can migrate up the common bile duct producing biliary obstruction and ascending cholangitis.

C/CHRONIC HEPATITIS, ALCOHOLIC DISEASE

Chronic hepatitis
  Aetiology
  Classification
Alcoholic liver disease
  Risk factors
  Fatty liver
  Alcoholic hepatitis
  Alcoholic cirrhosis

Chronic hepatitis

Chronic hepatitis can be defined as a condition in which inflammation of the liver continues without improvement for at least 6 months. This definition is too broad to be useful clinically, and the term is restricted to a group of conditions which are more precisely defined on the basis of aetiology and pathological features.

Aetiology

Autoimmune ('lupoid') chronic hepatitis—AI-CH

An autoimmune aetiology is suspected in many cases of chronic hepatitis. These typically occur in young women with a peak age at presentation of 10–20 years and female : male ratio of 3 : 1. Evidence for an autoimmune aetiology is based on the following.

Autoantibodies in the serum
Antinuclear antibodies are present in 80% of cases:

anti-smooth muscle antibodies in 70%; LE cells are found in 20%—hence the term 'lupoid' hepatitis. Liver–kidney–microsomal (LKM) antibodies, identify a subgroup of AI-CH, mainly occurring in children, and usually negative for the other autoantibodies. Antibodies to a soluble liver antigen (SLA) are sometimes also present.

Association with other autoimmune conditions
Chronic inflammatory bowel disease, Hashimoto's thyroiditis and Coombs'-positive haemolytic anaemia are all associated with AI-CH. In spite of the frequent presence of autoantibodies classically found in systemic lupus erythematosus (SLE) other manifestations of SLE are lacking and autoimmune chronic hepatitis is *not* thought to be part of the disease spectrum of SLE (see p. 96).

Response to immunosuppressive treatment
By steroids, azathioprine, etc.

Hepatitis viruses (see p. 231)
The incidence of hepatitis B surface antigen positivity in chronic hepatitis varies from 10% to 67%, but antigenaemia is low in the UK.

Non-A–non-B hepatitis is increasingly recognized as an important cause of chronic hepatitis following blood transfusion.

Response to immunosuppression in these cases is generally poor.

Drugs
Including α-methyl dopa, isoniazid and nitrofurantoin.

Other liver diseases
An element of chronic active hepatitis may be present in many other chronic liver diseases, including primary biliary cirrhosis, sclerosing cholangitis, alcoholic liver disease, Wilson's disease, and α_1-antitrypsin deficiency.

In most cases there are other features to indicate the underlying aetiology of liver damage in these conditions. In a minority, histological distinction from other causes of chronic hepatitis may prove to be impossible.

Pathological classification
The classification of chronic hepatitis is based mainly on morphological appearances; three main variants are recognized, although the distinction between these is somewhat blurred.

Chronic persistent hepatitis—CPH

Appearances
A mononuclear inflammatory cell infiltrate of lymphocytes, plasma cells and histiocytes is present in portal tracts, but the limiting plate between portal tracts and liver parenchyma is intact with no piecemeal necrosis.

Normal architecture is retained and lobular inflammation is absent or very mild.

Clinical course
This is usually a mild disease with a benign self-limited course, remaining static or resolving gradually over a period of months to years.

In a minority of cases—up to 10%, there is progression to chronic active hepatitis and cirrhosis.

Chronic lobular hepatitis—CLH

Appearances
Predominantly lobular inflammation similar to that seen in acute hepatitis (see p. 233). Portal inflammation is inconspicuous.

Clinical course
Generally regarded as a benign condition with favourable prognosis. *But* chronic non-A–non-B hepatitis frequently has a CLH-like picture and behaviour is unpredictable with progression to cirrhosis in up to 20% of these cases.

Chronic active hepatitis—CAH

Appearances
There is a portal mononuclear cell infiltrate as in CPH but with inflammatory spillover into periportal zones with necrosis of periportal hepatocytes—*piecemeal necrosis*.

In more severe cases inflammation and necrosis link portal tracts to hepatic venules—*bridging necrosis*.

Piecemeal necrosis and bridging necrosis are the features defining activity in CAH and the severity of these lesions is important in determining prognosis.

Fibrosis occurs in the wake of the necro-inflammatory lesions described above, and may progress eventually to cirrhosis.

There is variable lobular inflammation.

Clinical course

Clinical findings are highly variable. Some cases present as an acute hepatitis, others insidiously with vague non-specific symptoms. Biochemical abnormalities are almost invariably present.

Clinical course is unpredictable and prognosis depends on several factors, including underlying aetiology, histological severity and treatment given (see Table 13.2).

Overall there is a mortality rate of approximately 50% over 5 years.

Histological appearances in different forms of chronic hepatitis

With the exception of hepatitis B, it is not possible to be certain of the aetiology of chronic hepatitis on the basis of histological appearances. Components of the hepatitis B virus—surface antigen, core antigen and delta virus—can all be demonstrated in tissue sections by specific immunohistochemical and other staining methods. Features suggestive of other causes are listed below, but none of these can be regarded as specific.

Hepatitis non-A–non-B

Portal lymphoid aggregates with germinal centres, lymphoid aggregates around bile ducts, prominent lobular inflammation, fatty change.

'Autoimmune' CAH

Severe inflammation with prominent 'rosetting' of periportal hepatocytes.

Alcoholic liver disease

In countries where it is freely available, alcohol is the commonest cause of chronic liver disease.

There are three main effects.

1 Fatty liver.
2 Alcoholic hepatitis/fibrosis.
3 Cirrhosis.

There is a considerable overlap between these three patterns of damage, which are best regarded as different positions in a broad spectrum of alcohol-induced liver damage.

In addition to hepatotoxicity, alcohol also has undesirable effects on the heart (see p. 65) central nervous system (see p. 338) and pancreas (see p. 352).

Risk factors

Variations in individual susceptibility and problems in obtaining reliable accounts of drinking habits make it difficult to determine potentially 'toxic' levels of alcohol intake, but a number of factors have emerged as being important:

1 Alcohol is directly hepatotoxic, although other factors, e.g. malnutrition, may aggravate matters.
2 Severity of liver damage is related to amount and duration of intake.
3 Females are more susceptible than males.

A daily intake in excess of 50–60 g in males and 30–40 g in females is associated with a significant risk of liver damage. 10 g or 1 unit is roughly the equivalent of 0.5 pint of beer, one glass of wine or one measure of spirits.

Table 13.2 Prognostic factors in chronic hepatitis.

	Better prognosis	Worse prognosis
Histological type	CPH CLH	CAH
Histological severity (in CAH) Piecemeal necrosis Bridging necrosis	Mild Absent	Moderate or severe Present
Aetiology (untreated cases)	Hepatitis B	Hepatitis B with δ superinfection 'Autoimmune' CAH Hepatitis non-A–non-B
Treatment with immunosuppression	'Autoimmune' CAH	Hepatitis B Hepatitis non-A–non-B

Fatty liver

Appearances
Predominantly macrovesicular steatosis involving acinar zones 2–3. Rupture of fat cysts may evoke a granulomatous inflammatory reaction with formation of *lipogranulomas*.

However, fatty liver is a non-specific finding with many other possible causes (see p. 248).

Incidence
Very common—occurs in up to 90% of cases. Rapidly induced—within a few days. Readily reversible—complete disappearance within a few weeks of stopping drinking.

Clinical
Usually this is a 'benign' condition. Most patients are asymptomatic with normal or near-normal biochemical tests, though hepatomegaly is commonly present. Occasional fatal cases with severe microvesicular fatty change are described—*alcoholic foamy degeneration*.

Alcoholic hepatitis/fibrosis

Appearances
1 *Hepatocellular damage*: ballooning degeneration, Mallory's hyalin*, megamitochondria*, necrosis, and sometimes cholestasis. Mallory's hyalin is present as clumps of eosinophilic material in the cytoplasm of ballooned hepatocytes and is derived from intermediate filaments which form the cytoskeleton of liver cells. Megamitochondria are visible by light microscopy as rounded eosinophilic structures in the cytoplasm of hepatocytes.
2 *Inflammation*: predominantly polymorphonuclear leucocytes.*
3 *Fibrosis*: perivenular fibrosis*—fibrous thickening around hepatic venules and pericellular fibrosis*—'chicken-wire-like' pattern around individual hepatocytes.

Features marked with an asterisk are highly characteristic of alcoholic liver damage. When present in combination the diagnosis of alcoholic hepatitis is strongly suggested.

In common with fatty change the lesions of alcoholic hepatitis tend to be most prominent in perivenular areas, but in severe cases they may be dispersed throughout the liver parenchyma.

Incidence
About 30–35% of heavy drinkers develop alcoholic hepatitis, particularly when excess intake is prolonged over months or years. It is, however, still potentially reversible.

Clinical
Usually symptomatic, with biochemical abnormalities and with a significant mortality of 10–20% in the acute phase.

Inflammation, hepatocyte necrosis and fibrosis form the basis for subsequent development of cirrhosis.

Alcoholic cirrhosis

Appearances
The liver is usually large and micronodular in the early stages. A mixed or macronodular pattern supervenes in the late stages when the liver is also considerably shrunken.

Other features of alcoholic liver disease—fatty change, hepatitis—may persist in patients who continue to drink, but in those who have abstained from alcohol for a prolonged period of time, other effects of alcohol disappear and cirrhosis may be labelled incorrectly as 'cryptogenic'.

Incidence
Occurs in 10—15% of chronic alcoholics, particularly those with prolonged excess drinking, usually over a period of several years. By definition, alcoholic cirrhosis is irreversible.

Clinical
Some patients may be asymptomatic, even at such an advanced stage, but more commonly, one or more complications of cirrhosis develop (see p. 242)

Abstinence from alcohol can halt the progression of disease and improve prognosis, even in cases where cirrhosis has supervened.

D/CIRRHOSIS, CHOLESTASIS, BILE DUCTS

Cirrhosis
  Classification
  Appearances
  Biopsy diagnosis
  Complications
Cholestasis
Bile duct diseases
  Primary biliary cirrhosis
  Primary sclerosing cholangitis
  Extrahepatic biliary atresia

Cirrhosis

Definition
Cirrhosis is an irreversible condition affecting the entire liver. It represents the end stage of many disease processes which cause prolonged liver cell damage.

The diagnosis of cirrhosis is based on three morphological criteria:
1 loss of the normal architecture, with
2 nodules of regenerating hepatocytes, separated by
3 bands of fibrous tissue.

Classification
Cirrhosis can be classified on morphological appearances of the liver, or on an aetiological basis.

Morphological types
Morphological classification is based on the size of regenerating nodules.
1 *Micronodular*: small nodules of uniform size, < 0.3 cm, approximating to the size of normal hepatic lobules.
2 *Macronodular*: nodules of variable size, often greater than 1 cm diameter.
3 *Mixed*: small and large nodules present.

Aetiology
1 *Alcohol*: 50–70%—the commonest cause in the Western world.
2 *Postviral*: 5–10%—hepatitis B or hepatitis non-A–non-B.
3 *Biliary cirrhosis*: 5–10%—primary biliary cirrhosis—aetiology unknown; secondary biliary cirrhosis due to prolonged extrahepatic bile duct obstruction, sclerosing cholangitis, or biliary atresia.
4 *Metabolic diseases*: < 5%—haemochromatosis, Wilson's disease, α_1-antitrypsin deficiency, fibrocystic

disease of pancreas, galactosaemia, tyrosinaemia, glycogen storage disease.
5 *Vascular disorders*: very rare—Budd-Chiari syndrome, veno-occlusive disease or right heart failure.
6 *'Autoimmune'*: autoimmune CAH.
7 *Drugs*: methotrexate, isoniazid, iproniazid.
8 *'Cryptogenic'*: 10–25%—aetiology unknown. Formerly the commonest group, the number of cases in this category is falling with the use of sensitive methods for diagnosing other causes of cirrhosis.

Comparison of morphological and aetiological classifications
1 There is some correlation between aetiology and morphological patterns of cirrhosis; e.g. alcohol and biliary diseases tend to have a predominantly micronodular pattern whereas postviral cirrhosis typically has a macronodular pattern.
2 The value of morphological classification is becoming increasingly doubtful, particularly in end-stage disease where a mixed pattern commonly supervenes. Morphological classification is also difficult on needle biopsy specimens due to sampling problems.
3 An aetiological classification is most useful in determining prognosis and treatment.
4 The group of metabolic diseases are important to recognize, for two reasons:
  (a) They are a common cause of liver disease in children and young adults.
  (b) Many have a hereditary basis. This has important implications for screening of siblings, particularly as the prognosis can sometimes be considerably improved by early diagnosis and treatment.

Appearances

Diagnostic features
The main diagnostic features are discussed above.

Aetiology
Routine stains for iron—Perls' reaction, α_1-antitrypsin globules—PAS-diastase and hepatitis B surface antigen—orcein, may identify otherwise unsuspected aetiologies.

Activity
The presence of numerous inflammatory cells in fibrous septa with spillover and damage to periseptal hepatocytes indicates active progression of the cirrhotic process—*'active' cirrhosis*.

Biopsy diagnosis of cirrhosis

The diagnosis of cirrhosis on small needle biopsy samples is not always straightforward. The following problems may be encountered:

1 *'Early' cirrhosis*: in some cases a biopsy may show transitional features between potentially recoverable fibrosis and fully established cirrhosis. The terms 'early' or 'developing' cirrhosis are used to describe these cases.

2 *Sampling variation*: different parts of the liver may be affected to a different degree at the same time. A single needle biopsy cannot take account of this sampling variation.

3 *Macronodular cirrhosis*: in the absence of complete regeneration nodules, due to their large size, the diagnosis of macronodular cirrhosis is sometimes missed in needle biopsies.

Helpful pointers to a diagnosis of cirrhosis in these cases are: fragmentation of the biopsy, abnormal arrangement of cell plates, thickening of cell plates and disturbed relationships between portal tracts and hepatic venules.

Complications

Most patients with cirrhosis suffer complications, sometimes even death, related to hepatocellular failure and/or portal hypertension.

Approximately 10–15% of patients develop hepatocellular carcinoma as a terminal complication.

In a minority of cases—up to 10%, cirrhosis may be entirely asymptomatic and observed only as an incidental finding at post mortem.

Hepatocellular failure

Causes

Loss of liver cells and reduction in effective blood flow to surviving hepatocytes due to abnormal vascular relationships.

Effects

1 *Jaundice*: usually due to failure of hepatocytes to excrete bilirubin but may be obstructive in cases of biliary cirrhosis.

2 *Ascites and oedema*: reduced albumin synthesis and portal hypertension.

3 *Bleeding tendency*: reduced synthesis of clotting factors II, VII, IX, X and hypersplenism.

4 *Neurological disturbances—hepatic encephalo-pathy*: failure to detoxify nitrogenous substances from the gut.

5 *Endocrine*: gynaecomastia, testicular atrophy, palmar erythema, spider naevi. These are thought to be due to failure of hepatic inactivation of oestrogens.

6 *Renal failure*: hepatorenal syndrome (see p. 174).

7 *Spontaneous infections*, e.g. Gram-negative bacteria in bacterial peritonitis or septicaemia.

8 *Lung*: arteriovenous shunting with ventilation/perfusion mismatch—*hepato-pulmonary syndrome*—mechanism unknown. Pulmonary hypertension.

9 *Circulatory*: hyperkinetic circulation.

10 *Finger clubbing*: possibly related to pulmonary and circulatory changes above.

Portal hypertension

Causes

Compression of hepatic veins and sinusoidal blood flow by parenchymal regeneration nodules and obstruction of portal veins by fibrosis involving portal tracts.

Effects

These are described on p. 230.

Hepatocellular carcinoma—HCC

The incidence of HCC varies according to the underlying cause of cirrhosis, e.g. high in hepatitis B, low in biliary cirrhosis (see also p. 254).

In the UK, HCC usually develops as a late complication of long-standing cirrhosis.

Premalignant lesions are recognized in some cases of cirrhosis, though their natural history is uncertain:

1 *Liver cell dysplasia*: groups of hepatocytes with atypical nuclei showing enlargement, pleomorphism and hyperchromatism.

2 *'Adenomatous hyperplasia'*: large regeneration nodules—up to 8 cm diameter, with abnormally thick cell plates but without significant nuclear atypia.

Cholestasis

Definition

Cholestasis is defined as a disturbance in the normal bile secretory apparatus. As a result, substances normally secreted into bile accumulate within the liver and also appear in the blood.

Main features

1 *Clinical*: pruritus and jaundice.
2 *Biochemical*: elevated serum levels of conjugated bilirubin, alkaline phosphatase, cholesterol and bile acids.
3 *Histological*: deposition of bile pigments in liver tissue. Cholestasis tends to be most prominent in perivenular areas, probably reflecting functional differences between the different acinar zones. In some cases it exists in a so-called 'pure' form—i.e. without any other histological abnormalities, but more usually there are other changes present, depending on the underlying cause.

Causes

Extrahepatic cholestasis—large duct obstruction, 'surgical' cholestasis

Mechanical obstruction to the flow of bile in large ducts outside the liver or within the porta hepatis, due to:
1 *Gall stones*: impacted in the common bile duct.
2 *Tumours*, e.g. carcinoma of bile duct, periampullary carcinoma, carcinoma of pancreas.
3 *Strictures*: usually following surgery.
4 *Congenital diseases*: choledochal cyst, extrahepatic biliary atresia.
5 *Parasites*: fascioliasis, ascaris, opisthorcis, hydatid disease (rare).

Appearances

Parenchymal damage

The earliest damage, seen after a few days, is perivenular cholestasis. Bile pigment is present in the cytoplasm of hepatocytes, dilated biliary canaliculi and Kupffer cells. These appearances are non-specific but prolonged obstruction may lead to extravasation of bile from dilated canaliculi to produce characteristic 'bile infarcts'.

Portal tract lesions

These occur somewhat later than parenchymal lesions and are characterized by oedema, a mixed inflammatory infiltrate and proliferation of small ductular structures at the periphery of portal areas. If obstruction is prolonged there may be extravasation of bile from small intrahepatic bile ducts to produce 'bile lakes'. Like bile infarcts, these are almost pathognomonic of large duct obstruction.

Complications

Ascending cholangitis

Superimposed infection with multiple intrahepatic abscesses in severe cases.

Cirrhosis

Unrelieved biliary obstruction results in progressive portal fibrosis and may lead eventually to cirrhosis. Cirrhosis occurs only as a result of prolonged obstruction—months to years; it is thus relatively uncommon—less than 10% of cases, as biliary obstruction is usually relieved surgically.

Intrahepatic cholestasis

A failure of the bile secretory mechanisms located within the liver.

Intra-acinar cholestasis

Mechanisms are probably located in hepatocytes or biliary canaliculi.
1 Cholestatic viral hepatitis.
2 Cholestasis in alcoholic liver disease.
3 Cholestasis in cirrhosis.
4 Drug-induced cholestasis—e.g. anabolic and contraceptive steroids.
5 Cholestasis of pregnancy.
6 Benign recurrent intrahepatic cholestasis.
7 Cholestasis in sepsis.
8 Cholestasis in lymphoma—especially Hodgkin's disease.

In items 1–3 cholestasis is seen in association with other features of the respective diseases; in 4–8 cholestasis frequently occurs in a 'pure' form (see above) and the diagnosis is based on clinical circumstances.

Extra-acinar cholestasis

In these conditions the cause of cholestasis is damage to the intrahepatic bile ducts. The mechanism is presumably one of mechanical obstruction and many of the secondary changes are similar to those seen in large duct obstruction. Examples include:
1 Primary biliary cirrhosis.
2 Primary sclerosing cholangitis.
3 Cystic diseases of intrahepatic ducts—Caroli's disease, polycystic liver, congenital hepatic fibrosis.
4 Space-occupying lesions in liver.

Diseases of bile ducts

Primary biliary cirrhosis—PBC

Definition
A chronic cholestatic condition in which there is destruction of small intrahepatic bile ducts. True cirrhosis occurs only as a late manifestation, and the term primary biliary *cirrhosis* is thus inappropriate in many cases.

Aetiology
Many of the clinical, histological and immunological findings point to an autoimmune mechanism. The aetiology, however, is still not known.

Clinical
1 *Age/sex*: predominantly a disease of young to middle-aged women with peak incidence 30–60 years. Female : male, 10 : 1.
2 *Clinical features*: onset is usually insidious, with pruritus the most common presenting symptom. Jaundice occurs later with other manifestations of malabsorption, e.g. osteomalacia, osteoporosis. Eventually there are features of true cirrhosis resulting in death from liver failure or portal hypertension.
3 *Biochemistry*: elevation of serum alkaline phosphatase, cholesterol and bile acid levels. The bilirubin level is normal in the early stages but eventually rises.
4 *Immunology*: the most helpful diagnostic test is the demonstration of *antimitochondrial antibodies— AMAs*, which are present in more than 95% of cases. Nine subtypes of mitochondrial antibody have been identified; of these anti-M_2 is the most specific for PBC. Serum IgM level is increased.
5 *Associated diseases*: PBC is associated with several other diseases which are thought to have an immunological basis. These include: rheumatoid arthritis (see p. 100), autoimmune thyroiditis (see p. 128), systemic lupus erythematosus, scleroderma (see p. 98) and Sjögren's syndrome (see p. 103).

Microscopical
Four stages have been described. The distinction between these is somewhat artificial and it is probably best to regard PBC as a continuously evolving disease process with different parts of the liver being affected to variable degrees at different times.

Stage 1: bile duct lesions
Inflammatory portal lesions including granulomas are associated with destruction of small to medium-sized bile ducts. These lesions are rarely seen in needle biopsy specimens but, when present, are pathognomonic of PBC.

The number of small bile ducts is considerably reduced as the disease progresses—'*vanishing bile duct syndrome*'.

Stage 2: ductular proliferation; Stage 3: scarring—precirrhotic
Stages 2 and 3 are difficult to distinguish and are described together.

Bile ductular proliferation occurs at the margins of portal tracts and is associated with inflammatory cell infiltration and loose fibrous portal expansion. Portal–portal linkage may occur but normal lobular relationships are retained during these stages.

Cholestasis often becomes conspicuous.

Deposition of copper-associated protein—CAP—in periportal hepatocytes is a manifestation of chronic cholestasis and is also evident during these stages. It is present in lysosomal granules which stain black by the orcein method.

Stage 4: cirrhosis
Eventually the fibrotic process described above is associated with a true cirrhosis. This occurs as a late complication of PBC. Some patients develop end-stage disease without becoming truly cirrhotic.

Prognosis
Some patients have an asymptomatic benign form of the disease associated with prolonged survival.

Most patients, however, become symptomatic. There is no specific treatment for this form of the disease and death usually occurs within 5–10 years of presentation.

Liver transplantation offers the only effective method of cure. A minority of patients have developed features suggestive of recurrent disease after transplantation.

Primary sclerosing cholangitis—PSC

Nature
Primary sclerosing cholangitis is a fibrosing, inflammatory condition affecting extra- and intrahepatic bile ducts.

Aetiology

The aetiology is unknown but a similar pattern of bile duct damage can occur in association with traumatic, inflammatory and neoplastic diseases of the biliary system. PSC has to be distinguished from these cases of secondary sclerosing cholangitis.

Clinical

1 *Age/sex*: any age with peak incidence 20—50 years; male : female, 2–3 : 1.
2 *Clinical features*: progressive obstructive jaundice and recurrent acute cholangitis. Later manifestations are complications of cirrhosis and malignant transformation to cholangiocarcinoma which occurs in some cases (see p. 256).
3 *Biochemistry*: cholestatic pattern of liver function tests—as for PBC.
4 *Immunology*: AMA negative and normal IgM level—contrasting with PBC.
5 *Radiology*: the most important diagnostic test is endoscopic retrograde cholangiopancreatography (ERCP), which shows multiple strictures with 'beading' between narrowed segments.
6 *Associated diseases*: ulcerative colitis (UC); 50–70% of patients with PSC have UC. Conversely, approximately 5% of patients with UC develop PSC.

Crohn's disease—the association is less strong than with UC, but cases have been reported.

Other fibrosing inflammatory diseases—Riedel's thyroiditis (see p. 131), mediastinal fibrosis, retroperitoneal fibrosis.

Microscopical

There are many similarities between PSC and PBC, including a gradual progression to cirrhosis usually occurring over a period of several years.

Bile ducts

Bile ducts of all sizes are affected—in contrast to PBC which only affects small-to-medium sized ducts.
1 Extrahepatic ducts (see p. 262).
2 Large intrahepatic ducts—inflammation, ulceration and dilatation—*cholangiectasia*.
3 Medium-sized ducts—variable inflammation with characteristic 'onion-skin' periductal fibrosis progressing, in some cases, to complete replacement of ducts by nodular scars. These fibrosing duct lesions are thought to be diagnostic of PSC.
4 Small ducts—may show similar changes to medium sized-ducts. More commonly they disappear without trace—another example of a 'vanishing bile duct syndrome'.

Other features

These are very similar to those described for PBC. There is ductular proliferation, parenchymal cholestasis and progressive portal fibrosis leading eventually to a true cirrhosis.

Histological distinction between PBC and PSC is based on different patterns of bile duct damage. Diagnostic duct lesions are uncommonly seen in needle biopsy specimens and differentiation in these cases is made by the appropriate serological and radiological investigations.

Prognosis

This is very variable. Some patients have a relatively benign form of the disease, associated with prolonged survival, but most cases progress to cirrhosis within 5–10 years of presentation.

Cholangiocarcinoma is increasingly recognized as a terminal complication.

Extrahepatic biliary atresia

Nature

A congenital disorder in which there is failure of development of the extrahepatic bile ducts.

Aetiology

Cause unknown, but possibly related to intrauterine viral infection.

Clinical

Obstructive jaundice, presenting in the neonatal period.

Progressive jaundice leads to end-stage disease, usually within the first 2—3 years of life. Early surgical intervention with anastomosis of a loop of jejunum to the porta hepatis—*Kasai operation*—improves the outlook in some cases.

Appearances

The liver is relatively normal at birth but features of biliary obstruction rapidly supervene with progression to secondary biliary cirrhosis, in some cases within a few months.

E/METABOLIC, CHILDHOOD DISORDERS, PREGNANCY

Metabolic
  Iron
  α_1-Antitrypsin deficiency
  Wilson's disease
  Degenerative/storage
Liver disease in childhood
  Neonatal hepatitis
  Fibropolycystic diseases
  Reye's syndrome
Liver disease in pregnancy
  Cholestasis
  Acute fatty liver
  Eclampsia

Metabolic diseases of the liver

Iron overload in the liver

In normal physiological conditions iron is stored in the liver in the form of ferritin, which is dispersed throughout the cytoplasm of hepatocytes.

In states of iron overload, iron accumulates in the form of haemosiderin which is composed of polymerized ferritin admixed with protein. Haemosiderin is deposited in lysosomes, also known as siderosomes. Haemosiderin can he demonstrated in tissue sections as blue granules using Perl's Prussian blue reaction.

Excess iron deposition in the liver can be demonstrated either by histochemical staining, using Perl's reaction, or more accurately by biochemical analysis of liver tissue.

Terminology

1 *Siderosis* is any state in which excess iron is deposited in tissue.
2 *Haemochromatosis* implies excess iron storage in association with tissue damage.

Causes

1 *Primary haemochromatosis.*
2 *Secondary siderosis.*

Primary—'idiopathic'—haemochromatosis

Nature

A genetic defect of iron absorption, inherited as autosomal recessive and associated with HLA–A3, HLA–B14, HLA–B7.

In homozygotes there is excessive absorption of dietary iron in the gut. This occurs from birth and is associated with deposition of iron in many organs. The precise mechanisms involved are not certain.

The majority of disease—80–90%, occurs in males.

Appearances

Liver

In the early stages there is iron deposition in the liver without any other abnormalities—*simple siderosis*. As the disease progresses there is portal fibrosis with eventual progression to true cirrhosis—*haemochromatosis*. Development of cirrhosis takes place over a long period of time. Clinical presentation is rare before the age of 20, and many cases present between 40 and 60.

An increased risk of hepatocellular carcinoma is also described in haemochromatosis. It is not certain whether this is simply related to development of cirrhosis or whether iron deposition itself is carcinogenic.

Other organs

In genetic haemochromatosis deposition occurs in many other organs and is associated with varying degrees of damage, sometimes accompanied by fibrosis (see Table 13.3).

Course

Venesection and treatment with iron chelators effectively reduce the tissue iron deposits and considerably improve prognosis, especially if the diagnosis is made before significant tissue damage has occurred. Even in cases with established cirrhosis the outlook is improved with these treatments.

Secondary siderosis

Nature

Conditions in which iron overload is secondary to recognised causes:

Chronic anaemia

1 *Ineffective erythropoiesis*, e.g. thalassaemia, sideroblastic anaemia. In some cases with defective red cell production excessive iron is absorbed from the gut and deposited in the liver.

Table 13.3 Iron deposition in genetic haemochromatosis.

Organ involved	Site of deposition	Clinical features
Pancreas	Islets and exocrine acini	Diabetes mellitus*
Heart	Myocardium	Cardiac dysfunction (arrhythmias, cardiomyopathy)
Skin	Dermal macrophages and fibroblasts	Golden-grey skin pigmentation* (melanin also deposited in the dermis)
Endocrine glands	Thyroid, adrenal, pituitary	Hypogonadism (possibly related to pituitary involvement)
Joints	Synovial lining cells	Atypical arthritis

* In addition to hepatomegaly the two classical presenting symptoms of haemochromatosis are skin pigmentation and diabetes mellitus—'*bronzed diabetes*'.

2 *Tranfusional overload*: chronic anaemias which require regular blood transfusions, and haemolytic anaemias, result in excess tissue deposition of iron. In these conditions iron is mainly deposited in Kupffer cells, rather than hepatocytes.

Dietary overload
Ingestion of excessive amounts of iron is a rare but well-documented cause of hepatic siderosis. Two main situations are described:
1 Consumption of beer brewed in iron pots by South African Bantus—Bantu siderosis.
2 Prolonged ingestion of oral iron supplements in non-anaemic patients.

Chronic liver disease
Siderosis is commonly present as a secondary phenomenon in liver cirrhosis from any cause. The mechanism is uncertain but may relate to abnormalities in intrahepatic blood flow. Siderosis is usually mild but can occasionally be severe, particularly in alcoholic cirrhosis. In these circumstances distinction from primary haemochromatosis is sometimes difficult. Biochemical analysis of liver tissue may be required to make the distinction.

Appearances
A wide range of appearances can occur but, in general, siderosis tends to be less severe and less generalized than in the primary form. Except in cases which are secondary to cirrhosis other manifestations of liver damage are also less marked. However, in some cases there may be fibrosis and even cirrhosis—secondary haemochromatosis.

α_1-Antitrypsin deficiency

Nature
A genetically determined disease with a codominant autosomal inheritance.

The basic defect is a failure to release α_1-antitrypsin (α_1-AT), into the blood from hepatocytes and other cells which produce this protein.

Clinically significant disease is generally confined to homozygotes who have very low circulating levels of α_1-AT. Heterozygotes also have lower than normal levels of α_1-AT. This may predispose to tissue damage, particularly in combination with other factors.

Appearances

Liver
Varying patterns of liver damage occur in different age groups.
1 *Neonatal hepatitis*: often with a cholestatic picture.
2 *Chronic active hepatitis.*
3 *Cirrhosis*: this can occur in childhood—as early as 2 years, or in adults.

The diagnosis of α_1-AT deficiency is confirmed by the presence of characteristic eosinophilic globules in the cytoplasm of hepatocytes. The globules represent accumulates of the protein in endoplasmic reticulum and can also be demonstrated as purple globules by PAS-diastase staining or by immunohistochemical methods.

Lung
α_1-AT deficency is also associated with respiratory disease due to emphysema (see p. 378).

Wilson's disease—hepatolenticular degeneration

Nature
A genetic disease—inherited as an autosomal recessive. The primary defect is probably in the liver where there is:

1 Failure to excrete copper into the bile, associated with
2 Reduced synthesis of the serum copper-binding protein caeruloplasmin.

Deposition of copper occurs in various organs including liver, lenticular nuclei, eye and kidneys.

Appearances

Liver
A wide range of lesions may be produced in the liver including:

1 Fatty change.
2 Fulminant hepatitis.
3 Chronic hepatitis.
4 Cirrhosis.

Histological features are often indistinguishable from other conditions causing similar patterns of liver damage. Demonstration of excessive copper by histochemical staining of tissue sections, or biochemical analysis of fresh liver tissue, help in making the diagnosis.

Brain
Deposition of copper occurs in the basal ganglia leading to neuronal loss and symptoms of spasticity and tremor.

Eyes
Copper deposition in the cornea produces a characteristic greenish-brown discoloration—*Kayser-Fleischer rings*.

Kidney
Copper is excreted in the urine leading to tubular damage and aminoaciduria.

Course
Early treatment with the copper-chelating agent D-penicillamine can arrest many of the pathological processes described above, and greatly improve prognosis.

Miscellaneous degenerative/storage diseases of the liver

Fatty liver—steatosis
This is one of the commonest abnormalities seen in the liver and many causes are recognized. Two morphological patterns are recognized, although these are often mixed.

Macrovesicular steatosis
This is the more common form. Large fat droplets, usually solitary, are present in the cytoplasm of hepatocytes displacing their nuclei to the periphery. The main causes are:

1 Alcohol.
2 Diabetes mellitus.
3 Obesity.
4 Starvation—protein, energy malnutrition—*kwashiorkor*.

Microvesicular steatosis
This is the less common form but may be mixed with above. Multiple small cytoplasmic vacuoles are present in hepatocytes which have a normally positioned nucleus. Diagnosis can be difficult on light microscopy without the use of specific fat stains. The main causes are:

1 Reye's syndrome (see p. 250).
2 Acute fatty liver of pregnancy (see p. 250).
3 Some drugs—tetracycline, valproate.

Amyloidosis
The liver is commonly involved: deposits are mainly present in the walls of portal blood vessels and in the perisinusoidal spaces of Disse.

Granulomas
There are numerous causes of hepatic granulomas, which may be found in up to 10% of liver biopsies.

Infective
1 Bacteria, e.g. TB.
2 Fungi, e.g. *Cryptococcus*.
3 Viruses, e.g. CMV.
4 Parasites, e.g. schistosomiasis.
5 Rickettsiae, e.g. Q fever.

Hypersensitivity
1 Drugs, e.g. allopurinol, sulphonamides, phenylbutazone.

2 'Autoimmune' diseases, e.g. polyarteritis nodosa.

Neoplasms

1 Lymphoma: Hodgkin's disease, non-Hodgkin's lymphoma.
2 Epithelial: metastatic carcinoma.

Foreign bodies

For example, mineral oil.

Miscellaneous

1 Sarcoid.
2 Primary biliary cirrhosis.
3 Other chronic liver diseases, e.g. sclerosing cholangitis, cirrhosis.

Unknown

In up to 20–25% of cases no definite cause for granulomas is found—'idiopathic granulomatous hepatitis'.

Diabetes mellitus

Histological changes are commonly present in diabetes. These are rarely accompanied by significant clinical abnormalities (see p. 355)
1 *Fatty change*—common.
2 *Increased glycogen deposition*—common and often visible as glycogenation of hepatocyte nuclei, giving rise to a characteristic vacuolated appearance.

These two lesions are both non-specific and occur in many other conditions.
3 *Steatohepatitis*—rare. A picture closely resembling alcoholic hepatitis is sometimes seen in diabetics who strongly deny excess alcohol intake—'non-alcoholic steatohepatitis'.
4 *Cirrhosis*—very rare but an increased incidence of cirrhosis has been observed in diabetes. It is not clear whether this is a cause or effect of the disease.

Glycogen storage disease

The liver is involved in the inherited glycogen storage diseases I, II, III, IV, VI, VIII and IX.

The commonest histological finding is swelling and pallor of hepatocytes, due to abundant glycogen deposition. These histological features are non-specific and the diagnosis is based on the demonstration of a specific enzyme defect in peripheral blood or liver tissue.

Additional features seen in these diseases are development of hepatocellular adenoma or less commonly carcinoma (type I disease) and fibrosis leading to cirrhosis (type IV disease).

Lipid storage diseases

Many of these diseases involve the liver, usually as part of multisystem disorder. Examples include:
1 *Gaucher's disease*: glycosyl ceramide lipidosis.
2 *Niemann Pick disease*: sphingomyelin lipidosis.
3 *Wolman's disease*.
4 *Cholesterol storage disease*.

In these conditions abnormal lipids predominantly accumulate in the cytoplasm of Kupffer cells, which become enlarged and pale.

Liver disease in childhood

Many liver diseases occurring in childhood are discussed earlier, including extrahepatic biliary atresia (p. 245), α_1-AT deficiency (p. 247), Wilson's disease (p. 248), glycogen and lipid storage diseases (p. 249).

Neonatal hepatitis

This is a poorly defined condition in which there is inflammation of the liver associated with hepatocellular damage. A prominent feature in many cases is giant-cell transformation of hepatocytes which contain up to 40 nuclei. There is also variable cholestasis. In cases where cholestasis is prominent distinction from biliary diseases, including biliary atresia, can be difficult. Numerous causes of neonatal hepatitis are recognized including:
1 *Metabolic*: α_1-AT deficiency (see p. 247).
2 *Infective*: 'TORCH' agents—toxoplasmosis, rubella, cytomegalovirus, herpes simplex.
3 *Familial*: autosomal recessive inheritance.
4 *Idiopathic*: in up to 50% of cases no specific aetiological agent is identified.

Fibropolycystic diseases of the liver

A complex group of diseases with a broad spectrum of pathological appearances in which abnormal bile ductal structures are associated with varying patterns of fibrosis. Some are thought to represent disorders of remodelling of the fetal bile duct system—also called ductal plate malformations, but a unifying concept is still not available.

The abnormalities are thought to be present at birth, i.e. congenital, but in some cases may not present clinically until late childhood or adult life and in mild forms may even be asymptomatic throughout life.

In addition to the individual complications listed

below these diseases carry an increased risk of cholangiocarcinoma.

Congenital hepatic fibrosis

The liver parenchyma is divided into irregular islands by bands of fibrous tissue containing numerous irregular bile ducts. Normal lobular relationships are retained and the disease is thus not a true cirrhosis.

The main complication is portal hypertension with ascending cholangitis occurring more rarely. Many cases are associated with cystic disease of the kidneys which can be the presenting feature (see p. 162).

Polycystic disease

Childhood form

This is inherited as an autosomal recessive. Portal areas contain multiple biliary structures, some dilated, but gross cystic change is rarely evident macroscopically. The main complications are portal hypertension and cholangitis. Associated with renal cysts (see p. 162).

Adult form

Inherited as an autosomal dominant. The liver contains multiple, epthelial-lined cysts 0.1–10 cm diameter and bile duct microhamartomas—*von Meyenburg's complexes*. These are small nodules—less than 0.5 cm diameter, composed of irregular ductal structures embedded in a dense fibrous stroma. The main presenting feature is hepatomegaly, and liver function usually remains good. Cysts are also present in kidney (see p. 162).

Caroli's disease

In this condition there are numerous cystic dilatations of the intrahepatic biliary tree. Superadded infection with ascending cholangitis is the main complication.

Reye's syndrome

This condition is largely confined to children under the age of 15 years, although rare cases have been reported in adults.

Aetiology and pathogenesis

Most cases occur after a viral infection—most commonly influenza or varicella, and have received treatment with salicylates—usually aspirin.

Ultrastructural studies have shown mitochondrial abnormalities in many organs—liver, brain, kidney, heart, skeletal muscle. It is not clear whether these are a cause or an effect of the metabolic abnormalities which characterize this condition. The overall pathogenesis thus remains uncertain.

Clinical

The main features relate to cerebral oedema and liver failure. Death occurs in up to 40% of cases.

Liver

There is microvesicular steatosis which usually has a panacinar distribution. Fat droplets may be difficult to visualize by conventional light microscopy. Part of a liver biopsy should be frozen for fat staining if the diagnosis is suspected clinically.

Liver disease in pregnancy

Pregnant women are susceptible to the same liver diseases which affect non-pregnant women, and these account for most cases of liver damage which occur during pregnancy. Three uncommon diseases unique to pregnancy are:

Benign intrahepatic cholestasis of pregnancy

Clinical

Jaundice in the third trimester.

Appearances

'Pure' cholestasis, most prominent in perivenular areas.

Aetiology and pathogenesis

Uncertain. A familial tendency has been described. Some patients give a history of previous episodes of jaundice related to the oral contraceptive pill, suggesting an increased sensitivity to steroid hormones.

Acute fatty liver of pregnancy

Clinical

A serious condition presenting in the third trimester with jaundice and rapidly progressive liver failure. Untreated cases are associated with a high maternal and fetal mortality. Early recognition of the condition, and treatment by Caesarian section, has greatly improved the outlook.

Appearances

The histological appearances are characteristic, with severe microvesicular steatosis and ballooning involving perivenular hepatocytes which have a 'foamy' appearance. Varying degrees of cholestasis are also present.

Eclampsia

Clinical

Although the liver is commonly involved in eclampsia clinical features of hepatic damage are generally mild (see p. 178).

Appearances

The characteristic histological findings are irregular areas of necrosis and fibrin deposition in periportal areas. Fibrin thrombi are frequently deposited in adjacent portal vessels, in keeping with a DIC mechanism.

F/DRUG-INDUCED DAMAGE

Intrinsic hepatotoxins
Idiosyncratic hepatotoxins

Incidence

Drugs are increasingly recognized as an important cause of liver damage. Approximately 2.5% of hospital admissions for jaundice and up to 25% of cases of fulminant liver failure are ascribed to a drug aetiology.

Mechanisms

The mechanisms involved in drug-induced liver damage are complex and, in many cases, remain poorly understood. Two main pathways are recognized.

Intrinsic hepatotoxins

1 *Incidence of hepatic injury*: high.
2 *Dose dependence*: yes. Will produce liver damage in most individuals provided a sufficient amount taken—i.e. a *predictable* injury.
3 *Mechanisms*:
  (a) Direct hepatotoxicity;
  (b) Indirect hepatotoxicity—interference with metabolic pathways.
4 *Evidence of allergic reactions*: No.

Idiosyncratic hepatotoxins

1 *Incidence of hepatic injury*; low.
2 *Dose dependence*: no. Only produce liver damage in susceptible individuals and the amount required may be small, i.e. *unpredictable* injury.
3 *Mechanisms*:
  (a) hypersensitivity;
  (b) production of toxic metabolites—abnormal metabolism in susceptible individuals.
4 *Evidence for other allergic reactions*: common in hypersensitivity-related cases, e.g. fever, rash, eosinophilia, granuloma formation.

Morphological lesions

Almost all of the common patterns of liver damage that are described elsewhere in this chapter can be produced by drugs.

In most cases the histological features are indistinguishable from naturally occurring liver diseases, and the diagnosis of drug damage is usually one of exclusion.

It is impossible to list all of the drugs that can cause liver disease, but some examples of the lesions produced are:
1 *Fatty change*: large droplet—alcohol, methotrexate, corticosteroids; small droplet—tetracycline, valproate.
2 *Zonal necrosis*, e.g. paracetamol, carbon tetrachloride. These agents mainly involve acinar zone 3, probably because the enzymes responsible for converting them to toxic metabolites are present in highest concentration towards the acinar periphery. In severe cases necrosis can spread to involve acinar zones 2 and 1.
3 *Acute hepatitis*, e.g. isoniazid, halothane. The histological picture closely resembles that seen in viral hepatitis. Features pointing to a drug aetiology include eosinophilic infiltration, granuloma formation and fatty change, but these cannot be regarded as specific.
4 *Chronic hepatitis*, e.g. isoniazid, α-methyl dopa.
5 *Fibrosis/cirrhosis*, e.g. methotrexate. Long-term treatment with methotrexate has been associated with portal fibrosis and in some cases progression to cirrhosis.
6 *Cholestasis*:
  (a) 'Pure' cholestasis, e.g. oral contraceptive steroids.
  (b) Cholestatic hepatitis, e.g. chlorpromazine. In these cases there is prominent cholestasis with a variable inflammatory component. Distinction

from acute viral hepatitis can be difficult when the inflammatory element is prominent.

7 *Granulomas*, e.g. allopurinol, sulphonamides, phenylbutazone. Drugs are an important cause of unexplained liver granulomas—they may occur with or without other manifestations of liver injury.

8 *Vascular injury*:

(a) Veno-occlusive disease, e.g. cytosine arabinoside, 6-thioguanine, azathioprine.

(b) Peliosis hepatis, e.g. oral contraceptive steroids. Peliosis is characterized by areas of sinusoidal dilatation with formation of blood-filled cysts in the liver parenchyma.

9 *Tumours*:

(a) Liver cell adenoma, e.g. oral contraceptives.

(b) Hepatocellular carcinoma, e.g. anabolic steroids, oral contraceptives—rare.

(c) Haemangiosarcoma, e.g. thorotrast.

G/LIVER TRANSPLANTATION

Indications
Complications

Liver transplantation is now widely accepted as a method of treating various forms of irreversible liver disease. Advances in surgical technique and immunosuppression have greatly improved prognosis and many centres now report 1- and 3-year survival rates in excess of 70%.

Indications

1 *Chronic liver disease*: (a) primary biliary cirrhosis; (b) cirrhosis (other causes).

2 *Acute liver failure*: (a) fulminant viral hepatitis; (b) drug-induced liver failure.

3 *Primary liver neoplasia*: (a) hepatocellular carcinoma; (b) cholangiocarcinoma; (c) some vascular tumours.

The most common disease for which liver transplantation is carried out is primary biliary cirrhosis, which accounts for approximately one-third of cases in many centres. Approximately 10–20% of patients require a second or subsequent transplant as a result of complications relating to the previous operation(s).

Complications

A detailed account of liver allograft pathology is beyond the scope of this book, but the major pathological complications are listed below.

Rejection

Acute—'reversible'—rejection

Incidence
Sixty percent to 80% of patients, usually in the first few weeks after transplantation.

Histological features
There is a classical triad of:
1 Portal inflammation.
2 Bile duct damage.
3 Venous endothelial inflammation.

Outcome
Most cases respond to increased immunosuppression with high-dose steroids.

Chronic—'irreversible'—rejection

Incidence
Less common than acute rejection—5–20% of cases. Usually later—three to 12 months.

Histological features
There are two characteristic features:
1 Destruction of small and medium-sized intrahepatic bile ducts—'vanishing bile duct syndrome'.
2 Occlusive vascular lesions in the form of foamy histiocytes and/or fibrous tissue involving the intima of large and medium-sized arteries.

Outcome
Presents as a syndrome of progressive intrahepatic cholestasis. Most cases are unresponsive to immunosuppression and progress to graft failure. Retransplantation is the only effective method of treatment.

Ischaemia

Occlusive
Hepatic artery thrombosis.

Non-occlusive
Various factors may be responsible, including small vessels in donor graft, bleeding and hypotension.

Biliary tract problems

Biliary complications are quite common in the form of leaks and strictures usually occurring at the site of anastomosis between donor and recipient duct. In many cases these are thought to have an ischaemic aetiology. Secondary complications of obstruction and ascending cholangitis occur in some cases.

Opportunistic infection
In common with other allograft recipients there is a risk of infection with opportunistic organisms, including viruses, e.g. CMV, herpes simplex and fungi, e.g. *Aspergillus, Candida.*

Recurrent disease
Diseases known or suspected to recur in the liver allograft are:
1 Malignant neoplasms, especially cholangiocarcinoma.
2 Hepatitis B.
3 Budd–Chiari syndrome.
4 Alcoholic liver disease.
5 Primary biliary cirrhosis.
6 Non-A–non-B hepatitis (hepatitis C).

H/TUMOURS

Benign
  Epithelial
  Mesenchymal
  Tumour-like lesions
Malignant
  Epithelial
  Non-epithelial
Secondary

Benign

Benign epithelial

Liver-cell adenoma

Aetiology
Mainly occurs in women of reproductive age and is associated with oral contraceptive usage. Fairly common.

Macroscopical
Well circumscribed, yellow–brown nodule 2–30 cm diameter. Usually solitary, occasionally multiple.

Microscopical
Well-differentiated hepatocytes are arranged in thickened plates with no accompanying portal tract structures. They are often vascular.

Complications
Haemorrhage, infarction, rupture. Malignant change occurs very rarely, if ever.

Clinical
Often asymptomatic, a mass being discovered incidentally. May present with abdominal pain due to complications listed above.

Bile duct adenoma

Aetiology
Unknown but may be hamartomatous rather than a true neoplasm.

Macroscopical
A small (<1 cm) firm pale discrete nodule.

Microscopial
Multiple small bile ductular structures embedded in a fibrous stroma.

Clinical
Usually an incidental finding at laparotomy or post mortem but may be mistaken for a metastasis.

Bile duct cystadenoma

Aetiology
Unknown.

Macroscopical
Multiloculated cysts containing mucoid material and of variable size (5–25 cm diameter).

Microscopical
Cysts lined by columnar mucinous epithelium which may have surrounding mesenchymal stroma.

Clinical
Abdominal pain or swelling with large lesions. Small risk of malignant change.

Benign mesenchymal

Haemangioma—cavernous

Aetiology
Unknown but probably a hamartoma rather than a true neoplasm.

Macroscopical
Well circumscribed, red nodule usually solitary and quite small—<5 cm diameter. Rarely haemangiomas may be very large—up to 20 cm diameter—'giant cavernous haemangioma'.

Microscopical
Blood-filled spaces separated by fibrous septa.

Clinical
Most common benign tumour of liver and usually discovered as a incidental finding at post mortem. Larger lesions may present with abdominal swelling.

Fatty tumours
Lipoma, angiolipoma, angiomyolipoma all occur very rarely.

Benign tumour-like lesions
A collection of inflammatory, hyperplastic and hamartomatous lesions which may be mistaken on gross appearances for true neoplasms.

Focal nodular hyperplasia

Aetiology
Unknown but possibly a response to vascular malformation.

Macroscopical
Well circumscribed, often subcapsular with a central fibrous scar. Usually solitary and less than 5 cm diameter.

Microscopical
The central fibrous scar contains blood vessels and bile ducts and is surrounded by hepatocyte regeneration nodules.

Clinical
Mostly asymptomatic but may be mistaken for cirrhosis histologically. The localized nature of this lesion is an important diagnostic clue.

Mesenchymal hamartoma

Aetiology
Unknown.

Macroscopical
Usually well circumscribed, of variable size—3–21 cm diameter, and soft with cystic spaces.

Microscopical
Predominantly mesenchymal tissue admixed with blood vessels and irregular epithelial structures which are probably bile ducts.

Clinical
Presents with abdominal swelling.

Inflammatory pseudo-tumour

Aetiology
Unknown.

Macroscopical
Usually a solitary mass 2–25 cm diameter.

Microscopical
Numerous inflammatory cells—lymphocytes, plasma cells, macrophages, admixed with spindle cells and fibrous tissue.

Clinical
Usually presents in children and young adults with non-specific symptoms—fever, weight loss, abdominal pain and hepatomegaly. Is frequently mistaken for malignancy.

Malignant
Hepatocellular carcinoma is the commonest primary malignant liver tumour, accounting for 85–90% of cases: bile duct carcinomas account for 5–10%. The other tumours described below are all rare.

Epithelial

Hepatocellular carcinoma—HCC

Aetiological factors
1 *Cirrhosis*: between 70% and 90% of HCCs in the UK arise in a background of cirrhosis.

2 *Geographical*: uncommon in UK—2–3% of cancers, but common in parts of Africa, Far East—up to 40% of cancers. The risk of HCC supervening in cirrhosis is relatively small in the UK—5–15%, but considerably greater in 'high-incidence' areas—up to 50%.

3 *Hepatitis B*: There is increasing evidence to implicate hepatitis B as the major factor in the aetiology of liver cell carcinoma.

(a) *Epidemiological studies*: high-risk areas for HCC have high incidence of hepatitis B carriage.

(b) *Serological studies*: increased incidence of hepatitis B surface antigen seen in patients with HCC.

(c) *Prospective studies in chronic HBsAg carriers*: these have a much higher risk of developing HCC than non-carriers—200-fold in one study.

(d) *Molecular biology*: integration of HBV–DNA sequences has been demonstrated in HCC cells.

4 *Other viruses*: many patients with HCC have positive serological markers for hepatitis C infection. It is not clear whether hepatitis C is present as an 'innocent bystander', coexisting with hepatitis B, or whether it has a causative role.

5 *Mycotoxins*: aflatoxins produced by the fungus *Aspergillus flavus* can induce liver cell cancers in experimental animals. The fungus frequently contaminates foods stored in hot humid conditions and may account for some of the geographical variation noted above.

6 *Sex*: male : female, 8–9 : 1.

7 *Alcohol*: alcohol may act as a co-carcinogen with hepatitis B but is probably not a hepatic carcinogen *per se*.

8 *Other drugs*: anabolic/androgenic steroids and the oral contraceptive pill have both been reported in association with HCC but the risk, if any, is very small.

Macroscopical
May form a solitary large mass but often multifocal. Vascular invasion is commonly visible grossly and may be associated with portal vein thrombosis.

Microscopical
In the classical form tumour cells resemble hepatocytes and are arranged in thickened trabeculae mimicking the pattern of normal liver. The presence of bile pigment in the cytoplasm of tumour cells is pathognomonic.

Pseudoglandular, clear cell, and pleomorphic variants also exist.

Positive immunoperoxidase staining for α-fetoprotein—present in 60–80% of cases and/or α_1-antitrypsin—present in up to 75%, may be useful as an adjunct to conventional histological diagnosis.

Spread
HCC has a marked tendency to spread via intrahepatic veins, both portal and hepatic.

Lymphatic spread to nodes around the porta hepatis is also seen but metastasis to distant sites is relatively uncommon—less than half of cases at autopsy.

Prognosis
Prognosis is poor with a median survival of less than 6 months from presentation.

Variants of liver cell carcinoma
A number of variants of liver cell cancer have been recognized recently. These are worthy of note because they have a better prognosis than the conventional tumours. In some cases improved prognosis may relate to ease of resectability rather than intrinsic differences in behaviour.

Fibrolamellar carcinoma

Aetiology
Unknown, but *not* associated with the risk factors described above. It occurs in a younger age group than conventional HCC—90% of cases <25 years old.

Macroscopical
Solitary large tumour with a central stellate scar arising in non-cirrhotic liver.

Microscopical
1 Large, polygonal cells with abundant eosinophilic cytoplasm.
2 Abundant fibrous stroma with characteristic lamellar arrangement.

'Minute'—encapsulated HCC

Aetiology
Most are associated with cirrhosis and occur mainly in Southeast Asia.

Macroscopical
A solitary, small (<5 cm diameter), tumour with surrounding fibrous capsule.

Microscopical
Well-differentiated, but otherwise similar to conventional HCC.

Pedunculated HCC
Resembles the conventional HCC histologically but differs in having a superficial location, possibly related to origin in an accessory lobe.

Cholangiocarcinoma—CC

Aetiology
1 *Liver flukes*: Clonorchis sinensis, Opisthorcis viverrini.
2 *Primary sclerosing cholangitis.*
3 *Congenital cystic disorders of biliary tree*: Caroli's disease, polycystic liver disease, choledochal cysts.
4 *Drugs*: thorotrast.

Macroscopical
1 *Hilar CC*: this is a tumour arising in the vicinity of the porta hepatis and typically presenting with obstructive jaundice.
2 *Peripheral CC*: a tumour arising in the substance of the liver. Presenting symptoms are less specific but include abdominal pain and swelling.

Microscopical
The majority are well-differentiated adenocarcinomas associated with variable mucin production and an abundant fibrous stroma.

Distinction from metastatic adenocarcinoma can be difficult. Presence of *in situ* carcinomatous change in adjacent bile ducts is a useful pointer.

Course
Prognosis is similar to HCC. Most patients are dead within a few months of presentation.

Hepatoblastoma

Aetiology
Unknown, but many cases are probably congenital and most present in the first 2 years of life. One-third of cases have other congenital malformations.

Appearances
A solitary, well-circumscribed tumour 5–25 cm diameter. Composed of a mixture of primitive epithelial structures sometimes admixed with mesenchymal components. Epithelial elements usually predominate.

Course
Rapidly progressive in untreated cases and usually fatal from local invasion and/or metastases. Improved prognosis has been obtained with aggressive surgery, combined with radiotherapy and chemotherapy.

Non-epithelial

Angiosarcoma

Aetiology
1 *Thorotrast*: radiological contrast medium used until mid-1950s when it was discontinued because of cancer risk. Long latent interval. Cases related to thorotrast are still occurring.
2 *Vinyl chloride monomer*: in PVC workers.
3 *Arsenic.*
4 *Anabolic steroids.*
In the majority of cases no underlying cause is found.

Appearances
There are multiple haemorrhagic nodules throughout the liver containing pleomorphic spindle cells of endothelial origin. Growth along hepatic sinusoids with intact liver cell plates is highly characteristic. Tumour cells also form primitive vascular structures and solid masses.

Positive immunoperoxidase staining factor VIII-related antigen is a useful marker of endothelial origin.

Infantile haemangioendothelioma
A rare vascular tumour of children; of unpredictable behaviour but less aggressive than angiosarcoma. Often locally invasive and occasionally metastatic.

Epithelioid haemangioendothelioma
A rare vascular tumour of adults with a wide range of histological appearances, which can mimic metastatic adenocarcinoma and non-neoplastic liver diseases such as veno-occlusive disease.

Behaviour is unpredictable but generally less aggressive than angiosarcoma.

Malignant lymphoma

The liver is commonly involved as a secondary site in Hodgkin's disease and non-Hodgkin's lymphomas.

Lymphoma occurs more rarely as a primary liver tumour.

Secondary Tumours

The liver is a very common site for metastasis, particularly from epithelial tumours.

Forty–fifty per cent of cases of primary non-hepatic carcinomas have liver metastases at necropsy. Common sites are the gastrointestinal tract, pancreas, lung and breast. There is also a high incidence of involvement by lymphoma and leukaemia.

Tumour deposits tend to outgrow blood supply, causing central necrosis and producing a characteristic umbilicated appearance.

The incidence of liver involvement with metastatic tumour greatly exceeds that of primary hepatic neoplasms.

Chapter 14
Diseases of the Liver and Biliary Tract—Biliary Tract

A/GALL BLADDER

Congenital
Inflammations
Calculi
Cholesterolosis
Mucocele
Tumours
  Benign
  Carcinoma

Congenital

Congenital abnormalties of the gall bladder are numerous and include anatomical variations of:

1 Shape and size, e.g. hour-glass deformity, diverticulum formation.

2 Number—duplication, triplication.

3 Position, e.g. left-sided, intrahepatic, retroperitoneal, 'floating' gall bladder—abnormally long mesentery rendering the gall bladder excessively mobile.

In some cases there may be complete failure to develop—*agenesis*.

Most of these abnormalities are uncommon and. apart from an increased tendency to gallstone formation, have little clinical significance. They are often revealed during radiological examinations of the biliary system and may cause difficulties with gall bladder surgery.

Inflammations

Acute cholecystitis

Pathogenesis

Acute calculous cholecystitis
Gallstones are the most important factor predisposing to acute cholecystitis and are present in more than 90% of cases.

Calculous obstruction of the cystic duct or neck of the gall bladder is thought to be the primary event. Bile is sterile at this stage. The initial inflammatory damage is thought to be chemically induced.

Secondary bacterial infection occurs in the majority of cases—*E. coli*, other Gram-negative rods and clostridia are the main organisms involved.

Acute acalculous cholecystitis
In less than 10% of cases acute cholecystitis occurs without gallstones.

Predisposing factors include severe trauma, surgery, burns, systemic vasculitis and bacteraemia.

Bacteria can be cultured in most cases—transient bacteraemia with seeding of the gall bladder is suspected.

Appearances
Typical features of acute inflammation are present with ulceration of the mucosa, oedema and inflammation of the wall and a fibrinopurulent serosal exudate

Results
1 *Gangrenous cholecystitis*: in some cases there may be full-thickness necrosis of the gall bladder wall, analogous to gangrenous appendicitis. This is caused by severe inflammation resulting in vascular thrombosis and subsequent infarction.

2 *Perforation*: this major complication of gangrenous cholecystitis occurs in 5–10% of cases of acute cholecystitis and may be associated with localized abscess formation or a generalized peritonitis. The latter is usually very severe because of the irritant effect of bile.

3 *Empyema*: this is a variant of acute cholecystitis in which the organ is distended by pus, and is associated with duct obstruction.

Chronic cholecystitis

Pathogenesis
Gallstones are present in more than 95% of cases. Some cases occur as a result of repeated episodes of acute cholecystitis. More often, the onset is insidious and occurs without any clinically evident antecedent acute attacks.

Appearances
1 *Fibrosis*: the main pathological feature is thickening of the gall bladder wall. This is mainly due to fibrosis, although varying degrees of muscular hypertrophy may also be present. In some cases there is shrinkage of the organ.

An extreme form of fibrous scarring associated with dystrophic calcification may produce a rigid organ—'*porcelain gall bladder*'.

2 *Inflammation*: the great majority of cases are associated with a chronic inflammatory infiltrate of lymphocytes, plasma cells and macrophages, although the degree of inflammation is very variable. In some cases chronic inflammatory changes are very marked with formation of numerous lymphoid follicles—*follicular cholecystitis*.

3 *Glandular outpouchings*: the lining mucosa forms glandular outpouchings—Aschoff–Rokitanksy sinuses. The term *cholecystitis glandularis proliferans* has been used to describe cases where these glandular proliferations are particularly numerous.

Mucosal herniations often contain inspissated bile and, in some cases, may rupture to form bile granulomas—*cholegranulomatous cholecystitis*.

Eosinophilic cholecystitis
A rare condition in which the gall bladder wall contains an inflammatory infiltrate composed almost entirely of eosinophils.

In most cases this is a localized phenomenon and the underlying cause is unknown. Rarely eosinophilic cholecystitis occurs as part of a systemic eosinophilic disease, e.g. in parasitic infestation.

Gallstones

Incidence
Gallstones are very common, being found in 10–15% of post-mortems.

Composition

Cholesterol stones

Mixed cholesterol stones
Eighty per cent. Composed mostly of cholesterol with smaller amounts of calcium salts, bile pigments and protein also present. Usually multiple with a faceted surface and a characteristic laminated structure on sectioning. Only about 10% contain enough calcium to be visible on plain X-ray.

'Pure' cholesterol stones
Ten per cent. Usually solitary, pale yellow, up to 5 cm diameter with a radial arrangement of crystals on section.

Pigment stones
These form about 10% of calculi and are composed of calcium bilirubinate. They are usually multiple, small and dark in colour.

Aetiology
Predisposing factors are:

1 *Age*: increasing prevalence with age.

2 *Sex*: Female : male ratio approximately 2 : 1. The difference in sex incidence declines after the menopause. Multiple pregnancies may also increase the predisposition.

3 *Diet/obesity*: these may be important, by increasing cholesterol secretion from the liver.

4 *Drugs*: clofibrate and oestrogens.

5 *Gastrointestinal disease*: Crohn's disease, jejuno-ileal bypass and intestinal resection. These may all interfere with enterohepatic circulation of bile salts.

6 *Geographical*: high incidence of cholesterol stones in developed countries, e.g. Europe, North America and a high incidence of pigment stones in the Far East.

7 *Chronic haemolytic diseases*: including sickle-cell disease, thalassaemia, hereditary spherocytosis. These are associated with a high incidence of pigment stones.

Pathogenesis

Cholesterol stones
The precise mechanisms involved in the formation of cholesterol stones are not known but three main stages are probably involved:

1 *Abnormal bile composition—lithogenic bile*: cholesterol is virtually insoluble in water and is kept in solution by the combined detergent action of phospholipids and bile salts to form micelles.

Supersaturation of bile with cholesterol is an important factor predisposing to gallstone formation.

2 *Nucleation*: this is the process whereby cholesterol is precipitated to initiate stone formation. The factors involved in this critical stage are not known, but two main mechanisms have been suggested:

(a) Mucus hypersecretion with cholesterol deposition around mucus particles.

(b) Deficiency of antinucleating factors, possibly lipoproteins. Bacteria and parasites have also been proposed as possible nucleating agents but in most cases there is little evidence to implicate infection as an initiating factor.

3 *Growth of stone*: once the initial nucleus has been formed, subsequent growth occurs by a process of accretion. The mechanisms involved at this stage are also poorly understood but local factors such as infection and stasis are thought to be important.

Pigment stones

In normal bile, bilirubin is excreted in a conjugated form as bilirubin glucuronide. Pigment stones develop when there is an increased concentration of unconjugated bilirubin in the bile. Two main mechanisms are thought to be involved.

1 Hypersecretion of bilirubin in bile—this may account for the high incidence of pigment stones in chronic haemolytic states.

2 Secretion of glucuronidase with release of free bilirubin. The high incidence of pigment stones in the Far East is thought to be the result of bacterial infection.

Effects

1 *None*: many patients remain asymptomatic throughout life, with stones revealed as an incidental finding at autopsy.

2 *Acute cholecystitis*.

3 *Chronic cholecystitis*.

4 *Obstruction of cystic duct*: predisposes to cholecystitis (acute and chronic) and may cause biliary colic. If obstruction is complete and unrelieved it may lead to development of mucocele or empyema.

5 *Migration to bile duct*: causes obstructive jaundice and ascending cholangitis and predisposes to acute pancreatitis (see p. 352).

6 *Gallstone ileus*: a rare complication in which a large stone erodes through the wall of the gall bladder via a fistula into an adherent loop of small intestine. The stone then migrates and may cause intestinal obstruction, usually in the terminal ileum.

7 *Carcinoma of gall bladder*: most carcinomas of gall bladder occur in a background of cholelithiasis (see p. 261), but it is not clear whether there is a causal relationship.

Cholesterolosis

Collections of foamy, lipid-laden macrophages accumulate in the mucosa of the gall bladder to produce a characteristic macroscopic appearance with yellowish flecks and streaks in a reddish mucosa—'*strawberry gall bladder*'.

This is a symptomless condition, but commonly accompanies, and may predispose to, cholesterol stones.

In some cases the lipid deposits may increase in size to produce localized polypoidal lesions—*cholesterol polyps*.

Mucocele

This condition occurs when a stone impacts in the neck of the gall bladder or cystic duct without superadded infection. The gall bladder may be distended to several times its original size by thick mucinous secretions.

Tumours

Benign

'Adenomyoma'

A circumscribed usually fundal nodule composed of irregular glandular structures admixed with interlacing bundles of hyperplastic smooth muscle fibres.

The precise nature of this lesion is uncertain, but it is probably a localized hyperplastic phenomenon, possibly in response to obstruction, rather than a true neoplasm.

Adenoma

This is a true neoplasm arising from the gall bladder mucosa and usually presenting as a pedunculated polyp. Histologically it may be present in a papillary form—*papilloma*, or have a non-papillary pattern. Malignant transformation occurs in a minority of cases.

Cholesterol polyps

These are thought to represent localized forms of cholesterolosis and not true neoplasms (see above).

Connective tissue

Benign tumours may rarely arise from the wall of the gall bladder including leiomyoma, lipoma, fibroma and haemangioma.

Malignant

Carcinoma of the gall bladder

Incidence and aetiology

Occurs mainly in elderly people (60–70 years) with a female : male ratio of 2–3 : 1.

The majority of cases—80–90%, are associated with gallstones and chronic cholecystitis. It has been postulated that these factors predispose to the development of cancer, possibly by causing chronic irritation, but a causal relationship has not been proven. Approximately 0.5–1% of people with gallstones develop carcinoma of the gall bladder.

Appearances

Macroscopical

1 *Diffuse infiltrating*: gritty diffuse thickening with ulceration of mucosa and early serosal or liver invasion.
2 *Fungating*: protuberance into the lumen, usually with a papillary structure.

Microscopical

1 *Adenocarcinoma*: in 80–90% of cases. Mucus-secreting columnar cell type.
2 *Squamous carcinoma*: in 10%.
3 *Adenosquamous carcinoma*: mixed pattern and uncommon.
4 *Anaplastic carcinoma* of 'oat-cell' type.

Clinical features

Clinical presentation is often insidious and many cases are observed as an incidental finding in gall bladders removed for presumed chronic cholecystitis. Others present with symptoms related to local or systemic spread.

Spread

Most cases have spread by the time of diagnosis.
1 *Local*: direct invasion of liver, bile ducts, etc., commonly accompanied by jaundice.
2 *Lymphatic*: to lymph nodes in the porta hepatis.
3 *Blood*: most commonly to liver and lungs.

Prognosis

Tumours are rarely discovered at a resectable stage and 5-year survival rates are less than 1%.

Other malignant epithelial tumours

These are all very rare but include carcinosarcoma, malignant melanoma and carcinoid tumour.

Connective tissue

Rhabdomyosarcoma of embryonal type, malignant fibrous histiocytoma, and leiomyosarcoma are all extremely rare.

B/EXTRAHEPATIC BILE DUCTS

Congenital
Inflammatory
   Cholangitis
Stricture
Tumours
   Benign
   Carcinoma

Congenital

Accessory bile ducts

Rare, but can be of surgical importance.

Choledochal cyst

Cystic dilatation of the common bile duct, which may reach a diameter of up to 5–6 cm.

The majority of cases become symptomatic with complications related to obstruction, infection and stone formation. There is also a risk of malignant transformation, which occurs in up to 15% of cases.

Extrahepatic biliary atresia

This is a serious condition presenting as obstructive jaundice in the neonatal period. Secondary changes occur in the liver (see p. 245).

Inflammatory

Primary sclerosing cholangitis

Nature
A fibrosing, inflammatory condition affecting extra- and intrahepatic bile ducts (*see also* p. 244).

Appearances
Affected bile ducts are thickened by fibrosis and infiltrated by chronic inflammatory cells. The lumen is narrowed as a result of these changes. Areas of mucosal ulceration are commonly present.

Effects
1 Chronic biliary obstruction with secondary biliary cirrhosis (*see* p. 245).
2 Episodes of ascending cholangitis.
3 Malignant transformation—*cholangiocarcinoma*.

Benign stricture of bile duct

Aetiology
1 *Surgical*: most common, e.g. accidental ligature, surgical trauma during cholecystectomy and insertion of T-tube.
2 *Other causes*: rare but include perforated duodenal ulcer, chronic pancreatitis and gallstones.

Appearances
Fibrous thickening of bile duct wall, usually a variable-length segment. Some inflammatory changes may also be present.

Effects
1 *Obstructive jaundice.*
2 *Ascending cholangitis.*
3 *Biliary cirrhosis*: if obstruction is unrelieved, there is progressive portal fibrosis in the liver resulting eventually in cirrhosis (*see* p. 243).

Tumours of extrahepatic bile ducts

Benign
These are all rare. The most common presenting symptom is obstructive jaundice.

Epithelial
1 *Adenoma*: a polypoidal lesion growing into lumen of bile duct which often has a papillary pattern histologically. Malignant transformation is common.
2 *Cystadenoma*.

3 *Heterotopic pancreatic issue*: not a neoplasm.

Non-epithelial
Leiomyoma, lipoma and haemangioma occur rarely.

Malignant

Carcinoma of extrahepatic bile ducts

Aetiology
The predisposing factors are similar to those associated with carcinoma of the intrahepatic bile ducts (*see* p. 256).

Sites
Can occur anywhere along the biliary tree but approximately 50% arise in the upper third of the extrahepatic bile ducts.

Macroscopical
Three main types are recognized:
1 Fungating.
2 Intramural nodules.
3 Diffuse infiltrating.

Microscopical
1 *Adenocarcinoma*: more than 90%. Diffuse infiltrating types frequently have an abundant fibrous stroma giving rise to a characteristic scirrhous appearance. Tumours arising around the ampulla usually have a papillary pattern and form polypoidal masses.
2 *Squamous cell carcinoma*.
3 *Adenosquamous carcinoma*.
4 *Anaplastic carcinoma*.

Effects
The great majority of cases present with symptoms of bile duct obstruction. Superadded infection with ascending cholangitis occurs in a proportion of these.

Prognosis
The prognosis is variable and depends on the extent of spread at the time of diagnosis, but with an overall mean survival time of 6–12 months. Tumours arising in the vicinity of the ampulla of Vater may respond favourably to surgical resection by Whipple's procedure. Five-year survival rates in excess of 75% are reported for localized lesions in this region.

Other malignant tumours
Embryonal rhabdomyosarcoma, leiomyosarcoma and malignant lymphoma rarely occur.

Chapter 15
Diseases of the Lymphoreticular System

A/LYMPH NODES

Normal
Congenital
Acquired abnormal immune function
Reactive and inflammatory
  Non-specific reactive
  Non-specific inflammatory
  Specific reactive and inflammatory
Tumours
  Non-Hodgkin's lymphoma
  Hodgkin's disease
Secondary tumours

Normal

Anatomy

The lymph nodes and spleen are the principal lymphoid organs of the body. The main sites where lymph nodes are concentrated are neck, axillae, mediastinum, lung hilae, para-aortic, iliac and inguinal regions. Specialized lymphoid tissue or cells are also widely distributed in many other organs: the thymus is rich in T lymphocytes and mucosal tissues such as the gut, nasopharynx and lung have organ- or site-specific B lymphoid tissue known as mucosa-assiciated lymphoid tissue—MALT (*see also* p. 32).

Lymph node structure and function

Lymph nodes vary in size from less than 1 mm to over 2 cm. They contain a mixed population of cells including B lymphoid and T lymphoid cells, antigen processing and presenting cells of reticuloendothelial origin, macrophages, and stromal cells such as fibroblasts and endothelial cells. These cells may be static or circulate. Cells may enter the node via the afferent lymphatics—B cells, peripheral sinus or through paracortical high endothelial venules—T cells.

Lymph nodes are organized into three distinct zones (see Fig. 23):

Cortex

The cortex containing principally B lymphoid tissue is organized into *germinal follicles*. There is a surrounding *mantle zone* of small lymphocytes. The germinal centres contain a mixed population of two main types of transformed lymphoid cells:

1 *Centroblasts*: lymphoid cells with large rounded nuclei and multiple prominent nucleoli.
2 *Centrocytes*: lymphoid cells with small or large irregular nuclei and a dispersed nuclear chromatin.

Also present are:

3 *Dendritic reticulum cells*: antigen-presenting cells of the germinal follicle of reticuloendothelial origins.
4 *Tingible body macrophages*: responsible for removing cellular debris.

This zone undergoes rapid expansion during the humoral antibody response. The principal cellular processes involved in antigen processing, B lymphoid cell activation and transformation and plasma cell production are still speculative.

Paracortex

The interfollicular T zone or paracortex contains principally T lymphoid cells which are of two main types:

1 *Small T lymphocytes*: a large population of small T lymphocytes.
2 *Larger T immunoblasts*: a subpopulation of larger T immunoblasts, transformed large cells with rounded nuclei and central prominent nucleoli.

Also present are:

3 *Interdigitating reticulum cells*: specialized reticuloendothelial cells which are thought to have a role in antigen presentation or lymphoid cell communication.
4 *Specialized postcapillary venules*: these have large endothelial cells which are a distinctive feature of this region and T lymphocytes can usually be seen in the process of travelling between these endothelial cells. This area expands during the cell-mediated

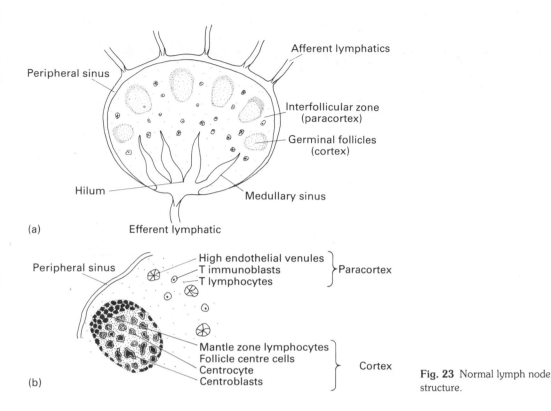

(a)

(b)

Fig. 23 Normal lymph node structure.

response. The precise mechanisms of T-cell activation transformation and proliferation are also still speculative.

Medulla

The medulla contains a mixture of:

1 B cells—predominantly plasma cells.
2 T cells.
3 Macrophages.

These are all arranged in cords with intervening sinusoid spaces. The efferent lymph-containing antibody, passes from the node via medullary sinus into the hilum and the efferent lymphatic. The macrophages present have a phagocytic function.

Lymphoid cell phenotype, maturation and transformation

Uncommitted lymphoid cells are presumed to originate in the bone marrow from stem cells and are thought to progress along a B cell or T cell lineage pathway after processing in bursa-equivalent Peyer's patches or thymus respectively.

Lymphocytes of all classes carry cell surface molecules which enable cell-to-cell recognition and interaction. They can be identified in the laboratory through immunofluorescence or immunocytochemical techniques using labelled antibodies specific for a particular molecular cell marker.

These markers, along with other reticuloendothelial cell markers, are now recognized by an international classification known as the *cluster differentiation system—CD*. They can be used to identify the lineage and particular class of lymphoid cells and are now widely used for lymphoid cell and lymphoma recognition and classification (*see* Table 15.1).

Both B and T lymphocytes undergo a specific process of DNA rearrangement following activation by appropriate novel antigen stimulus. In B cells this involves the immunoglobulin gene and results in the high specificity of the antigen-binding region of the antibody produced. Many different B cells will undergo transformation during the humoral response and a variety (polyclonal) of antibodies of different structure but similar antigen recognition specificity will be produced. Antibody can be identified by immunocytochemistry on the cell surface or in the

Table 15.1 Commonly used lymphoid cell phenotype markers.

Cell type	CD number	Name of molecule
All lymphoid cells	45	Common leucocyte antigen
B cells	19, 20, 22 Surface Ig	Surface pan B cell Immunoglobulin
T cells	1 3, 5 4 8	Thymocyte Pan peripheral T cell T-helper T-suppressor
Hodgkin's cells activated lymphoid cells	15 30	LeuM1 BerH2

cytoplasm in such B cells. Both specific heavy and light chain components will be produced with similar specificities in a reactive process depending on the stage of the reaction. One plasma cell can only produce one light chain type.

In a reactive process both kappa- and lambda-producing B lymphoid cells and plasma cells can be identified. B cell lymphomas will only have cells with one light chain class—monoclonal.

A similar process of rearrangement of the T cell receptor gene occurs during T cell transformation in the cell-mediated response. T cell receptors are similar in structure to immunoglobulins and are present on the surface of T cells.

At present antibodies to recognize various classes of these molecules are not available. Polyclonal and monoclonal T cell populations can be identified only by molecular DNA blotting technology, which requires specialist laboratory facilities.

Congenital

Inherited abnormalities of immune function

There are a variety of inherited abnormalities of immune function which are generally classified as defects of:

1 *Humoral immunity*, causing agammaglobulin-aemia or hypogammaglobulinaemia or abnormalities of a single immunoglobulin class.

2 *Cellular immunity*, which is usually associated with thymic hypoplasia.

The lymph nodes lack cortical or paracortical structures respectively and affected individuals usually die of either bacterial or viral respiratory infection in early childhood.

Acquired abnormalities of immune function

Treatment-associated immune deficiency

Both radiotherapy and chemotherapy can lead to immune suppression which can be associated with life-threatening opportunistic infections.

HIV infection

The human immunodeficiency virus HTLV–III is a lymphotrophic virus infection which affects T lymphocytes. Infection leads to reversal of T helper/suppressor cell ratio and a progressive lymphocytosis. The resulting immunodeficiency state predisposes affected individuals to a variety of opportunistic infections such as pneumocystis pneumonia, tuberculosis, cryptococcosis, herpes, candida and cytomegalovirus infection (see also p. 3).

HIV infection—lymph node effects

Following HIV infection a number of usually progressive changes may occur.

1 A significant proportion of individuals develop a form of generalized lymphadenopathy with fever and weight loss—*persistent generalized lymphadenopathy*. This often precedes overt evidence of AIDS. The lymph nodes show marked follicular hyperplasia, paracortical hyperplasia and additional florid reactive changes.

2 During progression to AIDS the lymph nodes undergo a process of involution with marked regression of follicles and fibrosis.

3 There is a transitional phase which has similarities to angioimmunoblastic lymphadenopathy.

4 AIDS patients have a very high incidence of malignant lymphoma, usually of high grade B cell type. Kaposi's sarcoma which is associated with AIDS may also arise in lymph nodes (see p. 419).

Reactive and inflammatory

Non-specific reactive

Lymph nodes may respond to various stimuli in a similar fashion. These are usually classified as follows:

Follicular hyperplasia

Enlarged prominent germinal centres demonstrating a hormonal type response usually to a bacterial infection, e.g. in lymph nodes draining an abscess. With persistent stimulation the follicles may expand to a large size—*'giant follicles'*—or may enlarge and break up with an intermingling of small lymphocytes—*'progressive transformation of germinal centres'*. This latter condition has been linked with lymphocyte-predominant Hodgkin's disease (see p. 276).

Paracortical hyperplasia

Expansion of the paracortex T zone without follicular enlargement indicating activation of cell-mediated immune response which is usually due to a viral infection. Infectious mononucleosis can result in very florid paracortical hyperplasia with numerous blast cells present which can lead to a misdiagnosis of malignant lymphoma.

Mixed

Most frequently a dual hyperplasia of both germinal follicles and the paracortex is seen indicating synchronous B and T cell responses.

Sinus and pulp histiocytosis

The sinuses or pulp of the node becomes filled with histiocytes—*activated macrophages*—which often show evidence of phagocytosis of debris. It occurs in response to a local or generalized tissue accumulation of macrophages which then migrate to the lymph nodes.

Specific patterns can be seen in dermatopathic lymphadenopathy (see p. 267) after lymphangiography when colloidal oils accumulate, in the lipid storage diseases such as Gaucher's disease (see p. 293), Niemann–Pick disease (p. 249) and Whipple's disease (see p. 35).

Non-specific inflammatory

Acute lymphadenitis

Various forms exist. Nodes draining sites of inflammation such as ulcers or abscess may show varying degrees. Changes range from mild with sinus dilatation by macrophages, to florid suppurative with neutrophil polymorphs present in peripheral sinuses and node parenchyma.

Staphylococcal infection can cause the most florid changes.

Some types of infection such as cat scratch disease (see p. 267) can give a picture of acute lymphadenitis with necrosis. Irregular areas of necrosis surrounded by macrophages is the typical picture.

A particular form of acute necrotizing lymphadenitis associated with malaise and slight fever, known as *Kikuchi's disease*, has more extensive nodal necrosis and inflammation.

Chronic lymphadenitis

An ill-defined entity. The lymph node shows variable changes including reactive hyperplasia, macrophage accumulation, collections of plasma cells and fibrosis. The picture is commonest in nodes from the inguinal region.

Granulomatous lymphadenitis

A wide variety of conditions can lead to granuloma formation in lymph nodes. The granulomas can range from small collections of histiocytes to confluence of large necrotizing granulomas. The character of the granuloma may relate to the underlying cause but cannot always be relied upon for diagnosis.

1 *Granuloma with bland necrosis*: tuberculosis, atypical mycobacterial infection, tularaemia, histoplasmosis, kala-azar.
2 *Acute necrotizing granuloma*: cat scratch disease, lymphogranuloma venereum, *Yersinia* infection.
3 *Small discrete granulomas*: sarcoidosis, Crohn's disease, berylliosis, malignant tumours, drug reactions.
4 *Single or small groups of macrophages*: toxoplasmosis, infectious mononucleosis.

Specific reactive and inflammatory

The type of reaction present in a lymph node, particularly if florid, can in some cases lead to identification of the underlying cause. Some of the more common are discussed below.

Sarcoidosis

A common disease of adults of all ages. It is seen much more frequently in Western populations and is of unknown aetiology. Lymphadenopathy is common and bilateral hilar lymph node enlargement is a very frequent finding in young adults (see p. 394). Other sites of involvement include lungs, skin, eyes, salivary gland and bone (see p. 15 and p. 19). The diagnosis is made by lymph node biopsy or cutaneous Kveim test.

Appearances

The nodes are enlarged but usually under 2 cm, firm and of a pale uniform colour. The node is variably but often extensively replaced by granulomas of small non-specific type (see above). These may coalesce but their discrete nature is still apparent. The residual lymph node tissue shows little reaction. Multinucleate giant cells are often present and may contain inclusions of a laminated calcified type—'Schaumann bodies'—or a star-shaped crystalline type—'asteroid bodies.

Significance

The disease may respond to steroids and is usually self-limiting. Other conditions, e.g. introduction of some types of foreign material such as beryllium, talc and zirconium used in antiperspirants, and Crohn's disease can give a similar appearance.

Dermatopathic lymphadenopathy

Nature

A form of pulp and sinus histiocytosis seen in lymph nodes draining sites of chronic skin disease, usually of inflammatory type such as psoriasis or eczema (see p. 413), and rarely of a neoplastic type—mycosis fungoides (see p. 419).

Appearances

The nodes are usually less than 2 cm diameter and may have a yellow or brown colour due to melanin accumulation. There is a characteristic, often pronounced, paracortical accumulation of interdigitating reticulum cells with a subpopulation of macrophages containing melanin pigment.

Significance

A benign reactive condition which can be mistaken clinically for malignant lymphoma. It can also occur in association with the skin lymphoma—*mycosis fungoides* (see p. 275).

Sinus histiocytosis with massive lymphadenopathy—Rosai—Dorfman disease

Nature

A dramatic reactive condition with changes identical to reactive sinus histiocytosis but leading to massive lymphadenopathy. It affects Negroes more frequently than Caucasians, presents usually in childhood and

causes massive painless bilateral enlargement of cervical glands or, less commonly, other groups.

Appearances

The lymph node shows marked sinusoidal accumulation of large distinctive histiocytes and giant cells, many showing phagocytosis of lymphocytes and other cells.

Significance

It is recognized as a distinctive clinicopathological entity. The natural history is of disease progression over months or years with phases of remission and relapse but eventual compete resolution. There is no effective form of therapy.

Cat scratch disease

Nature

Found where cats are kept as pets. A bacillary agent, probably chlamydial, has recently been identified in lymph nodes during infection. The disease typically occurs following a bite or scratch from a cat which is followed by lymphadenopathy of the draining nodes in a few days or weeks.

Appearances

The nodes are moderately enlarged. Areas of necrosis may be visible to the naked eye. There is a striking histological similarity to lymphogranuloma venereum and *Yersinia* infection (see below). The whole node shows a generalized mixed non-specific reactive picture with areas of histiocyte accumulation which progress to microabscesses with central necrosis. The histiocytes tend to be arranged around the necrotic irregularly outlined centre in a palisaded fashion. Bacillary organisms can be identified in histiocytes using silver stains, e.g. Warthin–Starry.

Significance

A self-limiting disease usually resolving within a few weeks or months and with no sequelae. A skin test using an antigen prepared from an infected lymph node may assist diagnosis.

Lymphogranuloma venereum

Nature

A sexually transmitted disease caused by *Chlamydia trachomatis* (see also p. 143). It is seen worldwide but is commonest in the tropics. The disease is usually most severe and persists longer in females than males. The primary lesion, a vesicle or ulcer, develops usually on the cervix or penis and may heal before lymphadenopathy, the principal lesion, develops. The groin and sometimes iliac and pelvic nodes enlarge, matt together, fix to the skin and break down forming sinuses. There may be associated constitutional symptoms.

Appearance

A picture virtually identical to that seen with cat scratch disease. The abscesses are often larger and may coalesce. Healing occurs with marked scarring.

Significance

A self-limiting disease but scarring is frequent. In females with severe disease vulval oedema due to lymphatic obstruction and vulval and rectal scarring can occur (see p. 203).

Yersinia infection—pseudotuberculosis

Nature

The organisms *Yersinia pseudotuberculosis* and *Y. enterocolitica* cause a form of enteritis frequently associated with marked mesenteric lymphadenitis. The organisms are carried by rodents and wood pigeons and are transmitted through eating contaminated, poorly prepared food. The diagnosis can be made from the appropriate history and clinical findings supported by serology.

Appearance

The mesenteric lymph nodes show an appearance virtually identical to lymphogranuloma venereum and cat scratch disease with large necrotizing areas of histiocyte accumulation in which Gram-negative acid-fast diplobacilli may be found. The presenting findings and involved lymph node site help to distinguish these conditions.

Significance

A self-limiting condition which may respond to broad spectrum antibiotics.

Infectious mononucleosis—glandular fever

Nature

A very common, often debilitating, disease of young adults in the Western world caused by the Epstein–Barr virus. The sexes are equally affected, transmission usually being mouth to mouth, hence the colloquial term 'kissing disease'. Symptoms are usually sore throat, fever and generalized lymphadenopathy. In addition splenomegaly and hepatic and CNS involvement may occur. The peripheral blood contains characteristic transformed lymphocytes. The diagnostic *Paul Bunnell test* recognizes sheep heterophil erythrocyte agglutinating antibodies in the serum.

It is interesting to note that the same virus is important in Burkitt's lymphoma (see p. 272) and nasopharyngeal carcinoma (see p. 361).

Appearances

Lymph node biopsy is rarely performed in suspected disease as simple serological tests are available for diagnosis. The nodes are enlarged to less than 3 cm and show a progressive enlargement of the paracortex which may efface cortical structures. The paracortex contains numerous large transformed T cells, 'immunoblasts', and smaller cells corresponding to the circulating cells. The changes can easily be mistaken for malignant lymphoma due to the active character of the changes and replacement of normal structures.

Significance

The disease is self-limiting but the course may be prolonged. Rare complications such as splenic rupture, jaundice and encephalomyelitis may occur.

Toxoplasmosis

Nature

The commonest human protozoal infection in UK and Europe caused by the organism *Toxoplasma gondii*. The usual route of infection is food contamination by cat faeces but other routes, including transplacental infection, are recognized (see p. 6). Lymphadenopathy, usually of the head or neck, is the most frequent presenting symptom, often with associated malaise and pyrexia.

Appearances

The nodes are seldom larger than 3 cm in size and show three distinctive histological features:
1 Follicular hyperplasia.
2 Epithelial cell aggregates.
3 Sinusoidal accumulation of 'monocytoid' stimulated B lymphocytes.

When these features are prominent the picture is said to be characteristic, but diagnosis should be supported by the appropriate serological tests.

Significance

The node appearances and clinical findings can be similar to infectious mononucleosis which can be excluded by toxoplasma complement fixation tests and Paul Bunnell testing. The disease is usually self-limiting although the lymphadenopathy may persist for many months. Severe infections may respond to antibiotic therapy.

Angioimmunoblastic lymphadenopathy—AILD

Nature

A clinicopathological entity of unknown origin usually affecting older individuals. Patients usually present with severe malaise, generalized lymphadenopathy, fever, hepatosplenomegaly and skin rash. Anaemia, often Coombs' positive, polyclonal hypergamma-globulinaemia, lymphopenia with leucocytosis and autoantibodies are usual. A wide variety of additional clinical and laboratory abnormalities may also occur.

Appearances

The lymph nodes are usually enlarged to 2–3 cm and tender. Histologically there is a characteristic expansion of the paracortical zone leading to effacement of the normal node structure. The proliferation includes prominent branching 'arborizing' small blood vessels lined by large endothelial cells and a mixed population of plasma cells, lymphoid cells and large transformed lymphoid cells.

Significance

A high proportion of cases progress to overt malignant lymphoma. It has been suggested that this condition may be an exaggerated form of hyper-immune reaction but recently clonal populations of lymphoid cells have been recognized in some cases, indicating that at least an underlying malignant lymphoma may be present (see p. 273).

Castleman's disease

Nature

A form of lymphoid proliferation of uncertain origin and significance described in three forms:

1 Localized hyaline vascular type.
2 Localized plasma cell type.
3 Multicentric type.

The latter is often associated with systemic symptoms and disturbances. Thoracic structures, particularly the mediastinum, are the commonest sites but it has been reported in many other tissues including mesentery, retroperitoneum and muscle.

Appearances

The lesions are usually well defined with a homogeneous cut surface. Microscopically the tissue resembles the structure of a lymph node but with absent sinuses. A prominent feature is the presence of numerous small follicular structures which have a centrally placed small vessel often with surrounding hyaline material. Small lymphoid cells are arranged in a concentric formation around these vessels. The interfollicular areas contain small lymphoid cells or abundant plasma cells in the plasma cell type.

Significance

Castleman's disease is generally regarded as an unusual reactive condition which is often self-limiting. In some patients immune suppression may occur leading to infection. There is an association with malignant lymphoma which is also currently poorly understood. Some cases have been shown to have a clonal population of cells which may represent an early lymphoma. Lymphoma developing after a diagnosis of Castleman's disease is also seen.

Tumours

Primary—malignant lymphoma, non-Hodgkin's lymphoma

Aetiology and epidemiology

The aetiology of most lymphomas is unknown but there are known associated factors with certain types:
1 *Radiation*: associated with general increase in incidence.
2 *Geographical*:
  (a) Burkitt's lymphoma in childhood associated with malarial and Epstein–Barr virus infections.
  (b) B cell lymphomas are more common in Western countries—80–90%.
  (c) T cell lymphoma predominant in some parts of Japan (see Table 15.2).
  (d) HTLV infection associated with specific types of

Table 15.2 Phenotype distribution (%) of malignant lymphomas in different countries.

	B	T	Not defined
Europe	80	6	14
USA	67	15	18
Japan	50	38	12

T cell lymphoma in the Caribbean and Japan.

3 *AIDS*: high incidence of malignant lymphoma virtually exclusively B cell (see p. 265).

4 *Autoimmune disorders*: includng Sjögren's syndrome (see p. 103) and Hashimoto's thyroiditis (see p. 128) are associated with lymphoplasmacytoid lymphomas.

5 *Chromosomal abnormalities*: particularly translocations involving the same break point on chromosome 14—Burkitt's lymphoma 8 : 14, follicular lymphoma 14 : 18, lymphocytic lymphoma 11 : 14.

Age and sex

Occur at all ages with a male predominance. There is an age variation between types and grades; children usually develop high-grade blast cell tumours whereas low-grade B cell tumours are virtually confined to adults.

Clinical

Presentation usually by painless enlargement of one or more lymph nodes, although malignant lymphoma is often more generalized and affects extranodal sites, e.g. Waldeyer's ring, gastrointestinal tract and skin, more often than Hodgkin's disease. Constitutional B type symptoms are uncommon.

Macroscopical

Enlarged lymph nodes or groups of adherent lymph nodes. The tumour has a fleshy, pale usually homogeneous appearance, although an indistinct nodular pattern may be seen with follicular lymphoma (see p. 272). Areas of necrosis or haemorrhage may be present in high-grade tumours.

Microscopical classification

Lymph nodes contain a wide variety of cell types with various forms of B and T lymphoid cells, specialized and non-specialized macrophages as well as stromal cells. Malignant lymphomas may develop from or show differentiation towards most of these cell types.

Modern classification of lymphoma is based on identification of the tumour cell phenotype (see Table 15.2), genotype with recognition of its normal nodal counterpart and the cellular organization in the tissues.

The Kiel classification is the most widely accepted

Table 15.3 The Working Formulation classification of malignant lymphomas.

Low grade	High grade
A Malignant lymphoma Small lymphocytic	H Malignant lymphoma Large cell, immunoblastic
B Malignant lymphoma, follicular Predominantly small cleaved cell	I Malignant lymphoma Lymphoblastic
C Malignant lymphoma, follicular Mixed, small cleaved and large cell	J Malignant lymphoma Small non-cleaved cell
Intermediate grade	*Miscellaneous*
D Malignant lymphoma, follicular Predominantly large cell	Composite Mycosis fungoides Histiocytic
E Malignant lymphoma, diffuse Small cleaved cell	Extramedullary plasmacytoma Unclassifiable Other
F Malignant lymphoma, diffuse Mixed, small and large cell	
G Malignant lymphoma, diffuse Large cell	

Table 15.4 The updated Kiel classification of non-Hodgkin's lymphomas.

B	T
Low grade	*Low grade*
Lymphocytic—chronic lymphocytic and prolymphocytic leukaemia; hairy-cell leukaemia	Lymphocytic—chronic lymphocytic and prolymphocytic leukaemia
	Small cerebriform cell—mycosis fungoides, Sezary's syndrome
Lymphoplasmacytic/cytoid (LP immunocytoma)	Lymphoepitheloid—Lennert's lymphoma
Plasmacytic	Angioimmunoblastic—AILD, LgX
Centroblastic/centrocytic	
follicular ± diffuse	T zone
diffuse	Pleomorphic, small cell (HTLV-I ±)
High grade	*High grade*
Centroblastic	Pleomorphic, medium and large cell (HTLV-I ±)
Immunoblastic	Immunoblastic (HTLV-I ±)
Large cell anaplastic (Ki-1 +)	Large cell anaplastic (Ki-1 +)
Burkitt's lymphoma	
Lymphoblastic	Lymphoblastic
Rare types/unclassified	*Rare types/unclassified*

modern classification in Europe and is dealt with in detail above. The Working Formulation is generally used in the United States (see Table 15.3).

Earlier classifications such as Rappaport's, used only cell size and cellular arrangement and have limited pathological relevance. More accurate understanding of the dynamic interactions and processes of lymphoid cell transformation during the immune response will undoubtedly lead to further modification of the current classifications (see Tables 15.3 and 15.4).

The updated Kiel classification

This classification separates B cell and T cell lymphomas into low and high grade types (Table 15.4).

B cell lymphomas—low grade

Lymphocytic/B chronic lymphocytic leukaemia

A common type of lymphoma in adults over middle age which is composed of diffuse sheets of small lymphoid cells. These cells have surface immunoglobulin and resemble mature small lymphocytes. The condition has an overlap with chronic lymphocytic leukaemia (CLL) and patients may have lymph node disease, lymphocytosis and bone marrow involvement. Lymphadenopathy when present is usually generalized. It is an indolent disease which progresses slowly. Death is from other coexistent disease, viral infection, anaemia or progression of the lymphoma.

Lymphoplasmacytoid

Similar to lymphocytic lymphoma but tumour cells have features of plasma cells and show cytoplasmic immunoglobulin synthesis. It presents as nodal disease, extranodal solitary tumour, leukaemia resembling CLL or 'hyperviscosity syndrome'. The latter is caused by tumour cell secretion of μ heavy chain immunoglobulin leading to a high IgM paraproteinaemia (very rarely IgG or IgA). In the node the tumour cells are arranged in diffuse sheets. They may contain intracytoplasmic Russell bodies or intranuclear Dutcher bodies—inclusions of immunoglobulin. Extracellular deposits resembling amyloid may be present. The behaviour is indolent, with death usually either from infection or disease progression. Transformation to high-grade lymphoma is rare.

Plasmacytic—plasmacytoma— extramedullary plasmacytoma

Similar to myeloma which involves the bone marrow, usually presenting as extranodal tumour deposits most commonly in the gastrointestinal tract. These deposits are composed exclusively of plasma cells which may be of mature or primitive morphology. The behaviour is generally indolent. Distinction from the extramedullary myeloma may be difficult and rests on the absence of marrow involvement.

Centrocytic

The tumour cells are small or large B lymphoid cells with characteristic irregular or cleaved nuclear contours resembling one type of centrocyte cell, putatively of the normal germinal centre. Presentation is by lymph node enlargement or commonly as extranodal tumour in sites such as the gut. The tumour cells are arranged in diffuse sheets with few admixed cells. Prognosis is usually worse than other B cell low-grade types, the disease progressing to widespread dissemination without blast cell transformation.

Follicular lymphoma—centroblastic/centrocytic, follicular or follicular and diffuse

Follicular lymphoma is one of the commonest types of malignant lymphoma. It is usually seen in older individuals being uncommon under age of 25. The female : male ratio is 1 : 1. Presentation with a single node enlargement or in extranodal sites is rare. The tumour architecture is distinctive with formation of follicular structures. In the pure follicular form the tumour cells, a mixture of follicle centre cells, centroblasts and centrocytes, are confined to these structures which resemble the normal germinal follicle. It can therefore be regarded as a well-differentiated tumour simulating the normal cortical zone of a lymph node. In some cases these follicular structures may condense to form diffuse sheets of tumour cells giving a mixed follicular and diffuse picture. Prognosis initially is good, with very slow progression to disseminated disease but cure is rare, with late blast cell (high-grade) transformation being a common outcome.

B cell lymphomas—high grade

Centroblastic

The tumour cells are round large blast cells resembling centroblasts of the follicle centre. They are arranged in diffuse sheets with few other cells present. This is a relatively common type of high-grade lymphoma presenting either as a primary tumour, usually in a single group of nodes, or as secondary blast cell transformation in a patient known to have follicular lymphoma. Prognosis prior to effective chemotherapy was very poor with rapid progression of the disease. Chemotherapy is now often effective with a good chance of cure.

Immunoblastic

This tumour is composed of large blast cells, mainly immunoblasts or blasts, showing plasma cell differentiation, arranged in diffuse sheets with few other cells present. They have a rounded nucleus with a central prominent nucleolus and some cytoplasm. Immunocytochemistry usually demonstrates evidence of immunoglobulin synthesis in the cytoplasm. They occur in adults, with peak incidence over the age of 50, as a primary tumour or secondary to previous low-grade lymphoma. The prognosis is generally poor even with modern chemotherapeutic regimes.

Lymphoblastic lymphoma and Burkitt's lymphoma

Burkitt in 1958 described an endemic form of lymphoma occurring in the malaria belt of tropical Africa and classically affecting young boys as a rapidly growing tumour in the jaw. Other sites of origin are recognized with the ovary being common in girls. Lymph node involvement is rare. The tumour is associated with Epstein–Barr virus infection, possibly in association with malaria infection and consistently shows 8 : 14 chromosomal translocations. The tumour is composed of small undifferentiated lymphoid blast cells of B cell origin arranged in confluent sheets. The tumours have high cell turnover with frequent mitotic figures and apoptotic cells present. The cell debris is phagocytosed by numerous large pale tingible body macrophages which give the histology its typical 'starry sky' appearance.

There has been much unresolved debate concerning the designation of other types of lymphoblastic lymphoma occurring outside Africa or without evidence of Epstein–Barr virus infection. These have been designated Burkitt-like or non-Burkitt. They have some significant differences with a later age of onset in childhood, a wider age range extending well into adult life and differing presentation with intestinal, mediastinal and nodal tumours being more common.

The prognosis of both types of disease is very poor if untreated, but response to modern chemotherapy is often dramatic with high rates of complete remission now being reported.

T cell lymphomas—low grade

T lymphocytic

This tumour is rare and analogous to B lymphocytic lymphoma/lymphocytic leukaemia. There is usually lymph node, marrow, blood and splenic involvement.

Small cerebriform cell

A form of skin lymphoma which can progress to systemic disease (see p. 420).

Lymphoepithelial lymphoma—Lennert's lymphoma

Originally thought to be a form of Hodgkin's disease, this entity is now recognized as a tumour of CD4 helper/inducer T cells. The tumour cell populations are predominantly small lymphoid cells, the characteristic features of the histology being an associated florid infiltration of epithelial cells throughout the tumour. The disease usually presents as localized lymphadenopathy most frequently in the neck and usually runs an indolent course.

T zone lymphoma

This tumour is the T cell equivalent of follicular lymphoma, the 'well-differentiated type' of B cell lymphoma (see p. 272). The tumour replaces but resembles the structure of the normal paracortical region of the node with preservation of the central follicular structures in early stages. The tumour is composed mainly of small and medium-sized T lymphoid cells with occasional larger transformed cells which may resemble Reed–Sternberg cells. There is associated proliferation of postcapillary venules and interdigitating reticulum cells. Other reactive cells such as macrophages and plasma cells may be present. Subsequent transformation into high-grade disease has been observed. Constitutional symptoms are frequent and involvement of the lung and pleura is common.

Angioimmunoblastic lymphadenopathy-like T cell lymphoma

Angioimmunoblastic lymphadenopathy (see p. 269) was originally described as a reactive condition with a characteristic clinicopathological picture which could progress to a high-grade lymphoma. Investigation of some cases has shown evidence of T cell receptor gene rearrangement indicating that at least a proportion of cases have an underlying form of T cell lymphoma. This disease, like AILD, has a variable poorly understood prognosis with progression to high-grade lymphoma in some individuals; however, the prognosis is generally regarded as better than many other types of T cell lymphoma.

Pleomorphic small T cell

This tumour has an association with HTLV-I infection and is then labelled adult T cell leukaemia/lymphoma (ATLL). The tumour may replace the node or involve the paracortex sparing the follicles. It is composed of small T lymphoid cells, usually CD4 positive, which vary in shape but not in size. The disease is normally a chronic progressive process but early acute transformation associated with a poor prognosis is seen. Some cases are associated with hypercalcaemia which confers a poorer prognosis.

T cell lymphomas—high grade

Lymphoblastic

This disease of children and adolescents is composed of primitive T lymphocytes of prothymocyte or thymocyte phenotype and classically presents with a large anterior mediastinal mass. The male : female ratio is 2 : 1. Nodal involvement, often of multiple sites, is commonly present and secondary involvement of the marrow with leukaemia frequently occurs. The cells are small and arranged in sheets with scattered pale macrophages present containing cellular debris and giving a starry sky appearance. This disease is very aggressive with rapid progression. Response to chemotherapy is usually observed but this may be short-lived with relapse often occurring.

Pleomorphic medium and large cell types

These tumours may also be associated with HTLV-I infection (see p. 270) and are similarly designated ATLL. This disease (ATLL) is usually of adults, mean age 57, with a male : female ratio of 1.4 : 1. It is endemic in some parts of Japan and also found in the Caribbean and in Caribbean migrants. The tumour replaces the node, and the tumour cells vary considerably in size and shape. There may be a mixture of plasma cells, eosinophils and macrophages. Vessels may be prominent but are not usually as branching as seen in AILD. Leukaemic circulation of cells is frequently found. The prognosis is generally poor with death from disease progression or infection. Hypercalcaemia is also seen in up to 50% and can lead to renal failure and death. Indolent chronic forms of the disease are recognized and associated with lower numbers of leukaemic cells.

Immunoblastic T cell

A tumour composed of sheets of large T lymphoid

cells of either CD4 or CD8 phenotype. They have rounded regular nuclei with single central nucleoli. There are few admixed cells or vessels present. There is also an association with HLTV-I infection (ATLL) when leukaemia may also occur.

Undifferentiated lymphomas

The cellular origin of some lymphomas cannot be identified by immunophenotyping or molecular gene rearrangement studies. These are generally high-grade large cell tumours. In some cases, although the phenotype (T or B cell) of the tumour cell population may be identified, the histological features do not fit any of the recognized subtypes. These tumours are designated as unclassified.

Within this group of tumours two relatively distinctive high-grade tumours are recognized.

Large cell anaplastic lymphoma Ki-1 lymphoma

This tumour is composed of sheets of large pleomorphic cells which may appear cohesive leading to misdiagnosis as undifferentiated carcinoma or melanoma. The cells express the CD30 (Ki-1) antigen which is present in activated B and T lymphoid cells. In some cases other T or B cells may be expressed and similarly T cell receptor or immunoglobulin gene rearrangement has been observed in some cases. A proportion of cases do not have a detectable B or T cell phenotype or genotype. The tumour tends to affect young adults and has a very poor prognosis.

Lymphoblastic—unclassified

This tumour is essentially similar to B or T cell lymphoblastic lymphoma but their phenotype cannot be identified. The prognosis is similar.

Non-lymphoid cell tumours

Histiocytosis X—Langerhans cell granulomatosis

Three diseases—eosinophilic granuloma, Hand–Schüller–Christian disease and Letterer–Siwe disease—are related to neoplastic proliferation of a particular form of histiocyte—the *Langerhans cell*. The most localized form of the disease, *eosinophilic granuloma*, is characterized by single or multiple destructive bone lesions but may present with, or progress to involve, lymph nodes (see p. 297). In

this instance the node sinuses are distended by large characteristic histiocytic cells with folded nuclei. Eosinophils are often present. *Letterer–Siwe disease* is an aggressive poorly responsive generalized condition usually occurring in children under the age of 3, with skin, bone, visceral and nodal infiltration by large histiocytic cells of the same origin (see p. 297).

True histiocytic lymphoma

The frequency of this condition has been overestimated in older classifications of lymphoma such as Rappaport's, by the assumption that all large cell lymphomas were of histiocytic origin. This tumour is now recognized to be very rare, and as a consequence of misclassification is poorly understood. The tumours which can be derived from macrophages and the specialized histiocytic cells of the normal lymph node, dendritic reticulum cells and interdigitating reticulum cells are recognized by their characteristic phenotype or cytoplasmic enzyme content. The cells have abundant cytoplasm, infiltrate the sinus or pulp and may show phagocytosis of red cells or cellular debris. The prognosis is variable.

Extranodal lymphoma

In general the Kiel classification is applied to both nodal and extranodal lymphomas. Although lymphomas may occur at virtually any extranodal site within the body they are more common at certain sites—gut, skin, lung, thyroid, testis, brain and salivary gland. There is, however, increasing recognition that some of these types of extranodal lymphoma are derived from specialized organ-specific types of lymphoid tissue. The most widely recognized is the lymphoid tissue of the gut and other mucosal sites such as salivary gland and lung, which has been called 'mucosa-associated lymphoid tissue—MALT'.

MALT lymphomas

Both low- and high-grade B cell lymphomas occur in mucosal sites. The low-grade tumours are composed of small irregular cells which resemble the centrocytes of the follicle centre. Characteristically they infiltrate mucosal epithelial tissue forming so-called lymphoepithelial lesions. They may progress to involve lymph nodes and other tissues. High-grade tumours are usually composed of cells resembling centroblasts or immunoblasts and have a prognosis similar to their nodal counterparts.

Cutaneous T cell lymphoma

Both B and T cell lymphomas may involve the skin as a manifestation of disseminated disease. However, a specific form of cutaneous T cell lyphoma—*mycosis fungoides*, is well recognized (see p. 419). It is composed of small to medium-sized T cells which have an irregular convoluted nuclear contour. These cells home to the skin and infiltrate the epidermis. Systemic progression—*Sezary syndrome*—may occur with lymph node involvement and leukaemic circulation of tumour cells.

Enteropathy-associated T cell lymphoma

A form of aggressive high-grade lymphoma of the small intestine is recognized which occurs in association with villous atrophy (see p. 37). The derivation of this tumour has led to much past speculation—previously known as *malignant histiocytosis of the intestine*, but it is now recognized as a form of intestinal T cell lymphoma. It has a poor prognosis.

Hodgkin's disease

Aetiology and epidemiology

Hodgkin's disease (HD) is a very well recognized clinicopathological entity but its aetiology is still poorly understood. In particular, the origin of the diagnostic Reed–Sternberg cell remains elusive, although some convincing evidence is now emerging.

There is recent molecular and immunophenotyping data showing that HD is not a single entity. Lymphocyte predominant HD is a disease of B lymphoid cell origin most probably arising in the germinal centre. It can follow the reactive process known as progressive transformation of germinal centres and progress in some patients after many years to a high-grade B cell lymphoma. The origin of other types of HD is less clear but molecular studies have shown T and more frequently B cell lymphoid rearrangement in some cases.

There is epidemiological evidence of an underlying infectious agent, probably viral, which may affect genetically susceptible individuals.

Age and sex

As a single entity, Hodgkin's disease is the commonest lymphoma—approximately 45%. There is a wide age range—2 to over 80 years—with a bimodal distribution, the peaks being in the third and seventh decades. The incidence is changing, mainly through increasing recognition by immunophenotypic and molecular studies of B and T cell lymphomas with similar morphological features to HD.

Overall there is a slight male predominance but with an equal sex ratio in the commonest nodular sclerosing subtype.

Clinical

The commonest presentation is painless enlargement of a lymph node. Cervical nodes are more frequently involved than axillary or regional. There may be underlying mediastinal and paracortex node involvement detectable through staging investigations.

Alcohol-induced node pain often occurs. Systemic symptoms designated as 'B symptoms' such as fever, night sweats and weight loss, may be observed. They confer a worse prognosis and are used for clinical staging.

Hodgkin's disease often appears to spread in a contiguous fashion via the lymphatics in a manner similar to metastatic dissemination of carcinoma, although blood-borne dissemination must explain spread to other organ sites such as liver, spleen and bone marrow.

Staging

The treatment of Hodgkin's disease is dependent on the measurable extent of disease spread. Staging has been improved by the availability of computerized axial tomography (CT) scanning and the need for staging laparotomy is reduced. The Ann Arbor staging system of 1971 is still widely used, with each stage being subdivided into A and B depending on the presence of associated B symptoms (see above)

Stage I   One single lymph node region or single extralymphatic site.
Stage II   Two or more lymph node regions on one side of the diaphragm (including spleen or localized extralymphatic site).
Stage III Lymph node involvement on both sides of the diaphragm (including spleen or localized extralymphatic site).
Stage IV   Diffuse or disseminated involvement of extralymphatic tissues.

Radiotherapy is generally given for lower stage disease, the field area being controlled by the extent of disease. Systemic chemotherapy is given for more widespread disease.

Macroscopical

Involved lymph nodes have a firm rubbery homogeneous consistency and may enlarge up to 10 cm. In nodular sclerosing disease the nodes tend to matt tightly together through fibrous tissue formation.

Microscopical

The diagnosis of Hodgkin's disease rests on identification of Reed–Sternberg cells or Hodgkin's cells in an appropriate cellular background. The precise diagnostic features differ with each subtype and variants of the Reed–Sternberg or Hodgkin's cells are recognized in the various subtypes. The classical Reed–Sternberg cell is large with abundant cytoplasm. The nucleus is lobed, double or multiple with each lobe or nucleus containing a single large prominent nucleolus with a clear surrounding chromatin zone.

Histological classification of Hodgkin's disease

Since the 1930s, classifications of Hodgkin's disease have been based on the proportion of lymphocytes present in the tumour with a relationship noted between high numbers and better prognosis and vice-versa. Currently the Rye classification with four groups is widely used, which is a simplification of Luke's classification described in 1960 (Table 15.5).

Lymphocyte predominant

Two forms of this disease are recognized—nodular and diffuse. The *nodular* type appears to arise from germinal centres giving the tumour its nodular character. The nodules are composed predominantly of small lymphocytes. The Hodgkin's cells seen in lymphocyte-predominant Hodgkin's disease have polylobulated nuclei and are often very scanty. Classical Reed–Sternberg cells are often not found. There may be small groups of macrophages present. The *diffuse* variant has a similar cellular composition often with more histiocytes and absence of nodular architecture. This is a rare but good prognosis type of Hodgkin's disease (see Table 15.5). Progression to high-grade B cell lymphoma may occur in some cases, usually after 10–15 years.

Mixed cellularity

This type of Hodgkin's disease has the most variable appearance. The cells present include lymphocytes, plasma cells, histiocytes, eosinophils and Hodgkin's cells, usually with easily recognizable Reed–Sternberg cells. A nodular arrangement is not seen. This type of Hodgkin's disease has an average prognosis. Death is from disease progression, infection or progression to lymphocyte depletion.

Nodular sclerosing

This is by far the most common type of Hodgkin's disease (Table 15.5). The lymph node structure is disrupted by wide bands of collagen-rich fibrous tissue separating nodules of lymphoid tissue. These nodules contain a variable—from lymphocyte predominance to lymphocyte depleted—composition of small lymphocytes and Hodgkin's cells. The nodular sclerosing Hodgkin's cell is known as the *lacunar cell* because of its abundant clear cytoplasm making the single or multilobed nucleus appear to be situated in a tissue space. Nodular sclerosing Hodgkin's disease is now often further classified into two grades, I or II, depending on the cellular content of the nodules, grade II disease having areas of lymphocyte-depleted histology. The prognosis and frequency of the two subtypes is different (Table 15.5).

Lymphocyte-depleted

In this variant the Hodgkin's cell dominates the histological picture. Although classical Reed–Sternberg cells are usually present the Hodgkin's cells vary widely in size and character, often with numerous large pleomorphic forms being present. Other cells, lymphocytes, plasma cells and histiocytes, are less prominent than in other types, although areas of necrosis may induce microabscess formation with an infiltrate of eosinophil and neutrophil polymorphs. There are two subtypes described—*the reticular form* with sheets of Hodgkin's cells and the *diffuse fibrosis*

Table 15.5 Frequency and behaviour of subtypes of Hodgkin's disease.

Rye classification	Percentage frequency in UK	Percentage 10-year survival
Lymphocyte-predominant	5	90
Nodular sclerosing	75	70
grade I	(55)	(80)
grade II	(20)	(50)
Mixed cellularity	18	55
Lymphocyte-depleted	2	20

form where the overall cellularity is reduced with deposition of collagen and hyaline material. Both are rare and have a very poor prognosis, usually with rapid disease progression (see Table 15.5).

Secondary tumours

Draining lymph nodes are often the first site of spread of metastases in carcinomas. Progression of nodal metastases tends to be sequential in the same direction as lymph flow, although reversal may occur following obstruction. Sarcomas tend to metastasize via the blood stream and nodal deposits are rare.

A wide variety of tumours can present as lymph node metastases but tumours such as breast, lung, nasopharyngeal carcinomas and malignant lymphoma are commoner. The primary site of origin may be indicated through the morphological appearances and features of the deposit, e.g. melanin production (melanoma), squamous differentiation (squamous cell carcinoma), mucin production (adenocarcinoma) and the site of the lymph node.

B/SPLEEN

Normal
Congenital
Atrophy
Trauma
Enlargement
Circulatory
Inflammations
  Non-specific
  Specific
Systemic disorders
Blood dyscrasias
Tumours

Normal

Structure

The spleen is an encapsulated vascular organ containing a high proportion of lymphoid tissue. Its normal weight is 120–200 g with weights over 250–300 g indicating an underlying abnormality. In functional and histological terms the spleen is divided into two distinct zones.

1 *Red pulp*: the largest volume of the spleen is made up of large sinusoidal spaces having a specialized fenestrated meshwork or sponge-like structure. Blood from the splenic artery circulates in this area, coming in contact with reticuloendothelial cells responsible for blood cell degradation.

2 *White pulp*: collections of lymphoid cells situated around specialized vascular structures.

The normal ratio of white : red pulp is 1 : 3 to 1 : 6. There is a progressive atrophy of white pulp with age and a consequent reduction in weight to approximately 100 g.

Function

The red pulp of the spleen serves as a filtration system for the blood. Effete circulating cells and other matter are trapped and taken up by the reticuloendothelial cells. The white pulp can be regarded as the 'lymph node of the blood stream' and provides an immune response role comparable to a peripheral lymph node.

Congenital

The spleen may be present as two or more separate structures—*splenunculae*. Complete absence is rare and sometimes associated with marrow hyperplasia.

Atrophy and removal

There is progressive atrophy of the spleen, predominantly of white pulp, with age. Vascular structures and trabeculae in the red pulp undergo hyalinization with age. Conditions leading to repeated infarction, in particular sickle cell anaemia and rarely thrombocytopenic purpura, can lead to progressive atrophy. Coeliac disease, other malabsorption states, alcoholism and some autoimmune diseases are associated with splenic atrophy.

Loss of the spleen through surgical removal or atrophy renders the individual more susceptible to bacterial infection, especially severe septicaemia, particularly from the pneumococcus. The risk is greater in children as the immune system, particularly humoral immunity, is less developed and may not have experienced such infection. Prophylactic antibiotics or pneumococcal vaccination is given to such individuals to reduce this risk.

Trauma

The splenic capsule is thick and rupture of a normal spleen requires considerable trauma, e.g.: involvement in a road traffic accident. An abnormal enlarged spleen, particularly when soft, e.g. in infectious mononucleosis or typhoid fever, may rupture with very little trauma, or rupture may occur spontaneously.

Peritonealneal seeding of splenic tissue may follow rupture and lead to return of splenic function after splenectomy.

Enlargement

The majority of conditions involving the spleen lead to its enlargement. This may be mild, moderate or massive. See Table 15.6 and the relevant sections below.

Hypersplenism

In some individuals with significant splenic enlargement a functional state of hyperactivity leading to a distinct clinical syndrome can occur. The features are anaemia, neutropenia and reticulocytosis. The syndrome is more common in patients with chronic infection such as malaria, kala-azar, tuberculosis and brucellosis, malignant lymphoma and lipoidoses.

Circulatory disorders

Portal hypertension

Aetiology

Hepatic cirrhosis is the commonest cause, with portal vein thrombosis and obstruction by tumour being rarer causes (see p. 241).

Appearances

The spleen is enlarged, firm, dark red or brown. There is fibrosis due to thickening of trabecular and sinusoid walls. The sinusoids are congested. Scattered firm areas of haemorrhage are present. Fresh haemorrhages appear dark red but with organization and scarring become brown. Haemosiderin pigment deposition in macrophages also gives the spleen a general brown colour—*brown induration*.

Results

Once established the change persists even if a portosystemic anastomotic circulation develops, e.g. between the splenic capsule and diaphragm through fibrous adhesions, or is formed by a surgical portosystemic anastomosis. Enlargement sufficient to cause features of hypersplenism may occur.

Congestive cardiac failure

Congestive right-sided heart failure leads to mild vascular engorgement of the spleen.

Appearances

The spleen is mildly enlarged—200–300 g, firm and dark red. The sinusoids are congested with red cells. There may be mild fibrosis and atrophy of the white pulp.

Table 15.6 Causes of splenic enlargement.

1 Infections
Bacterial: typhoid, tuberculosis, brucellosis, bacterial endocarditis
Viral: infectious mononucleosis
Parasitic*: malaria, kala-azar, schistosomiasis
2 Circulatory disorders
Portal hypertension
Congestive cardiac failure
3 Infiltration and connective tissue disorders
Rheumatoid arthritis (Felty's syndrome)
SLE
Amyloidosis
Lipid storage diseases
4 Tropical splenomegaly*
5 Blood dyscrasis
Leukaemia*: especially chronic myeloid
Haemolytic anaemia
Myelofibrosis*
Polycythaemia
6 Malignant lymphomas and Hodgkin's disease

* Indicates those conditions associated with massive splenomegaly.

Infarction

Aetiology and incidence
Splenic infarcts of varying size may occur after lodgement of emboli from mural, atrial or valvular cardiac thrombi (see p. 70) or from thrombosis of splenic arteries. Causes of local thrombosis include arteritis such as polyarteritis nodosa, local inflammation or in some conditions associated with splenic enlargement—lymphoma, leukaemia, sickle cell anaemia and malaria.

Appearances
Infarcts due to occlusion of an end artery are usually peripheral and wedge-shaped. Central infarcts may occur due to arteritis. Initially the necrotic area is congested and firm. It heals by fibrous scarring leaving a depressed scar puckering the capsule with a bland yellow amorphous central zone.

Inflammations

Non-specific

Acute generalized infection

Aetiology
Most forms of severe bacteraemia or septicaemia lead to splenic enlargement, e.g. bacterial endocarditis, abscess, acute pyelonephritis. Bacteria may be cultured from splenic samples.

Macroscopical
Moderate enlargement up to 500 g, with a pale soft red pulp—'septic spleen'.

Microscopical
Infiltration of red pulp by polymorphs and plasma cells. Hyperplasia of white pulp with germinal centre formation. Prolonged or severe infection, especially in children, may lead to depletion of white pulp.

Results
The spleen returns to normal after resolution of the infection. Peritoneal infection and some generalized infections can lead to a fibrous thickening of the splenic capsule in perisplenitis—'sugar-icing spleen'. Similar changes are seen following non-infective peritoneal exudation.

Chronic generalized infection

Non-specific
Chronic infections produce similar changes to the above, but to a lesser degree. Inflammatory conditions such as rheumatoid arthritis can lead to a marked prominence of the white pulp with large germinal centres.

Granulomatous
The spleen can contain granulomas in a wide variety of systemic granulomatous conditions, e.g. tuberculosis, sarcoidosis, brucellosis. The nature of the granulomas are more usually non-specific and may point to the diagnosis (see p. 248).

Specific

Typhoid and enteric fevers
The spleen responds to these severe infections in a similar fashion to other generalized acute infection (see p. 32). The spleen is enlarged, soft, deep red, the pulp resembling blood clot or blackcurrant jelly. There is a characteristic lymphoid and macrophage infiltration, the latter showing erythrophagocytosis. Neutrophil polymorphs are not prominent. Organisms may be detected and can be cultured (see p. 33).

Malaria
The spleen is enlarged in both acute and chronic malaria (see p. 5). In the acute form, there is marked congestion giving a haemorrhagic appearance. Malaria pigment—haemozoin—deposition is evident and malarial parasites can be found in lymphoreticular cells. In the chronic form, fibrosis, lymphoreticular hyperplasia and pronounced pigment deposition give the spleen a firm brown or black appearance.

Visceral leishmaniasis—kala-azar
This generalized infection of the lymphoreticular system by Leishmania donovani (see p. 6), results in marked splenic enlargement. The spleen is firm, congested and has a thickened capsule. There is expansion of lymphoreticular cells with organisms visible in macrophages.

Syphilis

Splenic enlargement is rare in syphilis but may occur through lymphoid hyperplasia in the secondary stage or the presence of gummata in tertiary syphilis.

Schistosomiasis

The adult trematodes in *Schistosoma mansoni* and *S. japonicum* infection migrate to the portal venous system and can cause splenic enlargement through portal venous obstruction (see p. 236).

Infectious mononucleosis

Variable enlargement of the spleen may occur due to expansion of the red pulp by the atypical mononuclear cells characteristic of the condition (see p. 268). The spleen may be very soft and can rupture, usually 3–4 weeks after the clinical onset of the disease.

Systemic disorders and infiltrations

Amyloid

The spleen is usually involved, often heavily, in secondary amyloidosis. Rarely, solitary or primary amyloidosis of the spleen may occur. Early deposition in secondary amyloidosis occurs around arterioles. More advanced involvement is recognized in two forms:

1 *Localized*: the commonest form producing a 'sago' spleen by deposition around white pulp arterioles producing multiple nodules 2–3 mm in diameter.

2 *Diffuse*: confluent deposition of amyloid throughout the red pulp sinusoidal system. The spleen is enlarged and has a characteristic waxy pale cut surface appearance.

Lipid storage diseases

There is accumulation of lipid material in macrophages in many sites in Gaucher's (see p. 293) and Niemann–Pick diseases. Involvement of the spleen may lead to enlargement.

Rheumatoid arthritis—Felty's syndrome

Enlargement of the spleen may occur in younger patients with rheumatoid arthritis leading to hypersplenism (see p. 100). The spleen shows hyperplasia of the white pulp with germinal follicle formation and hyperplasia of red pulp macrophages.

Blood dyscrasias

Idiopathic thrombocytopenic purpura

Autoimmune destruction of platelets can lead to mild enlargement of the spleen through hyperplasia of the white pulp and accumulation of macrophages containing lipid by-products of platelet phagocytosis and destruction. The spleen is often removed if other forms of treatment are unsuccessful.

Haemolytic anaemia

Being the site of red cell destruction, the spleen shows moderate (300–600 g) or sometimes more marked enlargement in this condition. There is congestion of sinusoids with accumulation of macrophages containing haemosiderin pigment. Infarction and fibrosis leading to a reduction in size may occur, and is common in sickle cell anaemia. In acquired autoimmune forms, hyperplasia of the white pulp may be seen.

Leukaemia

All forms of leukaemia produce splenic enlargement due to infiltration or accumulation of leukaemic cells. This is more pronounced in chronic forms, especially chronic myeloid leukaemia. Lymphoid cell leukaemias usually involve the white pulp but with progression may extend to involve red pulp. Myeloid leukaemia usually involves the red pulp with compression of the white pulp. In *hairy cell leukaemia*, a form of lymphocytic leukaemia, the infiltrate of characteristic 'hairy' cells is usually confined to the red pulp.

Myeloproliferative disorders and myelofibrosis

Bone marrow disorders leading to fibrosis of the marrow space or expansion of haemopoiesis lead to extramedullary haemopoiesis occurring in the spleen and other organs such as liver. Similar changes occur if the marrow is replaced in other conditions such as metastatic carcinoma.

Tumours

Benign

Hamartomas, cysts and haemangiomas occur rarely in the spleen and are usually identified as chance findings at splenectomy or autopsy.

Malignant

The spleen is a recognized but rare 'primary' site of occurrence of malignant lymphoma, but is frequently involved in disseminated malignant lymphoma and Hodgkin's disease. Low-grade lymphomas and Hodgkin's disease tend to involve the white pulp of the spleen initially. Focal large deposits without an obvious site of origin are more usual for high-grade tumours. Metastatic carcinoma may occasionally involve the spleen. Angiosarcoma is the commonest primary malignant stromal tumour of the spleen.

Chapter 16
Diseases of the Mediastinum

The mediastinum is that portion of the thoracic cavity located between the pleural cavities, extending antero-posteriorly from the sternum to the spine and sagittally from the thoracic inlet to the diaphragm. The majority of the lesions are masses of various types. The arbitrary division into anterior, superior, middle and posterior is useful since most of the lesions have a predilection for one compartment (see Fig. 24).

Effects of mediastinal masses

Most mediastinal masses/tumours are benign. Effects are:

1 *Asymptomatic*: incidental findings at X-ray or at surgery, e.g. neural tumours.

2 *Pressure effects*:

(a) *On the trachea*: causing cough, respiratory distress, stridor. These predispose to pulmonary infection, often recurrent.

(b) *On vessels*: superior vena caval syndrome.

(c) *On nerves*: voice changes due to recurrent laryngeal nerve involvement, spinal cord compression or intercostal nerve symptoms if a neural tumour.

(d) *On oesophagus*: produces dysphagia.

3 *Haemorrhage*: can cause rapid expansion and dangerous increase in size, especially with retrosternal goitre or cysts.

4 *Metastatic spread*: if the tumour is malignant effects from intrathoracic and extrathoracic spread can occur.

5 *Endocrine effects*, e.g. myasthenia gravis in thymoma, thyrotoxicosis in retrosternal goitre, hyperparathyroidism with parathyroid adenoma and Cushing's syndrome with carcinoid tumour. Diarrhoea, sweating and hypertension can occur with certain neural tumours, e.g. neuroblastoma.

Inflammations

Acute mediastinitis

Nature
Acute inflammation in the mediastinal tissues.

Causes
1 *Oesophageal perforation*: the commonest cause, e.g; foreign body such as bone or an endoscope, forceful vomiting—*Mallory–Weiss syndrome* (see p. 24), leakage of surgical anastomosis and carcinoma of oesophagus.

2 *Spread from infective foci*: in neck, retropharyngeal space, lung, pleura, pericardium or osteomyelitic foci in bone.

Appearances
Cellulitis and fibrinous, acute inflammation spreads through the loose connective tissues of the mediastinum. Abscess formation may occur.

Effects
1 *Systemic effects of infection.*
2 *Local effects of infection.*
3 *Death*: this condition has a high mortality.

Chronic mediastinitis

Definition
A chronic inflammation and fibrosing process of the mediastinum.

Causes
1 *Fungal infections*, e.g. histoplasmosis, especially in North America.
2 *Tuberculosis.*

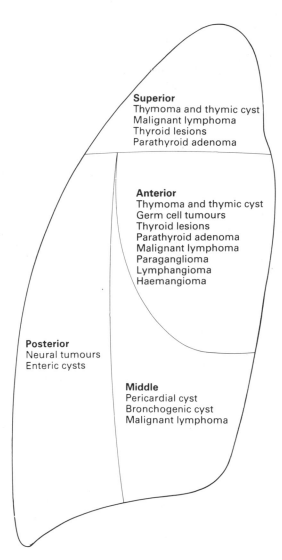

Superior
Thymoma and thymic cyst
Malignant lymphoma
Thyroid lesions
Parathyroid adenoma

Anterior
Thymoma and thymic cyst
Germ cell tumours
Thyroid lesions
Parathyroid adenoma
Malignant lymphoma
Paraganglioma
Lymphangioma
Haemangioma

Posterior
Neural tumours
Enteric cysts

Middle
Pericardial cyst
Bronchogenic cyst
Malignant lymphoma

Fig. 24 Mediastinal tumours—location.

3 *Fibrosing mediastinitis*: this condition can be idiopathic, often associated with Riedel's thyroiditis (see p. 131) or drug-induced (e.g. practolol and methysergide). Most causes of fibrosis of the mediastinum are secondary to *neoplastic infiltration* with an associated intense stromal reaction.

Appearances

Macroscopical
There is considerable fibrosis with compression of local structures.

Microscopical
There is intense fibrosis. Granulomas are seen in tuberculosis or fungal infection and a non-specific mononuclear infiltrate is seen in fibrosing mediastinitis. In cases due to malignancy the neoplastic cells can be identified but may be very sparse.

Developmental cysts

Nature
Benign fluid-filled cysts.

Types
1 *Pericardial*: attached to the pericardium and lined by mesothelium.
2 *Bronchial cysts*: are found along the bronchial tree usually in the posterior mediastinum and are lined by respiratory epithelium.
3 *Enterogenous*: attached to the oesophagus in the posterior mediastinum and are lined by glandular or squamous epithelium.
4 *Thymic*: (see below).

Thymus

Cysts

Site
These occur in the neck or anterior mediastinum.

Appearances
They are usually unilocular cysts lined by thymic tissue. The fluid may contain cholesterol crystals.

Aetiology
They are usually congenital but can be acquired due to degeneration within the thymus gland or within thymic neoplasms.

Follicular hyperplasia of thymus

Nature
This is generalized but usually slight enlargement of the thymus gland due to overgrowth of numerous reactive lymphoid follicles.

Associated disease
It is commonly associated with myasthenia gravis and is seen in 65% of patients with this condition (see p. 289). The autoantibodies are thought to be produced by the lymphoid tissue in some cases.

Thymoma

Nature
A primary epithelial tumour of the thymus gland. There are benign and malignant forms.

Incidence
Rare, but one of the commonest causes of mediastinal masses which occur mainly in adults above 50 years of age; M : F equal.

Associated diseases
1 *Myasthenia gravis*: 25% of patients with this condition have a thymoma; 40% of patients with thymoma have myasthenia gravis.
2 *Others*: hypogammaglobulinaemia, red cell aplasia and connective tissue diseases.

Site
Mainly in the anterosuperior mediastinum.

Appearances
Benign tumours are well circumscribed and encapsulated. They are solid, yellow/grey and divided into lobules by fibrous bands. Cystic degeneration is common. Malignant thymomas invade the local tissues. Histologically all benign and many malignant thymomas are basically epithelial and are of similar appearance, composed of uniform epithelial cells variably admixed with reactive lymphoid cells. The epithelial cells can be spindle-shaped or rounded and the lymphoid cells can be small and mature or activated blast forms.

Malignancy in thymoma
Ten per cent of thymomas are malignant.

Type 1
Histologically indistinguishable from benign thymomas but invade the local tissues, e.g. pericardium, lungs, pleura. They rarely spread outside the thorax.

Type 2
Rare types of primary malignant thymomas are recognizable histologically, e.g. squamous cell carcinoma, oat cell carcinoma.

Prognosis

Benign
Encapsulated benign tumours have an excellent prognosis after surgical removal.

Malignant
For type 1 invasive thymomas the prognosis depends on the extent of invasion and the adequacy of surgical excision. For type 2 tumours the prognosis is extremely poor.

Thymic carcinoid
A malignant tumour of similar morphology and clinical behaviour to other foregut carcinoids (see p. 36). One-third of cases are associated with secretion of ACTH causing Cushing's syndrome (see p. 117). The remainder are largely hormonally inactive.

Germ cell tumours
These are rare and account for 20% of primary mediastinal tumours but with a preponderance in young adult males. They are probably derived from misplaced germ cells during embryonic migration. Though found close to or within the thymus gland, they have no histogenetic relationship with true thymomas.

All types of germ cell tumours found in the gonads can occur as primary tumours of the mediastinum (see p. 225 and p. 119), particularly mature cystic teratomas—80% and seminomas/dysgerminomas.

They secrete the same substances as their gonadal counterparts, e.g. placental alkaline phosphatase, α-fetoprotein (see p. 200).

Malignant lymphoma
This occurs as part of a disseminated lymphoma or as a primary mediastinal tumour.

Primary Hodgkin's disease
Classically mediastinal Hodgkin's disease presents in young adult females and involves the thymus, lymph nodes or both.

The tumor is a smooth, solid thymic mass with enlarged solid lymph nodes but cystic changes can occur.

Microscopically the disease is often of the nodular sclerosing subtype (see p. 276), though other subtypes can occur.

Primary non-Hodgkin's lymphoma

Classically presents in young adult females with superior venal caval obstruction or respiratory distress involving the thymus, lymph nodes or both, usually appear as a solid mass of tumour with local invasion.

Histologically these are most commonly of either lymphoblastic T cell or centroblastic B cell types (see p. 271).

Thymolipoma

An encapsulated benign tumour composed of mature fat and thymic tissue.

Thyroid lesions

Intrathoracic thyroid lesions usually occur in the superior mediastinum (see p. 283).

Nodular colloid goitre

This is the commonest cause. It may arise from a retrosternal extension of a goitre in the neck or as the only manifestation of thyroid disease from the lower pole of the gland.

Nodular colloid goitre of congenitally ectopic tissue may also occur.

Parathyroid lesions

Seven per cent of parathyroid adenomas are found in the superior mediastinum and are usually small. If clinically manifest this is usually due to endocrine effects rather than their mass (see p. 138).

Neurogenic tumours

Tumours of the sympathetic nervous system

Ganglioneuromas, neuroblastomas and ganglio-neuroblastomas (see p. 110) occur in the posterior mediastinum arising from the sympathetic system.

Tumours of peripheral nerves

These have identical morphological and clinical features to those arising elsewhere (see p. 108) and include neurofibromas, Schwannomas and malignant nerve sheath tumours. These are most commonly related to intercostal nerves in the posterior mediastinum and can extend through the intervertebral foramina to form a partially intraspinal dumb-bell tumour.

Secondary mediastinal tumours

The involvement of mediastinal structures, especially lymph nodes, by metastatic tumour from a wide variety of primary sites is very common and results from direct or lymphatic spread.

Some secondary tumours can mimic primary mediastinal tumours with a minute primary lesion and huge mediastinal deposits, most typically bronchial oat cell carcinoma (see p. 404).

Other mediastinal masses

Connective tissue tumours

Most types of benign or malignant soft tissue and bone tumours can occur in the mediastinum but are rare, e.g. lipomas, leiomyosarcomas, chondromas and chondrosarcomas.

Vascular lesions

Aneurysms of the aortic arch or giant left atrium in mitral stenosis can produce pressure effects, e.g. vertebral erosion, dysphagia.

Chapter 17
Diseases of the Musculo-Skeletal System

A/NON-NEOPLASTIC MUSCLE DISORDERS

Muscle biopsy
General reactions
Classification
Congenital myopathies
Muscular dystrophies
Inflammatory myopathies
Secondary and metabolic myopathies
Neurogenic disorders
Disordered function
    Myasthenia gravis
    Periodic paralysis

Skeletal muscles are made up of striated muscle fibres that can be divided into two basic types by biochemical and physiological criteria:

Type 1 fibres: physiologically slow twitch. Contain abundant mitochondria and are adapted for aerobic metabolism.

Type 2 fibres: physiologically fast twitch. Contain abundant glycogen with capacity for anaerobic metabolism.

A normal muscle is composed of a mixture of these two basic types arranged randomly within the cross-section of the muscle. The proportion of each fibre type varies in different muscles: muscles involved in constantly maintaining posture are rich in type 1 fibres, muscles used for sudden bursts of power have a high type 2 fibre content. In postnatal life fibre type depends on innervation: change in innervation, e.g. by regeneration of severed axons, causes a redistribution of fibre types within a muscle.

Muscle biopsy

Muscle disease presents with clinical features of weakness, muscle wasting or muscle pain—*myalgia*. Biopsy of muscle may be performed to investigate neuromuscular disease and may be performed either as an open excision biopsy or a percutaneous needle biopsy. The muscle normally sampled is the vastus lateralis or occasionally the deltoid. Pathological evaluation requires preservation by snap-freezing in liquid nitrogen to allow sections to be cut for enzyme histochemical staining to permit delineation of fibre types, mitochondria and distribution of fibrosis. Electron microscopy is important in the evaluation of mitochondrial and structural changes which take place in congenital muscle diseases, so small portions need glutaraldehyde fixation.

General pathological reactions in muscle

There are several types of pathological reaction which take place in skeletal muscle affected by disease.

1 *Necrosis* of muscle may be either:

(a) Large areas—segments and fascicles, which are usually due to vascular pathology—atherosclerotic occlusion of major vessels or vasculitis of intramuscular branches.

(b) Single fibre necrosis which is seen in many of the primary muscle diseases.

2 *Fibre phagocytosis*: necrosis of a muscle fibre is followed by phagocytosis of the dead fibre by macrophages.

3 *Muscle fibre regeneration*: follows fibre necrosis. Regeneration takes place from a population of muscle stem cells—*satellite cells*, which are present in inactive form in skeletal muscles.

4 *Fibrosis of muscle*: occurs following organization of large areas of necrosis or as the end-result of prolonged single-cell necrosis, e.g. muscular dystrophy. This may also be accompanied by infiltration with adipose tissue.

5 *Inflammation of muscle*: is usually secondary to fibre necrosis. Primary inflammation occurs in a group of diseases termed *inflammatory myopathies*.

6 *Atrophy of muscle*: occurs with disuse, ischaemia, denervation and malnutrition. Macroscopically there

is loss of muscle bulk and, in severe cases, muscle is replaced by fibrous tissue and fat.

7 *Hypertrophy of muscle*: this occurs in individual fibres to compensate for loss or atrophy of other muscle fibres in disease. If fibres enlarge sufficiently then they may undergo fibre splitting to form smaller fibres.

8 *Change in fibre type distribution*: occurs with change in the innervation of muscle. In reinnervation following denervation, muscle fibres come to be arranged in groups rather than a random 'checkerboard' pattern. This is detected by histochemical stains.

Summary

In most diseases of muscle elements of atrophy, hypertrophy, necrosis, inflammation and fibrosis are present in variable proportions. A diagnosis of the type of muscle disease is based on evaluation of the relative presence of these factors. In general two main groups of disease are delineated on histological examination:

1 *Myopathic features*: hypertrophic and atrophic fibres with fibre degeneration, phagocytosis and variable amounts of fibrosis.

2 *Neuropathic features*: atrophic fibres seen in groups with intervening fibres showing fibre hypertrophy. Grouping of fibre types is seen in histochemical stains.

Classification of muscle diseases

Muscle disease can be divided into three main groups

Dystrophies

The muscular dystrophies are inherited diseases of muscle, often resulting in progressive deterioration of power.

Myopathies

1 Non-progressive congenital.
2 Inflammatory.
3 Secondary.
4 Metabolic.

The myopathies are a group of conditions of diverse aetiology grouped together because of a predominant impact of disease on the muscle. The congenital myopathies are distinguished from the dystrophies in that they are generally non-progressive.

Neurogenic disease

Disease of the nervous system, particularly of peripheral nerves or motor neurones, leads to atrophy of muscle groups in the neurogenic muscle diseases.

Non-progressive congenital myopathies

A group of disorders which generally present in childhood as hypotonia—*floppy baby*—or muscle weakness. They are generally non-progressive but may cause severe disability through secondary skeletal deformities or respiratory muscle involvement.

Many are named after specific *structural inclusions* seen on biopsy in muscle fibres, e.g. *nemaline body myopathy, central core disease, myotubular myopathy, congenital fibre-type disproportion*. They may be sporadic or associated with a genetic recurrence risk in siblings. Some are compatible with a long life expectancy.

Muscular dystrophies

Dystrophies are a group of genetically determined degenerative diseases of muscle. As a group they are characterized by the destruction of single muscle cells over a prolonged period of time with fibre regeneration and the development of fibrosis. There are many types which are classified according to the pattern of muscle groups involved, and pattern of inheritance. (see Table 17.1). Important subtypes are as follows.

Duchenne dystrophy

This is an X-linked recessive disorder with onset in early childhood. There is typically muscle weakness with a high serum creatine kinase (CK) level. Affected children show calf hypertrophy due to fatty replacement of muscle. The disorder has a poor prognosis with life expectancy only into the late teens. Cardiac muscle is also affected in the disease leading to cardiomyopathy (see p. 65). The molecular basis of the disorder is a mutation in the gene on the short arm of the X chromosome, coding for the protein *dystrophin*. This is a protein which is involved in anchoring the cell membrane of muscle to surrounding basement membrane, lack of this results in cell damage with contraction. A milder related type of dystrophy also due to abnormal dystrophin is *Becker dystrophy*.

Table 17.1 Classification of muscular dystrophies.

Type	Inheritance	Muscle involved in initial stages
Duchenne type	X-linked recessive	Pelvic girdle
Becker type	X-linked recessive	Pelvic girdle
Limb girdle	Autosomal recessive	Pelvic girdle
Facio-scapulo-humeral	Dominant	Face, shoulder girdle, arm
Scapulo-humeral	Autosomal recessive	Shoulder girdle and arm
Oculopharyngeal	Dominant	External ocular and pharynx
Myotonic dystrophy	Dominant	Face, respiratory, limbs

Limb girdle dystrophy

May become manifest either in childhood or adult life. It presents with weakness in pelvic girdle and proximal leg muscles or in shoulder girdle and proximal arm muscles. Cases are rare and most patients with this clinical pattern of weakness have metabolic or neurogenic muscle disease or have a late-onset Becker dystrophy. Nonetheless, if these disorders are excluded, the term limb girdle dystrophy appears a useful clinical syndrome, although it may have several different genetic bases which are at present unknown.

Facio-scapulo-humeral dystrophy

This presents with weakness in the face and shoulders with onset in the third decade and associated with a slow clinical progression. This clinical syndrome may be due to a variety of metabolic, inflammatory, neurogenic and myopathic disorders, and thorough investigation is required before the diagnosis is made.

Myotonic dystrophy

An autosomal dominant disorder characterized by muscle weakness, myotonia—inability to relax muscles—and other stigmata, including cataracts and frontal baldness in males, cardiomyopathy and low intelligence. The disease usually become apparent in adolescence with facial weakness and distal weakness in the limbs. Death in adult life is commonly due to involvement of the respiratory muscles.

Inflammatory myopathies

These are a group of diseases in which there is primary inflammation of muscle. The inflammatory infiltrate is usually composed of T cells and monocytes as part of an abnormal autoimmune response. As a group they are associated with a high ESR and raised serum CK levels. Important types are:

Polymyositis

This presents with weakness of proximal limb muscles, facial muscles—ptosis—and dysphagia. It may be associated with connective tissue diseases—SLE, rheumatoid disease, scleroderma (see p. 98) or malignancy, when it may be part of clinical syndrome of dermatomyositis (see p. 99)

Muscle biopsy shows lymphocytic infiltration in the perimysial connective tissue and around vessels with muscle fibre necrosis and phagocytosis. This disease responds to immunosuppressive treatment with steroids or azathioprine.

Inclusion body myositis

This is similar to polymyositis but occurs mainly in elderly patients. Pathologically there is evidence of inflammatory muscle destruction with the addition of inclusions composed of linear filaments seen within vacuoles in muscle by EM. This disorder is progressive with a poor response to immunosuppressive treatment.

Sarcoid

Muscle may be involved in sarcoidosis (see p. 394).

Secondary and metabolic myopathies

Many diseases of muscle are secondary to either systemic disease or metabolic abnormality. Common types are:

Type 2 fibre atrophy myopathy

This is the commonest abnormality seen in biopsy from patients with muscle weakness. The type 2 fibres are selectively reduced in size—atrophic. This abnormality is associated with a wide variety of conditions; causes include disuse, malignancy, steroid administration, Cushing's disease, thyroid disease and connective tissue diseases.

Endocrine myopathy

Steroids, therapeutic or in Cushing's disease, can cause wasting and weakness of proximal muscles with atrophy of type 2 fibres.

Similar changes occur with thyroid disease.

Carcinomatous myopathy

Carcinoma may cause non-metastatic manifestations in muscle through a variety of mechanisms.

1 Type 2 fibre atrophy myopathy.
2 Polymyositis or dermatomyositis.
3 Denervation with a paraneoplastic neuropathy.

In carcinomatous myopathy weakness is most common in proximal limb muscles.

Mitochondrial myopathy

This is due to genetic abnormalities in mitochondria which give rise to a group of diseases termed *mitochondrial cytopathies*, characterized primarily by muscle weakness, especially extra-ocular muscles, with or without other neurological and metabolic disturbances. Muscle biopsy reveals bizarre pleomorphic mitochondria often with crystalline inclusions. This is now recognized to be an important and common condition due to better recognition and investigation, and can have onset at all ages.

Glycogenosis

The main types of inherited glycogenosis affecting muscle are acid maltase deficiency (type 2), and McArdle's disease (myophosphorylase deficiency, type 5).

Neurogenic disorders

Clinically, weakness of muscle may be caused by denervation either due to disease of peripheral nerves or disease of anterior horn cells. Denervation is easily recognized on muscle biopsy as it causes atrophy of large groups of fibres. If reinnervation occurs, the normal random distribution of type 1 and 2 fibres is replaced by large groups of single fibre types—*fibre type grouping*.

Spinal muscular atrophy

An important group of neurogenic disorders of muscle, generally autosomal recessive and in which there is degeneration in the anterior horn cells in the spinal cord resulting in denervation of muscle. There are several clinical variants:

Werdnig–Hoffman disease

This disorder presents as a 'floppy baby' at birth and is due to congenital failure of innervation of skeletal muscle. Affected children have a very poor prognosis and usually die in the first year of life; this is therefore classed as the severe form of infantile spinal muscular atrophy. Muscle biopsy shows large areas of minute muscle fibres which have never been innervated, interspersed with small numbers of large innervated fibres.

Kugelberg–Wellander syndrome

This is a mild form of infantile spinal muscular atrophy with onset after birth in the first months of life. Affected children tend to have proximal limb girdle weakness with little tendency to deterioration with time. Muscle biopsy shows large groups of atrophic (denervated) fibres.

Juvenile spinal muscular atrophy

Affected children generally develop weakness of the legs around 8 months of age which is generally non-progressive and associated with a normal life expectancy. Muscle biopsy shows groups of atrophic fibres and fibre type grouping due to reinnervation.

Adult-onset spinal muscular atrophy

Generally presents with limb girdle weakness. Cases may have a dominant pattern of inheritance. Muscle biopsy shows features of neurogenic atrophy with fibre-type grouping indicative of reinnervation.

Disorders of muscle function

Myasthenia gravis

This a disease characterized by muscle weakness, proptosis and dysphagia. It is an autoimmune disease caused by autoantibodies to the acetylcholine receptor located in the postsynaptic membrane of muscle motor endplates. These antibodies cause failure of synaptic transmission by blocking receptor sites. Diagnosis is by administration of an anticholinesterase drug which increases acetylcholine concentrations and facilitates transmission, and treatment is with long-acting anticholinesterases.

Apart from non-specific aggregates of lymphoid cells in the interstitium, there is no pathology seen by light microscopy in muscle biopsy. There is a high incidence of thymic pathology associated with myasthenia gravis. Approximately 25% of cases have a thymoma (see p. 283). Other cases may show hyperplasia of the thymic gland. Thymectomy may improve the myasthenia in a proportion of cases.

Periodic paralysis
The periodic paralysis syndromes are characterized by paroxysmal attacks of paralysis and flaccidity of muscles. On muscle biopsy during an attack there are large vacuoles in fibres which develop from dilatation of the T tubules and sarcoplasmic reticulum. There are several types:

Hyperkalaemic periodic paralysis
Is most common in childhood and adolescence and is inherited as an autosomal dominant trait. Attacks occur after rest following a period of exercise, are short-lived (1–2 hours), and associated with elevation of serum potassium to between 5 and 7 mmol/l.

Hypokalaemic periodic paralysis
Is commonest in adult females and inherited as an autosomal dominant trait. Attacks typically occur on waking in the morning, and last for many hours. The serum potassium level in attacks falls to 2–2.5 mmol/l.

Normokalaemic periodic paralysis
Is commonest in adolescence and childhood, inherited as an autosomal dominant trait, and is characterized by severe prolonged attacks of paralysis in which the serum potassium level is in the normal range (3.5–5.3 mmol/l).

Thyrotoxicosis may also be associated with the development of periodic paralysis, a syndrome particularly seen in oriental males.

B/BONE—CONGENITAL, TRAUMATIC

Bone structure
Congenital
  Achondroplasia
  Dyschondroplasia
  Gargoylism
  Gaucher's disease
  Morquio's disease
  Melorheostosis
  Marfan's syndrome
  Marble bone disease
  Phocomelia
Traumatic
  Slipped epiphysis
  Osteochondritis
  Fractures

Bone structure
Bone is a connective tissue with specialized features which are relevant to an understanding of its pathology.

Cortex
There is a cortex composed of dense (compact) bone with Haversian systems.

Medulla
The centre of the bone is the medulla with trabeculae of cancellous bone between which there is marrow, active or fatty depending on the site.

Periosteum
External to the cortex is the periosteum which has an outer fibrous layer and an inner osteogenic layer.

Blood supply
The blood supply is derived from the nutrient artery which penetrates through to the medulla and supplies the inner portion of the cortex as well as the medulla. Periosteal vessels supply the outer layers of the cortex.

Regions
In growing bone there are the following regions which are illustrated in Fig. 25.
1 *Diaphysis* or shaft.
2 *Metaphysis*: the zone adjacent to, and on the shaft side of, the epiphyseal line.
3 *Epiphyseal line*: the zone of enchondral ossification.
4 *Epiphysis*: the portion of bone at the end of a long bone which ossifies separately.

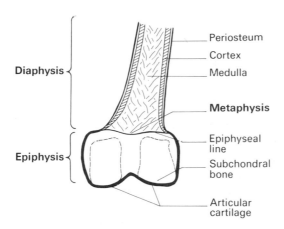

Fig. 25 Anatomical regions of a long bone.

Bone matrix

The organic matrix of bone—osteoid tissue, is composed of collagenous fibres separated by a muco-polysaccharide, chondroitin sulphate. The fibres are characteristically arranged in sheets—*lamellar bone*, which can be visualized with polarized light. In the embryo, young child and a range of pathological conditions irregular arrangement of fibres is a '*woven*' or *non-lamellar* pattern. There are three types of cell closely associated with osteoid tissue:

1 The mononuclear osteoblasts which lay down the osteoid tissue.
2 The multinucleated osteoclasts which are associated with bone resorption.
3 The osteocytes which are osteoblasts incorporated in lacunae in the bone matrix as bone cells, but which are no longer active in the formation of bone.

In health, bone matrix is not a static tissue, but is constantly changing due to osteoblasts laying down osteoid tissue and a balanced amount being removed by osteoclasts.

Bone mineral

This is the inorganic content of bone—'bone salt', which is composed of a complex of calcium and phosphates known as *hydroxyapatite*. This mineral is deposited in the osteoid tissue and renders it hard. Thus:

osteoid tissue + mineral = bone.

However, bone is not simply a rigid static structure, as there is a constant exchange of calcium and phosphates between the bones and the body fluids and tissues.

Ossification

There are many factors involved in the formation of bone including:
1 An adequate blood level of calcium and phosphorus.
2 Vitamin D in adequate amounts.
3 The bone matrix must be present.
4 The skeletal mesenchyme must be normal.
5 Weight-bearing and exercise stimulate bone growth.
6 Alkaline phosphatase, derived from osteoblasts, probably releases phosphates from organic combination and thus promotes the precipitation of the calcium × phosphate complex.
7 Parathormone is a major factor in the control of serum calcium levels and indirectly of the phosphate levels. Calcitonin is also important (see p. 127).
8 Hormones, especially thyroxine, adrenal hormones, oestrogens and pituitary hormones should be present in normal balance.
9 The pH of the tissue is important; normal ossification occurs in a slightly alkaline medium.

Bone growth

Growth of bone occurs by ossification of pre-existing tissues in two distinct ways:

Ossification in membrane

Osteoid tissue is formed in connective tissue by osteoblastic activity without the intervention of preformed cartilage, e.g. membrane bones of the vault of the skull.

Enchondral ossification

Ossification in preformed cartilage at epiphyseal lines and in the numerous separate ossification centres of bones, before and after birth.

Normal epiphyseal line

This is the site of enchondral ossification at the ends of long bones; enchondral ossification produces growth in length.

Macroscopical

A straight regular line with a white appearance due to a zone of calcification of cartilage and with a red vascular layer on the metaphyseal side.

Microscopical

An orderly structure composed of zones:

1 *Resting cartilage*: columns of regular, small, cartilage cells.

2 *Proliferating cartilage*: columns of large, hypertrophic, cartilage cells.

3 *Provisional calcification*: a zone of calcification of the cartilaginous stroma, the cartilage cells disappearing.

4 *Osteoid zone*: osteoblasts grow in from the vascular metaphysis to lay down osteoid tissue on the calcified matrix.

5 *Mineralization*: the osteoid tissue becomes mineralized to form bone.

6 *Remodelling*: the bone is altered by remodelling to produce compact cortical and cancellous medullary bone.

Congenital diseases of bone

Achondroplasia

Nature

A congenital disease of dominant inheritance affecting all the bones in which enchondral ossification occurs, e.g. the long bones, the base of the skull and the pelvis.

Macroscopical

Achondroplastic dwarfs are approximately 137 cm tall with normally developed trunks but short limbs.

1 *Long bones*: approximately two-thirds of the normal length with a 'dumb-bell' appearance due to a short shaft but normally developed epiphyseal bone.

2 *Spine*: lordosis.

3 *Pelvis*: reduced in all diameters.

4 *Head*: the base of the skull is small but the calvarium, which forms by ossification in membrane, is normal.

Microscopical

The abnormality is at the epiphyseal line where the epiphyseal cartilage is narrowed due to absence of the proliferating zone. As a result diminished growth in length occurs, the shaft is short but the epiphyseal bone is normally formed.

Dyschondroplasia

Nature

Developmental abnormalities of the epiphyseal line may result in persistence of cartilage inside or outside the bone.

Pathogenesis

There is persistence of epiphyseal cartilage into adulthood so that islands of cartilage are present within the bone—*enchondromas*, or on the cortical surface as cartilaginous masses growing away from the epiphyseal line—*ecchondromas*.

Macroscopical

1 *Enchondromas*: single or multiple masses of cartilage in any bone, e.g. femur, but most commonly found in the fingers—*Ollier's disease*.

2 *Ecchondromas*: cartilaginous nodules, frequently multiple, which are directed away from their epiphyseal line of origin; the most common site is adjacent to the knee joint. The disease has a familial tendency and is variously named—*diaphyseal aclasia*, *multiple exostoses*, or *cancellous osteomas*. The cartilage ossifies from the base to leave only a cap of cartilage covering the cancellous bone; this also eventually ossifies.

Results

1 *Enchondromas*: may slowly ossify with disappearance of the cartilage or may become cystic due to degeneration; some grow to produce benign chondromas within the bone. It is this type of lesion which is the probable site of origin of many chondrosarcomas.

2 *Ecchondromas*: produce protuberances, pain and deformity; a bursa may be formed superficial to the mass. Rarely, a chondrosarcoma may arise from the cartilage, an osteosarcoma from the bony base or a fibrosarcoma from the overlying fibrous tissues.

Gargoylism—lipochondrodystrophy

Nature

A rare autosomal or sex-lined recessive disease combining a chondrodystrophy with the storage of lipid material in the brain and viscera.

Appearances

There are irregularities of enchondral ossification with variation of the size, shape and density of the long bones and kyphosis due to deformed vertebrae with posterior displacement. The accumulation of gangliosides and cerebrosides in the nerve cells of the brain results in mental retardation and convulsions and similar lipid storage in the viscera produces hepatosplenomegaly and cardiomegaly.

Gaucher's disease

Nature

A familial disease mostly occurring in Jews and inherited as an autosomal recessive trait, due to accumulation of glucocerebrosides in histiocytic cells which are large (20–100 μm) and of characteristic 'crumpled' appearance of the cytoplasm.

Sites

Spleen, bone marrow, lymph nodes, brain, liver. Bones are often osteoporotic with a bubbly lytic appearance.

Chondro-osteodystrophy—Morquio's disease

Nature

A rare congenital autosomal recessive disease affecting predominantly the epiphyses and spine.

Appearances

There is a severe kyphosis due to wedge-shaped vertebrae with irregular calcification and deformity of the epiphyseal cartilages of the long bones resulting in enlargement of the ends of these bones.

Melorheostosis

Nature

A rare congenital disease manifested by cortical hyperostoses, which begins in childhood and slowly progresses.

Appearances

One or more bones of the limbs show thickened, flat, bony outgrowths from the cortex reminiscent of the appearance of wax solidifying from a candle. The causation of the disease is unknown but sometimes this extracortical bone has a cartilaginous cap, and the condition may thus be analogous to diaphyseal aclasia (see p. 292).

Marfan's syndrome

Nature

A developmental autosomal dominant disease affecting mesenchymal tissues and especially involving the skeleton, eyes and cardiovascular tissues.

Appearances

The affected individuals are tall and thin with long tapering fingers—*arachnodactyly*, subluxations of the lenses of the eyes, defects of the cardiac atrial septum and a predisposition to develop medionecrosis of the aorta and thus a dissecting aneurysm (see p. 81). The basic defect appears to be a biochemical abnormality of the connective tissue cement substance.

Marble bone disease—osteopetrosis; Albers–Schonberg's disease

Nature

An inherited disease, in severe form autosomal recessive, and in mild form dominant with increased density of all bones ossified from cartilage, especially the vertebrae, pelvic bones and ribs.

Appearances

The bones are extremely hard and yet brittle so that fractures readily occur. On section, the cortical compact bone extends into the medulla which is thus devoid of cancellous bone. The abnormality starts at the epiphyseal line where there is prominence and persistence of the zone of calcification. This becomes surrounded by dense compact bone and there is a failure of remodelling into a cortex and medulla.

Drug-induced—phocomelia

Nature

Failure or incomplete development of limbs due to interference with limb bud formation, e.g. as in thalidomide therapy during pregnancy.

Traumatic

Slipped epiphysis

Trauma is probably an important factor in the aetiology of slipped epiphysis but the precise mechanism remains unknown. Trauma may also affect the epiphyseal bone to cause osteochondritis juvenilis.

Osteochondritis juvenilis

Nature

This is a general term used to describe a number of

lesions at different sites but which have pathological features in common.

Aetiology

There is usually a history of trauma which probably interferes with the epiphyseal blood supply. This is then followed by an avascular bone necrosis.

Sites

The disease affects epiphyseal bone prior to epiphyseal line fusion.

Macroscopical

The epiphyseal bone is irregularly sclerotic and rarefied with fragmentation and deformity. In a weight-bearing site the deformity involves the articular cartilage, producing characteristic radiological appearances upon which the diagnosis is usually made.

Microscopical

The initial lesion is an avascular necrosis of bone and the subsequent changes are those of attempted repair, with bone regeneration, haemorrhages, organization, sequestration and callus formation.

Results

The lesion produces pain and the condition clinically mimics joint tuberculosis. The articular cartilage may become deformed as a result of the alteration of shape of the underlying bone and thus predisposes to osteoarthrosis, which is a common sequel, particularly in the hip.

Types

Named clinical types include:
1 Legg–Calve–Perthes—hip.
2 Osgood–Schlatter—tibial tuberosity.
3 Sever—calcaneum.
4 Kienböck—lunate.
5 Köhler—navicular.
6 Preiser—carpal scaphoid.

Fractures

Nature

A fracture is a break in the continuity of the bone and it may be complete or partial—greenstick, simple or compound, comminuted or impacted. A pathological fracture is one through an area of previously abnormal bone, e.g. through a tumour, cyst, etc.

Stages of healing

1 *Haematoma formation*: the fracture severs the blood vessels in the medulla, cortex and periosteum so that a haematoma is produced.
2 *Organization*: within 24 hours, capillary loops and fibroblasts begin to grow into the haematoma accompanied by an inflammatory cell infiltration. Thus, the area of blood clot is converted into vascular fibroblastic granulation tissue.
3 *Provisional callus*: by about the seventh day, islands of cartilage and osteoid tissue appear in this granulation tissue. The cartilage probably arises from metaplasia of fibroblasts and the osteoid tissue is laid down by osteoblasts growing in from the adjacent bone ends. The osteoid tissue, in the form of irregular spicules and trabeculae, mineralizes to form the provisional callus which is in three zones:
   (a) external callus—subperiosteal;
   (b) internal callus—medullary;
   (c) intermediate callus—cortical;
   This irregular new bone is rapidly formed and the provisional callus is largely complete by about the twenty-fifth day.
4 *Definitive callus*: the disorderly provisional callus is gradually replaced by orderly bone with Haversian systems—definitive callus.
5 *Remodelling*: the normal contour of the bone is reconstituted by the process of remodelling due to both osteoblastic bone formation and osteoclastic resorption. This occurs relatively slowly over a variable period of time but eventually all the excess callus is removed, and the original appearances and structure of the bone reconstituted.

Abnormalities of healing

Bones show great facility for healing but certain complications may occur:
1 *Malunion*: poor anatomical alignment of the fracture results in deformity, angulation or displacement.
2 *Delayed union*: this is common and is due to a large number of factors, many of which have in common the features of continued hyperaemia and decalcification:
   (a) *Infection*: Occurs most commonly following compound fracture with retardation of all stages of the repair process.
   (b) *Foreign bodies*, e.g. missiles, clothing, etc.
   (c) *Dead bone fragments*: especially in comminuted fractures.
   (d) *Inadequate immobilization*: results in damage to the reparative tissues.

(e) *Distraction of the fractured ends*: increasing the volume of repair tissue required.

(f) *Avascularity*: relative or absolute, e.g. avascular bone necrosis of the carpal scaphoid, head of the femur, etc.

(g) *Pathological fracture*, e.g. through tumours and cysts.

(h) *Age*: rapid healing occurs in young persons but is often retarded in the elderly. This is due in part to the presence of decreased vascularity and also from slowing of all metabolic processes.

(i) *Nutritional and metabolic disorders*: especially those affecting the basic materials required, e.g. calcium and phosphate; hypovitaminosis D; renal disease; parathyroid disorders; protein starvation, malabsorption syndromes or excessive protein loss as in albuminuria.

3 *Non-union*: bony union does not occur, the defect being filled by fibrous tissue. Occasionally, a false joint may form at this site—*pseudo-arthrosis*. The following factors may be responsible for non-union:

(a) Lack of immobilization.

(b) Interposition of soft tissues, e.g. muscle.

(c) Wide separation of fragments, e.g. patella.

(d) Pathological fracture, e.g. through a malignant tumour.

C/BONE—INFECTIONS, MISCELLANEOUS

Pyogenic osteomyelitis
Granulomatous osteomyelitis
Fibrous dysplasia
Paget's disease
Hypertrophic osteoarthropathy
Histiocytosis X

Bone infections

Pyogenic osteomyelitis

Pathogenesis

1 *Blood-borne*: usually in children and due to *Staphylococcus aureus*. In adults may complicate urinary tract infection—coliforms, sickle cell disease—*Salmonella* or intravenous drug abusers.

2 *Direct implantation*: complicating compound fracture wounds or surgery, particularly prosthetic joint replacements.

Appearances

When haematogenous, metaphyseal regions of long bones are most frequently involved, sometimes vertebrae in adults. Inflammation in the closed compartment of cancellous bone compresses vessels with necrosis of bone and bone marrow. Extension through the cortex elevates the periosteum which produces new bone to form an *involucrum*. Bone death may be extensive, forming a *sequestrum*.

Results

1 *Resolution*: when appropriate antibiotic therapy is quickly administered.

2 *Extension*: local destruction of bone may result in pathological fracture or sinus formation through skin. Joint involvement in continuity may result in suppurative arthritis.

3 *Chronic osteomyelitis*: late or inadequate therapy may result in recurrent clinical recrudescences of infection with sinus discharge. Drainage and removal of sequestra is then important. Bone sclerosis around pus is common—*Brodie's abscess*.

4 *Amyloid*: long-standing chronic bone infection is a significant cause of secondary AA amyloidosis (see p. 280).

Non-suppurative osteomyelitis—Garre's osteomyelitis

A rare condition, usually producing enlargement and increased density of the shaft of a long bone. Microscopically there is a chronic non-specific granulomatous reaction in the bone and associated new bone formation, but no pus is formed.

Granulomatous

Bone tuberculosis

Mode of infection

Haematogenous spread usually in children from a tuberculous focus elsewhere, most commonly from the lungs where the lesion may be either clinically active or healed.

Sites

The vertebral bodies are the commonest site (see p. 312) but long bones, fingers and joints (see p. 315) are also involved. In a long bone the tuberculous focus may start in the mid-shaft, at the metaphysis or in the subchondral bone.

Appearances

The bone becomes progressively and irregularly destroyed and shows extensive tuberculous granulation tissue but no new bone formation—*caries*.

Results

As long as the infection remains, active bone destruction continues. With antituberculous chemotherapy, healing occurs, firstly by fibrosis and subsequently by new bone formation.

Complications

These are frequent and include:

1 Extension through the periosteum into the soft tissues, sometimes with the production of a 'cold abscess'.

2 Sinus formation through the overlying skin.

3 Pathological fracture through the caseous material.

4 Joint involvement, especially with a subchondral focus (see p. 315).

5 Haematogenous spread to involve other organs.

6 Amyloid disease in very chronic cases.

Syphilis of bone

This is now a rare disease.

Congenital

1 *Osteochondritis* or *epiphysitis*.

2 *Periostitis*.

Acquired

1 *Periostitis*.

2 *Gumma*.

Miscellaneous bone disorders

Fibrous dysplasia—Albright's disease

Nature

In the complete and relatively uncommon syndrome there is a triad of fibrous dysplasia of bone, skin pigmentation and precocious puberty. This complete syndrome is rarely seen, but single bone involvement—monostotic fibrous dysplasia, is common.

Aetiology

Probably due to a developmental defect of mesenchyme with excess fibrous tissue in the bone.

Age

Young adults up to 40 years of age.

Sites

1 *Monostic type*: usually asymptomatic until a mass is found, e.g. jaw, ribs, femur or pathological fracture occurs.

2 *Polyostotic type*: presents with bone pain, fractures and bone deformities.

Appearances

The bone is expanded by firm, white, fibrous tissue containing palpable spicules of bone which fills the medulla and results in thinning of the cortex, so that pathological fracture is common. Avascular fibroblastic tissue replaces the bone. Spicules of woven bone, often of bizarre and unusual shape, mingle intimately with the collagenous stroma. Osteoblasts are inconspicuous.

Results

Local symptoms require curettage or resection. Osteosarcoma, chondrosarcoma or fibrosarcoma occasionally develops.

Paget's disease of bone—osteitis deformans

Nature

A disease occurring in both sexes above the age of 60 and associated with irregular thickening and softening of the bones. Consistent reports of viral-like inclusions in osteoclasts indicate a possible aetiology.

Bones affected

Isolated solitary lesions of the spine or pelvis are common radiological findings on routine examinations, but clinical disease produced by lesions in many bones is uncommon.

1 *Skull*: progressive increase in the size of the skull due to thickening of the bone which, on section, shows gross thickening of both tables and obliteration of the diploe. The base may also be involved to produce platybasia and pressure on nerves in their foramina.

2 *Spine*: thickening and softening of the bones resulting in kyphosis, shortening of the trunk and pressure on nerves in the intervertebral foramina.

3 *Femur*: increased in thickness with coxa vara and anterior bowing.

4 *Pelvis*: the bones are irregularly thickened, especially the iliac bones.

5 *Tibia*: anterior bowing with gross thickening and palpable irregularity of the bone contour.

6 *Clavicle*: thickened and unduly prominent.

On section, all the involved bones show gross and irregular thickening of cortical bone with loss of the normal sharp line of distinction between the cortex and medulla. The cortical bone encroaches upon the medulla in an irregular manner and there is softening and marked vascularity.

Macroscopical

There is increased osteoclastic activity absorbing bone on one side of bone trabeculae, but more dominant is marked osteoblastic activity laying down new bone on the other side. This new bone is irregular and there are well-marked 'cement lines' visible in the bone, producing the 'mosaic' or 'crazy-paving' appearance. The spaces between the thickened bone trabeculae are occupied by fibrous tissue containing large vascular channels. This latter feature is responsible for the marked vascularity evident macroscopically. The serum alkaline phosphatase is raised (see p. 302).

Results

This disease, which is slowly progressive but which, in severe cases, may be symptomatically improved by calcitonin, may produce:

1 *Deformities* of all the bones involved.

2 *Pain*: due to stretching of the periosteum.

3 *Pressure on nerves* as they pass through bony foramina, e.g. deafness, blindness, etc.

4 *Cardiac hypertrophy*: due to the grossly increased vascularity of the bones.

5 *Sarcomatous change* in approximately 1% of cases (see p. 303).

Hypertrophic pulmonary osteoarthropathy

Nature

Clubbing of the fingers associated with thickening of the terminal limb bones. Usually associated with chronic pulmonary disease or cyanotic heart disease.

Appearances

There is marked periosteal fibrosis and subperiosteal new bone formation of the distal phalanges to produce the clubbing. In severe cases this may also involve other bones of the hands, wrists or feet.

Histiocytosis X—Langerhans' cell granulomatosis

Nature

A range of disorders with infiltration of tissues, including bones, by Langerhans' cells, together with variable admixtures of eosinophils, giant cells, foamy cells and areas of fibrosis.

Langerhans' cells have lobulated, indented or grooved nuclei and contain on electron microscopy specific *Birbeck's granules*.

Types

1 *Solitary bone involvement*: this is the most common and is usually called *eosinophil granuloma*. Occurs mostly in young adults usually in cranium, jaw, humerus, rib or femur. These lesions normally spontaneously regress; this can be accelerated by low-dose radiation and long-term prognosis is excellent.

2 *Multiple bone involvement* (with or without skin involvement) usually called *Hand–Schüller–Christian disease*. Presents in childhood or young adults as multiple punched-out radiolucent areas of bones, particularly skull. The course is prolonged with alternating remissions and recrudescences and a normal favourable outcome. Strategically located deposits may cause proptosis or diabetes insipidus. Slight hepatosplenomegaly may be present.

3 *Multiple organ involvement*: usually called *Letterer–Siwe disease*. Skin, lungs, liver, spleen and lymph nodes are commonly involved in addition to bone. Some cases are aggressive and fatal in several months, particularly if under 18 months of age with anaemia and/or thrombocytopenia due to bone marrow involvement.

Histologically it is difficult to separate this type from the more indolent, though monomorphism, necrosis and high mitotic rate suggest a more rapid progression to death.

D/BONE—METABOLIC DISEASES

Bone rarefaction
Osteoporosis
Demineralization
Renal osteodystrophy
Hyperparathyroidism

Bone rarefaction

Rarefaction of bone is seen radiologically as decreased density and can be due to three completely different processes:

1 A deficiency of the bone matrix: *osteoporosis*.
2 Defective mineralization: *rickets* and *osteomalacia*.
3 Hyperparathyroidism: *osteitis fibrosa cystica*.

Osteoporosis

Definition

Osteoporosis is a reduction in the quantity of the bone matrix: the matrix which remains is fully mineralized. This is the result of a *relative* decrease in osteoblastic activity as compared with bone resorption by osteoclasts.

In osteoporosis the blood levels of calcium, phosphate and alkaline phosphatase are all within normal limits (*see* Table 17.2 on p. 302), although there is evidence of increased urinary calcium excretion.

Macroscopical

Osteoporotic bones are lighter in weight, less dense on radiography and show thinning of the cortex. This osteoporotic bone is weaker than normal and is, therefore, prone to fracture, e.g. in the spine.

Microscopical

The bone trabeculae are thinner than normal, but are fully mineralized. Usually there is a decrease in the number of osteoblasts resulting in a failure to lay down new bone matrix, although in some instances there may be an excess of osteoclastic activity absorbing the bone matrix.

Osteoporosis is found in the following conditions:

Scurvy

Nature

A generalized disease due to lack of vitamin C.

Aetiology

Ascorbic acid is water-soluble and is derived from the diet. It is rapidly absorbed and there is a long time lag before the appearance of signs of deficiency as there are large stores in many organs of the body. Scurvy arises due to inadequate intake of fresh fruit and vegetables, which are the main dietary source of the vitamin.

Action of ascorbic acid

Vitamin C is essential for:

1 The formation of collagen.
2 The formation of osteoid tissue.
3 The production of intercellular cement substances and maintenance of the integrity of blood vessels.

Thus, in scurvy, there is poor collagen formation, e.g. poor healing of wounds, lack of osteoid tissue so that normal bone matrix cannot be formed and haemorrhages from the abnormal blood vessels.

Macroscopical

Calcification is normal in scurvy and the zone of provisional calcification persists as a thick white line visible macroscopially and radiologically. There is decreased osteoid formation and haemorrhages occur in the vascular metaphysis and in the subperiosteal regions.

Microscopical

At the epiphyseal line the resting and proliferating zones are normal. The zone of provisional calcification is pronounced to form the 'scorbutic lattice', but osteoid deposition in this zone is deficient. Instead, there is a vascular, haemorrhagic and oedematous zone of myxomatous tissue. The bones also become generally osteoporotic as normal amounts of osteoid tissue cannot be formed by the osteoblasts, so that the whole skeleton becomes progressively deficient in bone matrix.

Disuse

Normal muscular activity is a stimulus for the preservation of normal bone structure, so that any prolonged immobilization or muscular paralysis induces osteoporosis. In the early stages, there is increased osteoclastic bone resorption resulting in thinning of the bone which may be associated with excessive mobilization of calcium, hypercalciuria and renal stone formation. Later, the bone becomes quiescent with diminution of both osteoclastic and osteoblastic activity. The bones return to normal when the patient resumes normal activity.

Hyperthyroidism

Thyrotoxicosis may be associated with mild osteoporosis, apparently due to increased osteoclastic activity.

Osteogenesis imperfecta

A congenital dominant disease in which the bones are slender and the trabeculae thinner than normal although normally mineralized. When severe, the condition may result in multiple fractures and gross deformities in the neonatal period.

A similar condition, producing multiple fractures and associated with blue sclerotics and otosclerosis, is known as *fragilitas ossium*.

Cushing's syndrome

Osteoporosis is a constant finding in this syndrome and is believed to be due to the suppression of osteoblastic activity by the excess glucocorticoids (see p. 117).

Corticosteroid therapy

The prolonged administration of prednisone and allied steroids frequently produces osteoporosis in a similar manner to Cushing's syndrome.

Impaired supply of proteins

Excessive loss of protein, e.g. the nephrotic syndrome; deficient production, e.g. cirrhosis of the liver; or malabsorption, e.g. malabsorption syndromes, may all result in osteoporosis. This is due to the inability to form osteoid tissue in protein-deficient states.

Primary, involutional, senile osteoporosis

Nature

The commonest type of osteoporosis with no known cause but with increasing frequency with age and presenting the features of an involutionary process.

Aetiology

Unknown mechanism but recent studies suggest a relative calcium deficiency to be important, perhaps with a failure of osteoblastic activity, through the involutionary process of the ageing body, to keep pace with skeletal loss. The widely held view that oestrogen deficiency, as in postmenopausal women, was important, has no support when unselected material is examined in which the sex incidence of porotic changes is roughly equal.

Sites

All bones except skull may be affected but particularly spine and upper femur.

Macroscopical

Affected bones are excessively fragile and prone to fracture or collapse, e.g. *codfish spine*, and very frequent fractures of femoral neck in the elderly.

Microscopical

The bone trabeculae are thinned and reduced in number but appear fully mineralized. The osteoblasts show little activity.

Demineralization

Definition

This second group of conditions causes bone rarefaction due to abnormalities of mineralization. The skeleton therefore contains osteoid tissue which is deficient of its mineral content. The group is characterized by lowered serum calcium and phosphate levels, the calcium × phosphate solubility product is reduced and the alkaline phosphatase is raised (see Table 17.2 on p. 302).

Rickets

Nature

A generalized bone disease due to deficiency of vitamin D and affecting the epiphyseal line and all other skeletal tissues.

Aetiology

Usually due to dietary deficiency, but sometimes may be caused by failure of absorption of vitamin D or by a low intake of calcium or phosphate.

Action of vitamin D

This fat-soluble vitamin has several actions including:
1 Aids in the absorption of calcium and phosphate from the intestine.
2 Utilization of calcium and phosphate and its deposition to mineralize osteoid tissue.

3 Excretion of phosphate.

Age
Young children, including infants more than 6 months old.

Incidence
The disease is now very rare in this and many other countries, but remains important in economically backward areas.

Macroscopical
1 *Enlarged epiphyseal lines*: these are widened, lengthened and irregular. This produces a clinical deformity commonly seen in the ribs where it is referred to as 'rickety rosary'.
2 *Softening of the bones*: the skeleton generally is poorly mineralized and soft. The resulting deformities vary according to the stresses at different sites, e.g. coxa vara, flattened pelvis, scoliosis, 'pigeon chest', etc.
3 *Stunted growth.*
4 *'Craniotabes'*: bossed appearance of the skull due to persistence of suture lines and fontanelles.
5 *Delayed dentition.*

Microscopical
The basic abnormality is a failure of full mineralization of osteoid tissue at all sites. The changes are thus:
1 The zone of provisional calcification is deficient, but there is continuation of growth of the proliferating cartilage cells so that areas of cartilage are found in the diaphysis away from the epiphyseal line.
2 The proliferating cartilage continues to grow to produce a thick, broad and irregular line.
3 Osteoid is laid down on the irregular foci of poorly calcified cartilage to produce a completely haphazard and irregular mass instead of the orderly arrangement of cells at the normal epiphyseal line.
4 The shafts of the bones are formed by osteoid tissue with gross deficiency of mineralization so that there is little true bone; this is the cause of the softening and resulting deformities.

Osteomalacia—adult rickets

Nature
This is the adult form of rickets and is relatively common in the very elderly (over 80 years) living alone and whose dietary intake is inadequate. Intest-

inal malabsorption syndromes also cause the condition (see p. 34).

Aetiology
Vitamin D deficiency and reduced calcium intake in adults, especially in women during pregnancy and lactation, when excessive demands are made upon relatively inadequate dietary supplies of calcium. Rickets or osteomalacia may occur in coeliac disease or idiopathic steatorrhoea, where there is failure to absorb both vitamin D and calcium. A gluten-free diet may markedly improve all aspects of the condition which is described on p. 34.

Appearances
There is an excessive amount of osteoid tissue surrounding the thin bone trabeculae with little evidence of mineralization. The lack of mineral results in softened bones and produces many of the changes seen in rickets, particularly the deformities. Some cases may also show areas of osteitis fibrosa cystica presumed to be due to secondary parathyroid hyperplasia following a lowering of the serum ionized calcium level (see p. 139). The biochemical changes are summarized in Table 17.2 on p. 302).

Renal osteodystrophy

Nature
The kidney is intimately involved in calcium and phosphate metabolism and, just as primary disturbances of mineral metabolism, e.g. in hyperparathyroidism, can cause renal disease, e.g. nephrocalcinosis, so some cases of renal disease will manifest skeletal changes. The part played by the kidney in maintenance of normal levels of calcium and phosphorus in the body is largely a tubular function. It follows, therefore, that skeletal abnormalities are most likely to occur in renal lesions associated with loss of tubular mass or with defective tubular function.

The bone changes due to renal disease, however, vary very widely according to the nature of the renal lesion, its duration and age of the patient, and renal rickets is not a term which describes the condition sufficiently accurately. Renal osteodystrophy is a preferred name for these secondary skeletal changes.

It should be noted that the changes are often patchily distributed and that the several types of change may occur together even in the same bone. In many cases of chronic renal disease significant bone abnormalities never occur but in a small proportion, particularly in progressive renal failure in childhood, the skeletal deformities may be the most striking clinical abnormality.

Bone changes
1 *Osteitis fibrosa*: due to reactive hyperplasia of the parathyroids—*secondary hyperparathyroidism*.
2 *Rickets or osteomalacia*: due to disturbance of vitamin D metabolism, probably due to an acquired insensitivity to its action.
3 *Osteosclerosis*: the cause of which is obscure but may be an unusual manifestation of parathyroid overactivity. In these cases there is markedly increased radiodensity of affected bones, particularly of the vertebrae. The bone adjacent to the intervertebral discs is affected in the first place—*rugger-jersey spine*. The cancellous trabeculae are grossly thickened with reduction of marrow space, remaining areas having a fibrocellular content.

Classification

Uraemic osteodystrophy
1 Juvenile form (renal dwarfism, renal rickets).
2 Adult form.

Associated with failure of tubular reabsorption
1 *Phosphaturia*: vitamin D-resistant rickets. A Mendelian dominant hereditary tubular disease characterized by defective tubular reabsorption of phosphates and hence increased urinary output. The bone changes are those of rickets or osteomalacia depending on the age of the patient and are resistant to normal dosage of vitamin D but respond to high dosage, which needs to be maintained in spite of the risk of hypercalcaemia and subsequent nephrocalcinosis.
2 *Renal tubular acidosis*: an intrinsic functional abnormality of renal tubules causing an inability to secrete an acid urine with resulting acidosis, high urinary calcium excretion and excess phosphate loss. The skeletal changes are those of osteomalacia. Potassium depletion also occurs and requires correction together with the acidosis: vitamin-D therapy improves the bone disorder. Osteomalacic changes may also be produced by the hyperchloraemic acidosis due to implantation of ureters in the colon.
3 *Fanconi syndrome*: a congenital autosomal recessive disorder of renal tubular function with a variety

of effects notably aminoaciduria, phosphaturia and glycosuria. The bone changes are those of osteomalacia. In some cases cystine crystals are deposited in the tissues—*Lignac–Fanconi syndrome*.

There is a *swan-neck* deformity of the proximal convoluted tubules which are shorter than normal. Treatment is by large doses of vitamin D together with correction of potassium depletion and acidosis.

Biochemical changes
These are summarized in Table 17.2 on p. 302.

Summary
Thus, bone matrix which is not fully mineralized is characteristic of osteomalacia and rickets. This may be due to:
1 *Dietary causes*: vitamin D deficiency.
2 *Intestinal malabsorption*, e.g. coeliac disease and idiopathic steatorrhoea.
3 *Renal causes*: congenital tubular defects; acquired loss of tubules.

When there is an associated lowering of serum ionized calcium level, the histological picture of osteomalacia may be complicated by secondary hyperparathyroidism with, in severe cases, osteitis fibrosa cystica.

Hyperparathyroidism

Osteitis fibrosa cystica— Von Recklinghausen's disease of bone

Primary hyperparathyroidism

Aetiology
Hypersecretion of parathormone by an adenoma, an adenocarcinoma or, more rarely, by hyperplastic parathyroid tissue (see p. 138).

Pathogenesis
The excess parathormone mobilizes mineral from the bone, followed by removal of matrix and subsequently by fibrous replacement and cysts.

Bone changes
Detectable bony changes occur in only 25% of cases of hyperparathyroidism.

Macroscopical
The bones become demineralized and, in advanced

Table 17.2 Metabolic changes in bone disease.

	Blood				Urine		
	Ca	P	Alk. Phos	Urea, etc.	Ca	P	Protein, etc.
Osteoporosis	N	N	N	N	N or Sl +	N	Nil
Osteomalacia	N or Sl low	Low	Raised	N	Low	Low	Nil
Hyperparathyroidism (uncomplicated)	Raised	Low	Raised or N	N	+ +	Raised	Nil
Uraemic oesteodystrophy	N or Sl low	Raised	N or raised	Raised	N or low	Low	Protein +
Phosphaturia	N	Low	N	N	Low	Raised	Nil
Tubular acidosis	N	Low	N	Low CO_2 High Cl Low K	Raised	Raised	Nil Raised K
Fanconi syndrome	N or Sl low	Low	N	N	Low	Raised	Protein + amino acid + glucose +
Paget's disease	N	N	Raised +	N	N	N	N

cases, so soft that they can be cut with a knife. Deformities follow the softening. In addition, there may be single or multiple expanded, haemorrhagic and cystic tumour-like areas in the bone—'*brown tumours*' (see p. 138).

Microscopical

The demineralized bone is removed by osteoclastic activity and replaced by vascular and cellular fibrous tissue containing many osteoclastic giant cells with cysts and areas of haemorrhage.

Effects

The appearances of the parathyroid glands, the nephrocalcinosis, metastatic calcification and the blood changes are described on p. 138. The important and diagnostic biochemical feature is a rise in the serum ionized calcium level.

Secondary hyperparathyroidism

As described above many examples of rickets and osteomalacia may contain areas of osteitis fibrosa cystica in the bones. This appearance is the result of excess parathormone due to secondary hyperplasia of the parathyroid glands induced by a low ionized serum calcium level. The conditions may thus follow disturbances of vitamin D metabolism, renal tubular lesions or malabsorption syndromes, or complicate regular renal dialysis.

E/BONE—TUMOURS

Osteoblastic tumours
Cartilage tumours
Fibrous tumours
Giant cell tumours
Giant-cell variants
Tumours of fat, vessels, nerves
Tumours of bone marrow cells
Chordoma
Secondary tumours

Secondary tumours in bone are common, but primary tumours of bone are comparatively rare. Malignant bone tumours account for approximately 0.6% of deaths from malignant disease. For the classification of bone tumours (see Table 17.3).

Bone tumours

These are osteoblastic tumours, i.e. tumours of osteoblasts.

Osteoma

Cancellous osteoma—osteochondroma

This is not a true tumour but is a manifestation of diaphyseal aclasia (see p. 292). The outgrowth of cancellous bone has a cartilaginous cap from which chondrosarcoma may rarely develop.

Table 17.3 Bone tumour classification.

Bone tumours	Cartilage tumours	Fibrous tumours	Giant-cell tumours
Osteoma (B)	Chondroma (B)	Fibroma (B)	True giant-cell tumour (M)
Osteoid osteoma (B)	Benign chondroblastoma (B)	Osteoblastoma (B)	Giant-cell 'variants' (B)
Benign osteoblastoma (B)	Chondromyxoid fibroma (B)	Non-ossifying fibroma (B)	
Osteosarcoma (M)	Chondrosarcoma (M)	Fibrosarcoma (M)	
		Malignant fibrous histiocytoma (M)	
Fatty tumours	**Vascular tumours**	**Nerve tumours**	**Bone marrow tumours**
Lipoma (B)	Haemangioma (B)	Neurofibroma (B)	Leukaemia (M)
Liposarcoma (M)	Angiosarcoma (M)	Schwannoma (B)	Ewing's tumour (M)
		Malignant nerve sheath tumours (M)	Primary lymphoma (M)
			Multiple myeloma (M)
Notochord tumour	**Epithelial tumour**		
Chordoma (M)	'Adamantinoma' of tibia (M)		

B, benign; M, malignant.

Ivory osteoma

A rare but true tumour of bone which almost always occurs in the skull in 40–50-year-olds. It is usually a spheroid of dense, compact bone and may cause pressure effects within the cranial cavity or in a nasal air sinus. Histologically, there is compact bone with Haversian systems. Symptoms are produced by pressure or by infection which may result in osteomyelitis of the adjacent bone.

Osteosarcoma—osteogenic sarcoma

Age

Maximal between 10 and 25 years of age but the tumour also occurs in an older age group arising in relationship to Paget's disease of bone.

Sites

May occur in any bone but most commonly found in the neighbourhood of the knee joint. They mostly arise in the metaphyses of long bones and rarely are multifocal in origin.

Predisposing factors

1 Paget's disease of bone.
2 Long-term effects of radioactive substances, e.g. painters of luminous watch dials.

In the majority of cases the causation remains completely unknown and trauma is almost certainly in no way an aetiological factor.

Macroscopical

A haemorrhagic, variegated tumour expanding the bone and destroying both medulla and cortex; spicules of bone may be palpable within the tumour substance. The periosteum is frequently raised to produce 'Codman's triangle' at the junction of the raised periosteum and the cortex. This is, however, in no way specific for an osteosarcoma and may be produced by any lesion which lifts the periosteum and is followed by subperiosteal new bone formation.

Microscopical

The essential feature is the presence of malignant osteoblasts which lay down spicules of irregular osteoid tissue. This osteoid tissue may or may not calcify, and this variable feature will determine the radiological appearances as being either osteolytic or osteosclerotic. The tumour osteoblasts are atypical, bizarre, show mitotic activity and frequently giant-cell forms. Small areas of cartilage may be present and secondary necrosis and haemorrhage are also frequently seen. It is common to find microscopical evidence of vascular invasion within the tumour tissue.

Spread

These tumours are rapidly growing, extend along the marrow cavity, destroy bone locally and often penetrate the periosteum to involve soft tissues. Lymphatic spread is unusual but vascular spread is common and early.

Prognosis
Until recently, amputation resulted in a 20% 5-year survival, but more local resections with prosthetic replacement and multidrug chemotherapy now show 50% survival at 5 years. Widespread blood-borne metastases occur, especially in the lungs. A better-differentiated variant, which develops on the external surface of a metaphysis, is the *juxtacortical osteosarcoma*. This type is bulky and slow-growing, with a 5-year survival of 80%.

Other osteoblastic tumours

Osteoid osteoma

Nature
A rare lesion occurring in the cortical area of any bone but especially in the femur and tibia. It arises in patients between 15 and 25 years of age and causes severe pain, especially at night.

Macroscopical
A central, pink, fleshy nidus of soft tissue of about 1 cm or less in diameter is surrounded by dense sclerotic bone.

Microscopical
The central nidus is composed of vascular tissue in which there is osteoblastic activity forming osteoid tissue and bone. A few osteoclasts may also be present.

Results
Incomplete removal may lead to a recurrence, but complete removal is curative. Nuclear magnetic resonance and computerized tomographic scans pre-operatively have markedly reduced the number of incomplete excisions.

Benign osteoblastoma—giant osteoid osteoma

Sites
Although most commonly seen in the neural arches of vertebrae, other bones in young adults may be the site of this very rare lesion.

Macroscopical
There is expansion of the medulla of the bone of origin by a mass with a translucent centre containing specks of calcification.

Microscopical
The appearances are somewhat similar to those of an osteoid osteoma but there is a more prominent fibrous stroma and the lesions are larger.

Results
Expansion of the bone of the vertebral arch may result in spinal cord compression (see p. 312). The histological appearance has to be distinguished from that of an osteosarcoma.

Cartilage tumours
These are tumours of cartilage cells.

Chondroma
Two types of chondroma are described:
1 *Ecchondroma—osteochondroma.*
2 *Enchondroma.*

The ecchondroma is the cartilaginous outgrowth which occurs in diaphyseal aclasia (see p. 292) and the enchondroma is the cartilage which persists within the bone in dyschondroplasia (see p. 292). The latter are single or multiple cartilaginous areas which may:
1 Ossify and disappear.
2 Remain as islands of cartilage.
3 Slowly grow as chondromas.

The most frequent site is the phalanges of the fingers, where they are usually multiple, but similar tumours may occur elsewhere, e.g. in the femur. Histologically, they are formed by regular, mature and comparatively acellular cartilage, with areas of ossification or mucoid degeneration in the stroma.

Results
Regression may occur at any stage or the lesions may continue to grow, producing pain or deformity. Pathological fracture through an enchondroma may occasionally occur and there is a risk of chondrosarcoma developing subsequently.

Chondrosarcoma

Nature
This tumour of cartilage cells is probably the most frequently encountered primary malignant tumour of bone.

Age
Mostly 30–60 years but also in children.

Sites
Pelvis and long bones, especially in the area of the knee.

Predisposing factors
Most of the tumours probably arise in pre-existing enchondromas or ecchondromas but some have been reported as occurring in association with Paget's disease in the older age groups.

Macroscopical
Bulky, lobulated, glistening and semitranslucent tumours. The tumour may be entirely within the bone but more usually extends outside or away from the bone to indent or invade adjacent soft tissues. White, gritty areas of calcification and areas of cystic degeneration are commonly seen.

Microscopical
A malignant tumour composed of cellular atypical cartilage with irregularity of the cells, many of which have double nuclei. Mitotic figures are usually scanty but areas of cystic change, calcification or ossification are frequently seen in the stroma.

Spread
These are more slowly growing than osteosarcomas and compress adjacent soft tissues in the early stages. Later, direct invasion occurs and blood, and occasionally lymphatic, spread may also be manifest.

Prognosis
Treatment is by wide local excision where feasible. Tumours can be histologically graded yielding 5-year survivals of 78%, 53% and 22% for low, moderate and high grades respectively.

Other cartilaginous tumours

Benign chondroblastoma—Codman's tumour
A rare tumour occurring in males at the age of 20 or younger. Epiphyseal bone with involvement of the epiphyseal line is the site of choice, especially at the knee or in the upper end of the humerus. Microscopically, this is a cellular tumour composed of chondroblasts. The cells frequently show mitoses and giant cells which, however, are much smaller than those seen in a giant cell tumour. In addition, there are areas of cartilage which may calcify and often areas showing some bone formation.

This is usually a benign tumour, but its chief importance is that the cellularity of the stroma may lead to a false diagnosis of malignancy, usually being designated as a malignant giant cell tumour. Occasional true cases behave locally aggressively, and rarely some metastasize without showing any significantly different histological features.

Chondromyxoid fibroma
An equally rare tumour occurring below the age of 30 and involving the epiphyseal line, especially at the upper end of the tibia and the small bones of the hands and feet; however, the epiphysis is spared. The tumour is firm and lobulated and composed of lobules of fibrous tissue separated by myxomatous tissue containing cells in lacunae, thus mimicking the appearances of cartilage.

This is a benign tumour and yet the cellularity and atypicality of some of the areas may result in an incorrect histological interpretation as a chondrosarcoma. Local recurrence (25%) is avoided by block excision.

Fibrous tumours
There are a number of fibroblastic lesions in bone:

Fibroma of bone
A rare lesion in bone producing a localized area of rarefaction with a clear-cut margin. Microscopically, it is composed of inactive, acellular, fibrous tissue, but its precise differentiation from fibrous dysplasia (see p. 296) is difficult to determine. The stroma may ossify to result in an 'ossifying fibroma' and the chief complication is pathological fracture.

Fibrosarcoma

Age
Occurs particularly in young adults and those of middle age, although the elderly are not exempt.

Sites
The metaphyses of long bones are the sites of election, 50% in distal femur or proximal tibia; some are periosteal.

Macroscopical

1 *Periosteal*: a white, firm, fibrous tumour firmly attached to the periosteum and involving the adjacent soft tissues to a greater extent than the bone.

2 *Endosteal*: the endosteal or medullary fibrosarcoma produces expansion of the bone with destruction due to replacement by firm, white, fibrous tumour extending within the medullary cavity and through the cortex.

Microscopical

These are fibroblastic tumours with variable collagen production. The medullary type destroys the bone as it progresses along the shaft and there is usually microscopic extension well beyond the macroscopic margins.

Spread

Spread occurs by direct invasion and also by lymphatics and by the blood stream.

Prognosis

The periosteal form has a better prognosis than the more common medullary type, whose low-grade examples have an 83% 10-year survival and high-grade ones 34%.

Other fibrous tumours

Malignant fibrous histiocytoma

Rather high-grade malignant bone tumours containing a mixture of spindle-shaped fibroblasts with histiocytic cells, some multinucleated. A 'storiform' pattern is characteristic (see p. 105).

Non-ossifying fibroma of bone—metaphyseal fibrous defect

This is a rare benign lesion which presents as a tumour in the subcortical region of the metaphysis of long bones of patients in the 12–20 year age group. The tumours are firm, fibrous and of yellow or brown coloration. They are composed of whorled fibrous tissue containing a variable number of foam cells and giant cells which contain haemosiderin pigment, but there is no bone formation. This is probably not a true tumour but a developmental aberration at the epiphyseal plate. The lesion, if followed radiologically over a period of time, gradually 'grows away' from the metaphysis towards the mid-shaft and eventually disappears.

Chondromyxoid fibroma

This is regarded by some authorities as essentially a benign fibrous tumour of bone displaying unusual myxomatous characteristics which simulate the appearance of cartilage. The lesion is described on p. 305.

Giant cell tumours—osteoclastoma

A tumour with many histological and clinical imitators—*giant cell variants*.

True giant cell tumours

Age

The common age is 20–35 years; they are rare below the age of 20. Most of the 'giant cell variants' occur in younger persons.

Origin

This is unknown, but is considered to be a tumour of mononuclear stromal cells which are the precursors of osteoclasts.

Sites

The epiphyses of long bones are the sites of election. They do not occur in mid-shaft regions or in the jaw, but the pelvis and vertebrae are rare sites. Bones around the knee joint account for over 50% of cases.

Predisposing factors

Apart from the few cases which arise from Paget's disease in the older age groups, there are no known predisposing factors.

Macroscopical

Present as eccentric expanding tumours destroying the bone and with little or no reactive bone formation. On section, the tumour is red and fleshy and expands the bone with thinning of the cortex. The tumour remains confined within the periosteum in most cases.

Microscopical

The essential diagnostic features are the presence of two types of cells:

1 The mononuclear cells which form the stroma of the tumour.

2 Giant cells of osteoclast type—20–30 centrally placed nuclei and abundant cytoplasm.

Fibrous tissue, cartilage and bone are not present in the stroma, and areas of haemorrhage and foam cells are seen only as secondary changes after trauma, fracture or attempted treatment. The mononuclear cells are tumour cells and are oval, round or spindle-shaped, often showing pleomorphism and mitoses. The giant cells do not show mitoses and are not phagocytic. It should be emphasized that the presence of significant amount of bone, cartilage, foam cells, fibrous tissue or large vascular spaces, excludes the diagnosis of a true giant cell tumour; these are the features of many of the 'variants'.

Spread

All giant cell tumours are locally malignant, and untreated they will progressively destroy the surrounding bone and may even penetrate a joint or surrounding soft tissue. Moreover, untreated, about 15% will eventually metastasize, still as a giant cell tumour, via the blood stream to the lungs.

Prognosis

Recurrence rates up to 35% occur with curettage, but only 7% or less if local excision is carried out *en bloc*. This may require allografts or prostheses to restore anatomical continuity and good function. Uncontrollable local recurrence or metastases occur in about 5%.

Giant cell variants

Solitary bone cyst—unicameral bone cyst

Simple cysts occur mostly in males before the age of 20 years and they frequently produce pathological fractures. Histologically, the fibrous wall contains giant cells of osteoclast type. They are not true tumours and, although their origin is obscure, they are probably congenital disorders.

Aneurysmal bone cyst

Large and often rapidly expanding lesions of long bones and vertebrae of young persons. Because of their rapidly increasing size they clinically imitate a malignant tumour. Macroscopically, they are extremely vascular lesions which microscopically show numerous, large vascular channels lined by a cellular fibrous tissue containing giant cells. Although superficially resembling osteoclasts, these giant cells are phagocytic and contain haemosiderin. The lesions are of uncertain origin but are often cured by curettage.

'Brown tumours'

These are the localized bone lesions of osteitis fibrosa cystica. The elevated serum calcium in this condition assists in arriving at the correct interpretation of these tumour-like masses containing giant cells, cysts and fibrous tissue (see p. 302).

Osteoblastoma

This fibrous lesion has been described on p. 304. It was formerly regarded as a fibrous, regressing or xanthomatous variant of giant cell tumour.

Benign chondroblastoma

The cellularity and the presence of giant cells in this tumour has resulted in misinterpretation of the appearances as those of a giant cell tumour (see p. 305).

Giant cell reparative granuloma

This benign lesion of the jaw contains giant cells and has frequently been misinterpreted as a true giant cell tumour (see p. 18).

Excessive osteoclastic activity

Any area of marked osteoclastic bone resorption may mimic a giant cell tumour. This appearance may be associated with osteoid osteoma, benign chondroblastoma, or with the edge of any rarefying bone lesion, e.g. fibrous dysplasia, in which osteoclasts may be profuse.

Summary

It will be noted that all the lesions mentioned above are benign, and if these are removed from any series of 'giant cell tumours' the remainder, which are the true giant cell tumours, only form a comparatively uncommon but important group. In all these variants, examination of the whole 'tumour' enables a correct diagnosis to be made, but considerable difficulties may occur in the interpretation of some biopsy material, especially if only small amounts are available for examination.

Fatty tumours

Lipomas can occur in bone, especially subperiosteally, but they are rare. Liposarcoma, which is described as occurring in the medullary cavity, is extremely rare.

Vascular tumours

Haemangiomas are common and are malformations most commonly seen in the bodies of vertebrae (see

p. 312). The malignant vasoformative tumour—*angio-sarcoma*, is rare and produces a large, very vascular tumour of high malignancy. Microscopically, it is composed of primitive and atypical blood vessels of capillary calibre and metastasizes rapidly.

Nerve tumours

Tumours of nerve tissue, neurofibroma, Schwannoma and malignant nerve sheath tumours, are occasionally found in bone but are extremely rare, except in the jaw (see p. 108).

Tumours of bone marrow cells

Nature

Tumours arising in haemopoietic and lymphoreticular cells of the bone marrow.

Leukaemia

This is by far the most common.

Ewing's tumour of bone

Nature

A tumour of characteristic appearance but of un-known cell type, though recent evidence suggests a primitive neuroectodermal origin.

Age

Children, nearly all below the age of 10 years, but occasionally in young adults.

Sites

The mid-shaft medullary region of long bones is the site of election, but it occasionally occurs in the pelvis and other flat bones.

Macroscopical

Fleshy, non-bone-forming tumours in the mid-shaft with reactive bone formation externally, producing the radiological 'onion-skin' appearance.

Microscopical

The tumour is composed of sheets of uniform, hyperchromatic, round cells, with little cytoplasm and virtually no stroma. Reticulin staining is negative and there is absence of fibrous tissue, cartilage or bone within the tumour matrix. The tumour cells contain abundant glycogen.

Spread

Local with destruction of bone. Early blood spread and pulmonary metastases are common.

Prognosis

Until recently, surgery and/or radiation resulted in 5-year survival rates of 5–8% but with high-dose irradiation and combined chemotherapy 5-year sur-vivals are now 75%.

Differential diagnosis

A secondary deposit in bone from a neuroblastoma of the adrenal or other sites in the sympathetic nervous system may closely simulate a Ewing's tumour and no example is acceptable unless an exhaustive search has excluded such a primary. A lymphoma may also show a similar picture, but can be identified by immuno-cytochemistry.

Primary lymphoma of bone

A rare primary B cell tumour of bone which typically occurs in young adults aged about 30 and presents as a radiotranslucent lesion in the diaphysis or meta-physis of a long bone. These are radiosensitive tumours: the prognosis is relatively good particularly if radiation and chemotherapy are combined. Survival for 5 years can be expected in at least 80%. This is almost always an isolated lesion and appears to differ from the generalized disease.

Multiple myeloma—myelomatosis

This uncommon tumour of marrow plasma cells most frequently involves the spine and flat bones.

Chordoma—tumour of the notochord

This occurs only in relation to notochord remnants, and is described on p. 312.

'Adamantinoma' of the tibia

This is a very rare primary tumour in bone, of epithelial appearance and which mimics an adam-antinoma of the jaw (see p. 16). The origin of this tumour is debatable but it is of low-grade local malignancy.

Secondary tumours in bone

Incidence

Secondary tumours are found in bones in 15–18% of

all fatal cases of malignant disease; they are thus much more common than all the primary bone tumours.

Sources

Metastases in bone most commonly arise from primary tumours of the prostate, breast, bronchus, kidney, stomach and thyroid or from a malignant lymphoma.

Macroscopical

Single or multiple, soft or hard deposits of tumours in bones; pathological fractures are common. In the spine there may be collapse of the vertebral bodies, but the discs are usually spared until an advanced stage.

Microscopical

Similar in appearance to the primary tumour but the bone reaction is variable:

1 In the early stages, the tumour grows between the bone trabeculae with no bone destruction and no visible radiological changes.

2 The tumour destroys and replaces the bone, producing the more usual appearance of osteolytic deposits.

3 The tumour cells may evoke an osteoblastic response resulting in osteosclerotic deposits. This occurs especially with prostatic carcinoma, but breast secondaries, Hodgkin's disease and other tumours may occasionally produce the same appearance.

F/DISEASES OF THE SPINE

Degenerative
Scoliosis
Kyphosis
Ankylosing spondylitis
Infections
Primary tumours
Secondary tumours

Degenerative diseases

Nature

Degenerative changes commonly occur in the spine with advancing age and may affect the synovial joints of the spine, the intervertebral discs or the bones.

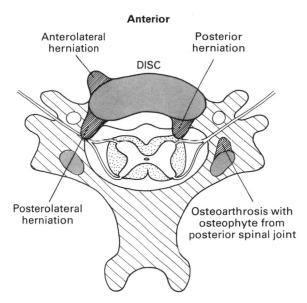

Fig. 26 Spine—sites of degenerative lesions.

Synovial joints—osteoarthrosis

Sites

The posterior and lateral spinal joints which have articular cartilages and synovial membranes, i.e. not the intervertebral discs.

Appearances

These joints are commonly affected by osteoarthrosis. There is degeneration of the articular cartilage with fibrillation and osteophyte formation is prominent (see p. 313).

Results

This degenerative joint disease may be associated with root pain and limitation of spinal movement, especially in the cervical region (see Fig. 26).

Intervertebral discs—degeneration

The central part of the intervertebral disc is composed of a myxoid, fluid-containing material—nucleus pulposus. This is bounded externally by the fibrocartilaginous annulus fibrosus and confined above and below by the vertebral bodies. The central nucleus pulposus is under constant pressure; if it escapes from its normal confines, pathological changes may result.

Vertical herniation

Herniation vertically results in protrusion of the nuclear tissue into the vertebral body above or below the disc. This becomes radiologically visible when reactive new bone surrounds the protrusion. This is extremely common and is called a *Schmorl's node* (see Fig. 27).

Posterior herniation

Posterior herniation of disc tissue produces bulging of the posterior longitudinal ligament which may cause pressure on the spinal cord. More frequently, the disc tissue herniates posterolaterally to one side of the mid-line to produce unilateral neurological pressure signs (see Fig. 26).

Annular herniation

As a result of desiccation of the nucleus pulposus, which is common with advancing years, the disc space becomes narrowed with resulting bulging of the fibres of the peripheral portion of the annulus fibrosus beyond the bony margins. This may occur posteriorly to produce the pressure symptoms of a disc syndrome, but more commonly occurs laterally or anterolaterally and eventually results in osteophytosis of the spine (see Fig. 27).

Osteophytosis or spondylosis

Osteophytosis of the spine is the condition of marginal bony lipping of the vertebral bodies at the disc margins. The disc tissue becomes narrowed following vertical prolapse or desiccation and the annulus fibrosus protrudes at the periphery thus raising the overlying periosteum from the adjacent vertebral margins. Reactive subperiosteal new bone formation results in bony spurs or osteophyte production but the line of the annulus fibrosus separates the bony spurs from each other. The osteophytes produced cause no clinical manifestations except in the posterolateral position where they may press on the spinal cord or nerve roots (see Fig. 26).

Adolescent kyphosis

The primary condition is herniation of the nucleus pulposus to produce Schmorl's nodes and narrowing of the disc space. The posterior portions of the vertebral bodies are supported by the posterior spinal joints but the anterior portions have no such support, so forward tilting of the vertebrae occurs leading to kyphosis. This deformity then interferes with normal growth of the vertebral bodies so that a permanent wedge-shaped deformity ensues. It was formerly considered that epiphysitis of the vertebral bodies produced this wedge-shaped deformity and this disease is still sometimes known as *Scheuermann's disease* (see Fig. 27).

Senile kyphosis

This is a common disease in the over-60 age group in which there is disc degeneration, especially of the anterior portion. The discs protrude in all directions with osteophyte formation and bony union occurs through the thinned anterior portions of the disc. Ossification then occurs between the vertebral bodies and the kyphosis is permanent.

Vertebral bone disorders

Primary, involutional, senile osteoporosis

This common type of osteoporosis causes decreased density of the vertebral bodies and predisposes to fractures. Many cases remain asymptomatic but pain, collapse and pressure on nerves at the intervertebral foramina may occur (see p. 298).

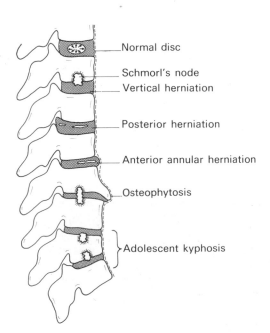

Normal disc

Schmorl's node
Vertical herniation

Posterior herniation

Anterior annular herniation

Osteophytosis

Adolescent kyphosis

Fig. 27 Spine—diagrammatic representation of the effects of disc degeneration.

Scoliosis

Definition
Lateral curvature of the spine associated with rotation of vertebrae.

Causes
1 *Congenital*: defects in development, or of ossification, of one or more vertebrae, may cause scoliosis, e.g. hemivertebra, absence of intervertebral disc with fusion of vertebral bodies, anomalies of ribs, etc.

2 *Paralytic*: following nerve paralysis there may be imbalance of the trunk muscles.

3 *Neurofibromatosis*: generalized neurofibromatosis is sometimes associated with other congenital abnormalities, including scoliosis or kyphoscoliosis due to failure of development of one side of the vertebral body (see p. 109).

4 *Neuropathic and myopathic*: rare causes of scoliosis are syringomyelia, Friedreich's ataxia and the muscular dystrophies.

5 *Pulmonary causes*: extensive unilateral pulmonary fibrosis following empyema or tuberculosis may produce scoliosis. Pneumonectomy or thoracoplasty may have similar effects.

6 *Vertebral destruction*: destruction or deformity of a vertebra by disease, e.g. rickets, tuberculosis, osteomyelitis, tumour or trauma.

7 *Compensatory*: scoliosis may follow compensatory rotation or tilting of the pelvis due to shortening of the leg bones, lesions of the hip, etc.

8 *Idiopathic*: this is the commonest variety of scoliosis and is not associated with any known or detectable disease; the diagnosis is made by a process of exclusion of the known causes.

Results
The vertebral bodies become deformed with a wedge-shaped appearance, the apices of which are directed towards the concavity. The intervertebral discs protrude and, by elevation of the periosteum, result in osteophytosis at the disc margins. In long-standing cases, fusion between the osteophytes across the disc tissue may produce permanent bony fixation of the spine in its deformed position.

Kyphosis

Definition
Flexion deformity of the spine. It may be associated with scoliosis—*kyphoscoliosis*.

Smooth kyphosis
A gradual exaggeration of the normal dorsal curvature of the spine.

Causes
1 *Disc disease*: adolescent and senile kyphosis (see p. 310).

2 *Faulty posture*: a doubtful aetiology.

3 *Early ankylosing spondylitis* (see below).

4 *Tuberculosis*: rarely.

5 *Paget's disease* (see p. 296).

Angular kyphosis
Sharp angulation of the spine produces a hump—*gibbus*.

Causes
1 *Congenital*: due to congenital 'wedge-shaped' vertebrae, to the narrowed 'cushion-shaped' vertebrae of Morquio's chondro-osteodystrophy or to gargoylism (see p. 292).

2 *Calvé's disease*: this was formerly regarded as a form of 'osteochondritis', but is now considered more likely to be a healed area of eosinophil granuloma (see p. 297) producing a plate of sclerotic bone in one vertebral body—*vertebra plana*.

3 *Trauma*: crush fracture may produce an acute angular kyphosis or the angulation may occur more slowly in Kümmell's disease. This occurs after trauma followed by bone rarefaction of the vertebra leading to collapse of the anterior portion of the body with wedge deformity. The process is probably due to progressive collapse of bone from weight-bearing at the site of a vertebral fracture.

4 *Vertebral body infection*: tuberculosis, or less frequently a pyogenic infection (see p. 312).

5 *Bone rarefaction*: rickets, osteomalacia, osteoporosis (see p. 298).

Results of kyphosis
The kyphosis results in deformity of the spine with compensatory curves above and below.

Ankylosing spondylitis—rheumatoid spondylitis

Nature
A disease characterized by a rigid spine due to ossification of the spinal joints and ligaments.

Aetiology

This remains unknown although a very large proportion of patients with the disease and close relatives have HLA antigen B27 present—more than 90%.

Incidence

Uncommon: Male : female, 2 : 1.

Appearances

There is a multiple arthritis affecting the spinal, costovertebral and sacroiliac joints. It starts as a proliferating synovitis with eventual fibrous replacement of the articular cartilages, fibrous ankylosis and subsequently bony ankylosis.

The intervertebral discs are of normal thickness but there is marginal ossification of the outer fibres of the annulus fibrosus. This results in fusion of the vertebral bodies at the periphery of the disc space—'bamboo-spine' appearance. Similar changes affect the spinal ligaments and sacroiliac joints, adding to the spinal rigidity see also p. 103.

Sometimes there is involvement of other joints, especially the hip and knee, by changes which are similar to those found in rheumatoid arthritis. Serological tests are, however, invariably negative;

Results

There is marked pain, stiffness of the spine and ultimately complete rigidity, often in a grossly deformed position. Rheumatoid aortitis may develop in long-standing cases (see p. 72), also iritis and conjunctivitis.

Infections

Pyogenic osteomyelitis

Blood-borne, or less commonly direct, pyogenic infection of the spine is largely due to *Staphylococcus pyogenes*, but occasionally from a wide range of microbial agents. The appearances are described on p. 295.

Spinal tuberculosis—Pott's disease

Now much less common, this disease still causes a high proportion of the cases of bone and joint tuberculosis, usually by haematogenous spread from a lung focus in children or the elderly.

Appearances are similar to those described on p. 295 with particular predilection for producing bony collapse, spinal cord compression and extra-spinal extension into adjacent muscles with formation of a 'cold abscesses' and tracking, e.g. psoas abscess to upper thigh.

Primary tumours of vertebrae

Incidence

With a few notable exceptions, primary tumours of the spine are extremely rare.

Types

All the primary bone tumours that are encountered elsewhere in the skeleton have been reported as occurring in the spine, e.g. osteosarcoma, chondrosarcoma, etc. These are considered on pp. 302–309 but certain lesions occur in the spine with sufficient frequency to merit special mention.

Benign tumours

Haemangioma

This relatively common hamartomatous vascular malformation is frequently asymptomatic and discovered incidentally by its characteristic radiological appearance of vertical bony buttresses in lumbar vertebral bodies.

Aneurysmal bone cyst

An uncommon bone lesion which occurs in the spine and long bones and is described on p. 307. Many examples of so-called giant cell tumour of the spine have been shown on subsequent review of the histological material to be aneurysmal bone cysts.

Benign osteoblastoma—osteogenic fibroma—giant osteoid osteoma

This rare tumour is most frequently found in vertebral neural arches of 15–25-year-olds. It is described on p. 304.

Malignant tumours

Chordoma

Origin

Arises from the remnants of the notochord.

Incidence

A very rare tumour.

Age
No age is exempt, but the cranial cases tend to present at a younger age group (35 years) than the sacral cases (50 years).

Sex
Male : female, 2 : 1.

Sites
Sacrococcygeal 50%; base of skull (sphenoid and basiocciput) 35%; vertebral column at various levels 15%. This tumour does not occur at any other site.

Macroscopical
Large, soft, mucoid, lobulated, locally destructive tumours. They extend by direct spread into adjacent tissues to produce large masses in the nasopharynx, retroperitoneal tissues, pelvis, buttocks or thighs. Frequently there are haemorrhagic, cystic or calcified areas in the tumour.

Microscopical
The tumour has a mucoid stroma in which there are clumps of polyhedral cells arranged in irregular groups. The cells have a characteristic vacuolated appearance—*'physalipherous cells'*. Multinucleate cells and foci of calcification are also commonly present.

Spread
Chordomas are slowly growing but invade directly into adjacent tissues:
1 Destroy the base of the skull and present as an intracranial space-occupying lesion.
2 Cord compression.
3 Produce sacral destruction and a pelvic mass.

Results
Unless diagnosed at a very early stage these tumours are not readily amenable to surgery but, because of their slow growth, many patients have lived for 5 years or more although long-term survivors are very few in number. A small minority, probably less than 10%, do metastasize to lymph nodes and via the blood to the lungs and liver.

Myelomatosis—multiple myeloma
The spine is the most common site of this usually generalized tumour of bone.

Secondary tumours
Secondary malignant deposits of tumour in the spine are common and approximately 4% of all spines examined at autopsy from elderly patients contain metastatic tumour.

G/DISEASES OF JOINTS

Normal
Osteoarthrosis
Rheumatoid arthritis
Suppurative arthritis
Tuberculous arthritis
Gout and pseudo-gout
Neuropathic
Osteochondritis dissecans
'Ganglion'
Osteochondromatosis
PVNS
Synovial sarcoma

Normal joints
A synovial joint has a lining of flattened synovial cells. The articular cartilages are normally closely apposed, smooth, resilient structures which glide over each other with every movement of the joint and are lubricated by the slightly viscid synovial fluid. The articular cartilage is an avascular structure which is demarcated from the subchondral bone by a calcified line and yet is moored to the underlying bone by fibres. The articular cartilage derives its essential nutrients from the synovial fluid.

Osteoarthrosis—osteoarthritis

Nature
An extremely common degenerative process of articular cartilage.

Age
Occurs spontaneously in the older age groups and is thus increasingly common above the age of 60 years. It may also occur in the joints of younger persons following any form of previous mechanical derangement, e.g. trauma, congenital dislocation of the hip, osteochondritis, etc.

Sites
Usually the large weight-bearing joints, e.g. the hip and knee also small joints in the hands.

Macroscopical

Loss of joint space due to thinning of the cartilage which shows loss of lustre and a velvety appearance from *fibrillation*. Later, the cartilage disappears in areas to produce ulceration and to expose the underlying subchondral bone. The bone becomes thickened as a buttressing effect and extends beyond the articular margins to form bony outgrowths—*osteophytes*. In some areas the subchondral bone is not thickened and may allow entry of the synovial fluid into the underlying bone to produce a radiological cystic appearance. The end result is an articular surface denuded of cartilage and formed by a highly polished surface of eburnated bone with marginal osteophytes, some of which may break off to form loose bodies in the joint.

Microscopical

The normal blue-staining cartilage (on haematoxylin and eosin staining) degenerates and becomes pink-staining with loss of mucopolysaccharide ground substance. The degenerate cartilage splits along the lines of the fibres, tangentially at the surface but vertically as the splits extend into the deeper layers, to produce fronds of degenerate cartilage—fibrillation. This cartilage falls off and the subchondral bone becomes thickened and compact. The osteophytes at the joint margins are formed by reactive new bone. The synovial membrane often shows fibrous thickening and may also contain small foci of degenerate cartilage. At a later stage no cartilage remains, articulation occurring between the two faces of eburnated, thickened, subchondral bone.

Results

The loss of cartilage results in radiological narrowing of the joint space; the osteophytes are also prominent radiologically. Pain is usually present and commonly severe and is due in part to the synovial reaction associated with phagocytosed fragments of degenerate cartilage. The end result is commonly a stiff and painful joint.

Rheumatoid arthritis

Nature

Although commonly a generalized disease of connective tissues (see p. 100), the polyarthritis due to disease of the synovial tissues is usually the dominant clinical and pathological feature.

Age

Usually presents in females between the ages of 20 and the menopause, and rather later in men. Children are not exempt—*Still's disease*.

Sites

Many of the small joints, particularly those of the fingers, hands and wrists are most commonly involved but the larger joints at the ankle, hip and knee are also frequently affected.

Macroscopical

The joints are painful, swollen and tender. The synovial membrane is thickened, with villous overgrowth, increased vascularity and a *pannus* or plate which grows over and replaces the articular cartilage.

Microscopical

The synovial membrane shows villous proliferation with an intense lymphocytic and plasma cell infiltration of the oedematous and vascular fronds. The subsynovial and the periarticular collagen shows swelling with oedema and degenerative changes in the collagen, including foci of fibrinoid necrosis. The proliferated synovial tissues extend over the surface of the articular cartilage as a pannus of fibrous tissue containing lymphocytes, eroding and gradually replacing the articular cartilage by a fibrous mass. This unites with similar fibrous tissue on the opposite side of the joint space to produce fibrous ankylosis.

Results

The periarticular collagenous changes produce pain and the fusiform joint swelling. The pannus and the fibrous ankylosis result in pain and limitation of joint movement. There is a disuse atrophy of the bone and muscles working affected joints. Any other connective tissue, especially muscles and blood vessels, may be involved by the rheumatoid process and subcutaneous nodules, composed of circular areas of necrotic collagen surrounded by histiocytes and giant cells, may also occur.

Suppurative arthritis

Origins

Pyogenic infection in joints was formerly common in children as a result of blood-borne infection or by extension of osteomyelitis in adjacent bones. This type is now uncommon, but increasing numbers of cases are seen in the elderly, as complications of rheumatoid joint disease, in the immunocompromised and intravenous drug abusers.

Appearances
The joint space is distended by pus and the synovial membrane oedematous and hyperaemic. Progressive destruction of articular cartilage follows from proteolytic enzyme action.

Results
The joint becomes rapidly disorganized unless antibiotic therapy and/or joint aspiration or drainage is quickly instituted. Ligaments in and around the joint may be destroyed and healing is by fibrous ankylosis followed by bony fusion.

Tuberculous arthritis

Nature
Previously a common presentation of tuberculosis, particularly in childhood, it is now relatively rare. The infection is by blood spread from lungs or less commonly intestine, often as a complication of the primary complex (see p. 375).

Sites
Spine—Potts' disease (see p. 312), hip, knee, wrist, ankle are the commonest sites.

Appearances
The synovium is thickened grey and gelatinous, distending the joint spaces and extending as a pannus across the articular cartilage and beneath the cartilage as subchondral granulations. The cartilage is thus dead and sequestrated. Fibrosis and caseation follow, with disorganization of the joint and ankylosis.

Gout

Nature
A disease due to abnormal purine metabolism whereby sodium biurate is deposited in many tissues, but particularly as subcutaneous tophi or in the periarticular tissues. The latter may involve the joint, producing mechanical derangements.

Age
Usually in middle-aged or elderly men although females may be affected, especially when there is a family history of gout.

Sites
The first metatarsophalangeal joint is the predominant site but many other joints, including those of the hands, may be affected.

Macroscopical
The joint is swollen and red and shows white 'chalky' patches in the skin, through which sodium biurate crystals can often be expressed. The periarticular tissues are distended by the deposition of these crystals and similar deposits may extend into the joint with disruption of bone and articular cartilage.

Microscopical
The affected areas show multiple foci of sodium biurate crystals surrounded by a fibrous and foreign body giant cell reaction.

Results
Joint function is disturbed by the presence of deposits and stiffness and pain result. Acute exacerbations are common which are exquisitely painful and are often associated with considerable constitutional upset. Deposition of the crystals in the kidney may lead to impaired renal function. Prophylactic treatment by allopurinol or related substances is very effective.

Pseudo-gout—calcium pyrophosphate deposition disease

Nature
Deposition of calcium pyrophosphate in synovial membranes sometimes causing secondary osteoarthrosis. When this occurs symptomatically before the age of 35 years it is usually inherited as an autosomal dominant pattern.

Appearances
Weakly birefringent small rectangular crystals and/or occasional non-crystalline deposits are present in synovium with foci of giant cell and histiocytic reaction. The characteristic crystals are also found in aspirated joint fluid.

Neuropathic arthritis—Charcot's joint

Nature
A degenerative joint disease which occurs due to loss of the sensory nerve supply.

Aetiology
This occurs most frequently in the knee or hip joints in tabes dorsalis and in the shoulder or elbow in syringomyelia. It may also follow nerve destruction in leprosy, but only rarely occurs with other causes of sensory nerve loss.

Appearances
The joint is swollen due to a large effusion and there is a rapid degeneration of the articular cartilage. The underlying bones show a mixture of decalcification and osteophyte formation and in some cases the capsular tissues may calcify.

Results
The large effusion associated with the loss of the subchondral bone results in stretching of the joint ligaments and in gross deformity. The deterioration is usually rapid and the joint becomes completely disorganized and unstable. Frequent dislocations occur but the condition remains painless throughout its course.

Osteochondritis dissecans

Nature
Due to necrosis of a segment of subchondral bone which sequestrates and is extruded into the joint space as a loose body. The aetiology is unknown, but trauma leading to an area of avascular necrosis is the most probable cause.

Age
Usually in children or young adults.

Macroscopical
There is a bony loose body in the joint with a cap of cartilage and a corresponding defect in the articular surface.

Microscopical
The loose body, usually triangular, is composed of dead bone but viable cartilage, as the cartilage continues to derive its metabolic needs from the synovial fluid.

Results
The condition predisposes to osteoarthrosis by trauma from the loose body and by the unevenness in the articular surface caused by the defect.

'Ganglion'

Nature
A cystic swelling most commonly found at the wrist, or less frequently at the ankle or foot, and always in close relationship to synovial membrane or tendon sheath.

Appearances
Small cystic swellings which may have a visible connection with the synovial membrane or tendon sheath and which contain mucoid, glairy fluid. All contain a myxomatous centre which originally may have been surrounded by synovial-type cells and a fibrous wall.

Pathogenesis
The majority are probably herniations of tendon sheath or synovial membrane which then become distended by modified synovial fluid to form the cystic spaces.

Cyst of semilunar cartilage

Nature
Multilocular cysts which occur in the semilunar cartilage of the knee joint, more commonly in the lateral cartilage.

Appearances
A multilocular cystic swelling containing mucoid material at the rim of the meniscus. The cystic spaces are lined by synovial cells and the mucoid contents may extend through the cyst wall in between the fibres of the fibrocartilage.

Pathogenesis
These are probably due to islands of synovial cells incorporated in the meniscus. The production of synovial fluid results in cyst formation.

Synovial osteochondromatosis

Nature
The presence of multiple nodules of cartilage in the synovial membrane.

Macroscopical
The synovial membrane, usually of the knee, shoulder or elbow, is studded by multiple nodules of translucent cartilage. Many of these protrude into the joint space

on a narrow pedicle or lie free within the joint cavity where they form loose bodies, sometimes several hundred in number.

Microscopical

The synovial tissues contain multiple foci of benign cartilage, some of which show areas of ossification. The cartilaginous loose bodies are viable and may continue to grow as they obtain their nutritional requirements from the synovial fluid.

Pathogenesis

This remains unknown; it is regarded by some authorities as a true tumour, but it is more probably a metaplastic or developmental abnormality of the synovial tissues.

Results

The condition produces progressive swelling of the joint with 'locking' due to the loose bodies. Synovectomy may be followed by recurrence but the lesion is entirely benign.

Pigmented villo-nodular synovitis—PVNS

Nature

A pigmented villous overgrowth of synovial membrane which may also be variably nodular. It is a benign self-limiting condition probably reactive in origin.

Types

Nodular—'tendon sheath tumour'—'giant cell tumour of tendon sheath'

Usually solitary small nodules on fingers or toes and related to tendon sheaths. They are slowly growing lobulated, yellow–brown and firm. Histologically they are polymorphic with synovial-type mononuclear cells sometimes arranged around cleft-like spaces and variable amounts of collagen, foam cells, haemosiderin-containing macrophages and giant cells. These nodules may be poorly encapsulated and enucleation may result in local recurrence. The lesion does not, however, behave as a tumour and the use of the term 'benign synovioma' should be avoided.

Large joint—villo-nodular

This type is less common and mostly occurs in knee or hip joints. The interior of the joint shows fronded, brown seaweed-like material, though occasionally only one or a few nodules are the sole manifestations. Extension into adjacent soft tissues and bone can occur and be mistaken for an invasive neoplastic lesion. The histological appearances are identical to those described above in the peripheral 'nodular' lesions. The lesion regresses spontaneously after a variable length of time.

Synovial sarcoma—malignant synovioma

Nature

A group of rare malignant tumours, mostly of high malignancy, with features suggesting origin in synovial cells.

Age

Usually present between 30 and 40 years of age.

Sites

Knee and hip most commonly but sometimes does not appear to be closely related to a main joint or bursa and may thus be of soft tissue mesenchymal origin.

Appearances

The joint-related tumours particularly may be well differentiated and biphasic, both types of cells present—one epithelial-like the other fibroblastic and stromal in appearance, resemble normal synovial cells. Cleft-like spaces may be seen. Many tumours are, however, monophasic and consist only of the fibrosarcoma-like cells, though electron microscopic features show identical appearances to the spindle cell component of the biphasic tumour.

Prognosis

The differentiated forms are slowly growing and wide local resection is curative. The more anaplastic tumours, which are more common, are extremely rapidly growing and produce pulmonary metastases at an early stage, so that there is only about a 5–10% 5-year survival.

Chapter 18
Diseases of the Nervous System

A/GENERAL, VASCULAR, TRAUMA

Response to injury
Vascular
    Disorders of vessels
    Hypoxia and ischaemia
    Infarction
    Laminar necrosis
    Venous sinus thrombosis
    Haemorrhage
Trauma

Several factors make pathology of the nervous system unique
1 While the nervous system is prone to general pathological processes, e.g. infection, inflammation and infarction, it is also the seat of specific diseases of specialized tissues of the nervous system, e.g. disease of myelin in demyelinating disorders.
2 The compact nature and anatomical complexity of the nervous system means that small lesions may produce effects out of proportion to their size.
3 Neuronal loss following damage cannot be compensated by regeneration of new nerve cells.
4 Repair in the nervous system is through proliferation of specialized support cells such as astrocytes, Schwann cells and perineural cells, rather than by granulation tissue and fibroblasts as in other tissues.

Brain structure in relation to pathology
Brain is composed of several distinct types of tissue which are the seat of specialized reactions to disease.

Neurones
These consist of a cell body with an *axon* and several short processes—*dendrites*. The axon is an extremely active part of the neurone and has a constant flow of

cytoskeletal filaments, mitochondria and vesicles to supply the distal parts of the nerve cell with energy and substrates for neural transmission. Severance of the axon by injury causes a distinct set of reactions to take place in the cell body but may not kill the neurone. Regeneration of the axon is possible after transection (see p. 319). Many axons are surrounded by myelin (see below).

Astrocytes
These are stellate-shaped cells which provide a support and transport function in the central nervous system. The foot processes of astrocytes ensheath blood vessels and form part of the blood-brain barrier.

Oligodendrocytes
These are the cells which form myelin, the lipid-rich insulating layer which surrounds axons in the central nervous system. Certain disease processes are particularly directed at either myelin or oligodendrocytes as typified in the demyelinating diseases such as *multiple sclerosis*. Failure of myelin formation is also seen in many of the inherited disorders of metabolism in a group of diseases mainly of childhood—*leukodystrophies*. When cell bodies die, or when axons are damaged, the myelin associated with the distal axons undergoes degeneration and this loss of myelin is a useful histological feature which can be utilized to identify old damage to neuronal pathways. Remyelination of axons may occur in the peripheral nervous system following loss of myelin due to a disease process.

Microglia
A population of resident cells of monocyte/macrophage type. Following damage to the central nervous system these cells undergo reactive hyperplasia and assist, along with macrophages and lymphoid cells

recruited from the blood, in mounting local immunological and phagocytic responses. These cells play
central roles in immune-mediated damage such as in
multiple sclerosis, as well as in mounting responses to
viral infections of the brain.

Meninges

Divided into three layers—*pia, arachnoid* and *dura*,
covering the brain and spinal cord. They are composed of collagen, fibroblasts and specialized epithelial cells—*meningothelial cells* which can give rise
to tumours—*meningiomas*. The meninges delineate
several tissue planes in which intracranial bleeding
may take place in the form of extradural, subdural
and subarachnoid haemorrhages (see p. 323). The
meninges may also act as a physical barrier in
which infective processes may be limited to form a
meningitis.

Responses of the nervous system to injury

Neuronal chromatolysis

Following damage to the axon, the neuronal cell body
swells associated with peripheral migration of the
Nissl substance (rough endoplasmic reticulum), and
nuclear swelling. This *chromatolysis* is part of a
cellular mechanism for affecting repair and regeneration of the axon, which begins to take place as the cell
recovers.

Phagocytosis

Following death of neurones there is necrosis with
degeneration of the axon and associated myelin. The
dead tissues are removed by phagocytotic macrophages which are derived from blood monocytes
as well as microglia. These cells become vacuolated
by accumulated lipid as a result of the high lipid
content of myelin—*foamy macrophages* or foam
cells.

Gliosis

Collagenous scarring is not the usual pattern of
repair in the central nervous system. Damaged areas
are replaced by proliferation of astrocytes which form
a *glial scar* in the process of *gliosis*. In areas of
extensive tissue damage gliosis may not completely
repair the defect and a partly cystic, partly gliotic area
remains.

Cerebral oedema

Nature
Cerebral swelling as a result of excess tissue fluid
accumulating in the brain.

Causes
This is frequently seen with damage to the central
nervous system from many different causes. It is also
the final common pathway by which many disorders of
the nervous system cause death. Oedema and swelling
are usually the result of breakdown of the blood–brain
barrier and common causes are:
1 Ischaemia—infarction.
2 Trauma—head injury.
3 Inflammation—encephalitis or meningitis.
4 Around cerebral tumours—primary or secondary.
5 Metabolic disturbances—e.g. hyponatraemia, hypoglycaemia.

Outcome
Cerebral swelling is associated with a rise in the
pressure within the rigid skull vault—*raised intracranial pressure*—and if it progresses this will eventually result in an intracranial pressure which is greater
than the perfusion pressure of blood entering the
brain. When this point is reached there is global death
of brain tissue.

Cerebral herniation

Nature
The intracranial compartment is divided into three
spaces by the dural membranes of the falx and
tentorium cerebelli. Cerebral herniation is movement
of a part of the brain from one space to another with
resultant damage.

Pathogenesis
Cerebral swelling is particularly dangerous when it
causes local expansion of one part of the brain. Under
these circumstances there may be movement of this
part within the meningeal compartments in the skull
resulting in compression of vital structures.

Types
1 Herniation of the medial part of the temporal lobe
pushing down over the tentorium cerebelli to compress the upper brain stem—*transtentorial herniation*.
2 Herniation of the lower part of the cerebellum

(cerebellar tonsils) which push down into the foramen magnum and compress the medulla—*coning*.

3 Herniation of the cingulate gyrus beneath the falx cerebri.

Outcome

Cerebral herniation gives rise to characteristic clinical signs as vital structures become first stretched and later compressed by shifts in the brain substance. This is a common end stage in many cerebral pathologies as a prelude to brain death.

Vascular disorders of the central nervous system

Disorders of cerebral blood vessels

Congenital

Arteriovenous malformations are maldevelopmental connections between cerebral arteries and venous channel which are composed of leashes of fragile vessels. They may cause epileptic fitting but the major problem is that they bleed, causing secondary cerebral damage. Haemangiomas also occur in the brain as cavernous or capillary lesions (see p. 333).

Atherosclerosis

Atheroma of cerebral vessels mainly affects the main named cerebral arteries. It is generally most severe in the vertebral and basilar arteries compared to the anterior and middle cerebral vessels. Atherosclerotic *aneurysms* of cerebral arteries may develop, and these are generally fusiform and affect the basilar artery.

Arteriolar sclerosis

Arteriosclerosis of small vessels penetrating the brain substance is usually associated with long-standing hypertension or diabetes (see p. 83). The vessels develop replacement of their walls by acellular hyaline material which predisposes to the development of intracerebral haemorrhage, commonly into basal ganglia, pons or cerebellum, and also may produce chronic reduction of flow to the deep white matter and lead to ischaemic loss of myelin resulting in dementia—*Binswanger's disease* (see p. 335).

Amyloid

Amyloid derived from β (A4) protein, as seen in Alzheimer's disease plaques (see p. 335) may be deposited in the cerebral vessels of the elderly, causing *congophilic angiopathy*. This may predispose to lobar intracerebral haemorrhage affecting the periphery of the cerebral hemisphere in contrast to the deep haemorrhages seen in arteriolar sclerosis.

Aneurysms

Berry

These are due to developmental defects in the internal elastic lamina of vessels which allows herniation of intima to form small saccular aneurysms which resemble small berries (see p. 85). These occur particularly at the branch points of vessels around the circle of Willis. Approximately half arise in the region of the anterior communicating cerebral artery, a third at the point where the middle cerebral artery divides deep in the Sylvian fissure, and one-fifth arise in the region of the internal carotid arteries usually at the point of origin of the posterior communicating artery. These aneurysms are prone to rupture with consequent subarachnoid haemorrhage.

Infective—mycotic

Occasionally, in cases of endocarditis (see p. 70) infective aneurysms may develop in cerebral arteries as a result of inflammatory destruction of a small segment of arterial wall by local bacterial infection from a small septic embolus.

Atherosclerotic

Most common in relation to disease of the basilar artery.

Hypoxic and ischaemic damage

Nature

Damage to the brain through failure of supply of oxygen or nutrients

Pathogenesis

1 *Failure of blood oxygenation*: in respiratory disease and asphyxiation.

2 *Failure of blood flow*: which may be either *focal*, as occurs in thrombosis of a specific cerebral artery leading to regional cerebral infarction, or *generalized*, for example following a cardiac arrest and resulting in diffuse cerebral cortical damage.

Outcome

Failure of blood oxygenation leads to widespread

death of neurones in the brain, especially vulnerable sites are hippocampus and cerebellar cortex.

Focal cessation of blood flow leads to *cerebral infarction* in the territory supplied by the artery involved. Occlusion of the carotid arteries results in infarction in the territory of supply of the middle and anterior cerebral vessels comprising frontal, parietal and superior temporal lobes, usually also involving the internal capsule. Occlusion in the vertebrobasilar system leads to infarction in the brain stem, cerebellum and occipital lobes.

Cerebral infarction

Nature
Death of cerebral tissue following interruption of vascular supply

Aetiology
1 *Embolism from the heart*: mural thrombus following myocardial infarction, atrial fibrillation, endocarditis (see p. 70). This occurring principally to the anterior and middle cerebral arteries.
2 *Embolism from complicated atheromatous plaques*: particularly from carotid arteries in the neck and aortic arch.
3 *Thrombosis of arteries supplying the brain*: usually as a result of pre-existing atheroma and occurring principally in the carotid artery in the neck and in the vertebrobasilar system.
4 *Arteriolar sclerosis*: when affecting small penetrating deep cerebral vessels, in hypertension, results in small (less than 1 cm) areas of infarction in basal ganglia, internal capsule, hemispheric white matter and brain stem—*lacunar infarcts*. In addition there may be ischaemic loss of myelin from cerebral hemispheric white matter—*Binswanger's disease*, commonly associated with development of dementia.
5 Hypotension may cause poor blood flow in the boundary zone between arterial territories causing infarction.
6 *Mechanical obstruction*: when vessels are trapped following cerebral herniation, e.g. occipital lobe following trans-tentorial herniation.
7 *Vasculitis*: this uncommon condition may also cause cerebral infarction (see p. 83).

Macroscopical
In the early stages of infarction changes are limited to blurring of the normal demarcation between grey and white matter and focal swelling; later the infarcted area becomes macroscopically soft—*pale or anaemic infarct*. If a thrombus which has occluded a cerebral artery undergoes lysis then the infarcted area may become reperfused with blood resulting in marked haemorrhage into the infarcted territory—*haemorrhagic infarct*. Large cerebral infarcts may be associated with swelling sufficient to cause cerebral herniation.

Microscopical
Histological early changes become evident at about 18 hours and neurones become shrunken and pink-stained with pyknotic nuclei. Repair of the infarcted area begins when monocytes enter the brain from the blood and begin to phagocytose dead tissues. Phagocytic cells accumulate lipid and develop pale foamy cytoplasm. Astrocytes around the area enlarge and divide and the infarcted territory becomes replaced by proliferation of astrocytes—*gliosis*—becoming particularly evident 14–18 days after infarction. If the infarcted area is small, a few millimetres, then gliosis may obscure the area of damage. Larger areas of infarction invariably heal as fluid-filled cystic spaces bounded by gliosis.

Cortical necrosis

Nature
Death of neurones throughout areas of the cerebral cortex.

Pathogenesis
Generalized failure of blood flow or oxygenation, e.g. following cardiac arrest, results in widespread damage to the cerebral cortex with death of the majority of cortical neurones. Cortical necrosis also results from severe hypoglycaemia.

Appearances
Phagocytosis of dead neurones and gliosis occurs as with regional infarction. In severe cases, there is extensive loss of axons from the brain as a result of this massive neuronal loss and the affected cortex becomes atrophic and shrunken.

Outcome
This is the usual pathology in the brain as a result of cardiac arrest or anaesthetic disaster. Those affected by global severe cortical necrosis are generally left

with severe residual brain damage in a vegetative state. Lesser degrees of hypoxia or hypoglycaemia result in similar damage limited to specially vulnerable areas of the hippocampus and cerebellar cortex.

Venous sinus thrombosis

Nature
Occlusion of the venous sinuses and cerebral cortical veins by local thrombosis.

Pathogenesis
Predisposing factors include dehydration in children and in adults, disorders which cause hypercoaguability of blood, particularly polycythaemia.

Appearances
Macroscopically thrombosis of venous sinuses or cortical veins result in venous infarction of the adjacent brain which is typically extremely haemorrhagic.

Intracranial haemorrhage
1 *Extracerebral haemorrhage*: which occurs in relation to the coverings of the brain.
2 *Intracerebral haemorrhage*: which occurs within the brain.
   Intracerebral haemorrhages can be either large and expansile—*haematomas*—or small and diffuse—*petechial haemorrhages*.

Intracerebral

Cerebral haematoma

Nature
An expansile haematoma within the brain parenchyma.

Pathogenesis
Most intracerebral haematomas arise in patients who have been hypertensive. Prolonged hypertension results in arteriosclerotic change as well as the development of small microscopic dilatations—*microaneurysms*, also termed Charcot–Bouchard aneurysms, in small cerebral vessels which predispose to vessel rupture. Less common causes include bleeding into a tumour, vascular malformations, cerebral vasculitis, bleeding associated with disordered coagulation, bleeding occurring in association with leukaemias, and that which occurs in association with cerebral vascular amyloid (*see* p. 320).

Macroscopical
The common sites for intracerebral haematoma are sites supplied by fine perforating vessels, notably basal ganglia and internal capsule area, thalamus, cerebellum and pons. They appear as a large blood clot which results in compression, distortion and necrosis of surrounding brain. It is not uncommon for bleeds in the basal ganglia or thalamus to rupture into the ventricular system.

Outcome
Large bleeds which cause raised intracranial pressure or those which rupture into the ventricular system are almost invariably fatal. Smaller haemorrhages may not be fatal but are removed by phagocytic cells to leave a gliotic cystic cavity and persistent permanent neurological dysfunction.

Diffuse petechial haemorrhages

Nature
Multiple small pinpoint haemorrhages scattered throughout the brain.

Pathogenesis
Disruption of the walls of small cerebral blood vessels with extravasation of red cells leading to widespread petechiae in the brain.

Causes
1 Vasculitis of small cerebral vessels.
2 Cerebral malaria.
3 Acute hypertensive encephalopathy.
4 Fat embolism.
5 Acute haemorrhagic leucoencephalitis—allergic vasculitis of cerebral vessels.
6 Head injury.

Outcome
Petechial haemorrhages into the brain are usually part of the end stage of severe cerebral damage associated with general decline in conscious level, cerebral swelling and cerebral herniation.

Extracerebral
Extracerebral intracranial haemorrhage is divided into different types according to the anatomical space in which it occurs in relation to the meninges (Fig. 28).

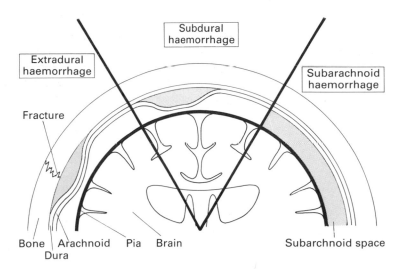

Fig. 28 Extracerebral intracranial haemorrhages.

Extradural haemorrhage

Location
Bleeding into the extradural space, i.e. between the skull and the dura.

Cause
Trauma to the skull, usually with fracture, which causes tearing of arteries or a venous sinus running outside the dura, in particular the middle meningeal artery associated with injury to the temporal bone.

Effects
The haematoma appears as a gelatinous layer of blood clot outside the dura which causes compression of the underlying brain with consequent trans-tentorial herniation manifest by decline in conscious level and upper brain stem compression. These are commonly fatal unless diagnosed early and treated by surgical evacuation.

Subdural haemorrhage

Location
Bleeding into the subdural space, i.e. between the dura and the arachnoid.

Cause
These types of haematoma are caused by bleeding from venous vessels which traverse the subdural space and are generally caused by trauma.
1 *Acute subdural haematomas*: commonly seen fol-

lowing head injury caused by falls or assaults, when they may be associated with other types of injury to the brain or skull (see p. 324).
2 *Chronic subdural haematomas*: may be seen as a result of minimal trauma and are mainly seen in the very young, including non-accidental injury to children, and the elderly. They may become apparent weeks or months after an apparently trivial injury. Blood escapes slowly and becomes partly organized by a fibrovascular granulation tissue membrane. This may increase in size as a result of further bleeding or osmotic effects of degenerating blood clot.

Effects
The haematoma appears as a layer of gelatinous blood clot (acute type) or an organized layer of granulation tissue and clot (chronic type). Compression of underlying brain occurs and causes decline in conscious level plus other neurological signs such as hemiparesis. Untreated progressive cases result in death due to cerebral herniation and brain stem compression. The most important aspect of treatment is suspicion of the diagnosis followed by scan confirmation and surgical evacuation.

Subarachnoid haemorrhage

Location
Bleeding into the subarachnoid space, i.e. between the arachnoid and the pia.

Causes
1 *Traumatic*, in association with head injury.
2 *Spontaneous*:
   (a) rupture of a cerebral arterial aneurysm,
   (b) rupture of a vascular malformation,
   (c) rupture of an intracerebral haematoma into the subarachnoid space.

Effect
There is a layer of blood over the cerebral surface in the subarachnoid space and blood is present in the CSF. Sixty per cent of cases die immediately: others present with headache and signs of meningeal irritation. Surgical intervention in those who survive includes attempts to clip the bleeding aneurysm.

Trauma to the central nervous system
Brain damage due to head injury is one of the most frequent causes of disability and death, particularly in young males, the main cause being road traffic accidents. Injury to the brain is divided into *primary*—that which takes place as a result of impact damage, and *secondary*—that which occurs as a result of brain swelling.

Pathogenesis
The main damage to the brain occurs as a result of acceleration/deceleration creating rotational and shearing forces which act on the mobile brain which is anchored within a rigid skull by tough dural membranes (falx and tentorium cerebelli).

Patterns of damage
Two main patterns of injury occur.

Cerebral contusions
Sustained when areas of the brain are crushed by coming into contact with the skull. The commonest sites are the underside of the frontal lobes, the tips and inferior aspects of the temporal lobes, the occipital poles and the cerebellum. Early contusions are visible as areas of petechial haemorrhage into cortical grey matter and underlying white matter; however, with time, oozing of blood occurs and contusions become haemorrhagic. Severe contusional damage may be associated with virtual rupture of a temporal lobe with extensive subarachnoid and subdural haemorrhage.

Diffuse axonal injury
A pattern of damage to the white matter tracts in the brain in which there is shearing of axons as a result of acceleration/deceleration/torsional forces. The majority of changes are usually only detectable histologically but useful pointers to its occurrence are petechial haemorrhage in the corpus callosum and cerebellar peduncles. Patients who have sustained diffuse axonal injury and survive are generally severely disabled.

Effects
Head injury is frequently associated with other trauma and is frequently complicated by the development of hypoxic cerebral damage. Severe head injury is complicated by the development of cerebral oedema which may cause impairment of cerebral perfusion. Damage in survivors is repaired by gliosis.

B/INFECTIONS

Patterns
Meningitis
Cerebritis
Encephalitis and myelitis
Viral
Fungal
Protozoal
Metazoal
Important disorders
   Tuberculosis
   Syphilis
   AIDS

Patterns of infection
The nervous system is prone to many infective processes which develop in five main patterns:
1 *Meningitis*: inflammation of the leptomeninges.
2 *Cerebritis*: focal inflammation of the brain.
3 *Cerebral abscess*: a fibrous capsule forms around a focus of cerebritis to form an abscess containing pus.
4 *Encephalitis*: diffuse infection of the brain or *myelitis*, diffuse infection of the cord.
5 *Meningo-encephalitis*: combination of meningitis and encephalitis/cerebritis.

Meningitis

Causes

Acute purulent meningitis
1 Neonates—*Escherichia coli* and enteric organisms.
2 Children—*Haemophilus influenzae, Neisseria meningitidis, Streptococcus pneumoniae.*

3 Adults—*Neisseria meningitidis, Streptococcus pneumoniae, Haemophilus influenzae*.
4 Elderly—*Listeria monocytogenes, Streptococcus pneumoniae, Neisseria meningitidis*.

Lymphocytic meningitis
No organism detected in many cases.

Mumps, coxsackie, ECHO, Epstein–Barr, lymphocytic choriomeningitis and polio viruses.

Granulomatous and chronic meningitis
1 *Mycobacterium tuberculosis*.
2 *Treponema pallidum*—syphilis.
3 *Cryptococcus neoformans*.
4 *Borrelia burgdorferi*—Lyme disease.

Routes of infection
1 *Blood-borne* as part of a bacteraemia or septicaemia.
2 *Direct spread* from infection in middle ear, mastoid, nasal sinuses, dural venous sinuses, osteomyelitis of vertebra or skull.
3 *Penetrating wounds* including fracture of skull.

Effects
1 *Acute purulent meningitis* is a severe life-threatening infection almost invariably caused by bacteria. The CSF typically shows abundant neutrophil polymorphs and a low sugar.

Macroscopically there is a cream-coloured exudate in the subarachnoid space and histologically this is composed of an acute inflammatory exudate. Secondary thrombosis of superficial vessels leads to secondary damage to the brain or spinal cord. When treated early there is resolution.

Organization of the inflammatory exudate may lead to obstruction of the drainage pathways for CSF and cause hydrocephalus (see p. 330).
2 *Lymphocytic meningitis* is a benign self-limiting disease caused by some viral infections. The CSF contains a small increase in lymphoid cells and may show a mild elevation of protein.
3 *Granulomatous and chronic meningitis* are severe inflammatory types of meningitis typified by chronic or granulomatous inflammation. The CSF shows an increased lymphocyte count with plasma cells and monocytes exhibiting evidence of phagocytic activity.

Macroscopically there may be slight thickening and opacity of the leptomeninges; however in some cases they become markedly thickened and fibrosed. In tuberculous meningitis, granulomas are visible and mycobacteria may be visible on ZN staining. In cryptococcal infection the fungi are usually clearly visible. In other conditions there may be only lymphocytic infiltration of the meninges and cuffing of meningeal vessels by lymphocytes and plasma cells. Meningeal fibrosis is common and may lead to obstruction of the drainage pathways for CSF and cause hydrocephalus (see p. 330).

Cerebritis

Nature
Focal inflammation of the parenchyma of the brain.

Causation
The organisms causing purulent or chronic meningitis commonly also spread into the brain to cause an associated focal cerebritis. Cerebritis may also occur as a result of septic emboli, e.g. from bacterial endocarditis, lodging in the brain. Localized areas of cerebritis also occur in fungal infection of the brain, e.g. *Aspergillus, Candida* and with *Toxoplasma* infection.

Appearances
There is diffuse congestion of the meningeal vessels commonly associated with brain swelling caused by cerebral oedema. On cut surfaces there are haemorrhagic foci and small areas of yellow–grey softening in the brain at the sites of cerebral inflammation. Histologically foci of cerebritis appear as areas of necrosis infiltrated by neutrophils and smaller numbers of mononuclear inflammatory cells. There is swelling of adjacent astrocytes.

Outcome
Many cases are fatal because of extensive sepsis, associated meningitis or involvement of critical brain areas. Focal areas of cerebritis may become loculated as a cerebral abscess.

Cerebral abscess

Nature
A cerebral abscess is a zone of infection (cerebritis) which has been walled off from adjacent brain. In contrast to other forms of injury in the nervous system which are walled off by gliosis, cerebral abscesses develop a tough collagenous fibrous capsule derived

from granulation tissue sprouting from cerebral blood vessels.

Causes

Cerebral abscesses arise from three main routes:

1 *Local extension*: usually from sepsis in the middle ear or mastoid cavities (see p. 112).

2 *Blood spread*: especially with bacterial endocarditis, cyanotic congenital heart disease and pulmonary bronchiectasis (see p. 373).

3 *Trauma*: following open skull fracture.

Common organisms involved in cerebral abscess include staphylococci and *Streptococcus viridans*. Microbiology usually reveals mixed organisms and it is not uncommon to find anaerobic bacteria involved. Tuberculosis may form a localized caseous mass— *tuberculoma*. Cerebral abscesses may also be caused by fungal infection, e.g. *Candida*, *Aspergillus* and *Amoebae*.

Effects

An abscess appears as a rounded cavity filled with pus. Early lesions are surrounded by reactive astrocytic cells and oedematous brain. With time, fibroblasts derived from tissue adjacent to blood vessels proliferate and cause development of a wall of vascular and fibrous granulation tissue. Abscesses may occur in preferential sites according to aetiology:

1 Temporal lobe or cerebellum from infection related to the middle ear.

2 Frontal lobe from nasal sinuses.

3 Frontal lobe in association with chronic lung sepsis.

Cerebral abscesses often cause dramatic problems of raised intracranial pressure because of massive surrounding oedema. If they are not excised or drained surgically then they may rupture to cause meningitis or ventriculitis.

Encephalitis and myelitis

Nature

In contrast to cerebritis, encephalitis describes diffuse inflammation of the brain while myelitis is that affecting the cord.

Causes

Encephalitis and myelitis are usually caused by viral or Rickettsial infections although certain bacterial organisms, for example *Listeria*, *Treponema* and *Borrelia*, may also elicit this pattern of disease. Details of diseases are described in the section on viral diseases of the nervous system, see below.

Macroscopical

In fatal cases there is usually hyperaemia of the meninges with brain swelling. On cut surfaces there may be petechial haemorrhages in the brain. Encephalitis due to herpes simplex is characterized by extensive necrosis of the temporal lobes.

Microscopical

The histological hallmarks of an encephalitis or myelitis are:

1 Death of neurones with phagocytosis of dead cells.

2 Cuffing of cerebral blood vessels by lymphoid cells.

3 Activation and enlargement of astrocytic cells.

4 Increase in the number and size of microglial cells in the brain.

In addition to these features evidence of specific infection may be seen in the form of a characteristic cellular inclusion body, e.g. cytoplasmic Negri bodies in rabies, and nuclear viral inclusion bodies in herpes encephalitis.

Viral diseases of the nervous system

Herpes simplex virus—HSV

HSV-I causes necrotizing encephalitis particulariy affecting temporal lobes of the brain. HSV-II causes herpetic meningitis and also neonatal necrotizing encephalitis if transmitted from maternal genital herpes.

Herpes zoster

Causes shingles in peripheral nerve dermatomes and may be latent in dorsal root ganglion cells. May cause a vasculitis of the central nervous system particularly in immunosuppressed patients.

Arthropod-borne infections

Eastern and western equine encephalitis, Venezuelan encephalitis, Japanese B and Murray Valley encephalitis caused by RNA viruses of the Toga and Bunya groups, which have vertebrate hosts and mosquito vectors and cause epidemic encephalitis with a high mortality.

Poliovirus

This is a picorna enterovirus. Many cases of infection result in a lymphocytic meningitis which resolves without effects. It may also cause poliomyelitis which is characterized by two clinical stages of infection: a preparalytic prodromal phase of viraemia followed by a paralytic phase in which motor neurones are killed. Spinal disease causes flaccid paralysis and may involve neurones innervating the diaphragm. Bulbar disease causes problems with speech and swallowing.

Rabies virus
Rhabdo virus is transmitted by animal bite and travels in peripheral nerves to CNS where it causes a severe meningoencephalitis with a high fatality rate. Negri bodies are present and viral inclusions are histologically visible in nerve cells.

Cytomegalovirus
Causes encephalitis with necrotizing lesions in immunosuppressed patients, e.g. AIDS, transplant recipients. Also causes congenital infection of the CNS *in utero*, resulting in microcephaly and cerebral calcification.

HTLV-1
Associated with development of tropical spastic paraparesis, a form of demyelination of the spinal cord.

HIV-1
The causative virus of AIDS may cause several primary types of pathology in the nervous system independent of any opportunistic infections which may develop as a consequence of immunosuppression (see p. 329).

Measles
Infection of brain by measles virus causes subacute sclerosing panencephalitis characterized by neuronal death and gliosis. Viral inclusion bodies are prominent.

JC virus
A papova virus which is the cause of progressive multifocal leucoencephalopathy. Infection causes multiple foci of demyelination of the brain in immunosuppressed patients but may also rarely affect those who are otherwise normal.

Creutzfeld–Jakob disease
The transmissible agent is uncertain but suspected to be an abnormal structural variant of a normal cell protein—*prion protein or PrP*. The disease is associated with a rapidly progressive dementia in humans with histological vacuolation in the cerebral cortex—*spongiform encephalopathy*. The disease is similar to kuru in humans, scrapie in sheep and bovine spongioform encephalopathy (BSE) in cattle. Most cases are sporadic but human cases have resulted from inoculation with tissue from an affected person. The disease can be transmitted by inoculation of affected tissue into animals.

Experimentally, and in the rare human transmission cases, the disease has a long incubation period hence was termed a *'slow virus disease'*. Identical and transmissible disease results from a hereditary mutation in the gene coding for the prion protein in humans—*Gerstmann Straussler syndrome*—causing familial cases of cerebellar ataxia and dementia. Because it is highly likely that the agent is not a virus but an abnormal protein this disease is unique in being both inheritable and transmissible.

Fungal infection of the nervous system

Nature
Infection of the nervous system by fungal agents. This is frequently in the context of an immunocompromised state, for example chemotherapy, steroid treatment or AIDS.

Causative organisms
1 *Candidiasis* affects the central nervous system as part of systemic septicaemia caused by primary *Candida* infection elsewhere, e.g. gastrointestinal tract, endocarditis. The pattern of infection is generally that of multiple small cerebral abscesses.
2 *Phycomycoses: mucormycosis, zygomycosis*, generally arise as a primary infection related to the nasal sinuses with vascular spread to the brain. Fungi spread along vessels causing vascular thrombosis and extensive associated infarction. May be seen as a complication of diabetic ketoacidosis.
3 *Aspergillosis* frequently affects immunosuppressed patients either by blood spread from systemic or pulmonary disease or from direct spread of infection of the paranasal sinuses. The pattern of disease is the formation of large fungal abscesses with vascular invasion by fungi giving rise to secondary infarction.
4 *Cryptococcosis* is due to a yeast-like organism

which most commonly causes a fungal meningitis in immunosuppressed patients (see p. 4).

Protozoal infection of the nervous system

Nature
Infection of the nervous system by protozoa.

Causative organisms
1 *Amoebae* infect the nervous system in two main patterns. *Entamoeba histolytica* infection of the gut and liver may spread to brain by the blood to cause an amoebic abscess (see p. 236). Primary meningitis may be caused by free-living soil and water amoebae such as *Naegleria* and is usually acquired by swimming in pools containing large numbers of organisms.
2 *Toxoplasma* is a protozoal organism which may cause congenital infection leading to hydrocephalus and cerebral calcifications, but is now frequently seen in immunosuppressed patients as secondary infection causing cerebritis with necrosis of affected brain regions.
3 *Malaria* caused by a variety of *Plasmodium*, particularly *P. falciparum*, may affect the brain (see p. 5). In fatal cases of cerebral malaria the brain is swollen and there are numerous petechial haemorrhages seen on cut surfaces. Small blood vessels show thrombosis, extravasation of red cells—*ring haemorrhages*, and there may be a glial reaction to the haemorrhages (see p. 322).
4 *Trypanosomiasis* may be associated with an encephalomyelitis in the acute disease (see p. 7).

Metazoal infection of the nervous system

Nature
Infection by metazoal parasites.

Common causative organisms
1 *Hydatid disease*, caused by *Echinococcus granulosus*, is associated with development of cysts in the brain in 2–5% of cases (see p. 236).
2 *Cysticercosis* is caused by the larval form of the pork tapeworm *Taenia solium* with the development of brain cysts following ingestion of ova (see p. 9).

Other important infective disorders

Tuberculosis

Nature
Infection of the CNS by *Mycobacterium tuberculosis*. The bacteria reaches the CNS by blood spread from the site of primary infection, usually the lung. Tuberculosis of the CNS may also frequently develop in the setting of AIDS.

Patterns
There are two main types of infection:

Granulomatous meningitis
In tuberculous meningitis numerous granulomas develop in the meninges and these may be seen as small white spots macroscopically. Clinically patients develop confusion, headache, cranial nerve palsies or general malaise with pyrexia. The CSF typically shows a raised cell count composed of mononuclear cells, particularly lymphocytes and plasma cells. CSF protein is raised and there may be slight reduction in CSF glucose. Mycobacteria can be identified in and cultured from the CSF.

Tuberculous abscess—tuberculoma
These appear as rounded masses up to several centimetres in diameter walled off by fibrous tissue with a granulomatous inflammatory infiltrate and central caseous necrosis. There may be considerable mass effect due to cerebral oedema in response to the lesion. These lesions occur within the cerebral hemispheres and are also common within the cerebellum.

Outcome
Even when treated with appropriate antibacterial agents there is frequent development of meningeal fibrosis which can cause obstruction of CSF flow leading to hydrocephalus.

Neurosyphilis

Nature
Infection of the central nervous system with *Treponema pallidum*.

Patterns
In secondary syphilis there may be a lymphocytic meningitis.

In tertiary syphilis there are three main patterns of disease:

1 *Meningovascular syphilis* is a form of chronic meningitis typified by plasma cell infiltration of the meninges, meningeal fibrosis and endarteritis of blood vessels. This causes secondary ischaemic damage to the brain—infarction—and also leads to the development of cranial nerve palsies. Occasionally a localized gumma forms in relation to the meninges.

2 *Tabes dorsalis* affects only 2–5% of those who contract syphilis, is caused by damage to sensory nerve roots and leads to degeneration, loss of nerve fibres and myelin, of the posterior columns of the spinal cord. Clinically there are 'lightning' pains in the limbs, ataxia, loss of vibration sense and proprioception, and neuropathic degenerative joint disease.

3 *Parenchymal neurosyphilis* causes neuronal death in the cerebral cortex and leads to cerebral atrophy. Clinically there is early loss of frontal lobe function progressing to severe dementia—*general paresis of the insane*—GPI.

Diagnosis

Neurosyphilis may be manifest by a mixed pattern of damage to the nervous system, e.g. taboparesis, a mixture of tabes dorsalis and parenchymal neurosyphilis. CSF examination usually shows a mild increase in lymphoid cells, an increased protein and normal CSF sugar. Serological tests for syphilis are usually positive in the CSF.

Acquired immunodeficiency syndrome—AIDS

Primary infection

Infection with the retrovirus HIV-1 causes the syndrome of AIDS. In the nervous system HIV-1 infection is associated with several patterns of disease:

1 *Lymphocytic meningitis* occurs at around the time of seroconversion.

2 *HIV encephalitis* is a form of encephalitis characterized by formation of multiple nodules of microglial cells including the formation of multinucleate giant cells. There may be associated myelin loss and slight hyperplasia of astrocytes—HIV leucoencephalopathy. This cerebral involvement is common in AIDS and probably accounts for the symptomatology of so-called AIDS dementia.

3 *Vacuolar myelopathy* is characterized by vacuolation and loss of myelin from the spinal cord, most

marked in the lateral columns of the thoracic cord.

4 *Diffuse poliodystrophy* shows reactive astrocytes and microglia in cerebral grey matter.

5 *Demyelination of peripheral nerves* is seen in some AIDS cases.

Secondary infections

AIDS results in several opportunistic infections of the CNS, including:

1 Cryptococcal meningitis.

2 Cytomegalovirus, and herpes zoster encephalitis.

3 Toxoplasmosis.

4 Progressive multifocal leucoencephalopathy.

AIDS patients may develop primary cerebral lymphomas (see p. 345).

C/DEVELOPMENTAL, DEMYELINATING, NEURODEGENERATIVE, METABOLIC, TOXIC

Developmental
Perinatal
   Hydrocephalus
   Syringomyelia
   Phacomatoses
   Inborn metabolic
Demyelinating
Neurodegenerative
Heredofamilial
Metabolic and toxic

Developmental abnormalities

Nature

Abnormalities of the nervous system present at birth.

Pathogenesis

Developmental abnormalities of the CNS are common—1% of newborns, and can be divided into:

1 *Primary*: where they are the direct result of a genetic abnormality.

2 *Secondary*: where they are due to disruption of development by an intra-uterine disease process such as infection, ischaemia or toxins including drugs.

Types

The main types of developmental abnormality of the CNS are listed in Table 18.1.

Table 18.1 Developmental abnormalites of the CNS.

Porencephaly and schizencephaly	Cystic cavities in the brain due to gliosis following infarcts caused by intra-uterine vascular occlusion
Ulegyria	Gliotic shrunken gyri as a result of hypoxic necrosis
Agyria and pachygyria	Brain is smooth or with few gyri; due to failure of migration of neuroblasts into developing brain
Heterotopia	Ectopic foci of grey matter due to premature arrest of migrating neuroblasts in developing brain
Holoprosencephaly	Single large ventricle with non-division of forebrain
Microcephaly	Small brain; may be due to many causes
Diastematomyelia	Duplication (splitting) of cord
Anencephaly	Absent cranial vault and failure of development of cerebral hemispheres
Encephalocele/encephalomeningocele	Herniation of brain and meninges due to abnormal neural tube fusion; occipital, frontal, orbital, nasal types
Myelomeningocele/meningocele	Herniation of cord and/or meninges as part of a defect in neural tube fusion
Arnold–Chiari malformation	Type II commonest; displacement of cerebellum and brain stem into the foramen magnum and upper cervical canal; commonly associated with meningocele and hydrocephalus

Causes

Although the majority of developmental abnormalities of the nervous system have no identifiable causative factor there are many known causes shown in Table 18.2.

Perinatal abnormalities of the nervous system

Nature

The neonatal brain is predisposed to a variety of abnormalities which may be the cause of neurological abnormality in childhood, e.g. the development of cerebral palsy. The two main abnormalities found are haemorrhage and necrosis.

Intraventricular haemorrhage

Nature

Bleeding into the ventricular cavity

Pathogenesis

1 *Germinal matrix haemorrhage*: bleeding into the germinal matrix, the mass of developing neuroblasts overlying the head of the caudate nucleus from which nerve cells migrate into the brain. This is particularly common in premature infants.

2 *Choroid plexus haemorrhage*: bleeding from the parenchyma of the choroid plexus.

Outcome

In survivors, hydrocephalus is the most common sequel.

Periventricular leucomalacia

Nature

Areas of necrosis in the white matter of the neonatal brain characteristically in the deep parieto-occipital white matter.

Risk factors

Congenital abnormalities, endotoxaemia, low socio-economic status of mother.

Effects

Associated with cases of cerebral palsy.

Hydrocephalus

Nature

Hydrocephalus is a condition in which there is increase in the CSF volume within the brain with expansion of the cerebral ventricles. This most com-

Table 18.2 Causes of developmental abnormalities of brain.

Chromosomal abnormalities	
Down's syndrome (trisomy 21)	Abnormal gyral formation and defective arborization of neuronal processes
Trisomy 13–15 (Patau's syndrome)	Forebrain abnormalities with midline facial clefts
Trisomy 17–18 (Edwards syndrome)	Gyral maldevelopment
Single gene abnormalities	
Autosomal recessive gene	Meckel syndrome (encephalocele)
	Roberts syndrome (encephalocele)
Multifactorial	
Genetic and environmental	Anencephaly, meningocele, encephalocele
Infections	
Rubella	Microcephaly, focal necrosis of brain areas
Cytomegalovirus	Necrosis and developmental failure
Toxoplasmosis	Necrosis and developmental failure
Teratogens	
Thalidomide	Anencephaly and meningomyelocele
Aminopterin	Anencephaly and encephalocele

monly occurs as a disease of childhood but may be acquired in later life.

Classification

There are two main types
1 *Non-communicating hydrocephalus*: implies blockage of the CSF pathway from the ventricles to the subarachnoid space.
2 *Communicating hydrocephalus*: due to impairment of resorption of CSF at the arachnoid villi along the dural venous sinuses.

Causes

1 *Congenital malformations*: stenosis of the aqueduct of Sylvius, Arnold–Chiari malformation.
2 *Tumours*: particularly located in the brain stem, cerebellum or pineal region.
3 *Scarring*: postinflammatory fibrosis of exit foramina at base of brain.
4 *Haemorrhage*: intraventricular or in the posterior fossa.
5 *Genetic*: X-linked inheritance.

Macroscopical

There is dilatation of the ventricular cavities of the brain. In cases of stenosis of the cerebral aqueduct this does not involve the fourth ventricle.

In children, before fusion of the skull bones there is progressive enlargement of the head circumference.

In adults where the skull is rigidly fused there is thinning of the skull vault with prolonged disease.

Microscopical

With long-standing disease there is axonal damage and gliosis in the white matter, especially that beneath the ependymal lining of the ventricles.

Effects

If the onset of the CSF obstruction is sudden then signs and symptoms of raised intracranial pressure occur. If the onset of the obstruction is slow then a chronic rise in intracranial pressure takes place which, in adults, produces dementia with gait disturbance and incontinence as prominent associated features. Operative shunting of CSF into the peritoneal cavity may relieve signs and symptoms.

Syringomyelia

Nature

A tube-shaped cystic cavity which develops in the spinal cord causing compression of the white matter tracts and consequent neurological disability.

Appearances

Syringeal cavities are most common in the cervical spinal cord and may extend up and down over many segments. The affected spinal cord appears fluctuant and on cut surfaces there is a slit-shaped cavity which replaces much of the cord volume. The cavity typically occurs at the junction between the anterior third and posterior two-thirds of the cord and extends across the mid-line to efface the anterior commissural fibres.

Histologically the cavity is lined by dense astrocytic gliosis, *not* by ependyma, but the syrinx may communicate with the central canal of the spinal cord.

Similar disease of the medulla is termed *syringobulbia*.

Causes

Most cases of syrinx formation are secondary to trauma, ischaemia or in association with tumours of the spinal cord. Less commonly, a syrinx may be a primary phenomenon when it is assumed to be developmental.

Effects

The cavity causes compression of the spinal cord fibre tracts. Early effects cause pain in the arms, wasting of the intrinsic muscles of the hand and spastic weakness in the legs. There is typically loss of pain and temperature sensation with preservation of touch due to interruption of crossed pain and temperature fibres in the commissural region.

Phacomatoses

Nature

These are familial disorders in which developmental abnormalities are associated with the growth of tumours which are either hamartomatous or neoplastic.

Types

Neurofibromatosis

This is one of the most common inherited disorders of the nervous system. Until recently this was thought to be one entity, but genetic techniques now show two distinct syndromes.

Neurofibromatosis 1 (NF1) was formerly called *von Recklinghausen's syndrome* and is an autosomal dominant disorder affecting 1 : 4000 individuals. The main clinical features include peripheral neurofibromas, hamartomas of the iris, café-au-lait spots in the skin; less prominent are optic nerve gliomas, learning difficulties, macrocephaly and bone abnormalities—dysplasia of the sphenoid and thinning of long bone cortex. There is a risk of development of neurofibro-

sarcomas derived from the benign neurofibromas. The gene defect in NF1 is located on chromosome 17.

Neurofibromatosis 2 (NF2) was formerly called *bilateral acoustic neurofibromatosis (BANF)* and is an autosomal dominant disorder affecting 1 : 100 000 individuals. The clinical features are development of bilateral Schwannomas of the eighth cranial nerve—acoustic neuromas, as well as a propensity to develop meningiomas, gliomas, other Schwannomas and posterior lens opacities. The gene defect for NF2 is located on chromosome 22.

Tuberose sclerosis

An autosomal dominant condition with a frequency of around 1 : 100 000 The clinical features are epilepsy (88%), mental retardation (60%), skin lesions (90%) and retinal hamartomas (50%).

Skin lesions are facial angiofibromas—*adenoma sebaceum*, fibromas, connective tissue hamartomas—*Shagreen patches*, and café-au-lait spots. Retinal hamartomas are nodules of astrocytes which grow in the retina and appear as flat grey patches obscuring the vascular pattern on fundoscopy.

Cardiac lesions may occur in the form of benign rhabdomyomas in around 30% of cases. Renal tumours in the form of angiomyolipomas occur (see p. 183). In the lung there may be abnormal overgrowth of smooth muscle in vessels causing lymphangioleiomyomatosis (see p. 396). In the bones there may be foci of fibrous dysplasia (see p. 296).

The brain in affected individuals may show microcephaly or be enlarged. The characteristic lesion, from which the syndrome is named, consists of nodules of overgrown neurones and astrocytes in the cortex—*tubers*. These appear as large (1–3 cm) firm white nodules typically occupying the crest of a gyrus. In the ventricular system of the brain there is focal proliferation of astrocytes beneath the ependyma which appear as linear rows of bead-like protrusions 3–4 mm in width resembling candle-wax drips—*candle guttering lesions*. These may enlarge and form tumours termed *subependymal giant cell astrocytomas* (see p. 341). As a result of incomplete expression, *formes frustes* of the condition are common, for example children with mental retardation and epilepsy but no other stigmata.

Von Hippel–Lindau disease

This is a familial disorder in which there are multiple benign tumours of the brain and spinal cord—

haemangioblastomas (see p. 345). Angiomas of the retina may also be present and there is predisposition to development of carcinoma of the kidney (see p. 184).

Sturge–Weber syndrome

A non-familial syndrome characterized by large angiomas of skin of the head and underlying brain. The angiomatous involvement of the brain may cause secondary ischaemic changes.

Inborn errors of metabolism and the nervous system

Nature

The nervous system is involved in several inborn errors of metabolism, either primarily or as a consequence of systematized disease.

Leucodystrophies

Nature

These are a group of disorders characterized by a genetically determined metabolic abnormality in the metabolism of myelin, generally as a result of an enzyme defect. They are usually manifest in childhood as motor impairment and intellectual failure and can also rarely occur in adult life.

Main types

1 *Metachromatic leucodystrophy*: caused by arylsulphatase A deficiency. Autosomal recessive.
2 *Krabbe's disease*—globoid cell leucodystrophy. Galactocerebroside B galactosidase deficiency. Autosomal recessive.
3 *Adrenoleucodystrophy*: peroxisomal enzyme deficiency in oxidation of long-chain fatty acids. X-linked recessive.

Diagnosis

Diagnosis in life is made by assay of enzymes on either blood leucocytes or cultured fibroblasts.

Storage disorders

Nature

Inborn errors of metabolism characterized by storage of abnormal material, particularly in the tissues of the nervous system. They arise mainly in childhood and present with failure of normal development of motor and intellectual milestones.

Main types

1 *Gangliosidoses*: autosomal recessive conditions associated with neuronal storage of gangliosides. Examples are *Tay–Sachs disease* and *Sandhoff's disease*.
2 *Ceroid lipofuscinoses*: disorders with unknown enzyme defects causing neuronal storage of lipofuscin-like lipids, e.g. *Batten's disease*.
3 *Niemann–Pick disease*: due to deficiency in sphingomyelinase activity and has several variants with or without neurological involvement (see p. 249).
4 *Gaucher's disease*: due to a deficiency of β-glucocerebrosidase, is associated with intellectual deterioration in childhood and storage of glucocerebroside in macrophages in CNS (see p. 293).
5 *Mucopolysaccharidoses*: may affect the brain and stored material may be seen in perivascular macrophages. The main types are *Hurler's syndrome—gargoylism*, *Scheie's syndrome*, *Hunter's syndrome*, *Sanfilippo syndrome*, *Morquio's syndrome* and *Maroteaux–Lamy syndrome*.

Diagnosis

Diagnosis is made by demonstrating abnormal enzyme activity in lymphocytes or cultured fibroblasts in addition to demonstrating excess storage product in tissues. Batten's disease is not associated with a known enzyme defect and diagnosis is made by demonstration of abnormal lipid material in the rectal ganglion cells on rectal biopsy.

Wilson's disease

Nature

This is an autosomal recessive disorder in which excessive copper accumulates in the brain, liver and kidneys (see p. 248).

Appearances

In severe cases there is shrinkage of the basal ganglia which histologically show loss of nerve cells and gliosis.

Course

Neurologically the disease usually presents in adolescence with spasticity, rigidity, dysarthria and painful muscle spasms. It may also present as psychiatric disease. Laboratory tests show low serum copper concentrations, reduced caeruloplasmin levels and increased urinary copper excretion. Treatment with chelating agents prevents progression of disease.

Demyelinating diseases

This is a group of diseases which have the common factor of primary damage to myelin within the nervous system.

Multiple sclerosis

Nature

A disease of uncertain aetiology characterized by relapsing episodes of immunologically mediated demyelination within the central nervous system. Loss of myelin from critical sites leads to disturbance of neurological function. Early clinical symptoms are blurring of vision as a result of disease of the optic nerves, incoordination as a result of disease of cerebellar peduncles or abnormal sensation from disease affecting long sensory tracts. Late stages of the disease commonly involve blindness, paraplegia and incontinence as a result of spinal tract involvement, ataxia as a result of spinal and cerebellar involvement and also intellectual dysfunction caused by loss of hemispheric white matter.

Aetiology

It has a peak incidence between the ages of 20 and 40 years with a slight female predominance. The aetiology of the condition is uncertain. Viral and immunological mechanisms have been postulated and it is possible to demonstrate an active immunological response in the affected areas of the CNS with activation of cell-mediated immune responses. However there are at present no firm clues as to cause. It is likely that the disease is the result of a genetic susceptibility predisposing to mounting an inappropriate immune response to viral infection.

Macroscopical

Macroscopically, areas of active demyelination appear as salmon-pink granular areas of softening in the white matter; however, it is unusual to see the active lesions. It is more common to see the end-result of previous healed areas of myelin loss which appear as sharply demarcated areas of firm grey discoloration of white matter termed *plaques*. In addition, less well defined areas may be visible termed *shadow plaques*.

The plaques are best seen at the angles of the lateral ventricles, in the cerebellar peduncles, and in the brain stem, although can be found at any site in the brain or spinal cord.

Microscopical

Histologically active plaques show myelin loss associated with lymphocytic cuffing of small vessels and the presence of foamy macrophages. Enlargement of astrocytic cells is also seen, particulariy at the periphery of the lesions. With time, active plaques show little in the way of mononuclear inflammatory cells and are populated by large astrocytic glial cells— *burnt-out plaques*. Axons traversing a plaque are mostly preserved but there is some definite loss of axons from plaque areas.

Diagnosis

Diagnosis is based on clinical evaluation and, increasingly, the use of CT scanning and magnetic resonance imaging to show the areas of demyelination within the brain and spinal cord. CSF examination commonly shows a mild increase in lymphoid cells, a mild increase in protein and a normal glucose level. It is possible to show activation of the immune system in the CNS by the demonstration of *oligoclonal bands* of immunoglobulin in the CSF by electrophoresis. The diagnosis remains essentially clinical and by exclusion of other causes of focal neurological disease.

Perivenous encephalomyelitis

Nature

Acute immune-mediated demyelination often occurring after viral infection or immunization.

Pathogenesis

These are uncommon disorders and are felt to represent immune complex-mediated vascular damage localized to the brain. Patients present with deteriorating conscious levels 1–2 weeks after a viral illness, vaccination or vague respiratory tract infection.

Appearances

Loss of myelin is seen from around small venules within the brain and there may be associated brain swelling. In postinfectious encephalomyelitis there is a lymphocytic infiltrate in association with the demyelination. In acute haemorrhagic leucoencephalitis there is necrosis of vessel walls with neutrophil and lymphocytic cells in association with the demyelination.

Central pontine myelinolysis

Demyelination in the pons in association with abnormal serum sodium levels. This pattern of demyelination occurs in association with rapid correction of hyponatraemia by intravenous infusion of sodium salts.

Loss of myelin is seen from the pons and occasionally from the corpus callosum. The precise mechanism of the myelin loss is uncertain.

Myelin loss in other diseases

Myelin is lost following many diseases as a secondary phenomenon and, although there is marked loss of myelin, these are traditionally separated from the primary demyelinating disorders

1 *Binswanger's disease* is characterized by loss of hemispheric myelin through arteriosclerotic ischaemic damage (see p. 320).

2 *Inborn errors of metabolism* may cause abnormal formation or metabolism of myelin—*dysmelination*, e.g. metachromatic leucodystrophy due to arylsulphatase A deficiency (see p. 333).

3 *Progressive multifocal leucoencephalopathy*, in which demyelination is caused by infection by papova virus (see p. 327).

Neurodegenerative diseases

These are a group of disorders which increase in incidence with ageing, particularly after the age of 65. They are of unknown cause, may in some instances be familial, and result in degeneration of specific groups of neurones or brain areas giving rise to characteristic clinical syndromes. Only the main types are given here.

Alzheimer's disease

Nature

A neurodegenerative disease which is the commonest cause of dementia. Clinically there is failure of memory and frequently disturbances in emotion. As disease progresses there is physical decline with poor food intake and inability to walk. Death is commonly due to the development of a pneumonia.

The cause of the disease is unknown; however, there are well-defined familial cases which are providing important clues in hunting for specific gene defects leading to disease.

Appearances

There is loss of neurones from the cerebral cortex and consequent reduction in size of the brain—cerebral atrophy. Atrophy in Alzheimer's disease is particularly seen in the temporal, parietal and frontal lobes.

Histologically there are three main abnormalities seen in Alzheimer's disease:

1 *Amyloid* is deposited extracellularly in the cerebral cortex in spherical deposits called *senile plaques*. The amyloid precursor protein is termed A4 or β protein, and although it has been found to have homology with a protease inhibitory substance its role in disease is uncertain. Similar plaques are also seen in Lewy body dementia (see p. 336), the dementia seen in the brains of elderly Down's syndrome cases, and in the dementia associated with boxing—*dementia pugilistica*.

2 Abnormal protein filaments accumulate in neurones of the cerebral cortex forming structures called *neurofibrillary tangles*. These are comprised of several protein components which physically form paired helical filaments. Tangles are frequently flame-shaped and occupy much of the space within the neuronal cytoplasm.

3 Dendritic processes and axons in the cerebral cortex become distorted, twisted and dilated—*neuropil threads*. This is also seen particularly around the amyloid deposits and the resulting *dystrophic neurites* form part of senile plaques.

In severe cases these changes are widespread in the cerebral cortex but in early cases are mainly seen in the temporal lobe of the brain.

Parkinson's disease

Nature

A neurodegenerative disease marked by disturbance of movement in which patients have rigidity, slowness of voluntary movement and a rest tremor. The disease is associated with loss of nerve cells from the substantia nigra in the mid-brain which causes disease by reducing the amount of dopamine in the basal ganglia. The cause of the disease is unknown. The disease characteristically affects the elderly but may be symptomatically treated by administration of drugs which correct this neurotransmitter imbalance such as L-DOPA. Eventually there is failure of response to treatment, and patients die from wasting and poor nutritional intake.

Appearances

There is loss of pigment from the substantia nigra as a result of death of the melanin-containing dopaminergic cells.

Surviving cells in the substantia nigra contain pink-staining spherical inclusion bodies based on accumulations of neuronal intermediate filaments—Lewy bodies.

Lewy body dementia

Nature

A neurodegenerative disease which is the second commonest cause of dementia, having clinical features which overlap between Alzheimer's disease and Parkinson's disease. Affected patients have a cortical dementia with mild features of rigidity and bradykinesia. A proportion of patients present with otherwise typical Parkinson's disease but develop dementia after a few years.

Appearances

The brain shows atrophy of temporal and parietal regions. In addition there is loss of pigment from the substantia nigra.

Histologically, Lewy bodies (see above) are seen in the remaining neurones of the substantia nigra as well as in neurones in the cerebral cortex. Amyloid plaques similar to those seen in Alzheimer's disease are present, but in 70% of cases no neurofibrillary tangles are present.

This disease has been variably termed Lewy body dementia, diffuse Lewy body disease or Lewy body variant of Alzheimer's disease. It has only recently been recognized as a major cause of dementia and its relationship to Alzheimer's disease and Parkinson's disease is still under investigation.

Pick's disease

This is an infrequent disease resulting in dementia which is most common in women. Macroscopically the frontal and temporal lobes of the brain are particularly affected, resulting in the development of severe memory impairment in combination with a syndrome of disinhibition notable for the emergence of frontal lobe primitive reflexes.

Appearances

Pathologically affected neurones become swollen and contain spherical inclusion bodies—Pick bodies—composed of abnormal cellular filaments with some similarities to the filaments seen in Alzheimer's disease. Neurones die and the cerebral cortex becomes progressively gliotic. It is of unknown cause.

Dementia of frontal lobe type

Clinically this is a syndrome similar to Pick's disease but without inclusions. The brain shows frontal and temporal atrophy with neurone loss, gliosis and vacuolation in the outer layers of the cerebral cortex. This condition has been suggested to account for between 5% and 10% of cases of dementia. Many cases develop degeneration of motor neurones in the brain stem and cord in the late stages of the disease. It is of unknown cause.

Motor neurone disease—amyotrophic lateral sclerosis

A progressive neurodegenerative disease in which there is selective loss of motor neurones from spinal cord, brain stem and motor cortex.

The cause of the disease is unknown and it is predominantly a disease of old age, but occasionally affecting those in middle age. It typically begins with mild weakness or clumsiness in one limb, or may present with dysarthria or difficulty with swallowing. There is usually progression to severe paralysis with loss of swallowing and respiration leading to death in 2–3 years. For uncertain reasons the motor nerves to the sphincter muscles and the eyes are not affected.

Different clinical subtypes have been distinguished depending on the motor neurones involved.
1 *Progressive muscular atrophy*: involvement of spinal lower motor neurones.
2 *Progressive bulbar palsy*: involvement of brain stem motor neurones.
3 *Amyotrophic lateral sclerosis*: involvement of cortical motor neurones.

In practice, although a patient may present with one pattern of disease, with time most patients show features of generalized loss of motor neurones giving a mixed clinical picture.

Appearances

Macroscopically there is atrophy of the anterior (motor) nerve roots of the spinal cord. Histologically there is loss of motor neurones with replacement gliosis. Loss of myelin is seen from the pyramidal (motor) tracts in the brain stem and cord. Inclusion bodies composed of filamentous material of unknown composition can be seen in surviving neurones.

Progressive supranuclear palsy

This condition presents with features similar to Parkinson's disease but is also characterized by the development of supranuclear ophthalmoplegia. In contrast to idiopathic Parkinson's disease, neurones in the substantia nigra, as well as in many brain stem nuclei, contain large neurofibrillary tangles with many molecular similarities to those seen in Alzheimer's disease. The disease predominantly affects elderly males and results in progressive extrapyramidal rigidity, paralysis of gaze and usually mild dementia over a period of 5–10 years. Treatment with L-DOPA is generally ineffective.

Multi-system atrophies

Nature

Several degenerative disorders of the central nervous system are characterized by loss of groups of neurones in the brain, brain stem and spinal cord, and are given names according to the pattern of involvement. Although of undoubted clinical and genetic heterogeneity, these can be grouped together pathologically as multisystem atrophies.

The clinical effects depend on the structures involved in each syndrome but prominent effects are: extrapyramidal rigidity and tremor—nigral involvement, cerebellar ataxia—Purkinje cell loss, with areflexia, spasticity, loss of pain sensation, loss of touch sensation and loss of vibration/proprioception occurring with spinal tract involvement. Orthostatic hypotension occurs with loss of spinal sympathetic neurones.

Types

1 *Spinocerebellar degenerations*: a group of familial diseases of diverse aetiology and inheritance in which there is loss of cerebellar cortical neurones together with degeneration of tracts in the spinal cord. The most common of these is *Friedreich's ataxia*, which is a spastic cerebellar ataxia in which there is degeneration of the posterior columns, corticospinal and spinocerebellar tracts in the spinal cord. There is also commonly a cardiomyopathy (see p. 66).

2 *Cerebellar cortical atrophies*: a group of familial diseases presenting with cerebellar ataxia typically with onset in the third decade. Pathology is dominated by loss of Purkinje cells from the cerebellar cortex with secondary loss of neurones from the inferior olivary nuclei.

3 *Olivopontocerebellar atrophies*: a group of diseases with inconsistent clinical and pathological features in affected families, many being autosomal dominantly inherited. Features of cerebellar ataxia, extrapyramidal rigidity and bulbar paresis reflect loss of neurones from the pons, cerebellar cortex and substantia nigra. Investigation of genetic and metabolic features in affected families will lead to a better classification of disease as there is poor correlation between pathology and clinical features even within single affected families.

4 *Idiopathic orthostatic hypotension—Shy–Drager syndrome*: a disorder characterized by orthostatic hypotension, which occurs mainly in men in the sixth decade. This may occur in isolation or as part of a more widespread multi-system atrophy involving the substantia nigra, motor neurones or cerebellar cortex. Pathologically there is loss of neurones from the intermediolateral column in the thoracic spinal cord. Some cases are often accompanied by formation of Lewy bodies as seen in idiopathic Parkinson's disease.

Heredofamilial degenerative disorders

These are a group of familial neurodegenerative diseases. Though many of the multi-system atrophies discussed above are also heredofamilial degenerations other main types are presented below:

Huntington's disease

Nature

A neurodegenerative disease characterized by abnormal choreiform movements and dementia with onset in middle life.

The disease is due to an autosomal dominant gene disorder with a prevalence of around one in 20 000. Recombinant DNA techniques can now be used to probe the region of the gene on the short arm of chromosome 4 in affected families and to predict affected individuals.

Appearances
There is macroscopic atrophy of the caudate and putamen due to cell loss.

Outcome
Affected individuals develop movement disorder following by progressively severe dementia and die as a result of severe mental and physical incapacity.

Lafora body disease
This is a progressive degenerative disease with onset in childhood, with myoclonic epilepsy and subsequent dementia, patients dying before the age of 30. Pathologically neuronal cell bodies contain large spherical inclusions—Lafora bodies—composed of glucose polymers.

Mitochondrial cytopathies
Mitochondrial cytopathies may present with neurological disease as well as muscle disease (see p. 289). Cases of myoclonus epilepsy, certain cases of optic atrophy and cases with degeneration of cerebral white matter have now been shown to be due to heritable defects in mitochondrial DNA.

Metabolic and toxic disorders

Pernicious anaemia
Deficiency of vitamin B_{12} (see p. 27) may result in neurological disease marked by paraesthesiae, ataxia and sensory abnormalities. This is due to degeneration of the lateral and posterior columns of the spinal cord—subacute combined degeneration of the cord.

Hepatic encephalopathy
Patients who have hepatic failure develop impaired consciousness due to the onset of hepatic encephalopathy thought to be due to the presence of excitatory transmitter substances in the blood which have not been detoxified by the liver (see p. 242). Histologically, enlarged astrocytes may be seen in the brain characterized by vacuolated nuclei—Alzheimer type 2 astrocytes.

Carbon monoxide poisoning
If death does not occur immediately following carbon monoxide poisoning then there may be delayed damage to the brain characterized by necrosis of the globus pallidus, frequently associated with demyelination of the hemispheric white matter and also with cortical necrosis (see p. 321). Neurological signs usually become apparent 24–36 hours after exposure to carbon monoxide.

Metals and the brain
1 *Aluminium* in dialysate fluid can cause dementia in patients undergoing treatment by haemodialysis. Aluminium has also been implicated in the pathogenesis of Alzheimer's disease as it can be found in the amyloid centre of senile plaques, but any role in causing the disease is doubtful.
2 *Lead* ingestion may result in an encephalopathy as well as a peripheral neuropathy.

Alcohol and the brain
Chronic alcoholism may cause degenerative changes in the central and peripheral nervous system.
1 *Cerebellar degeneration* may occur with atrophy of the cerebellar cortex and the clinical development of a cerebellar ataxia.
2 *Wernicke's encephalopathy* is due to thiamine deficiency which is commonly seen in chronic alcoholism. Because thiamine is necessary for carbohydrate metabolism encephalopathy may be precipitated in an alcoholic by intravenous therapy with glucose. It is manifest clinically by a triad of mental confusion, ataxia and abnormal eye movements with ophthalmoplegia. Pathologically there is disruption of the walls of small vessels in the regions of the mamillary bodies, floor of the fourth ventricle and adjacent to the walls of the third ventricle. This is manifest by petechial haemorrhages and necrosis seen macroscopically in mamillary bodies. This may be fatal unless treatment is given by administration of B complex vitamins including thiamine. If recovery occurs there may be permanent impairment of recent memory—*Korsakoff's psychosis*.

Alcohol may also cause a peripheral neuropathy (see p. 348).

D/TUMOURS

Neuroepithelial
   Astrocytic
   Oligodendroglial
   Ependymal
   Choroid plexus
   Uncertain histogenesis
   Neuronal
   Pineal
   Embryonal
Meningeal
   Haemopoietic and lymphoid
   Germ cell
Cysts and tumour-like conditions
Regional extensions
Secondary

Although they account for only 2.2% of all deaths from cancer, primary neoplasms of the central nervous system are important in that they affect younger age groups compared to most of the other common primary tumours. Primary CNS tumours account for 22% of cancer deaths in those under the age of 15 years, being second only to the leukaemias, and account for about 10% of cancer deaths in those between 15 and 35 years of age.

Brain tumours present with either focal neurological signs or as a consequence of space-occupancy with features of raised intracranial pressure. Tumours are derived from the various tissues which make up the CNS and are classified according to their cell of origin. There are seven main groups:
1 Neurepithelial origin.
2 Meningeal origin.
3 Haemopoietic origin.
4 Germ cell origin.
5 Cysts.
6 Local extension of regional tumours.
7 Metastases.

Tumours of neuroepithelial origin
These tumours are also broadly grouped under the term *gliomas* in recognition of their main origin from glial cells of the nervous system, and comprise astrocytic tumours, oligodendroglial tumours, ependymal tumours, choroid plexus tumours, neuronal tumours, pineal tumours and embryonal tumours.

Grading of gliomas
The histological grade of glial tumours shows a close relation with prognosis. The features assessed in grading are:
1 *Cellularity*: low/high.
2 *Mitoses*: none/few/many.
3 *Pleomorphism*: none/moderate/marked.
4 *Proliferation of vascular endothelium in tumour*: absent/present.
5 *Necrosis of tumour*: absent/present.

Low-grade tumours
These have a low cellularity, no mitoses, no nuclear pleomorphism, no vascular endothelial proliferation and no necrosis.

High-grade—anaplastic—tumours
These have high cellularity, nuclear pleomorphism, and vascular endothelial proliferation
Necrosis in a glial tumour is an index of a high degree of malignancy.

Tumours of astrocytic origin

Astrocytoma

Nature
A glioma derived from astrocytic cells with no histological features of atypia.

Macroscopical
Astrocytomas appear as ill-defined pale areas of softening in the tissue of the nervous system, which blend into adjacent normal brain. They may arise in the cerebral hemispheres, brain stem, spinal cord or cerebellum.

Microscopical
Tumours are composed of astrocytic cells with no atypical histological features—i.e. low cellularity, no pleomorphism, no mitoses, no vascular endothelial proliferation. There are several histological variants depending on the cytology of the neoplastic astrocytes:
1 *Fibrillary*: stellate cells with numerous processes full of glial filaments.
2 *Protoplasmic*: less processed cells, rounded nuclei, fewer glial filaments.
3 *Gemistocytic*: swollen, brightly pink-stained cytoplasm of cells.
4 *Mixed*: mixture of above types.

These types do not have a bearing on prognosis which is related to grade as assessed above.

Behaviour

These tumours may arise in adult life as well as in childhood. Most tumours present with focal neurological signs or those of raised intracranial pressure. Because of the ill-defined nature of most astrocytomas surgical removal is rarely possible and treatment by surgical debulking and radiotherapy is usual. Low-grade tumours are associated with many years survival. It is possible for a low-grade tumour to evolve into a high-grade tumour with time. Tumours do not metastasize but recur locally and by spread within the brain substance.

Anaplastic-malignant-astrocytoma

Nature

A tumour derived from astrocytic cells with histological features of atypia.

Macroscopical

Anaplastic astrocytomas appear as ill-defined pale areas of softening in the tissue of the nervous system which blend into adjacent normal brain. They most commonly arise in the cerebral hemispheres and less commonly in the brain stem, cerebellum or spinal cord.

Microscopical

Tumours are composed of astrocytic cells with atypical histological features of high cellularity, cell pleomorphism, frequent mitotic figures and vascular endothelial proliferation. Histological variants occur as described above for astrocytoma.

Behaviour

These tumours may arise in adult life as well as in childhood, and present with focal neurological signs or those of raised intracranial pressure. Surgical removal is rarely possible as above, and the treatment is similar for astrocytomas. Tumours do not metastasize but spread locally. Evolution to a glioblastoma may occur with time.

Glioblastoma

Nature

A primitive malignant form of glial tumour with astroglial differentiation.

Macroscopical

Tumours appear as necrotic haemorrhagic masses often apparently circumscribed from adjacent brain. They generally arise in the cerebral hemispheres, less frequently in the brain stem and only very rarely in the cerebellum or cord.

Microscopical

Tumours are composed of a mixture of primitive small cells with rod-shaped nuclei, larger cells with astrocytic morphology, often gemistocytic, and frequently multinucleate tumour giant cells. There is vascular endothelial proliferation, numerous mitoses and necrosis. The necrosis delineates this type of lesion from the anaplastic astrocytoma. Despite the apparent circumscription of many of these tumours histological examination usually reveals widespread tumour in adjacent brain tissue. Gliosarcomas are a subtype of glioblastoma in which cells assume a spindle-shaped morphology more usually seen in a sarcoma of soft tissues.

Behaviour

These tumours may present as glioblastomas de novo or may evolve as a glioblastoma from a pre-existing lower-grade glial tumour. They are the commonest form of primary cerebral tumour and are most frequent in those over the age of 60 years, although may occur at any age. They present with signs of raised intracranial pressure or focal neurological deficit depending on tumour site. They commonly spread within the neuroaxis and, unlike most other glial tumours, have been documented to metastasize outside the brain, albeit very rarely. These tumours carry a dismal prognosis despite treatment with surgery and radiotherapy, with a median survival of around 10 months from diagnosis.

Pilocytic astrocytoma

Nature

A tumour derived from astrocytic cells which histologically have a bipolar spindle-shaped morphology—hence hair-like or pilocytic.

Pathology

These lesions are most commonly seen as tumours of the cerebellum in childhood, where they are frequently macroscopically cystic and have an excellent prognosis following surgical removal. Another site for this type of tumour is in the optic nerve where it also has a favourable prognosis. The pilocytic astrocytomas arising around the third ventricle and the hypothalamic region, while being characterized by slow growth, usually cause death in 5–8 years because of their deep site in a critical brain area.

Pleomorphic xanthoastrocytoma

A tumour derived from astrocytic cells which assume a pleomorphic giant cell pattern including intracellular lipid deposition. Tumours appear to arise from superficial astrocytic cells and form circumscribed rounded lesions. They behave as good prognosis lesions after surgical removal and their importance is that they can be confused with glioblastoma because of the presence of giant cells and cellular pleomorphism. In contrast to glioblastomas these lesions show no necrosis and no mitoses.

Subependymal giant cell astrocytoma

A rare tumour composed of giant astrocytic cells almost invariably associated with tuberose sclerosis (see p. 332). They are located mainly in the walls of the anterior part of the lateral ventricles at which site they grow and obstruct the foramen of Monro, resulting in obstructive hydrocephalus.

Tumours of oligodendroglial origin

Oligodendroglioma and anaplastic-malignant-oligodendroglioma

Nature
Glial tumours composed of cells resembling oligodendrocytes.

Macroscopical
These tumours are very similar to astrocytomas in macroscopic appearance, being ill-defined grey–white lesions which merge with adjacent brain. They arise in the cerebral hemispheres and have only rarely been described in the brain stem, cerebellum or cord. The temporal lobe is a frequent site of occurrence. Tumours are frequently calcified.

Macroscopical
Tumours are composed of cells with rounded nuclei and pale vacuolated or pink-staining cytoplasm resembling oligodendrocytes. Despite the cytological resemblance, cell biological investigation of these tumours shows no markers in common with those expected in normal oligodendrocytes. Despite this fact the name remains in use from long tradition. These lesions may be divided into low-grade and anaplastic oligodendrogliomas on the basis of cellularity, mitoses, pleomorphism and vascular proliferation. It is not uncommon to find mixed glial lesions with both astrocytic and oligodendroglial features—oligo-astrocytomas.

Outcome
Low-grade tumours in the temporal lobe have a favourable prognosis. High-grade tumours recur locally and also have a propensity for invasion of the meninges and spread in the neuroaxis via CSF pathways. These lesions may progress to form tumours histologically identical with glioblastomas.

Tumours of ependymal origin

Ependymoma and anaplastic-malignant-ependymoma

Nature
Tumour derived from ependymal cells. Several histological variants exist—*cellular, papillary, epithelial, clear cell*.

Appearances
Ependymomas are commonest in the first two decades of life and comprise around 10% of all intracranial tumours in childhood.

The commonest site for ependymomas is in the region of the fourth ventricle in childhood, where they generally behave as locally recurrent lesions despite surgery and radiotherapy. Ependymomas of the spinal cord are also common and are generally amenable to local resection.

Histologically these tumours appear as sheets of cells which form tubules resembling the central canal of the spinal cord. Electron microscopy shows cilia, microvilli and desmosomes on cells confirming their epithelial type. Anaplastic-malignant-ependymoma is characterized by the presence of mitoses, high cellularity, pleomorphism and vascular endothelial proliferation.

Myxopapillary ependymoma

This is a variant of ependymoma seen in the region of the filum terminale of the spinal cord. Histologically, cells secrete extracellular mucinous material and this gives rise to the myxoid nature of these tumours. They behave as locally infiltrative lesions which may not be surgically resectable because of infiltration amongst nerve roots of the filum.

Subependymoma

A rare low-grade tumour of ependymal cells, commonly densely calcified, seen in the elderly, and most commonly in the region of the fourth ventricle. May be an incidental finding at autopsy but may also block the cerebral aqueduct and cause hydrocephalus.

Tumours derived from choroid plexus

Choroid plexus papilloma and carcinoma

Nature
Tumours derived from the epithelial cells of the choroid plexus.

Appearances
Choroid plexus papillomas are commonest in the first decade of life, most usually arising in the lateral ventricle. They appear as frond-like tumours and histologically almost exactly replicate the normal structure of the choroid plexus, being made up of vascular stromal cores covered in a cuboidal and columnar epithelium.

Choroid plexus carcinomas are also commonest in childhood and are invasive malignant epithelial tumours derived from the choroid plexus epithelium. They are characterized by solid foci macroscopically and cellular pleomorphism, mitoses, with invasion of brain histologically.

Glial tumours of uncertain histogenesis

Gliomatosis cerebri
A neoplastic proliferation of small rod-shaped cells which spread diffusely through the white matter and grey matter of the brain, presenting with prominent features of raised intracranial pressure. The histological origin of the neoplastic cells is uncertain as they do not stain with markers of mature glia. The prognosis for this diffuse type of glial neoplasm is very poor despite treatment.

Tumours containing neuronal elements
There are several tumours of the nervous system which contain neuronal differentiated cells, either alone or in combination with neoplastic proliferation of glial elements.

Gangliocytoma and ganglioglioma

Nature
Rare neoplasms of the early decades of life, containing mature neurones.

Appearances
These appear as well-circumscribed lesions, frequently calcified and often located in the temporal lobe region where they give rise to symptoms of temporal lobe epilepsy.

Histologically, gangliocytomas are composed of large misshapen ganglion cells with open nuclei, large nucleoli and Nissl substance. Gangliogliomas are composed of the same type of misshapen ganglion cells but, in addition, contain neoplastic astrocytes as seen in astrocytomas.

Central neurocytoma

Nature
Neoplasms occurring in the ventricles of young adults, composed of small mature neurones. This was recently recognized as a distinct entity, and prior to 1986 most would have been misdiagnosed as intraventricular oligodendrogliomas.

Appearances
These lesions appear as a mass within the lateral ventricles, frequently calcified. Histologically they are composed of sheets of uniform small cells with round nuclei, no mitoses and a pink-staining fibrillar background almost indistinguishable from an oligodendroglioma. Electron microscopy shows neurosecretory granules in cells and confirms their neural type. The prognosis of this type of tumour is favourable.

Rare neurone-containing tumours
Histological investigation of CNS tumours, particularly those arising in childhood, using sophisticated histological methods including immunochemistry, has revealed neuronal differentiation in several tumours usually associated with a favourable prognosis, e.g.

the desmoplastic ganglioglioma of infancy and dysembryoplastic neurepithelial tumour of infancy which currently appear in the WHO classification of tumours of the CNS.

Tumours derived from pineal cells

Pineocytoma and pineoblastoma

These tumours may occur in childhood and in adult life, and present as masses in the pineal gland which result in early compression of the superior and inferior colliculi giving rise to paralysis of upward gaze and compression of the cerebral aqueduct resulting in hydrocephalus.

Pineocytomas are composed of mature-appearing pineal parenchymal cells—a type of neurosecretory cell (see p. 36)—which recapitulate the lobulated architecture of the normal gland on histology. Pineoblastomas are composed of small anaplastic cells and have been grouped in some classifications as a primitive neuroectodermal tumour.

These lesions typically behave aggressively and have a propensity for spread through the neuraxis by CSF dissemination.

Embryonal tumours of the CNS

Nature

These are a group of tumours composed of primitive small cells which closely resemble the primitive cells found in the developing brain, hence embryonal. They may be differentiated into one cell type or may be composed of cells with multipotential differentiation. The term *primitive neuroectodermal tumour* (PNET) has been proposed as a unifying term in which to group all of these lesions, but in the WHO classification, tumours with one line of differentiation are given specific names, while the term PNET is used to describe types of tumour with either multipotential or no apparent differentiating features. These lesions are commonest in childhood when they form a large proportion of primary tumours.

Neuroblastoma

An embryonal neoplasm of the cerebral hemispheres in childhood presenting with features of a rapidly growing tumour. Histologically composed of necrotic sheets of highly cellular mitotically active small cells forming rosettes and ultrastructurally containing neurosecretory granules. This is a highly malig-

nant tumour with a dismal prognosis despite treatment.

Ependymoblastoma

An embryonal neoplasm of the cerebral hemispheres and ventricular regions in childhood presenting with features of a rapidly growing tumour. Histologically composed of sheets of highly cellular, mitotically active, small cells forming ependymal tubules and ultrastructurally composed of epithelial cells with cilia, desmosomes and microvilli similar to ependyma. This is also a highly malignant tumour with a dismal prognosis.

Primitive neuroectodermal tumours—PNETs

Medulloblastoma

Nature
A tumour composed of primitive small cells with multiple lines of differentiation arising in the cerebellum.

Appearances
These lesions are commonest in childhood and become much less frequent after the first two decades of life. They present with features of a rapidly growing space-occupying lesion of the cerebellum.

Macroscopically, tumours appear as soft fleshy masses, most usually in the vermis of the cerebellum and less commonly in the lateral lobes. Necrosis and haemorrhage are common.

Histologically, tumours are made up of sheets of small anaplastic cells with rod-shaped and rounded nuclei. Evidence of neuronal maturation is seen by the formation of rosettes similar to those found in neuroblastoma and pale-staining islands of cells with a fibrillar stroma. Glial differentiation is seen by special staining which shows structural proteins typical of astrocytic cells—*glial fibrillary acidic protein (GFAP)*.

Treatment with surgery, radiotherapy and chemotherapy results in frequent long-term survival with 10-year survival being in excess of 50% in some series. Irradiation of the whole neuroaxis is required as these tumours have a propensity for spread via CSF pathways.

Central or spinal PNETs

Nature
Tumours seen in the cerebral hemispheres or spinal cord composed of anaplastic small cells with no morphological evidence of differentiation.

Appearances
These lesions are almost exclusively seen in childhood and present as rapidly growing space-occupying lesions.

Macroscopically these lesions appear as soft fleshy tumours within the brain or cord. Necrosis and haemorrhage are common.

Histologically they are composed of sheets of anaplastic small cells with no rosettes, tubules or special staining characteristics to point to a line of differentiation. Ultrastructural study of many tumours reveals subtle neuronal differentiation below that normally seen in the neuroblastoma.

These lesions have a dismal prognosis with early local recurrence and spread via CSF pathways.

Medulloepithelioma
A rare lesion composed of anaplastic cells which form epithelial-like structures resembling the early stages of development of the embryonal nervous system and associated with a very rapid rate of growth.

Tumours of the meninges
There are several subgroups of tumours which arise from tissues forming the meninges. The main groups are:

1 *Meningiomas*: derived from meningeal epithelial—meningothelial cells.
2 *Mesenchymal-derived* tumours.
3 *Melanocyte-derived* tumours.
4 *Tumours of uncertain histogenesis*.

Tumours derived from meningothelial cells

Meningiomas

Nature
Tumours derived from the epithelial cells—meningothelial cells, which line the leptomeninges.

Macroscopical
The most frequent sites for intracranial lesions are parasagittal, cerebral convexities, sphenoid wing, olfactory groove, optic nerve sheath and foramen magnum. Meningiomas are usually solitary lesions but may be multiple. They are typically spherical or rounded lesions which arise from a flat base from the dura and grow over many years to compress underlying brain. Less frequently meningiomas arise as plaque-like lesions, especially those over the sphenoid ridge. The majority of lesions are fleshy and rubbery in consistency but a minority are tough and fibrous. Infiltration of the skull by tumour is not uncommon and may cause local bony thickening. This invasion is not a sign of malignancy but is part of the pattern of growth of this type of tumour.

Microscopical
Tumours are composed of meningothelial cells which may adopt a variety of histological patterns. The main types are:

1 *Syncytial meningiomas*: composed of sheets of plump epithelial cells.
2 *Fibroblastic meningiomas*: composed of spindle-shaped cells and are frequently collagenous.
3 *Transitional meningiomas*: composed of a mixture of fibroblastic and syncytial patterns.
4 *Psammomatous meningiomas*: characterized by the formation of spherical whorls of epithelial cells which surround balls of collagen which undergo calcification forming *psammoma bodies*—meaning grains of sand.

There are three grades of tumour:

1 *Benign meningiomas*: slow-growing expansile lesions which gradually compress underlying brain and present with focal neurology or gradual onset of signs of raised intracranial pressure. This is the most common type.
2 *Atypical meningiomas*: present in the same way as benign meningiomas but are characterized by atypical histological features of mitoses, pleomorphism and necrosis, and are associated with an increased risk of local recurrence after surgery.
3 *Malignant meningiomas*: rapidly growing expansile lesions which mainly compress but also invade underlying brain. They have highly atypical histological features and behave as locally aggressive malignant tumours resembling sarcomas.

Outcome
Benign and atypical meningiomas are amenable to surgical resection and have an excellent prognosis

although, as mentioned above, lesions with atypical histology have a tendency to local recurrence, albeit at a slow pace after several years. Lesions in critical sites, e.g. foramen magnum, that cannot be excised are associated with a poor prognosis despite a slow growth rate.

Malignant meningiomas recur locally with rapid growth but are fortunately the least common type of meningioma.

Tumours derived from melanocytic cells

The meninges have a normal population of melanocytic cells which may produce tumours. Benign proliferations of melanocytic cells occur as well as primary malignant melanomas. These are rare lesions.

Tumours derived from cells of uncertain origin

Haemangiopericytoma

This tumour presents as a mass lesion with the macroscopic features of a meningioma (see above) but is histologically composed of cells which resemble haemangiopericytes of blood vessels. These lesions are histologically identical to haemangiopericytomas elsewhere (see p. 91) and at this site behave as locally aggressive lesions. They have a typically high mitotic rate,

Haemangioblastoma

This tumour is commonly part of the inherited condition of Von Hippel–Lindau syndrome (see p. 332) and most commonly arises in the cerebellum but also rarely in the spinal cord and brain stem. They are benign tumours composed of a mixture of cell types including astrocytes, stromal cells of uncertain origin and a rich capillary vascular supply. Excision of tumours is usually curative; however, multiple new tumours occur in affected persons. These tumours may secrete erythropoietin and cause polycythaemia.

Tumours of haemopoietic and lymphoid cells

Malignant lymphomas of nervous system

Primary lymphoma of the nervous system, previously called *microgliomas*, has recently become a common tumour, formerly being rare. The lesions are usually high-grade non-Hodgkin's lymphomas of B-cell type (see p. 271) but rare T-cell tumours are described. Importantly, these lesions are associated with immunosuppression and are particularly seen in the context of patients with AIDS (see p. 329).

Macroscopically lesions are ill-defined, usually deep-seated in the hemispheric white matter and may be multifocal. A curious histological feature is a tendency for tumour to grow into and along cerebral blood vessels.

Despite treatment with radiotherapy and chemotherapy these tumours have a bad prognosis, with the majority of patients dead at 5 years after diagnosis.

Plasmacytoma

Rare solitary plasmacytomas (see p. 271) may arise in the brain. They are composed of sheets of plasma cells and may be associated with a monoclonal light chain in serum.

Germ cell tumours

Germ cell tumours identical to those seen in the ovary and testis may also arise in the brain. Most of these arise in the pineal gland with a minor proportion arising just above the pituitary gland—*suprasellar germ cell tumours*. The main types seen in the brain are:

1 Germinomas—histologically identical with seminoma (see p. 199).
2 Embryonal carcinoma.
3 Yolk-sac tumour.
4 Choriocarcinoma.
5 Teratomas.
6 Mixed germ cell tumours.

The histological appearances of these tumours is described in the section on testicular tumours (see p. 199).

These lesions behave as malignant germ cell tumours and require treatment by radiotherapy and chemotherapy. Yolk-sac tumours may be followed up from serum or CSF levels of α-fetoprotein, secreted by the tumour.

Cysts and tumour-like conditions

Numerous different types of cysts and tumour-like lesions involve the CNS:

1 *Dermoid and epidermoid cysts*: these are lined by squamous epithelium and form cysts filled with keratin. They behave as slowly expanding space-occupying lesions.
2 *Colloid cysts of the third ventricle*: cysts lined by

epithelium similar to that covering the choroid plexus. They occur in the third ventricle where they may obstruct the outflow into the cerebral aqueduct and produce hydrocephalus.

3 *Enterogenous cysts*: rare developmental lesions in the vertebral canal which are lined by intestinal epithelium.

4 *Granular cell tumours*: may arise in the nervous system, the commonest site being in relation to the hypothalamus.

5 *Hamartomas of the nervous system*: may occur composed of a mixture of neuronal and glial cells.

Extensions of regional tumours into the central nervous system

Craniopharyngioma

Craniopharyngiomas are epithelial tumours believed to be derived from embryological rests of cells from Rathke's pharyngeal pouch which forms the anterior pituitary gland (see p. 122).

They account for 3% of intracranial tumours, and are commonest in childhood but also occur in adults. They arise in the suprasellar region and grow to compress the underlying pituitary gland as well as the overlying hypothalamus and optic chiasm. Because of their site they generally present with either endocrinopathy or visual problems.

Macroscopically, tumours vary in appearance with both cystic and solid components. Tumour may grow into adjacent brain where it excites a dense astrocytic gliotic response as well as up into the third ventricle, and also surround major blood vessels at the base of the brain. The cysts frequently contain a brown fluid with cholesterol-lipid likened to engine oil.

Histologically, sheets of epithelial cells are seen forming solid areas as well as lining cysts. The epithelium is essentially squamous in type and varies between sheets of basal type cells through to a squamous pattern associated with keratinization. Calcification is a very common feature.

These lesions are benign but their infiltrative tendency into the hypothalamus, third ventricle and around major vessels means that local recurrence is a problem.

Other local tumours

The central nervous system is also frequently involved by local extension of paragangliomas (see p. 113), chordomas (see p. 312) and chondroid tumours (see p. 304) from the skull base.

Metastatic tumours

Metastases to the nervous system are equally common as primary CNS tumours and clinically account for the bulk of neoplastic involvement of the CNS outside specialist centres.

Extradural metastases compress the spinal cord, and common primary lesions arise in prostate, kidney, breast and lung together with lymphoma and myeloma.

Metastases to brain cause signs of space occupancy, or focal neurology. Primary sites of origin in order of frequency are lung, breast and skin melanoma, but most carcinomas have the capability.

Tumours of cranial and spinal nerves

The cranial and spinal nerves may develop nerve sheath tumours, the pathology of which is described in pp. 108–110. The main types are Schwannomas, neurofibromas and malignant peripheral nerve sheath tumours.

Schwannomas of the eighth cranial nerve—*acoustic neuromas*—may present with a distinct clinical syndrome due to space occupancy in the cerebellopontine angle.

E/PERIPHERAL NERVES

Normal
Pathological reactions
Hereditary neuropathies
Compression
Vascular disorders
Toxic neuropathy
Metabolic neuropathy
Immune demyelination
Vasculitic neuropathy
Infections
Paraneoplastic neuropathy
Tumours

Normal peripheral nerve

A normal peripheral nerve is made up of several nerve fascicles. Each fascicle is surrounded by a special layer of perineural cells to form the perineurium. Within the perineurium are Schwann cells, axons and endoneurial collagen. The Schwann cells may form myelin or may simply support nonmyelinated axons. A nerve derives blood supply through vasa nervorum which are branches of local main arterial vessels.

Pathological reactions in nerve

There are three main pathological types of damage to peripheral nerves:

1 Primary axonal degeneration.
2 Primary demyelination.
3 Destruction of both axon and myelin.

The type of damage depends on the nature of the disease process, e.g. demyelination is commonly due to autoimmune processes; axonal degeneration is usually due to toxins and destruction of both axon and myelin occurs with compression, ischaemia or infection of a nerve trunk.

Providing that the cell body of the nerve remains intact, damage to the peripheral axon or myelin may be repaired by regeneration.

Diseases of peripheral nerves—neuropathies—result in abnormalities of sensory as well as motor transmission. Because motor nerves are generally larger and myelinated while sensory axons are smaller and commonly non-myelinated, a disease of peripheral nerve may be predominantly motor or sensory in character depending on which type of fibre is preferentially affected by the disease process.

Clinically, several terms are used to describe peripheral nerve disease:

1 *Polyneuropathy*: refers to symmetrical involvement of several peripheral nerves.
2 *Mononeuritis*: refers to disease affecting one peripheral nerve.
3 *Mononeuritis multiplex*: refers to disease of several nerves in an asymmetrical manner.
4 *Radiculopathy*: refers to disease affecting a nerve root.

Although the term *neuritis* is used it does not necessarily imply an inflammatory pathology.

Nerve biopsy

Disease of peripheral nerve is usually investigated clinically and by electrophysiology. In unusual circumstances it may be necessary to biopsy a nerve when investigations have failed to reveal a cause for peripheral nerve disease. The commonest site at which a nerve biopsy is taken is from the sural nerve, which has the advantage of leaving no clinically significant neurological deficit. Because pathological changes in disease are frequently subtle, it is not sufficient to fix a biopsy of the nerve in formalin and perform conventional histology, nerve biopsies require fixation and preparation for electron microscopy for diagnostic interpretation.

Axonal degeneration

In axonal degeneration the damaging stimulus causes metabolic derangement to the whole nerve cell which becomes unable to maintain the long axonal process. The result is degeneration of the axon which starts at the axon terminal and, with time, progresses up the nerve towards the neuronal cell body. This process is sometimes termed *'dying back' neuropathy*, and is commonly seen in neuropathies with toxic and metabolic causes (see p. 348).

Demyelination

Certain disease processes spare the axon but cause damage to Schwann cells with loss of myelin. When this occurs over a small length of an axon it is termed *segmental demyelination*. This pattern of nerve damage is associated with marked slowing of conduction in large axons which can be detected by electrophysiology. It is particularly seen in Guillain–Barré syndrome and chronic demyelinating polyradiculoneuropathy (see p. 349)

Regeneration in the peripheral nervous system

An area of segmental demyelination can recover by regrowth of Schwann cells and re-forming of myelin. Such areas of myelin repair are characterized by smaller lengths of myelin between nodes of Ranvier.

The sequence of events which follows sectioning of axons in a nerve—*Wallerian degeneration*—is a process that under favourable conditions leads to axonal regeneration. If an axon is severed or damaged then the axon and myelin distal to the injury degenerates and both the myelin and axon distal to the injury are destroyed within phagocytic vacuoles in Schwann cells, with a contribution from local macrophages. The Schwann cells in the distal nerve swell and proliferate within the basement membrane tube normally enclosing them. The stump of the proximal axon swells and from it several small axon sprouts grow and make contact with the swollen Schwann cells which then guide the growing axon sprouts down the route of the nerve at a rate of 2–3 mm per day to the point where the axon would synapse. The axon is then remyelinated.

While this process of regrowth is occurring the

nerve cell body changes in morphology, becoming swollen with displacement of the RER–Nissl substance—to the periphery of the cell and increase in the quantity of cytoplasmic cytoskeletal filaments. This change in the nerve cell—*central chromatolysis*—reflects metabolic demands for regenerative growth.

This facility for regrowth is the basis for surgical repair of peripheral nerves, however, axons cannot grow down a portion of nerve that is replaced by collagenous scar. In this instance surgical excision of the scar and insertion of a nerve graft provides the Schwann cells in basement membrane 'tubes' which allow axons to grow in a linear and directed fashion.

Hereditary peripheral neuropathies

This is a group of neuropathies which have a familial basis and typically have a slowly progressive course. In some cases the neuropathy has a known metabolic disorder, in others the metabolic abnormality is unknown (Table 18.3).

Entrapment and compression

Compression or entrapment of a nerve or nerve root may occur at several sites. The commonest are:

1 Nerve roots in the intervertebral foramen by osteophytes in osteoarthritis of the spine.
2 Median nerve in the carpal tunnel at the wrist.
3 Ulnar nerve in the flexor carpal tunnel at the medial epicondyle of the humerus.
4 Common peroneal nerve at the neck of the fibula.

At the site of entrapment or compression, nerves undergo segmental demyelination with clinical slowing of conduction. With long-standing or severe compression there is axonal degeneration in addition

Table 18.3 Hereditary neuropathies.

Known metabolic effect
  Porphyria
  Abetalipoproteinaemia
  Fabry's disease
  Leucodystrophies
  Familial amyloidosis

Unknown metabolic defect
  Hereditary motor and sensory neuropathies (HMSN)
    (includes Charcot–Marie–Tooth disease)
  Hereditary sensory and autonomic neuropathies
    (HSAN)
    (includes Riley–Day syndrome)
  Giant axonal neuropathy (GAN)

to demyelination. Regeneration of the axon or myelin may occur if the compression is relieved by operation.

Morton's neuroma is a particular clinical syndrome in which the plantar interdigital nerve undergoes repeated subclinical trauma resulting in an exquisitely painful swelling of the nerve. Patients develop paroxysmal severe pain in the foot, mostly between the third and fourth toes.

Vascular disorders

Marked loss of myelinated axons occurs in the main nerve trunks of patients who have critical ischaemia of lower limbs due to atherosclerosis.

Vasculitis, e.g. in polyarteritis nodosa (see p. 102), may cause focal infarction of nerve trunks and give rise to a mononeuritis multiplex.

Toxic neuropathies

Many substances cause toxic damage to peripheral nerves and both drugs and industrial exposure to chemicals are common causes. The drugs isoniazid, sulphonamides, vinca alkaloids, e.g. vincristine, dapsone and chloroquine, have all been well documented as causes of peripheral neuropathy as are exposure to lead, arsenic, mercury and acrylamide. Chronic alcohol abuse is an important cause of peripheral neuropathy and may be very severe, although in some cases it is uncertain what is due to direct toxic effects of alcohol and what is due to vitamin deficiency. Very many more substances are implicated, and full lists are provided in specialized texts.

Pathologically, most toxins produce a 'dying back' pattern of axonal damage that results in symmetrical sensory/motor neuropathy. The sensory signs appear in a *'glove and stocking'* distribution, reflecting loss of the ends of the longer axons. Lead produces segmental demyelination in addition to axonal degeneration.

Metabolic diseases and neuropathy

Diabetes mellitus is associated with four patterns of neuropathy:

1 Symmetrical predominantly sensory peripheral polyneuropathy.
2 Autonomic neuropathy.
3 Proximal painful motor neuropathy.
4 Cranial mononeuritis, mainly third, fourth and sixth nerves.

The sensory and autonomic neuropathy is due to axonal degeneration as well as segmental demyelination. Motor neuropathy and cranial mononeuritis are as a result of vascular occlusion in the blood vessels supplying nerves.

Vitamin deficiency is an important cause of peripheral neuropathy, particularly B_1 (thiamine) and B_{12}.

Amyloid may infiltrate peripheral nerves and cause a neuropathy. This occurs in cases of secondary amyloid, such as due to myeloma—light-chain-derived—and chronic inflammation—serum amyloid A protein-derived. In addition there are several types of familial amyloid causing neuropathy due to a gene defect in the gene coding for transthyretin (pre-albumen) or gelsolin (an actin-associated protein), which become deposited as amyloid in nerves.

Immune demyelination

Acute postinfectious polyneuropathy—Guillain–Barré syndrome

This is an immune-mediated demyelination of peripheral nerves seen after a variety of infective processes but usually 2–4 weeks after a viral illness. It is the commonest form of acute neuropathy. Affected patients develop motor neuropathy with lesser sensory changes, due to widespread demyelination in peripheral nerves.

Histologically, there is focal infiltration of nerves by lymphoid cells with phagocytic macrophages ingesting degenerate myelin.

In about half the cases patients develop respiratory failure due to involvement of nerves suppling intercostal and diaphragmatic muscle, and require ventilation for several weeks. Remyelination over a period of 3–4 months is associated with recovery in the majority of cases.

Chronic demyelinating polyradiculoneuropathy

This is a chronic form of immune-mediated demyelination histologically characterized by marked proliferation of Schwann cells around axons which have been repeatedly demyelinated and remyelinated. The Schwann cells form an onion skin-like arrangement around axons and cause physical swelling of peripheral nerves giving rise to the term *hypertrophic*

neuropathy. Hypertrophic neuropathy also occurs in some hereditary neuropathies.

Vasculitic neuropathy

Mononeuritis multiplex is frequently part of the clinical picture in systemic vasculitis such as occurs in polyarteritis nodosa, SLE, Wegener's granulomatosis, rheumatoid disease (see p. 100). This is due to segmental necrosis of nerves as a result of lesions in the vasa nervorum.

Infections

Two infections particularly affect peripheral nerves.

1 Herpes zoster may lie dormant in dorsal root ganglia and recur in later life as a pustular skin rash localized to the dermatome of the sensory segment—*shingles*.

2 Leprosy affects peripheral nerves, particularly in its tuberculoid form when there is destruction of cutaneous nerves by granulomatous inflammation leading to anaesthetic areas, trophic ulceration and loss of digits (see p. 3).

Paraneoplastic neuropathy

A peripheral neuropathy may occur as a paraneoplastic phenomenon. Recently, several cases have been shown to be due to generation of autoantibodies to tumour which cross-react with components of myelin.

Tumours of peripheral nerve

Tumours of peripheral nerve—Schwannomas, neurofibromas and malignant peripheral nerve sheath tumours—are described on pp. 108–110.

Post-traumatic neuroma—amputation neuroma

Severing of a nerve, either by surgery during amputation or through trauma, results in collagenous scar formation at the site of the lesion. In most cases this scar is entirely asymptomatic. In other cases there is overgrowth of collagenous scar tissue, Schwann cells and regenerating axons to form a nodule—neuroma.

Some of these nodules may be very painful to pressure while others are pain-free. They represent a regenerative hyperplastic phenomenon and are not truly neoplastic.

Chapter 19
Diseases of the Pancreas

Normal pancreas

Development

The pancreas is formed by dorsal and ventral buds. These grow from the duodenum and are drained by two separate ductal systems. The two buds subsequently fuse to form a single organ in which the ductal systems also fuse.

Structure and function

There are two components.

Exocrine

This forms 80–85% of the organ.

The functional unit of the exocrine pancreas is the acinus, the cells of which have numerous granules containing digestive enzymes. The digestive enzymes are released as inactive precursors, which subsequently become activated in the duodenum. They have three main functions:

1 Protein digestion, e.g. trypsin, elastase.
2 Fat digestion, e.g. lipase, phospholipase.
3 Carbohydrate digestion, e.g. amylase.

Pancreatic acini are aggregated into lobules which are separated by fibrous septa. The latter contain blood vessels which supply pancreatic lobules and contain interlobular ducts through which secretory products drain to reach the main pancreatic duct.

Endocrine pancreas

This forms a very small proportion of the organ—less than 5%.

The great majority of endocrine cells are grouped together into the islets of Langerhans, microscopical structures measuring 50–250 μm in diameter. The average adult pancreas contains roughly 1 million islets dispersed throughout pancreatic lobules.

Pancreatic islets have four main cell types which have different secretory functions (Table 19.1). The four cell types can be identified by immunohistochemical staining with specific antibodies to the individual hormones. This technique is very useful in the identification and classification of islet cell tumours (see p. 357).

Congenital

Ectopic pancreas

Incidence

Found in 2% of post mortems.

Sites

In order of frequency: stomach and duodenum; jejunum; Meckel's diverticulum; ileum.

Size

Usually small—<0.5 cm diameter, although rarely up to 3–4 cm diameter.

Effects

Nearly always asymptomatic but inflammation, intestinal obstruction and development of islet cell tumours are rare complications.

Table 19.1 Types of cell in pancreatic islets.

Cell Type	Humoral secretion	Percentage of total
A (alpha)	Glucagon	15–20
B (beta)	Insulin	75
D (delta)	Somatostatin	5–10
PP	Pancreatic polypeptide	1–2

Annular pancreas

A rare abnormality in which the head of pancreas encircles the duodenum as a collar and may cause obstruction. This is due to failure of the ventral bud to rotate properly.

Duct abnormalities

These are fairly common but generally of little clinical significance, though they may cause problems to the surgeon in accidental ligation and, in some cases, predispose to attacks of acute pancreatitis. Examples include:
1 Persistent accessory duct of Santorini.
2 Main duct drains into bile duct instead of ampulla.
3 Main duct enters duodenum above the ampulla.

Congenital cysts

These are thought to result from anomalous development of the ductal system—*dysgenetic cysts*.

These are unilocular, ranging in size from microscopic to a few centimetres in diameter, and are usually lined by a single layer of cuboidal epithelium. They can be solitary or multiple, when they may be associated with cystic disease of other organs, e.g. liver, kidney (see p. 250).

Other causes of pancreatic cysts

1 *Inflammatory pseudocysts*: in acute pancreatitis (see below).
2 *Retention cysts*: with duct obstruction.
3 *Neoplastic cysts*: cystadenoma and cystadenocarcinoma (see pp. 354–5).

Diseases of the exocrine pancreas

Cystic fibrosis

Nature

A generalized disease of exocrine glands with production of abnormally viscid mucus secretions—*mucoviscidosis*.

Incidence

Approximately one in 2000 births in Caucasian populations but very uncommon in Asians and Africans.

Aetiology and pathogenesis

Inherited as an autosomal recessive: 5% of the population in the UK are heterozygous carriers. The cystic fibrosis gene has been identified on the long arm of chromosome 7.

The underlying nature of the disease remains unknown, but the evidence points to a defect of anion transport across epithelial cells.

Appearances

The pathological changes are due to:
1 Obstruction of ducts by inspissated secretions.
2 Secondary changes in the parenchyma drained by the affected ducts.

Pancreas

Involved in 85–90% of cases. There is obstruction of ducts by mucus plugs with atrophy, fibrosis and inflammation of pancreatic acini. Islets are relatively spared. The changes are similar to those occurring in chronic pancreatitis (p. 353).

Effects. Pancreatic insufficiency with steatorrhoea and malabsorption syndromes (see p. 34).

Lungs

Involved in at least 90% of cases (see p. 373). Viscid secretions accumulate in the mucous glands of large bronchi and in the lumina of bronchioles with superimposed inflammatory changes causing chronic bronchitis, bronchiectasis and, in some cases, lung abscesses.

Effects. Recurrent chest infections, often with unusual organisms especially *Pseudomonas aeruginosa*, leading to respiratory failure.

Small intestine

Secretions accumulate in the lumen of the small intestine.

Effects. Intestinal obstruction by inspissated meconium in the neonatal period—*meconium ileus*.

Liver

The classical histological appearance is the presence of mucus plugs in dilated cholangioles at the periphery of portal tracts, associated with periportal fibrous scarring—*'focal biliary fibrosis'*.

In some cases these focal biliary lesions may extend and coalesce resulting eventually in a *true cirrhosis*.

Effects. Although histological abnormalities are

present in up to 50% of cases, clinical disease is apparent in only 10–15%.

Salivary glands
Changes are similar to those occurring in the pancreas.

Vas deferens
This is also obstructed, resulting in azoospermia and infertility in those males who survive to adulthood.

Diagnosis
The most useful diagnostic test is the presence of increased NaCl in sweat. The finding of a positive sweat test in the presence of one or more of the main clinical syndromes listed above is good evidence for the diagnosis of cystic fibrosis.

The gene responsible for causing cystic fibrosis can be identified prenatally by the detection of a characteristic pattern of restriction fragment length polymorphism (RFLP) in chromosomal material obtained from amniotic fluid or chorionic villus biopsy.

Course of the disease
There are considerable variations in the severity and time of presentation of the disease.

Approximately 10–15% of cases present in the neonatal period with meconium ileus.

The remainder present in early infancy with complications related to pancreatic and/or pulmonary disease.

With improvements in medical management many patients are now surviving into early adult life. The mean life expectation is now approximately 25 years.

Inflammations

Acute pancreatitis

Nature
An acute inflammatory process caused by destructive effects of enzymes released from pancreatic acini.

Aetiology

Main factors
Present in up to 80% of cases.
1 Gallstones.
2 Alcohol.

Other contributory causes
3 Congenital abnormalities of pancreatic ducts.
4 Trauma.
5 Hyperparathyroidism.
6 Viral infections, e.g. mumps and viral hepatitis.
7 Vascular lesions—shock, vasculitis (e.g. polyarteritis nodosa) thrombosis and embolism.
8 Hypothermia.
9 Septicaemia.
10 Drugs—including corticosteroids, thiazide diuretics, azathioprine and sulphonamides.

Unknown
In some cases no predisposing factors can be identified, i.e. idiopathic.

Pathogenesis
Two main pathways are probably involved:

Duct obstruction
This mechanism is likely to be involved in pancreatitis associated with gallstones. As the main pancreatic duct and common bile duct join together at the ampulla of Vater, impaction of a gallstone at this site has two effects which may lead to pancreatic damage:
1 Reflux of duodenal contents including bile, resulting in toxic injury to pancreatic acini.
2 Increased intraductal pressure leading to enzymatic leakage from pancreatic ducts.

The initial obstructive event may be transient and short-lived. However, once acinar damage has occurred a vicious circle of events is started in which enzymatic release results in further acinar damage and so on.

An obstructive mechanism may also be involved in acute alcoholic pancreatitis. Chronic alcohol ingestion results in the production of a protein-rich pancreatic fluid which can form solid plugs in smaller pancreatic ducts.

Direct acinar injury
Some of the less common causes of pancreatitis, e.g. viruses, bacteria, drugs, ischaemia, trauma may result in direct acinar damage.

In cases associated with ischaemia, including hypothermia where hypotension is frequently present, pancreatic damage has a characteristic pattern involving the periphery of lobules—perilobular necrosis. This is the site most prone to the effects of ischaemia.

Appearances

Many of the pathological changes in the pancreas and surrounding tissues can be explained on the basis of the enzymes released from damaged acini:

1 *Fat necrosis*: due to release of lipases. Characteristic yellow flecks are present in the pancreas, mesentery and omentum, often with secondary calcium deposition.

2 *Proteolytic destruction*: due to release of proteases. This results in widespread destruction of the pancreatic parenchyma and further enzymatic release.

3 *Vascular damage*: due to release of elastase and other enzymes. This causes haemorrhage into the pancreas and blood-staining of peritoneal fluid. In severe cases haemorrhage may be very extensive—*acute haemorrhagic pancreatitis*.

Biochemical changes

1 *Hyperamylasaemia*: caused by release of amylase from damaged acini The serum and urine amylase levels are elevated during the acute phase (first 24 hours) but fall to normal levels later.

2 *Hypocalcaemia*: this is due to deposition of calcium in areas of fat necrosis.

3 *Hyperglycaemia*: due to associated damage to pancreatic islets.

4 *Hyperbilirubinaemia*: a mild degree of jaundice is common and is probably due to external compression of the bile duct by oedema.

Complications

Local

1 Abscess formation.

2 Pseudocyst formation: this is a localized collection of fluid, necrotic inflammatory debris and blood-stained material occurring in the wake of acute pancreatitis. It differs from 'true' cysts in having no epithelial lining, being surrounded instead by a zone of inflammatory granulation tissue. Pseudocysts measure up to 10 cm diameter, and are found either within the pancreas itself or, more commonly, in the adjacent tissue, particularly of the lesser sac. They communicate into the pancreatic duct system.

3 Duodenal obstruction.

4 Fistula formation.

5 Chronic pancreatitis: although acute and chronic pancreatitis share common predisposing factors, most cases of chronic pancreatitis are *not* preceded by any acute episodes.

Systemic

The main systemic complication is *shock*, which in severe forms leads to multiorgan failure. Two mechanisms are probably involved:

1 Peritonitis leading to intestinal damage and endotoxin release.

2 Septicaemia due to secondary bacterial infection, either in the pancreas or peritoneum.

Outcome

The mortality depends on the severity of the initial episode, being negligible in mild cases and up to 50% in cases with a severe haemorrhagic pancreatitis. The overall mortality is approximately 20%.

Chronic pancreatitis

Aetiology

Main factors

1 Alcohol.

2 Biliary tract disease—due to gallstones or anatomical abnormalities of pancreatic ducts, e.g. pancreas divisum.

Other contributory causes

3 Hypercalcaemia.

4 Hyperlipidaemia.

5 Tropical pancreatitis.

6 Familial pancreatitis—autosomal dominant.

7 Infections, e.g. mumps, tuberculosis.

Unknown

In 40–50% of cases no predisposing factors can be identified, i.e. idiopathic.

Pathogenesis

The pathogenetic mechanisms are thought to be similar to those involved in acute pancreatitis (see above), the chronic disease probably being the result of repeated subclinical episodes of mild acute pancreatitis. The mechanisms involved in 'tropical' pancreatitis are unknown, although protein-calorie malnutrition is thought to play a role.

Appearances

Macroscopical

The gland is firm and shows loss of the normal lobulation. Focal calcification is frequently evident. In some cases pancreatic ducts are dilated and contain calculi.

Microscopical

The main features are atrophy and loss of exocrine acini which are replaced by fibrous tissue. In some cases the glandular structures are considerably distorted by fibrous scarring and distinction from pancreatic carcinoma may be very difficult. Variable infiltration by chronic inflammatory cells is also present. The islets are relatively spared and often appear unusually prominent. Varying degrees of calcification are commonly present and when extensive may cause 'chronic calcifying pancreatitis'.

Effects

1 *Abdominal pain*: recurrent episodes of vague upper abdominal pain are the most common presenting symptom. In mild cases these may be the only manifestation of chronic pancreatitis.
2 *Malabsorption*: deficient production of pancreatic enzymes, usually as a consequence of extensive scarring, results in steatorrhoea, hypoalbuminaemia and weight loss (see p. 34).
3 *Diabetes mellitus*: this tends to be a late manifestation of the disease, but when it occurs may be difficult to control.
4 *Jaundice*: fibrous scarring in the head of pancreas may produce external compression of the common bile duct and cause obstructive jaundice. Distinction from a malignant stricture can be difficult.
5 *Pseudocyst formation*.
6 *Pancreatic calcification*: in severe cases this may be so extensive as to be visible radiologically.

Tumours of the exocrine pancreas

Benign

Epithelial

1 *Mucinous cystadenoma*: large, multiloculated cysts lined by columnar mucin-producing epithelium mostly occurring in young/middle-aged women. Focal malignant change is commonly present.
2 *Serous cystadenoma*: multiloculated cysts lined by cuboidal glycogen-rich epithelium. They occur in a more elderly population than do mucinous neoplasms. The cysts are sometimes very small— *microcystic variant*. These tumours may cause

problems due to biliary obstruction, but malignant change is very rare.
3 *Acinar cell adenoma*.

Non-epithelial

Mesenchymal: lipoma, haemangioma, lymphangioma are all extremely rare.

Malignant

Epithelial—carcinoma of pancreas

Incidence

This is a fairly common tumour causing 3–5% of cancer deaths in the UK.

Aetiological factors

1 Cigarette smoking.
2 High-fat diet.
3 Diabetes mellitus.

Site

The most common site is the head—60% of cases, followed by the body—15–20% and tail—5–10%. In 10–20% the gland is involved diffusely and the site of origin cannot be determined.

Macroscopical

Typically tumours are solid, irregular, firm and white.
Rarely they may have a prominent cystic appearance—*cystadenocarcinoma*—which may represent the malignant counterpart of benign cystadenoma.

Microscopical

1 *Ductal adenocarcinoma*: the majority of tumours are adenocarcinomas, usually moderately or well differentiated and composed of glandular structures which are thought to arise from pancreatic ducts. Mucin production is commonly evident. Production of an abundant fibrous stroma is typical, giving rise to the characteristic 'scirrhous' gross appearance. In some cases this feature may cause problems in distinction from chronic pancreatitis. The presence of perineural invasion is diagnostic of malignancy.
2 *Other types*: these are all uncommon but include:
(a) *Adenosquamous carcinoma—mucoepidermoid carcinoma*. Mixed glandular and squamous areas of variable proportions.
(b) *Pleomorphic carcinoma*: giant cell and small cell types exist. They form about 7% of exocrine pancreatic tumours.

(c) *Spindle cell carcinoma*.
(d) *Acinar cell carcinoma*: arise from exocrine secretory cells—1% of exocrine tumours.
(e) *Cystadenocarcinoma*.
(f) *Pancreaticoblastoma*—infantile carcinoma. Rare bulky tumours occurring under 7 years of age with a mixture of epithelial and mesenchymal elements.

Effects

1 *Biliary obstruction*: tumours arising in the head of pancreas usually obstruct the common bile duct and cause obstructive jaundice. This may progress to biliary cirrhosis if survival is for a sufficient length of time (see p. 243).
2 *Pancreatic obstruction*: obstruction to the main pancreatic duct produces features of chronic pancreatitis. This is rarely clinically important but may cause further problems in biopsy diagnosis, if tissue is taken from the margin of a tumour.
3 *Non-metastatic effects*: pancreatic tumours are associated with various non-metastatic syndromes of uncertain aetiology, including recurrent venous thrombosis, peripheral neuropathy and myopathy.

Spread

1 *Direct*: to adjacent organs including, stomach, transverse colon and retroperitoneal space.
2 *Lymphatic*: occurs early to involve peripancreatic, gastric, mesenteric and omental nodes.
3 *Blood*: also occurs early, with the liver being the most common site.
4 *Peritoneum*: carcinomatosis peritonei.

Pancreatic carcinoma tends to have an insidious presentation. This particularly applies to tumours in the body and tail, which are often clinically silent until metastases have occurred.

Prognosis

This is poor, with overall 5-year survival less than 5%. Most of the tumours which are resectable are low-grade ampullary lesions.

Non-epithelial

Mesenchymal

Primary malignant soft tissue tumours of the pancreas are extremely rare but include liposarcoma, leiomyosarcoma and fibrosarcoma.

Malignant lymphoma

Hodgkin's and non-Hodgkin's lymphoma frequently involve the pancreas and peripancreatic lymph nodes.

Secondary tumours

Infrequent, except by direct spread from stomach or transverse colon or blood-borne from breast, bronchus or malignant melanoma.

Diseases of the endocrine pancreas

Diabetes mellitus

Nature

A metabolic disease caused by a deficiency of insulin.

Incidence

Diabetes is a common disease affecting 1–2% of the population.

Classification of diabetes mellitus

Primary diabetes

In 95% or more of cases diabetes is due to a primary disorder of pancreatic islets. Two main types are recognized which differ in terms of clinical presentation, aetiology and pathogenesis.

Type I diabetes
Also known as *insulin-dependent diabetes mellitus* (IDDM) or *juvenile-onset diabetes*.

Incidence. Forms 10–20% of primary diabetes: Male : female equal.

Clinical features
1 Early age of presentation, usually <20–25 years.
2 Body weight usually normal or reduced.
3 Commonly develop ketoacidosis.
4 Insulin required for treatment.

Aetiology and pathogenesis
Three main factors are thought to be involved:
1 *Genetic predisposition*: common association with HLA-DR3, HLA-DR4—present in 98% of cases. There is a familial tendency—5–10% incidence in first-order relatives and 40–50% concordance rate in identical twins.
2 *Autoimmunity*. There is considerable evidence to suggest that autoimmune mechanisms are involved, particularly in the early stages of the disease.

(a) *Islet cell antibodies*: found in 85—90% of cases at the time of presentation. In some cases antibodies develop months or years before clinical presentation.

(b) *Insulitis*: intense lymphocytic infiltration of pancreatic islets is seen during the early stages of type I diabetes. The lymphocytic infiltrate includes both T and B lymphocytes, and particularly occurs around islets containing residual beta cells.

(c) *'Aberrant' HLA-DR expression*: in normal individuals major histocompatibility complex (MHC) class II antigens are not expressed on the surface of pancreatic islets.

Aberrant expression of class II antigens (HLA-DR) is present in pancreatic islets in the early stages of the disease. Cells which express these antigens may be recognized as 'foreign' by lymphocytes, thus triggering immune destruction.

3 *Environmental factors—viral agents*: these may act as a trigger for the autoimmune processes described above.

(a) *Evidence for viral infection in diabetes*: there is a seasonal variation in onset of diabetes and a temporal association with known viral infections. Antibodies to viruses are commonly found in newly diagnosed cases.

(b) *Possible viral agents*: congenital—rubella; acquired—mumps, measles, Coxsackie B, infectious mononucleosis.

(c) *Possible mechanisms of viral aetiology in diabetes mellitus*: viruses may cause the release of cytokines, e.g. gamma-interferon, from mononuclear cells, resulting in enhanced MHC expression by islet cells, or be directly toxic to islets.

Type II diabetes

Also known as *non-insulin-dependent diabetes mellitus (NIDDM)* or *maturity-onset diabetes*.

Incidence. Constitutes 80–90% of primary diabetes: Male : female, 1 : 4.

Clinical features
1 Older age of presentation, usually >40 years.
2 Weight: patients are usually obese.
3 Ketoacidosis is rare.
4 Insulin is not required for treatment.

Aetiology and pathogenesis. There is no evidence for any of the immunological mechanisms described

in islets in Type I disease.

The pathogenesis of this form of diabetes is unclear, but the following mechanisms are thought to be involved.

1 *Genetic factors*: there is a familial tendency with > 90% concordance rate amongst identical twins. An autosomal dominant inheritance has been demonstrated in some cases.

There are *no* HLA associations.

2 *Relative insulin deficiency*: the amount of insulin circulating in these patients is normal or increased in contrast to Type I diabetes in which insulin levels are invariably reduced. However, the insulin fails to perform the usual functions and hyperglycaemia occurs. The mechanisms involved in this relative deficiency are poorly understood but two factors may be involved:

(a) Reduced secretion compared to amounts required, possibly related to islet cell 'ageing'.

(b) Peripheral resistance to insulin, due to reduced numbers of receptors on target cells.

Secondary diabetes

In less than 5% of cases, diabetes is secondary to various other diseases. These can be considered in two groups:

Pancreatic diseases
Acute pancreatitis—transient hyperglycaemia rather than true diabetes, chronic pancreatitis, haemochromatosis (see p. 246), rarely pancreatic carcinoma.

Diseases interfering with actions of insulin
1 Hypercortisolism—in Cushing's syndrome or iatrogenic (see p. 117).
2 Acromegaly—from pituitary tumours (see p. 125).
3 Pancreatic islet cell tumours—glucagonoma and somatostatinoma (see p. 357).

Organ changes

Pancreas

Macroscopical
The pancreas appears normal in cases of primary diabetes.

Microscopical
Type I diabetes.
1 *Early disease*: the early stages of the disease are

characterized by inflammatory damage to islets—*insulitis*.

2 *Late stages*:

(a) Reduction in number and size of islets.

(b) Marked reduction in number of B cells.

(c) Hyalinization and fibrosis of islets. This is a non-specific finding probably due to ischaemic damage caused by diabetic vascular disease.

Type II diabetes. The changes in type II diabetes are generally much more mild and, apart from the secondary changes of fibrosis and hyalinization, there may be no detectable abnormalities in islets on light microscopy.

Cardiovascular system

Large vessels

Diabetes is an important risk factor in the development of atheroma (see p. 79).

Complications of atherosclerosis—myocardial infarction, cerebrovascular disease and peripheral vascular disease—account for 80% of deaths in diabetics.

Small vessels

1 Arterioles: hyaline arteriolar sclerosis.

2 Capillaries: thickening of basement membranes.

Kidneys

Kidneys are almost invariably abnormal in diabetes (see p. 167). Renal failure accounts for approximately 10% of deaths and up to 50% of deaths in the juvenile-onset group. Lesions seen include the following:

1 Pyelonephritis and papillary necrosis—due to the general predisposition to infections.

2 Diabetic glomerulonephropathy—diffuse or nodular glomerulosclerosis or exudative lesions (see p. 167).

3 Glycogen vacuolation of tubular epithelium.

4 Benign nephrosclerosis—from renal artery atheroma and hyaline arteriolar sclerosis.

Eyes

Cataracts and retinopathy with microaneurysms, arteriolar hyalinization and proliferative changes (see p. 151).

Nervous system

Cerebrovascular disease, autonomic neuropathy and peripheral neuropathy (see p. 348).

Skin

1 Trophic changes, due to neuropathy and/or micro-angiopathy.

2 Peripheral gangrene due to vascular disease.

3 Boils and carbuncles from increased susceptibility to infection.

4 Xanthelasmas (see p. 141).

Liver (see p. 249)

1 Fatty change.

2 Nuclear glycogenation of hepatocytes.

3 Non-alcoholic steatohepatitis.

4 Cirrhosis.

Lungs

1 Miscellaneous bacterial infections.

2 Tuberculosis—increased risk of TB, which is often rapidly progressive.

Haemochromatosis

The pancreas is commonly involved in genetic haemochromatosis (see p. 246). Haemosiderin pigment is deposited in islets and exocrine acini with associated atrophy of parenchymal cells and interstitial fibrosis. The main clinical complication is diabetes mellitus, which is present in over 50% of cases—'bronzed diabetes'.

Islet cell tumours

These are rare in comparison with tumours of the exocrine pancreas, and mostly occur in the 30–50-year age group. Many islet cell tumours are hormonally functional and are thus classified according to the hormone(s) produced. In some cases the hormones produced are ectopic, i.e. not normally formed in the pancreas.

Types and effects

1 *Insulinoma*: 70–75% of cases. Derived from pancreatic β-cells. This has the classical clinical triad of:

(a) hypoglycaemia which is related to;

(b) fasting or exercise and relieved by;

(c) feeding or parenteral administration of glucose. The majority are solitary non-metastasizing lesions—10% multiple, 10% malignant.

2 *Gastrinoma*: 20–25% of cases. Clinically excess gastrin production is associated with the *Zollinger–Ellison syndrome* of gastric hypersecretion, multiple peptic ulcers and diarrhoea.

These tumours are multiple in 50% of cases and

clinically malignant in 60–70%. Approximately 10–20% occur in other sites, e.g. duodenum.

Gastrinomas, and occasionally other islet cell tumours, may be part of the MEN I syndrome with adenomas also present in other endocrine glands, particularly the parathyroid and pituitary (see p. 139).

3 *Vipoma*: associated with production of vasoactive intestinal polypeptide (VIP) resulting in the syndrome of watery diarrhoea, hypokalaemia and achlorhydria—WDHA— also known as the *Verner Morrison syndrome*.

4 *Glucagonoma*: these are derived from pancreatic alpha cells. Excess glucagon production is associated with diabetes mellitus (usually mild), necrolytic migratory erythema and uraemia.

5 *Somatostatinoma*: derived from pancreatic delta cells and associated clinically with diabetes mellitus, cholelithiasis and steatorrhoea.

6 *Pancreatic polypeptide secreting—PPOMA*: very rare and asymptomatic endocrinologically, even when high levels of circulating hormone are present.

Appearances

Islet cell tumours are usually solitary but may be multiple in up to 20% of cases. They are usually present as small, firm. circumscribed yellow–brown or red nodules which can occur anywhere in the pancreas. Some tumours may be so small as to be difficult to find.

Tumours have similar histological appearances, irrespective of the cell of origin. They generally consist of small nests and ribbons of cells which closely resemble normal pancreatic islets. Cytological characteristics are not reliable in predicting malignant behaviour, and malignancy can be determined with confidence only in the presence of metastases. Even if metastasis does occur. the clinical progression of these tumours is often surprisingly slow.

Although histological appearances are not specific the precise nature of an islet cell tumour can often be determined in tissue sections by immunoperoxidase staining with specific antisera to pancreatic hormones.

Chapter 20
Diseases of the Respiratory System

Upper respiratory tract—nose and nasal sinuses

Rhinitis
Sinusitis
Polyps
Midfacial granuloma
Tumours

Acute rhinitis

Acute infective rhinitis

Organisms
The common cold—acute coryza—is by far the commonest cause of acute rhinitis, usually with additional nasopharyngitis and sinusitis. It is usually due to rhinovirus (over 100 serotypes).

Other viral causes include corona, respiratory syncytial, parainfluenza and adenoviruses. It is a prodrome of some systemic viraemias, e.g. measles. Bacterial superinfection often occurs.

Appearances

Macroscopical
There is oedema, erythema and swelling of the nasal mucosa with a mucoid or watery fluid exudate. Bacterial superinfection results in ulceration and mucopurulent exudate formation.

Microscopical
Oedema, vascular congestion and a mild inflammatory infiltrate initially. Polymorph infiltration occurs when there is bacterial superinfection. There is often loss of lining epithelium.

Effects
1 *Complete resolution*: the usual result.
2 *Bacterial superinfection*: common—usually resolves but can spread to cause sinusitis.
3 *Chronic sinusitis* (see below).
4 *Tracheobronchitis and bronchopneumonia*: may occur in debilitated patients.

Allergic rhinitis—hay fever
Due to an IgE-mediated hypersensitivity response to an allergen, e.g. pollen. The mechanism is similar to allergic asthma (see p. 382). Morphologically characterized by oedema and an infiltrate of mast cells, lymphocytes, histiocytes and numerous eosinophils. Recurrent attacks are often complicated by nasal polyp formation.

Irritant rhinitis
Working in a dusty environment or with irritant chemicals can cause recurrent acute or chronic rhinitis.

Chronic rhinitis
Can be due to recurrent attacks of acute rhinitis or more rarely it can be due to a specific granulomatous infection, e.g. rhinosporidiosis, tuberculosis, leprosy.

Acute sinusitis

Aetiology

Nasal infection
Usually due to spread of infection from the nose. The common upper respiratory viral infections are the usual precipitating factors (see above).

Dental infection
Spread from infected teeth or following dental extraction can occur in the maxillary sinus.

Organisms
Haemophilus influenzae, Strep. pneumoniae and *Strep. pyogenes* are the commonest causes.

Appearances
The morphological changes are of typical acute inflammation.

Effects
1 *Resolution*, without sequelae, is the result in many cases.
2 *Mucocele—empyema*: blockage of ostial outlet results in accumulation of secretions and mucus retention, which occasionally forms a tumour-like mass. If infected it becomes purulent to produce an empyema.
3 *Chronic sinusitis*: a sequel of local structural damage and continued infection. Kartagener's syndrome is associated with chronic sinusitis (see p. 373).
4 *Osteomyelitis*: can occur in acute and chronic sinusitis.
5 *Orbital cellulitis*: usually bacterial and serous but can be fungal in diabetics.
6 *Intracranial complications*: spread to the intracranial cavity can occur, causing meningitis, intracranial abscess or suppurative thrombosis of the cavernous sinus.

Nasal and sinus polyps
These are bilateral inflammatory hypertrophic polypoid nodules, are not true neoplasms, and are associated with allergic rhinitis, infection or cystic fibrosis.

They can become very large and histologically are composed of loose oedematous stroma containing inflammatory cells, rich in eosinophils. Can cause nasal/sinus obstruction with secondary infection.

Midfacial granuloma syndrome
These are a group of conditions often midline and presenting with progressive ulceration and destruction of structures in the upper respiratory tract, i.e. nose, nasopharynx, palate, sinuses. The three main conditions are:

Wegeners's granulomatosis
Upper respiratory tract disease can be part of either the systemic or limited forms (see p. 395).

Lethal midline granuloma—Stewarts's granuloma
Characterized histologically by an angiocentric dense polymorphous infiltrate of small lymphocytes, plasma cells, blast cells and atypical large lymphoid cells. Granulation tissue, ulceration and fibrosis are also seen.

Lethal midline granuloma is now considered to be closely related to *lymphomatoid granulomatosis*. These are regarded as peculiar types of T-cell lymphoma. In some cases overt large cell lymphoma develops (see p. 273). The condition can remain localized or become disseminated.

If untreated, death occurs from systemic disease, from erosion of blood vessels, superadded local infection or development of pneumonia.

Malignant lymphoma
Malignant large cell lymphomas, usually T cell, of conventional appearance can present in this manner.

Nasal papilloma
The commonest benign tumour of the region and more common in men. Usually unilateral and associated with HPV infection—types 6 and 11 (see p. 210). There is usually an exophytic mass with delicate fibrous fronds covered by columnar or squamous epithelium, but some examples are endophytic—*inverted papillomas*.

Recurrences, often multiple, are common—one-third of cases. Carcinomatous transformation occurs in approximately 3%.

Squamous cell carcinoma

Sinonasal squamous cell carcinoma
Typical squamous cell carcinomas are the commonest malignant tumours in the upper respiratory tract. They invade local structures extensively and often

present late with effects on adjacent structures, e.g. cranial nerve palsy. Lymph node metastases occur early and may be the presenting feature, but tumours often remain localized to the head and neck.

Prognosis is poor with a less than 10% 5-year survival.

Nasopharyngeal carcinoma—lymphoepithelioma

This specific subtype of squamous cell carcinoma is the most common primary malignant tumour in the Far East. It is strongly associated with Epstein–Barr virus infection, the virus being demonstrable in tumour cells in most cases (see p. 268).

Early metastasis to cervical lymph nodes is common, the primary nasopharyngeal mass being silent. Local spread also occurs. Histologically it is distinct from typical squamous cell carcinomas, being composed of uniform large cells with prominent nucleoli growing diffusely or in nests and associated with an intense mononuclear inflammatory cell infiltrate. Prognosis is relatively good. With radiation therapy there is an 80% 5-year survival rate for localized disease and 50% for advanced disease.

Glandular tumours

Salivary type tumours (see p. 19) arise in the mucus glands in the nasopharynx, palate and sinuses. Adenoid cystic carcinoma and mucoepidermoid tumours are relatively more common than pleomorphic adenomas. Adenocarcinomas of no specific type are more common in woodworkers. Long-term prognosis for malignant tumours is often poor.

Nasopharyngeal angiofibroma

A benign neoplasm arising from nasal erectile tissue of the posterior nasal space/nasopharynx which occurs almost exclusively in males between 10 and 25 years.

Macroscopically it forms a polypoid mass which will bleed markedly on manipulation and can grow to a large size.

Histologically it is composed of large and small vessels within an often cellular fibrous stroma.

This is hormonally responsive to testosterone. It will often regress incompletely after puberty.

Plasmacytoma

A malignant neoplasm composed of a monomorphic population of plasma cells (see p. 271) which presents as a soft haemorrhagic nasal/nasopharyngeal mass with invasion of local structures.

These can be solitary, but many patients subsequently develop disseminated myeloma, often after many years (see p. 313).

Other tumours

A wide range of other tumours can occur. The most common are of vascular or neural origin.

Upper respiratory tract—larynx

Laryngitis
Singers node
Papilloma
Keratosis
Carcinoma in situ
Carcinoma
Other tumours

Acute laryngitis

A common disease in adults and children

Aetiology

Infection
Acute laryngitis usually follows an upper respiratory tract infection involving nose, sinuses, etc. and is rarely primary. Organisms include viruses—e.g. rhinovirus, influenza, bacteria—e.g., *Strep. pyogenes*, *Haemophilus influenzae*, *Corynebacterium diphtheriae*. *H. influenzae* can cause a very severe and life-threatening acute epiglottitis in children.

Diphtheria is now very rare but very serious (see p. 362).

Irritants
Ingestion or inhalation of irritant gases or fluids can cause severe laryngitis with oedema, e.g. ammonia.

Appearances

Macroscopical
Usually red, smooth, oedematous swollen mucosa.

Corrosive substances or severe bacterial infections cause ulceration and fibrinous exudate.

Microscopical
A typical acute inflammatory reaction.

Results

1 *Resolution*: infective causes usually resolve without sequelae.
2 *Extension*: spread of infection can occur throughout the respiratory tract. Tracheobronchitis, bronchopneumonia or lung abscesses may develop.
3 *Airway obstruction*: can occur particularly in children—where the larynx is narrow, suffering from *H. influenzae* epiglottitis, or in cases of corrosive chemical ingestion. This is due to laryngeal oedema.

Diphtheria

This is a very rare but serious upper respiratory tract infection by *Corynebacterium diphtheriae* affecting the pharynx, larynx and nose. There is severe local ulcerative acute inflammation classically with formation of a '*membrane*'. Death may be caused by myocardial damage due to release of exotoxins.

Chronic non-specific laryngitis

Found in smokers and drinkers, town-dwellers, with overuse of voice, exposure to irritant chemicals or physical agents and in relation to chronic infection of the respiratory tract.

There is a non-specific chronic inflammatory cell infiltrate in the submucosa. There may be mucosal squamous metaplasia.

There are no serious effects.

Tuberculosis

Occurs secondary to active pulmonary tuberculosis due to spread via the airways (see p. 374). Macroscopically there is swelling and ulceration of the laryngeal mucosa, particularly the vocal cords, with histologically typical granulomatous inflammation (see p. 375).

Laryngeal nodule—singers node

A benign nodular lesion occurring on the anterior part of the vocal cords due to excessive use of the voice, and is characterized by squamous epithelium overlying oedematous connective tissue showing fibroblastic proliferation. Late stages are characterized by fibrosis, fibrin deposition and prominent vascularity.

Papilloma

Nature
A benign squamous papillary lesion.

Incidence
Uncommon. Occurs mainly in children but also in adults.

Aetiology
Caused by human papilloma virus—HPV. Specific subtypes 6 and 11 are involved (see p. 210).

Appearances

Macroscopical
Friable fronded papillary nodules rarely greater than 1 cm diameter. Often multiple, especially in children.

Microscopical
Papillary finger-like projections of fibrous tissue covered with a layer of stratified squamous epithelium. Vacuolation, mitotic activity and nuclear pleomorphism occur due to the effects of the virus (see also p. 210).

Effects

Children
The papillomas are usually multiple—*juvenile laryngeal papillomatosis*—and recur over a long period of time. They can cause *respiratory tract obstruction*. Carcinomatous transformation is rare and usually follows irradiation therapy.

Adults
Usually solitary with less tendency to recur.

Keratosis

Seen in smokers and excessive voice users. Characterized by thickening of the vocal cords due to hyperkeratosis and acanthosis of the squamous epithelium (see p. 415).

Coexisting epithelial dysplasia may be seen—mild, moderate or severe (i.e. carcinoma *in situ*) as at other sites (see p. 211).

There is a small risk of development of squamous cell carcinoma—3% of all patients. This is related to the degree of cellular dysplasia.

Carcinoma *in situ*

Histologically the features are the same as at any other site, e.g. cervix, skin (see p. 416), notably the presence of atypical cells throughout the whole thickness of the epithelium.

Approximately 20% of patients will develop invasive carcinoma, often taking many years to develop after initial diagnosis and treatment. It can be seen adjacent to an invasive carcinoma or in isolation. If a diagnosis of carcinoma *in situ* is made on biopsy a diligent search for invasive tumour should be made. Recurrences occur after treatment.

Squamous cell carcinoma of the larynx

Incidence
Accounts for 2% of all cancers and 90% of all laryngeal malignancies.

Affects mainly men aged 40–70 years with a peak incidence at 55–65 years.

Aetiology
1 *Smoking* is the main risk factor showing a linear dose-response relationship. The risk is exacerbated by *heavy alcohol consumption*.
2 *Radiation* to the head and neck carries a small increase in risk.
3 *Carcinoma in situ and keratosis* can precede invasive carcinoma (see above).

Sites
1 *Glottic*: arising from the vocal cords—60%.
2 *Supraglottic*: involves false cords, ventricle and/or laryngeal surface of the epiglottis—30%.
3 *Subglottic*: tumours arise below the vocal cords and above the tracheal rings—5%.

Appearances
Ulcerated, diffuse, grey, solid or papillary masses. Early glottic tumours often appear as indurated plaques. Histologically they are typical squamous cell carcinomas.

Spread

Local
Spread occurs to local laryngeal structures and then into the soft tissues around the larynx. The tumour is often confined by the laryngeal cartilages for a considerable time. Glottic tumours are often less extensive than in other sites.

Lymphatic
Once tumour has spread to extralaryngeal tissues, metastases to the regional nodes occur rapidly. Tumours confined to the glottis have a low incidence of nodal disease.

Blood
Occurs late if at all. Lungs are the commonest site.

Effects
1 *Local invasion* of vital structures, e.g. blood vessels.
2 *Localized infection* of ulcerated tumour.
3 *Bronchopneumonia*: due to aspiration of infected material.

Prognosis
Overall, 80% of patients with glottic tumours, 65% with supraglottic tumours and 40% with subglottic tumours survive 5 years. This depends on the location of the tumour, the extent of tumour spread—particularly extralaryngeal spread—and the presence of lymph node metastasis.

Other laryngeal tumours
Tumours other than typical squamous cell carcinomas are rare but many types of tumour can occur. They include:
1 Carcinomas: verrucous carcinoma (see p. 15), oat cell carcinoma (see p. 404), basosquamous carcinoma (see p. 417) and adenoid cystic carcinoma (see p. 20).
2 *Others*, e.g. haemangiomas, angiosarcoma (see p. 91), granular cell tumours (see p. 15), chondromas.

Respiratory tract—lungs

A/EMBRYOLOGY, ANATOMY, FUNCTION, DIAGNOSTIC METHODS

Lung development
Anatomy
Lung function
  Gas exchange
  Defence mechanisms
  Surfactant
Tissue diagnostic methods
  Histological
  Cytological

Development of the lung

The lung is endodermal in origin, arising from a midline foregut diverticulum which bifurcates to form two lung buds. These grow into the splanchnic mesoderm which develops into the connective tissue elements of the lung.

Growth and branching of the airways occur to produce a *pseudo-glandular* appearance by 15 weeks. Flattening of the lining epithelium and increased vascularity characterize the *canalicular* phase by 25 weeks. From 25 weeks there is development of alveoli and alveolar ducts. Alveolar development continues after birth.

Macroscopic anatomy

The lower respiratory tract is that portion distal to the larynx. The lungs weigh between 350 and 425 g and are divided into three lobes on the right and two on the left by the visceral pleura. The tract comprises:
1 *The conductive airways.* Consist of the trachea, main lobar, segmental and subsegmental bronchi, then bronchioles including terminal bronchioles. These give rise to:
2 *The respiratory component.* Includes the respiratory bronchioles, alveolar ducts and alveoli.

The right main bronchus is more vertical than the left—important in aspiration (see p. 370).

Bronchi distal to the lobar bronchi with the corresponding pulmonary artery, supply *bronchopulmonary segments*—important surgically.

The lung has a dual *blood supply.* The bronchial arteries arising from the aorta are systemic and supply the bronchi. The pulmonary arteries divide to produce a network of capillaries in the lung. These eventually become the pulmonary veins and pass centrally in the interlobular septa.

Lymphatics drain the pleura, lung parenchyma and airways. The parenchymal channels originate in the respiratory bronchioles and follow the bronchi centrally to drain into the peribronchial, hilar and mediastinal lymph nodes. These then drain via the main lymphatic ducts into the great veins. Pleural lymphatics drain centrally with the pulmonary veins.

Microscopic anatomy and definitions
(*see* Fig. 29)

Bronchioles
Are distal airways in which no cartilage or mucous glands are present within the walls.

Terminal bronchioles
Are those distal airways immediately proximal to the first-order respiratory bronchioles.

Respiratory bronchioles
Are those distal bronchioles in which alveoli are seen within the wall. They form the link between the conducting airway and the respiratory apparatus.

Lung lobule
Is that area of lung tissue supplied by three to five terminal bronchioles which radiate from the centre and are accompanied by muscular pulmonary arteries. It is a hexagonal area bounded by connective tissue septae and measures 1–2 cm diameter.

Respiratory acinus
Is that portion of the lung tissue formed by the branching from a single terminal bronchiole. The

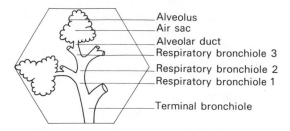

Fig. 29 Normal lung lobule.

respiratory bronchioles arising from this may branch 3 to 5 times and end in alveolar ducts and alveoli. The number of alveoli in the wall of such respiratory bronchioles increases with each division.

Airway histology

Lining epithelium
The conducting airways are lined by ciliated columnar epithelium. Mucus-secreting *goblet cells* are seen in the bronchi but not bronchioles. Other cells in the epithelium include *neuroendocrine cells* containing dense core granules and regulatory peptides, e.g. bombesin. *Clara cells* are present in bronchioles only and secrete mucin-poor protein.

Mucus-secreting glands
Are seen in the subepithelial connective tissue in the bronchi but not in bronchioles.

Cartilage and muscle
The trachea and main bronchi have C-shaped incomplete cartilage rings in their walls. Smooth muscle is present in the remaining part of the wall. Bronchi distal to this have a prominent circumferential muscle coat and discontinuous cartilage plates in the wall. This is important in asthmatic bronchoconstriction (see p. 381).

Alveolar structure
This is important in gas exchange. The alveolar wall is 5–10 μm thick. It is composed of:
1 *Capillary endothelial cells.*
2 *Basement membrane* of alveolar lining cells and endothelium.
3 *Interstitial connective tissue*: this is absent in most parts of the alveolar wall but where present contains fibroblasts, muscle cells, elastic tissue and collagen.
4 *Alveolar lining cells*: 90% of the alveolar surface is covered by flat thin plate-like *type 1 pneumocytes*. *Type 2 pneumocytes* line the remainder and these are important in production of surfactant and repair of alveolar epithelium after damage.

Alveolar macrophages are present in the lumen or on the alveolar surface.

Aspects of lung function

Gas exchange
The primary function of the lung is gas exchange,

supplying oxygen (O_2) and removing carbon dioxide (CO_2) from the blood. This involves:
1 *Ventilation*: the flow of air through the airways into the alveoli.
2 *Diffusion*: the passage of O_2 and CO_2 between the alveolar air and the blood.
3 *Perfusion*: the flow of blood through the alveolar capillaries.

Disorders affecting ventilation, diffusion or perfusion lead to respiratory impairment and can cause *respiratory failure*, which is when the lung cannot adequately oxygenate the arterial blood or prevent CO_2 retention at rest. It can be defined as an arterial $Po_2 < 8$ kPa and/or a $Pco_2 > 7$ kPa at rest, and may be due to:
1 *Ventilatory abnormalities*:
   (a) *Restrictive diseases* are those in which expansion of the lung is impaired due to alterations in parenchyma, e.g. pulmonary fibrosis; failure of chest wall expansion, e.g. neuromuscular disease; or pleural disorders, e.g. pleural fibrosis.
   (b) *Obstructive disease* is due to impaired airflow through the airways, chronic obstructive airways disease—COAD (see p. 379).
2 *Perfusion abnormalities*: as in pulmonary embolism causing decreased area available for gas exchange.
3 *Diffusion abnormalities*: occur when alveolar walls are thickened, e.g. cryptogenic fibrosing alveolitis (see p. 392) or when the sizes of the 'alveoli' are increased as in emphysema.

Pulmonary defence mechanisms
Every individual inhales a large number of foreign particles. Those over 10 μm in diameter are deposited in the nose, those 5–10 μm reach the large airways and those 1–5 μm reach the alveoli. Particle size is important in pneumoconiosis (see p. 387) and infection.

Mechanisms that normally maintain lung sterility are:
1 *Nasal clearance*: the hairs and nasal anatomy result in nasal deposition of most inhaled particles. These are cleared by the mucus-covered ciliated epithelium to the throat to be swallowed or expectorated.
2 *Tracheobronchial clearance*: particles deposited in the trachea or bronchi are cleared by the mucociliary apparatus.
3 *Alveolar clearance*: particles in the alveoli are engulfed by macrophages which either migrate to the bronchioles and are removed by the mucociliary apparatus, or pass into the lymphatic system.

Surfactant

Surfactant is a complex phospholipid-rich substance secreted by type 2 pneumocytes. It lines the alveolar walls, lowers the surface tension and increases compliance, maintaining alveolar expansion. Deficiency is important in hyaline membrane disease of the newborn (see p. 401).

Diagnostic methods—tissue diagnosis in pulmonary disease

Tissue is commonly obtained from the lung and pleura for pathological examination to aid the diagnosis and prognosis of pulmonary diseases. This includes tissue for histology, cytology, electron microscopy and microbiology. The types of sample/biopsy are:

Histological assessment

By examination of cells *and* tissue architecture.

1 *Bronchial biopsy*: small samples of bronchial wall are taken via a rigid or flexible bronchoscope, e.g. for diagnosis of a bronchial mass or tumour.

2 *Transbronchial biopsy*: a small sample of alveolar parenchyma is taken through the bronchial wall with a bronchoscope. This is most useful in the diagnosis of some interstitial diseases, e.g. sarcoidosis.

3 *Open lung biopsy*: this is surgical resection of a peripheral wedge of lung tissue approx. 2 cm diameter. This method results in the highest diagnostic yield for diffuse pulmonary diseases. It is also useful in diagnosis of 'coin' lesions (see p. 406).

4 *Frozen section*: during surgery a piece of tissue can be rapidly examined and often diagnosed by the pathologist. The information may be used in deciding the extent of surgery.

5 *Needle biopsy*: this is a sample of tissue obtained using a cutting needle—'trucut'. Most useful for parenchymal mass lesions.

6 *Pleural biopsy*: often useful in the investigation of pleural effusions, e.g. diagnosis of tumour or tuberculosis.

7 *Lung resection*: removal of a whole lobe or lung in the treatment of malignant disease is examined to determine prognostic factors, e.g. tumour involvement of lymph nodes.

Cytological assessment

By examination of cells only.

1 *Sputum*: sputum samples, i.e. from the lower respiratory tract, can be useful in the diagnosis of suspected malignant disease and in infectious condi-

tions including pneumocystis (see p. 372).

2 *Bronchial brushing*: brushing of the bronchial wall or tumour during bronchoscopy, e.g. useful in diagnosis of suspected neoplasm.

3 *Fine needle aspiration*: aspiration of cells using a fine-bore needle inserted into the lung under radiological control is useful in the diagnosis of deep parenchymal lesions.

4 *Pleural fluid aspiration*: examination of aspirated fluid is useful in investigation of its causes, e.g. identification of malignant cells.

5 *Broncho-alveolar lavage*: aliquots of warm saline are instilled into a segmental bronchus during bronchoscopy. This is aspirated and samples can be prepared for cytological assessment. Differential counts of cell types present are useful in the differential diagnosis of certain interstitial diseases, e.g. cryptogenic fibrosing alveolitis and extrinsic allergic alveolitis.

Electron microscopy

This is sometimes used as an ancillary investigation, e.g. typing tumours or tissue infiltrates and identification of types of mineral fibres in suspected pneumoconiosis.

Microbiology

Direct examination and culture are important techniques on tissue samples.

B/INFLAMMATIONS

- Acute tracheobronchitis
- Pneumonia
- Lung abscess
- Bronchiectasis

Acute tracheobronchitis

Definition

An acute infection of part or all of the tracheobronchial tree.

Incidence

Very common, usually mild and self-limiting but can be very severe in the elderly, debilitated or in children.

Causes and predisposing factors

1 *Viral*: including rhino virus, influenza and parainfluenza viruses.

2 *Bacterial*: including *Streptococcus pneumoniae* and *Haemophilus influenzae*. Prior upper respiratory tract infection is common. Bacterial superinfection frequently complicates viral tracheobronchitis. Severe ulcerative bronchitis can complicate bronchiectasis or bronchial tumours.

3 *Predisposing factors*: as for pneumonia (see below).

Appearances

Macroscopical
The mucosa is swollen and red with a surface exudate producing a catarrhal, fibrinous, membranous or purulent appearance.

Microscopical
Typical acute inflammation with loss of epithelium.

Course
1 *Resolution*.
2 *Bronchopneumonia*: due to spread into the adjacent lung parenchyma.

Pneumonia

Definition
Consolidation of lung tissue by the presence of an intra-alveolar inflammatory exudate of infective origin.

Incidence
One of the commonest infective causes of death in developed countries. It is more common in the very young, elderly, those in hospital and in influenza epidemics. Pneumococcal infections are more common in the winter and *Legionella* in the autumn (see p. 370). It occurs in previously healthy individuals as well as being a frequent terminal complication of many systemic diseases.

Classification
Pneumonia may be classified by:
1 *Anatomy*: lobar pneumonia, bronchopneumonia.
2 *Clinical*: community-acquired pneumonia, hospital-acquired pneumonia, recurrent pneumonia, aspiration pneumonia, pneumonia in immmunocompromised host and rare pneumonias.

3 *Aetiology*: bacterial, viral, fungal, rickettsial, chlamydial, protozoal.

The aetiological classification is definitive but the clinical classification is probably the most useful in practice.

Predisposing factors
1 *Suppression of cough reflex*: e.g. coma, anaesthesia, neuromuscular disorders.
2 *Impaired mucociliary apparatus*: e.g. cigarette smoke; inhalation of hot or corrosive gases; viral diseases—e.g. influenza; genetic conditions—e.g. immotile cilia.
3 *Impaired alveolar macrophages*: e.g. alcohol, cigarette smoke, oxygen toxicity.
4 *Impaired systemic immunity*: e.g. drugs—cytotoxics and immunosuppressives, AIDS, congenital immunodeficiencies, leukaemias.
5 *Pulmonary oedema*: e.g. in cardiac failure.
6 *Retention of secretions*: e.g. bonchial tree obstruction, bronchiectasis.
7 *Instrumentation*: e.g. endotracheal tube, mechanical ventilation.
8 *Drugs*: e.g. previous broad-spectrum antibiotics, cytotoxics.
9 *Prior viral respiratory tract infection*: e.g. postinfluenza.
10 *Other*: e.g. hospitalization, general debility, immobility, postoperative.

Mode of infection
Pathogens may reach the lung parenchyma by:
1 *Inhalation* from the environment, e.g. nebulizer circuit.
2 *Aspiration* of oropharyngeal flora.
3 *Colonization* of diseased lower respiratory tract, e.g. bronchiectasis.
4 *Direct spread* from adjacent focus of infection.
5 *Blood spread*: bacteraemia and septicaemia.

Organisms
1 *Bacteria*: *Streptococcus pneumoniae* (pneumococcus), *Staphylococcus aureus*, *Haemophilus influenzae*, coliforms—e.g. *Klebsiella* and *Pseudomonas*, anaerobes—e.g. *Bacteroides*, *Fusobacteria*, *Legionella pneumophilia*, mycobacteria.
2 *Tuberculosis* (see p. 374).
3 *Viruses*: influenza, parainfluenza, adenovirus, measles, etc.

Anatomical types

Lobar pneumonia

Nature
This is pneumonia characterized by large areas of uniform consolidation of a part of a lobe or entire lobe of lung.

Incidence
The commonest type of community-acquired pneumonia. Usually it affects healthy adults and rarely the very young or old.

Aetiology and pathogenesis

Organism
Ninety per cent are due to the pneumococcus. The pathogenicity of subtypes depends on microbial products—e.g. pneumolysin, resistance to phagocytosis—capsular polysaccharide, and ability to incite inflammatory exudates.

Other organisms
Include *Klebsiella*, *Staphylococcus aureus*, streptococci, *Haemophilus influenzae* and *Legionella*.

Mode of infection
Via the bronchial tree.

Appearances
The classical description is for pneumococcal infection.

Site
Sharply confined to the lobe(s) which are diffusely affected.

Stages
Stage 1—congestion. Grossly the lungs are heavy, red and boggy. Microscopically there is alveolar wall congestion and early acute inflammatory changes with bacteria in alveoli.

Stage 2—red hepatization. The lungs are firm, deep red and airless. A fibrinous pleurisy is often seen. There is an intense intra-alveolar exudate of fibrin, polymorphs and phagocytosed organisms with some red cell extravasation.

Stage 3—grey hepatization. The lungs are firm, grey/brown and airless. The intra-alveolar exudate is still present but red cells have lysed and alveolar walls are no longer congested. Lung architecture is preserved.

Stage 4—resolution. The exudate is digested and absorbed rapidly so that the lungs return to normal without parenchymal destruction. Pleural inflammation often organizes with fibrosis and adhesions.

Staphylococcal and *Klebsiella* pneumonias may suppurate with abscess formation. *Klebsiella* also produces a mucoid appearance on cut surface and thick bronchial secretions.

Results
1 *Resolution*: in the majority of cases.
2 *Bacterial dissemination*: blood spread of organisms with meningitis, arthritis, endocarditis or pyaemic abscesses. Direct spread occurs to the heart and pericardium (see p. 60).
3 *Empyema*: extension of infection to the pleural cavity.
4 *Abscess formation*: parenchymal destruction and suppuration are rare with pneumococcal infection but abscess formation does occur with staphylococci and *Klebsiella*.
5 *Incomplete resolution*: resolution may be incomplete with fibrous organization of exudate resulting in pleural and/or parenchymal fibrosis.
6 *Pleural effusion*: a non-infected effusion is common.
7 *Death*: overall mortality for pneumococcal pneumonia is higher in those with bacteraemia, and is also related to the organism—subtype IV is more pathogenic, age and the presence of other illnesses.

Bronchopneumonia

Nature
Patchy infective consolidation of the lungs in a predominant bronchial/peribronchial, 'lobular' distribution.

Incidence
An extremely common form of pneumonia, particularly in hospital populations and as a terminal event complicating numerous other diseases.

Aetiology and pathogenesis

Organisms
Include Gram-negative bacteria—e.g. *Klebsiella*, *Pseudomonas*, *Escherichia coli*, *Proteus*, *Streptococcus pneumoniae*, influenza and anaerobes. The organism involved usually depends on whether the pneumonia is hospital- or community-acquired.

Predisposing factors
As for pneumonia in general (see p. 367).

Mode of infection
Usually from pre-existing infective bronchitis which spreads to cause bronchiolitis and then extends to the adjacent lung parenchyma.

Appearances

Site
Usually bilateral: the lower and apical segments of the lower lobes are most frequently involved.

Macroscopical

Externally fibrinous or purulent pleuritis is seen. Multiple firm areas of consolidation are distributed around bronchi and bronchioles, the bronchial mucosa is inflamed and their lumina are filled with mucopus. The consolidated areas are pale grey, ill-defined and of variable size. These may become confluent.

Microscopical
A suppurative bronchitis and bronchiolitis with acute inflammatory exudate or pus within the lumen. The peribronchial alveoli are filled with polymorphs, fibrin and organisms, and show destruction of alveolar walls and suppuration—cf. lobar pneumonia. Patchy collapse is also seen, associated with bronchial obstruction.

Results
1 *Resolution*: this occurs only if treatment is instituted early and before there is structural damage.
2 *Lung fibrosis*: usually the exudate is not completely absorbed but becomes organized with repair to the central area of suppuration and residual fibrous scarring.
3 *Bronchial damage*: resulting in scarring of the bronchial wall. Imperfect restitution of the mucosa predisposes to further infection and to bronchiectasis (see p. 373).
4 *Suppuration*: single or multiple abscesses may form.
5 *Empyema*: extension of infection to the pleural cavity.
6 *Pericarditis*: direct extension to the pericardium can occur.
7 *Death*: bronchopneumonia is a very common cause of death, occurring frequently as a terminal manifestation of many diseases.

Community-acquired pneumonia

Organisms
Pneumococcus is by far the commonest cause, resulting in classical or antibiotic-modified lobar pneumonia (see p. 368).
  Other causes include *Haemophilus influenzae*, *Legionella*, *Staphylococcus aureus*, *Mycoplasma*—in 10–20%, and viruses with bacterial superinfection in 10–20%. Gram-negative bacterial infection is unusual.

Recurrent pneumonia
This means three or more separate attacks of pneumonia in one patient and, if localized to one area of lung, it suggests a localized bronchopulmonary abnormality, e.g. tumour, foreign body.
  If it occurs in more than one area of lung it suggests a more generalized disorder, e.g. bronchiectasis, chronic sinusitis, recurrent aspiration—e.g. in neuromuscular disorders or an immune deficiency state.

Hospital-acquired pneumonia— nosocomial

Nature
Pulmonary infection developing 2 or more days after hospital admission for some other reason.

Incidence
Between 0.5 and 5% of hospital patients develop pneumonia.

Predisposing factors
As listed on p. 367 these usually underlie the development of hospital-acquired pneumonia, which is usually of bronchopneumonic distribution.

Organisms
Gram-negative bacteria cause over 50% of cases.

Staphylococcus aureus, S. pneumoniae, anaerobes and *Legionella* are the other organisms implicated.

Aspiration pneumonia

Nature
Pneumonia resulting from aspiration–inhalation of extraneous material into the lung, e.g. gastric contents (acid), oropharyngeal secretions—infected or non-infected—or food.

Predisposing factors
Include depressed cough reflex—e.g. post-surgery anaesthesia or neuromuscular disease—oesophageal stricture, persistent vomiting, near-drowning, chronic infective sinusitis or alcoholism.

Organisms
Infections are often mixed and include anaerobes from gingiva—e.g. *Bacteroides*, fusobacteria, Gram-negative bacteria and staphylococci.

Effects
1 *Sterile aspiration* is often complicated by secondary pneumonia.
2 *Infected aspiration*: often results in extensive necrotizing bronchopneumonia with abscess formation.
3 *Other effects* include:
  (a) *asphyxial death* due to massive aspiration—e.g. gastric contents,
  (b) *diffuse alveolar damage* from gastric acid,
  (c) *bronchiolitis obliterans* from recurrent gastric acid aspiration,
  (d) *bronchiectasis*,
  (e) *localized pneumonia*—large foreign bodies,
  (f) *diffuse nodular granulomatous inflammation*—small organic particles,
  (g) *lipid pneumonia* (see p. 400).

Infection in immunocompromised host
This is described on p. 397.

Bacterial pneumonias—individual types

Pneumococcal
This is usually community-acquired and of lobar type. There are several serological subtypes.

Klebsiella
Usually community-acquired. Strongly associated with poor oral hygiene and common in alcoholic males.
1 *Acute*: lobar with mucoid appearance with necrosis.
2 *Chronic*: extensive fibrous scarring, abscess formation and necrosis.

Legionella pneumonia

Organism
Legionella pneumophilia is the usual subtype.

Source
From the environment, especially piped hot-water systems, water reservoirs and cooling units of air-conditioning systems. These are all colonized by *Legionella* and overgrowth of the organism is probably important. Inhalation of water droplets is related to outbreaks. There is no case-to-case transmission.

Clinical
Legionella causes a range of illness from subclinical infection to Pontiac fever—a flu-like illness—or pneumonia. It occurs in immunocompetent individuals but the incidence is increased in bone marrow and renal transplant patients. Mortality is related to therapy used and prior health of the individual.

Appearances
The pneumonia is of lobular bronchopneumonic distribution with a tendency to become confluent and appear lobar. Fibrinous pleuritis and abscesses are common in cases coming to post mortem. Histologically the changes are of an acute fibrinopurulent pneumonia rich in mononuclear cells. There is often considerable lysis or necrosis of the exudate and alveolar walls

Staphylococcal pneumonia

Source
Humans are the main reservoir of infection as carriers. It is acquired in the community or in hospital and is commonly secondary to a prior viral upper respiratory tract infection. It is an important cause of death in influenza epidemics.

Clinical
It complicates the postoperative state (e.g. tracheal intubation, impaired coughing), prolonged intravas-

cular cannulation, occurs in debilitated patients and can be secondary to blood-borne spread from a distant infective focal site.

Appearances
It is nearly always a severe bronchopneumonia becoming confluent early. Abscess formation is common.

Results
There is a high mortality, e.g. 70% in patients over 70 years of age.

Haemophilus influenzae *pneumonia*

Source
Most infections by this Gram-negative bacterium are caused by encapsulated forms. Infection occurs by inhalation from carriers or from aspiration from an infected upper respiratory tract. It is a common complicating infection in pre-existing lung disease, especially COAD (see p. 379).

Appearances
The pneumonia is lobar or bronchopneumonic in distribution.

Other Gram-negative bacterial—coliforms
A wide range of Gram-negative bacteria, e.g. *Escherichia coli*, *Pseudomonas*, *Klebsiella*, *Proteus* and *Serratia*, are important causes of hospital-acquired pneumonia (see p. 369). These organisms occur particularly in those patients who are debilitated, postsurgical, on ventilation or immunosuppressed.

Anaerobic bacteria
Bacteroides, fusobacteria, anaerobic cocci and clostridia usually occur secondary to aspiration (see p. 370).

Other bacteria
Rare causes of bacterial pneumonia include plague, tularaemia, anthrax.

Viral pneumonias

Incidence
Viruses are a common cause of pneumonia in early childhood but they are much less frequent in healthy adults. They are, however, important in certain groups of immunocompromised patients, e.g. organ transplants.

Aetiology
True pneumonias may be due to: influenza which can occur in healthy adults; respiratory syncytial virus mainly in young children; adenovirus in previously healthy adults; cytomegalovirus—CMV—in immunocompromised patients only; varicella zoster—chicken pox; herpes simplex and measles.

Appearances
Changes are largely based on fatal cases.

Macroscopical
Multiple small foci or extensive often haemorrhagic consolidation of both lungs. The areas are firm and congested. There is congestion of the trachea and bronchi.

Microscopical
1 *Trachea and bronchi*: intense vascular congestion with mononuclear inflammatory cell infiltrate.
2 *Lungs*: dependent on severity, ranging from interstitial congestion and oedema to widespread changes of diffuse alveolar damage—DAD (see p. 386). In some cases viral inclusion bodies are seen—e.g. CMV, or giant cells—e.g. measles.

Effects

Primary
Clinical disease ranges from extremely mild pulmonary involvement to fulminating lethal forms. Influenzal pneumonia is particularly serious.

Secondary infection
Secondary infection with pyogenic bacteria transforms the disease into a severe suppurative bronchopneumonia. This is particularly common in influenza.

Mycoplasma pneumonia
This accounts for 15–20% of community-acquired pneumonia. It can affect any age group, is more common between 5 and 15 years, but is more serious in adults.

Infection is usually restricted to the upper respiratory tract and the pneumonic illness is usually mild. Complications are rare and fatalities are unusual. The lungs show peribronchial and interstitial mononuclear cell infiltrates similar to that seen in viral infections.

Chlamydial and rickettsial pneumonia

Pneumonia can complicate a number of chlamydial and rickettsial infections particularly typhus, psittacosis and Q fever. Except in psittacosis, fatal cases are rare.

Fungal pneumonia

Invasive fungal pneumonia has a high mortality and is nearly always seen in immunocompromised hosts (see p. 398).

Parasitic and helminthic pneumonia

The patients are almost always immunosuppressed. The commonest parasitic infection is *Pneumocystis*, and *Strongyloides* is the most frequent worm causing pulmonary problems. Both are important in AIDS (see p. 398).

Pneumocystis

Organism
Pneumocystis carinii.

Incidence
Extremely common in AIDS where it affects 30–50% of cases.

Source
A high percentage of the population is exposed to *Pneumocystis* and infection results from activation of latent organisms.

Appearances
Macroscopical. There is a bilateral, diffuse, pale tan, firm, slightly mucoid infiltrate filling the parenchyma.

Microscopical. There is a foamy intra-alveolar exudate with a usually minimal mononuclear interstitial pneumonitis. Organisms are seen in the exudate particularly with silver stains.

Results
Recurrence after treatment is common with a 10–30% mortality rate in AIDS.

Lung abscess

Nature
A localized area of pulmonary parenchymal suppurative necrosis due to infection by pyogenic organisms.

Causes

Aspiration
Oropharyngeal secretions normally contain a large number of organisms. Inhalation of this material into the lung predisposes to infection. The infections are often mixed, usually contain anaerobes and occur in the following situations:
1 *Inhalation of infected material*—e.g. from nasal sinuses.
2 *Impaired conscious state*—e.g. head injury, alcohol intoxication, anaesthesia, epilepsy and stroke.
3 *Disturbance of swallowing*—e.g. strictures of the oesophagus—benign and malignant, achalasia and pseudobulbar palsy in motor neurone disease. Secretions cannot be swallowed so accumulate and spill over into the lungs, particularly at night. They can become infected either within the lung or within the oesophagus.

Infections
1 *Pneumonia*: abscess can occur as a complication of a primary necrotizing pneumonia, e.g. *Staphylococcus aureus*, *Klebsiella*, *Streptococcus milleri*.
2 *Local spread*: from spinal or subphrenic abscess, empyema.
3 *Blood-borne*: from any infectious focus, can localize in the lung by septicaemia, bacteraemia or septic embolism.

Pre-existing lung disease
1 *Tumours*: obstruction of a bronchus by a tumour produces retention of secretions, parenchymal collapse and colonization by organisms and resulting suppuration. This is common in bronchial carcinoma (see p. 404).
2 *Others*: including bronchiectasis and congenital abnormalities, e.g. bronchogenic cyst.

Cryptogenic
In many cases no identifiable predisposing cause is discovered.

Appearances

Abscesses associated with aspiration are usually solitary, occur more so on the right (vertical right main bronchus) and involve predominantly the posterior segment of the upper lobe and the apex of the lower lobe. Postpneumonic and bronchiectatic abscesses are often multiple and basal. Pyaemic abscesses tend to be scattered. Their size varies from a few millimetres to many centimetres. They are filled with pus, sometimes air and tissue debris, and when chronic have fibrous walls.

Results

There are several possible outcomes:

1 *Scarring*: the abscess may resolve with fibrous obliteration.
2 *Empyema*: due to extension of infection or rupture into the pleural cavity.
3 *Bronchopleural fistula*: with serious effects.
4 *Haemoptysis*: due to erosion of vessels in the abscess wall.
5 *Pneumonia*: by local extension into the adjacent parenchyma.
6 *Metastatic abscesses*: due to blood spread, e.g. to brain (see p. 326).
7 *Amyloidosis*: rare and of the reactive systemic type when chronic abscesses persist.

Bronchiectasis

Nature

Abnormal and irreversible dilatation of bronchi.

Incidence

Is now relatively uncommon in Western countries due to the decline in predisposing childhood infections, particularly whooping cough and measles, but is still important in other parts of the world and in other predisposing circumstances.

Aetiological factors

1 *Bronchial obstruction*: by intraluminal foreign bodies, inflammatory exudates, tumours, fibrous strictures of wall and extrinsic bronchial wall compression—e.g. enlarged lymph nodes, from tumour, tuberculosis.
2 *Major congenital abnormalities*: cystic disease and intralobar sequestration with repeated infections (see p. 402).

3 *Cystic fibrosis*: bronchiectasis is the most serious complication of this condition resulting from retention of abnormally viscid mucus due to mucous gland dysfunction (see p. 351).
4 *Abnormal ciliary function*: ciliary abnormalities due to structural defects in dynein arms result in failure of clearance of mucus and bacteria as in *Kartagener's syndrome*—bronchiectasis, sinusitis and situs inversus.
5 *Immunodeficiency states* (see p. 265).
6 *Necrotizing pneumonia*: bronchiectasis complicates necrotizing pneumonias, most commonly after severe childhood chest infections, particularly whooping cough and measles.
7 *Post-allergic*: following allergic bronchopulmonary aspergillosis (see p. 398).

Pathogenesis

Bronchial obstruction leads to collapse of lung tissue by absorption of air from the distal lung. Retained mucus becomes infected and inflammation extends into the bronchial wall. Bronchial dilatation occurs as the effects of inspiratory pressures transmitted to the damaged bronchi combine with distension due to retained secretions. Irreversible dilatation develops with structural, inflammatory changes and fibrosis.

Appearances

Macroscopical
In two-thirds of cases both lungs are involved, particularly the lower lobes. Segmental and subsegmental bronchi are predominantly involved. These are dilated with mucus or pus and the walls are non-specifically inflamed. Adjacent lung parenchyma shows variable inflammation, fibrosis, collapse and scarring.

Results

1 *Recurrent infections*: including sinusitis, acute bronchitic exacerbations, pneumonia, lung abscesses and metastatic systemic abscesses, particularly to the brain.
2 *Haemoptysis*: slight to massive from erosion of enlarged bronchial vessels.
3 *Pulmonary hypertension and cor pulmonale*: with respiratory failure, where there is extensive destruction of lung tissue.
4 *Amyloidosis* of the secondary systemic reactive type.

C/TUBERCULOSIS, ATYPICAL MYCOBACTERIA

Tuberculosis
  Primary
  Post-primary
Atypical mycobacterial infection

Pulmonary tuberculosis

Nature

Tuberculosis—TB—is a chronic granulomatous infective disease caused by *Mycobacterium tuberculosis*.

Incidence

This is a very important disease worldwide, although much less common now in Western populations. There were seven cases per 100 000 population of England and Wales in 1984, i.e. 8000 cases, but in parts of Africa prevalence rates approach 500 per 100 000.

In developed countries clinical disease now generally affects the older and immigrant populations: 15% of patients with active tuberculosis in UK died in 1983. The lung is by far the most common important clinical site of infection.

Pathogenesis

Organism

Mycobacterium tuberculosis is a slender acid-alcohol-fast rod on Ziehl–Nielsen (ZN), staining

Mode of infection

Tuberculosis is commonly acquired as a result of infection from 'open' cases due to inhalation or ingestion of infected material in the form of droplets in dust, food or milk. Routes of entry are:

1 *Respiratory tract*—by inhalation.
2 *Intestinal tract*—by ingestion.
3 *Skin*—by inoculation.
4 *Placenta*—congenital—by transplacental spread.

Predisposing factors

A number of factors predispose to the development of TB and many cases have more than one category.
1 *Access of organism:* close contact with open cases of disease, e.g. crowded and unhygienic working and living conditions.
2 *Susceptibility:* the old, very young, Black and Asian populations have an increased susceptibility.
3 *Nutrition:* often a disease of the undernourished and underprivileged.
4 *Occupation:* there is increased incidence of tuberculosis in some types of pneumoconiosis, particularly silicosis and in health workers.
5 *Other disease:* pre-existing chronic lung disease, corticosteroid and other immunosuppressive and cytotoxic drug therapy, diabetes mellitus, alcoholism and most immunodeficiencies, particularly AIDS, are predispositions.

Types

Primary

The pattern of disease is due to first infection with the organism and consists of a small parenchymal peripheral focus with a large response in the draining lymph nodes.

Post-primary

The pattern of disease is due to reactivation or possibly reinfection of a previously infected individual. In this type there is a large localized parenchymal reaction with minimal lymph node involvement.

Mechanisms

In primary disease the organism causes a minimal acute polymorphonuclear inflammatory response in the tissues during the first 10 days. During the first 24 hours the polymorphs phagocytose organisms but do not kill them, and they drain these viable organisms into the regional lymph nodes.

At approximately 10 days a type 4 hypersensitivity cell-mediated immune reaction develops to the bacillary cell wall constituents. Due to the release of various lymphokines from stimulated T cells, including *macrophage chemotactic factor*, *macrophage inhibitory factors*, *IL-1*, *TNF-α*, cells which form the constituents of the tubercle (see below) accumulate. There is activation of macrophages with enhanced killing of intracellular bacteria and surrounding tissue necrosis, both within the lesions at the primary site and in the involved lymph nodes.

The mycobacteria do not produce exotoxins or toxic enzymes and thus reactions are all due to hypersensitivity to cell wall constituents. These include several glycolipids, some of which, including cord factor, are related to virulence. They cause decreased fusion of lysosomes and phagosomes and increased intracellular survival of organisms in macrophages.

The basic lesion—the tubercle

Macroscopical

The basic lesion of tuberculosis is the tubercle; this appears as a pinhead-sized white or greyish minute focus in the tissues. They can coalesce to form larger lesions (see below).

Microscopical

There are several layers (see Fig. 30).

1 A central zone of acellular cheesy necrosis—*caseation*.

2 A surrounding zone of large pale pink-staining cells which are modified histiocytes—*epithelioid cells*.

3 *Langhans' giant cells* derived from the fusion of epithelioid cells with a characteristic peripheral distribution of the nuclei in a 'horseshoe' arrangement.

4 A lymphocytic rim of variable thickness.

5 A peripheral zone of fibroblastic tissue merging with the surrounding structures and increasing in amount with the age of the lesion.

Ziehl–Nielsen staining reveals *M. tuberculosis*. A tuberculous lesion in the tissues is composed of many such tubercles which have amalgamated to form the characteristic granulomas. This process may heal or spread. Healing is a slow process with progressive fibrosis and later calcification. The central portion remains caseous for a long time and viable

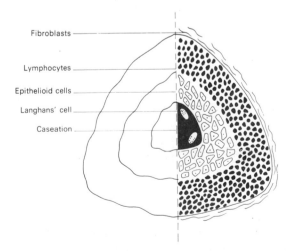

Fibroblasts

Lymphocytes

Epithelioid cells

Langhans' cell

Caseation

Fig. 30 Diagrammatic representation of a tubercle.

organisms may remain in this apparently inactive healed lesion. Reactivation—post-primary tuberculosis, may develop from this.

Primary tuberculosis

Nature

This is due to first infection of an individual with *M. tuberculosis*.

Appearances

The lung is by far the commonest primary site of infection. Other sites include pharynx, larynx, skin and intestine.

The primary parenchymal focus—*Ghon focus*—is usually situated subpleurally at the apex of the lower lobe or the base of the upper lobe. This appears as a small circumscribed grey or white nodule with a soft necrotic caseous centre. It is associated with enlarged caseous hilar lymph nodes. The lung and lymph node lesions constitute the primary or *Ghon complex*.

Results

Healing

The vast majority of cases heal with fibrosis and eventual calcification and only 10% are symptomatic. Organisms may remain viable long term within the cells in the centre of the resulting scar.

Spread

Direct. Progressive primary tuberculosis is the result of continued enlargement of the primary complex with local destruction of parenchyma. Pleural involvement can occur to produce an *effusion* or *empyema*. The lymph nodes can enlarge, obstruct bronchi and cause *collapse* and *bronchiectasis* of the distal lung.

Bronchial. Erosion into the bronchial tree with spread of infectious material can produce:

1 *Foci of infection in other parts of the lung.*

2 *Tuberculous bronchopneumonia.*

3 *Laryngeal tuberculosis,* from coughed infected sputum.

4 *Intestinal tuberculosis,* from swallowing infected sputum.

Haematogenous. Erosion into blood vessels can produce:

1 *Foci of infection in other parts of the lung.*

2 *Miliary tuberculosis*—generalized.
3 *Single-organ tuberculosis*, e.g. bone, kidney, joint, brain.

Post-primary (secondary) tuberculosis

Tuberculous infection occurring in a previously sensitized individual and due to: (1) *reactivation* of quiescent but viable organisms, or (2) inhalation of further organisms—*reinfection*.

Appearances

Post-primary tuberculosis usually begins in the apical segments of the lungs and consists of confluent caseous granulomas which spread directly and locally, but without lymph node lesions. This can either heal spontaneously with fibrosis and calcification—though viable organisms remain without producing any clinical symptoms—or spread to produce various types of progressive tuberculosis.

Spread

Apical cavitating fibrocaseous tuberculosis. As a result of direct extension and continuing caseation, a progressive area of lung destruction ensues. If the caseous material is expectorated through an eroded bronchus a cavity results. There is often considerable fibrosis in the wall of the cavity which is lined by tuberculous granulation tissue. This lesion can heal at this stage but may spread further.

Progressive cavitating pulmonary tuberculosis. The initial apical infection may continue to spread by direct extension involving progressively more pulmonary parenchymal tissue and often with little fibrous reaction. Further spread may then occur into the bronchi, blood stream or directly into the pleura.

Tuberculous bronchopneumonia. Spread into the bronchial tree may establish new foci of infection throughout the lung or, in highly sensitized individuals, produce tuberculous bronchopneumonia. Infected material may also be coughed with healing or give rise to *laryngeal* or *intestinal* infection.

Miliary tuberculosis. Erosion of a blood vessel or lymphatic involvememt may disseminate the organisms into the blood to produce numerous systemic miliary tubercles within multiple organs including the lung, spleen, liver, kidney and meninges.

Progressive isolated organ tuberculosis. When spread via the blood or lymphatic system occurs it may result in miliary dissemination, but many or most organisms are rapidly destroyed by immunological mechanisms. The organisms may persist in specific isolated organs to produce continued progressive disease at those sites: subsequent secondary dissemination can then occur. Organs commonly involved are cervical lymph nodes, meninges, kidneys, adrenals, bones, Fallopian tubes and epididymis.

Pleural tuberculosis. Infection may spread to involve the pleura to produce effusions or empyema. Healing produces fibrosis or adhesions.

Chronic results

Pulmonary fibrosis

The lung lesions may heal with fibrosis at any stage, particularly with treatment. This ranges from minor apical scarring to extensive and severe widespread fibrosis producing localized to widespread honeycombing (see p. 392) and is particularly seen in relapsing and progressive untreated disease. This is complicated by respiratory failure and cor pulmonale.

Pleural fibrosis

Fibrosis commonly obliterates the pleural space.

Bronchiectasis

Damage to the bronchial walls and scarring can cause distal pulmonary collapse, secondary infection and bronchiectasis.

Infection in immunocompromised individuals

Mycobacterial infections of all types are increased in immunocompromised individuals (see p. 397), in most cases due to reactivation of latent infection.

Features are similar to infection in immunocompetent individuals but disease usually progresses more rapidly due to decreased host response.

Atypical mycobacterial infection

Organisms

A group of non-tuberculous mycobacteria of which the more important types are *M. avium intracellulare* and *M. kansasii*.

Source

The organisms are widely distributed in soil and water. Infection is acquired directly from the environment and *not* by case-to-case contact.

Clinical pattern

Immunocompetent

These patients usually have pre-existing chronic lung disease, particularly chronic bronchitis and emphysema. Morphological changes are identical to *M. tuberculosis*.

Immunocompromised

Particularly seen in AIDS (see p. 397). Pulmonary involvement is usually part of a systemic infection and there is often little host response to the organism.

Fungal infections

Because they are most clinically relevant in relationship to the immunocompromised host, they are described on pp. 398–399.

D/OBSTRUCTIVE AIRWAYS DISEASE

Chronic bronchitis
Generalized emphysema
Small airways disease
   Smoking-associated
COAD
Emphysema—other types
Asthma

Chronic bronchitis—chronic large airways disease

Definition

Chronic cough with production of sputum on most days for at least 3 months in the year and for at least 2 consecutive years.

Appearances

Macroscopical

There is 'webbing' and swelling of the mucous membrane of the bronchi accompanied by excess mucus and/or mucopus within the dilated lumina.

Microscopical

An increase in size and number of mucus-secreting glands in the large bronchi and trachea, and of single goblet cells in distal bronchi. The respiratory epithelium may show squamous metaplasia and usually sparse chronic inflammation and dilated vessels. Infective exacerbations are marked by an increase in polymorphs within the lumen and in bronchial tissues.

Aetiology

The irritant effect of cigarette smoke inhalation and atmospheric pollution, e.g. by SO_2 and NO_2, or dusts, e.g. coal, result in the production of mucous gland enlargement and in damage to the respiratory epithelial cells resulting in the squamous metaplasia.

Effects

Chronic effects

Chronic cough with viscid mucus production.

Acute exacerbations

Recurrent acute infective exacerbations occur, usually bacterial, particularly by *H. influenzae* and pneumococci.

Association with chronic obstruction airways disease—COAD

Simple chronic bronchitis, i.e. large airways disease, does *not* cause significant airflow obstruction (COAD) alone. When chronic large airways disease is associated with small airways disease and emphysema, induced by cigarette smoking, these two conditions are the cause of clinically significant airways obstruction (see p. 379).

Generalized emphysema

Definition

Permanent abnormal enlargement of the air spaces distal to the terminal bronchioles, accompanied by destruction of their walls and without obvious fibrosis.

Types

The main types are illustrated in Fig. 31.

Centriacinar/centrilobular

Macroscopical

In advanced cases the lungs are voluminous and pit on

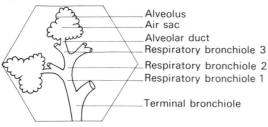

(a) Lobule

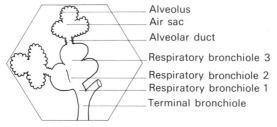

(b) Centrilobular emphysema

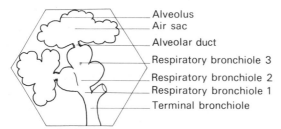

(c) Panacinar emphysema

Fig. 31 Diagrammatic representation of generalized emphysema.

pressure due to loss of elasticity. There may be large peripheral bullae, i.e. greatly dilated air spaces. On the cut surface of distended fixed lungs, clusters of dilated air spaces are seen in the centre of each lung lobule with preservation of alveoli at the periphery. The changes are most severe in the apices.

Microscopical
There is enlargement and destruction of the respiratory bronchioles with preservation of alveolar ducts and alveoli in the earlier stages. As the disease advances more tissue is destroyed and the appearances come to simulate panacinar emphysema (see below). Chronic inflammatory changes are seen in the bronchiolar walls.

Other changes
The morphological lesions of chronic bronchitis and small airways disease usually coexist.

Panacinar/panlobular

Macroscopical
The lungs are voluminous and pit on pressure. There are widespread irregular dilated air spaces involving nearly the whole of each lung lobule. Little normal alveolar tissue is recognized in these areas. The changes are widespread but more severe in the lower lobes, particularly at the base. Peripheral bullae are also seen.

Microscopical
There is destruction of alveoli, alveolar ducts and respiratory bronchioles. Few alveoli are seen and these are greatly dilated.

Aetiology

α_1-Antitrypsin deficiency
There are several alleles for the antiprotease α_1-antitrypsin, inherited co-dominantly, and certain phenotypes are associated with a predisposition to develop emphysema (see also p. 247). Phenotype Pi-protease inhibitor MM is normal. Phenotype Pi ZZ is most commonly associated with the development of severe spontaneous emphysema. Other phenotypes are associated with lesser degrees of α_1-antitrypsin deficiency and develop significant emphysema at a later age. Patients with α_1-antitrypsin deficiency develop more severe emphysema and at an earlier age if they smoke cigarettes. The emphysema is of *panacinar* type.

Cigarette smoking
This is the main risk factor for the development of *centrilobular* emphysema.

Pathogenesis

The protease—antiprotease hypothesis
This is the currently favoured pathogenetic mechanism for the development of emphysema. Normally neutrophils are the main source of protease in the lung. This enzyme causes destruction of lung tissue. Some neutrophils which are normally sequestered in the lung gain access to the air spaces and, if activated,

they release the proteases (mainly elastase) and reactive oxygen metabolites. Circulating antiproteases, mainly α_1-antitrypsin, produced by the liver, are present in the interstitial tissues of the lung and these inhibit the action of the neutrophil elastase.

α_1-Antitrypsin deficiency

The elastase released from polymorphs is incompletely inactivated due to the low levels of α_1-antitrypsin resulting in tissue destruction with consequent emphysema.

Smoking

Cigarette smoking causes an increase in the number of polymorphs and macrophages in the alveoli, partly by the stimulation of release of chemotactic factors from macrophages. It also stimulates the release of polymorph, mast cell and macrophage elastase and polymorph-derived, oxygen-derived free radicles. Reactive oxygen species in the smoke and the oxygen derived free radicles inhibit α_1-antitrypsin. There is thus an imbalance between the proteases and the antiprotease activity resulting in tissue damage and emphysema.

Effects

COAD

The patient with pure emphysema typically has type A or 'pink puffer' clinical features (see p. 380). Centrilobular emphysema is usually associated with coexistent chronic bronchitis and small airways disease due to smoking.

Small airways disease

Smoking associated

Definition

This is inflammatory and fibrous alteration of the bronchi and bronchioles less than 0.2 cm diameter.

Aetiology

This is due to the toxic effects of inhaled cigarette smoke.

Appearances

Early lesion

In the terminal and respiratory bronchioles an infiltrate of lymphocytes, macrophages (some pigmented) and occasional neutrophils are seen.

Late changes

There is some loss of airways, severe fibrous scarring, muscle hypertrophy, distortion of the walls and an increase in goblet cells with excessive luminal mucus.

Effects

This produces COAD, in association with emphysema and chronic bronchitis.

Small airways disease—other causes

Similar changes in small airways can be seen in the various pneumoconioses, cystic fibrosis and bronchiectasis.

Chronic obstructive airways disease—chronic bronchitis and emphysema—COAD

Definition

The above terms are used synonymously and describe 'a clinical syndrome characterized by persistent and relatively irreversible airflow limitation, i.e. obstruction, with chronic productive cough for at least 3 months of a year and for more than 3 years. This is associated with hyperinflation of the lungs and frequently a degree of arteriolar hypoxaemia with or without carbon dioxide retention.'

This definition *specifically excludes bronchial asthma*, but a poorly defined 'overlap' syndrome between asthma and chronic bronchitis and emphysema does exist. Such patients experience longer survival, a greater component of reversibility of the airways obstruction and a more complete recovery from acute exacerbations.

Patients with COAD have anatomical emphysema, small airways disease and chronic bronchitis in varying degrees.

Aetiology

Age

COAD is rarely clinically significant in patients less than 50 years of age, due to its long natural history.

Cigarette smoking

There is overwhelming evidence to implicate smoking as the most important factor in the production of all three of the anatomical lesions of COAD. These are produced as independent effects. COAD is common in smokers, rare in non-smokers and the severity of clinical disease is related to the number of cigarettes smoked.

Environmental
The morbidity and mortality of COAD is related to the degree of general atmospheric pollution, but this effect is only significant in smokers in whom the degree of effect is proportional to the number of cigarettes smoked.

Infection
Viral and bacterial infections are important in the production of acute exacerbations of COAD and may be important in the progression of disease but they are not causative.

Allergic predisposition
Evidence suggests that allergic factors *per se* have a minor role in the aetiology of *persistent* airflow limitation.

Hereditary factors
α_1-antitrypsin deficiency (see p. 378) is a rare but important predisposition to develop emphysema.

Individual susceptibility
Only 15% of individuals who smoke develop significant COAD, for reasons which are unclear.

Socioeconomic factors
COAD is more prevalent in lower social groups. This is related to smoking habits, general pollution exposure and occupation.

Occupation
Coal mining is probably causally associated with COAD but there is little evidence to indicate that other occupations are significant. Simple chronic bronchitis, i.e. without airways obstruction (see p. 377), is seen as a consequence of chronic exposure to a wide variety of dusts.

Appearances
These are discussed on pp. 378–379.

Clinicopathological correlation
Patients with COAD form a heterogeneous clinical

group. The ends of the spectrum are 'pink puffers' (type A) and the 'blue bloaters' (type B), but most patients have a mixed pattern of clinical disease between the two extremes.

Pathologically these patients are also heterogeneous with a mixture of chronic bronchitis, emphysema and small airways disease, and there is imperfect correlation between clinical and functional changes. Type A patients have the most severe emphysema and type B the least.

Most cases corresponding to the mixed clinical picture have a combination of anatomical emphysema, small and large airways disease.

Structural and functional correlation

Cough and sputum production
Is due to chronic large airways disease, i.e. chronic bronchitis.

Hyperinflation of chest
Correlates with anatomical emphysema. There is loss of elastic recoil from loss of alveolar walls, air trapping and a reflex reaction where the patient breathes at a higher functional residual capacity to maintain small airways patency.

Impaired maximal respiratory airflow
Due to:
1 *Small airways narrowing*: from irreversible distortion and fibrosis and from the more reversible changes of inflammation, mucus production and oedema.
2 *Emphysema*: loss of elastic recoil from loss of alveolar wall support leads to increased or earlier airways closure for any expiratory pressure.

Impaired gas exchange
Due to:
1 *Emphysema*: loss of alveolar capillary units and ventilation/perfusion imbalance due to air space enlargement.
2 *Small airways disease*: ventilation/perfusion imbalance due to altered ventilation of lung segments.
3 *Impaired ventilatory control and drive*: some patients with COAD suffer worse hypoxia and hypercapnia during sleep. They are usually a subgroup of 'blue bloaters'.

Results
1 *Respiratory dysfunction*: progressive decline in

respiratory function eventually leading to *respiratory failure and death*.

2 *Cor pulmonale* (see p. 73).

3 *Pneumothorax*: due to rupture of large peripheral emphysematous bullae.

4 *Infections*: acute infectious exacerbation is common particularly in type B—blue bloaters. Bacterial infections are the most severe, particularly *H. influenzae*. This causes acute acceleration of air flow obstruction.

Emphysema—other types

The term emphysema has been used to describe a variety of conditions which fall outside the definition of generalized emphysema given on p. 377, but it is retained due to long-standing common usage.

Destructive emphysema

Irregular or scar emphysema

Dilated air spaces at the periphery of scars in the lung parenchyma due to any cause, e.g. tuberculosis, sarcoid, pneumoconiosis. Large bullae may form as a result of traction forces. This type is focal and of no functional significance, but pneumothorax due to rupture may occur.

Paraseptal

Emphysematous spaces distributed around lobular septae, bronchi, blood vessels and deep to the pleura. This is a cause of spontaneous pneumothorax in young adults, often occurs alone and is of no functional significance.

Senile

In the elderly there is some dilatation of alveoli and respiratory passages with a mild decrease in respiratory function. This may decrease the 'reserve' of the elderly and can effect ability to withstand other significant lung disease.

Unilateral emphysema—McCleod's syndrome

Unilateral hypertransluscent lung. Rare and usually asymptomatic.

Non-destructive emphysema

Focal dust emphysema

Most commonly relates to coal dust exposure. Dust ingested by macrophages collects in alveoli and lymphoid tissue with a minimal reticulin reaction. There is resulting dilatation of the second- and third-order respiratory bronchioles giving a centrilobular distribution of the emphysema. Destruction of pulmonary parenchyma is minimal and there is no significant disability *per se* (see p. 390).

Compensatory emphysema

This is due to overdistension of alveoli around areas of collapsed lung, e.g. during acute attacks of asthma, or in the remaining lung tissue after surgical resection of lung.

Infantile lobar emphysema

A rare disorder confined to a lobe or segment of lung. Causes include atresia of bronchial cartilages and extrinsic bronchial compression.

Interstitial emphysema

This is air within the interstitial tissue of the lung caused by tearing of alveolar walls.

Common causes include violent coughing, especially in patients with asthma, chronic bronchitis and emphysema and whooping cough. Other causes include surgical or traumatic injury.

Bubbles of air may reach the mediastinum and may extend to the neck to produce 'surgical emphysema', but rarely produce significant sequelae.

Asthma

Definition

A condition characterized by widespread variation over short periods of time in resistance to air flow in intrapulmonary airways. This may occur spontaneously or in response to treatment.

Incidence

An extremely important condition with an increasing prevalence to about 5% in Western populations.

Asthma affects all age groups and can develop at any time, though onset is commonly in childhood.

Classification and aetiology

Asthma is heterogeneous aetiologically and in severity. There is overlap and blurring of the various subtypes and many patients do not fit neatly into any one type. Classification can be based on the principal stimuli inducing an attack or whether there is an allergic basis, but exact mechanisms are often uncertain.

Immunulogical status

Extrinsic asthma
The most common type triggered by environmental allergens, e.g. pollens, etc. A positive family history of atopy is usual. Serum IgE levels are raised and an immediate type 1 hypersensitivity to allergen is produced on skin challenge.

Intrinsic asthma
Often triggered by an upper respiratory tract infection. A family history is uncommon and IgE levels are normal. There is no atopy and skin testing is negative.

Precipitating factors
All asthmatics have an increased responsiveness and hyperirritability of the airways to non-specific irritants and bronchoconstrictor substances, as well as to any specific allergen. Precipitating factors are:
1 *Exercise*: including association with cold air and hyperventilation.
2 *Upper respiratory tract infection*: can exacerbate symptoms in known asthmatics but is not generally causative.
3 *Air pollution*: irritant gases, e.g. SO_2, NO_2 and smoke particles.
4 *Psychological factors*: can exacerbate attacks but are rarely dominant.
5 *Drugs*, e.g. aspirin, β-blockers, penicillin, etc. (see p. 398).
6 *Occupational factors*: this is asthma caused by specific exposures in the workplace. There are a very large number of potential substances (see Table 20.1). Prognosis is usually good if exposure ceases, but some allergens can trigger persistent asthma despite complete cessation of exposure. The mechanism is often unclear and frequently does not involve an IgE-mediated mechanism.
7 *Allergens*: a large number of potential allergens can precipitate asthma by IgE-mediated mechanisms. The main allergens are: house dust mite; feathers; pollens; animal proteins; foods, e.g. milk and eggs; occupational agents (see Table 20.1) and drugs (see p. 398).

Appearances

Macroscopical
The lungs may appear normal, but in patients dying of asthma lungs are classically overinflated with patchy collapse. This results from occlusion of the bronchi and bronchioles by thick tenacious mucus.

Microscopical
The changes vary but in severe cases:
1 There is marked bronchial muscle hypertrophy.
2 The submucosa is oedematous with vascular dilatation and an inflammatory cell infiltrate of eosinophils, polymorphs, lymphocytes, mast cells and macrophages.
3 The subepithelial basement membrane is thickened by collagen.
4 Epithelial damage is seen and there is considerable denudation.
5 Submucosal glands are enlarged and there is an increase in the number of goblet cells in the bronchi and extension to bronchioles.
6 Luminal mucus plugs are present and contain epithelial cells and eosinophils. *Curschmanns' spirals* are seen—densely coiled mucus strands, and *Charcot–Leyden crystals* are produced from eosinophil proteins.

Pathogenesis
The exact mechanisms leading to clinical asthma remain uncertain in many types of asthma, but *generalized airway hyper-responsiveness* to specific and non-specific bronchoconstrictor trigger factors is central to the pathogenesis, probably due to persistence of inflammatory cells in the bronchial wall.

Immunological model of asthma
Asthma due to inhaled allergen has three phases:
1 *Early*: rapid-onset bronchoconstriction (15–20 minutes).

Table 20.1 Examples of occupational asthma.

Substance	Occupation
Animal proteins	Vets, laboratory workers, farmers
Grain, flour	Millers, bakers, farmers
Hardwood dusts	Carpenters
Epoxy resins	Chemical workers
Isocyanates	Paint and plastics workers
Formaldehyde	Hospital workers
Drugs (penicillins, etc.)	Pharmaceutical industry

2 *Late*: second wave of bronchoconstriction 4–6 hours after recovery from early phase (hours).

3 *Hyper-reactivity*: increased non-specific airways responsiveness to specific and non-specific trigger substances (days).

Exposure of atopic individuals to allergen results in production of IgE antibodies which bind mast cells. Re-exposure results in binding of antigen (allergen) to mast cell IgE with release of mediators such as histamine producing the *early reaction*. Activation of macrophages occurs, with release of chemotactic factors for neutrophils and eosinophils which accumulate in the bronchial wall. Release of inflammatory mediators from the macrophages, polymorphs and eosinophils causes bronchoconstriction, microvascular leak with mucosal oedema causing the *late reaction*.

Persistence of inflammatory cells in the bronchial wall with damage and loss of epithelial cells results in *prolonged airway hyper-reactivity*. An exaggerated response of the airway then occurs on further re-exposure to allergen or other bronchoconstrictor trigger factor(s) over ensuing days.

Effects and complications

Disease remission
Fifty per cent of children with asthma or wheezing resolve spontaneously. Persistence is related to severity and the presence of atopy. There is a risk of relapse in adulthood. Remission in adult-onset asthma is less likely to occur.

Acute severe asthma—status asthmaticus
Progression of asthma to breathlessness at rest with signs of cardiac stress. This can be sudden or occur over several hours.

Death
Occurs in 0.2% of asthmatics, usually but not always preceded by an acute severe attack.

Chronic severe asthma
A small percentage of patients develop increasingly severe and increasingly irreversible asthma in middle or old age.

Cor pulmonale
Right ventricular hypertrophy occurs but clinical cor pulmonale due to asthma alone is rare (see p. 381). Smokers with airways hyper-responsiveness are particularly at risk of developing irreversible COAD.

Other complications
Pneumothorax and cough-induced rib fractures can occur.

Associated conditions
Asthma is a component of some other conditions, e.g. allergic bronchopulmonary aspergillosis (see p. 398).

E/VASCULAR DISORDERS

Thromboembolism
Infarction
Non-thrombotic embolism
Oedema
Pulmonary hypertension
Haemorrhage
Diffuse alveolar damage

Pulmonary thromboembolism

Nature
Obstruction of part or whole of the pulmonary arterial tree by thrombus that has become detached from its site of formation—usually in the peripheral venous system, and carried to the lung.

Incidence
A very important condition which accounts for 1% of hospital deaths but rising to 30% in patients with severe burns or trauma.

Predisposing factors
Over 95% of pulmonary emboli arise from thrombi in the large veins of the leg or pelvis. Factors predisposing are:
1 Venous stasis,
2 Increased blood coagulability.
3 Damage to vessel endothelium.

Conditions producing these include immobility, surgical or accidental trauma, heart disease, pregnancy and puerperium, oral contraceptives, obesity and intravascular catheters.

Appearances

Emboli
Large emboli. Impact in the major pulmonary arteries or sit astride the bifurcation in both the left and right main trunks—*saddle embolus.*

Small emboli. Lodge in the smaller more peripheral segmental or subsegmental arteries.

Lung parenchyma
May appear normal, or show intense haemorrhagic change or infarction.

The heart
Acute right ventricular dilatation in massive obstruction of the pulmonary artery or right ventricular hypertrophy in cases of recurrent pulmonary thromboembolism causing pulmonary hypertension.

Pathophysiology

Lungs
Hypoxia and hypercapnia due to ventilation/perfusion mismatch secondary to underperfusion of ventilated lung, reflex bronchoconstriction and vasoconstriction. Fever, tachypnoea and tachycardia due to effects of tissue infarction

Cardiac
Acute right ventricular failure due to acute major obstruction of the pulmonary circulation. Systemic shock is due to decreased pulmonary blood flow leading to decreased left ventricular filling and output. There is an additional effect of hypoxia on heart muscle function.

Right ventricular hypertrophy with slowly progressive obstruction of the pulmonary vascular tree can occur with multiple small emboli.

Results
These are highly dependent on the *size of the embolus* and the *status of the cardiopulmonary system.*
1 *Silent*: up to 80% of emboli are clinically silent because they are small and are often lysed by fibrinolysins. Infarction does not normally occur in these circumstances, and in the absence of significant myocardial disease because of adequate collateral bronchial circulation.

2 *Infarction.*
3 *Recurrent emboli*: episodes of embolism, small or large, produce increasing problems sometimes ending in death.
4 *Sudden death*: massive embolism with obstruction of a large artery can result in sudden death or acute right-sided heart failure followed by death.
5 *Circulatory shock*: with massive emboli.
6 *Chronic pulmonary hypertension*: an uncommon but important cause which may be very difficult to diagnose (see p. 94).
7 *Abscess*: some infarcts become secondarily infected and form abscesses. Alternatively the embolus may be septic (see below).

Prognosis
Overall mortality of diagnosed embolism in patients without pre-existing cardiovascular disease is 8% and approximately 50–60% in those with pre-existing disease.

Pulmonary infarction

Cause
Usually associated with embolism but may rarely occur due to a primary vascular thrombosis associated with an abnormal circulation, e.g. in pulmonary hypertension (see p. 94).

Appearances

Macroscopical
The lower lobes are involved in 75% of cases. The infarcts are pyramidal in shape and haemorrhagic with their base on the pleural surface, over which there is a fibrinous reaction.

Microscopical
Haemorrhagic tissue necrosis with an inflammatory reaction at the margins.

Results
These vary with size and multiplicity.
1 *Pulmonary dysfunction*: due to loss of lung tissue.
2 *Pulmonary vascular obstruction.*
3 *Pleurisy and pleural effusion*: often haemorrhagic.
4 *Healing*: resulting in a fibrous scar.

5 *Septic infarction*: primary septic embolism or secondary infection leading to abscess formation.

Non-thrombotic embolism

Fat embolism
Following fracture of bones and sometimes fatal but clinically usually overshadowed by cerebral signs.

Amniotic fluid embolism
Release of amniotic fluid into the circulation in labour can result in sudden cardiovascular collapse or diffuse alveolar damage (see p. 386). Fetal squamous cells are seen in the pulmonary vessels

Air embolism
Air can enter the circulation after trauma or surgery to the great veins, or by faulty apparatus or techniques with intravascular therapy. If quantities are large, sudden cardiovascular collapse occurs due to functional obstruction to the pulmonary circulation and acute right heart failure.

Decompression sickness—Caisson disease
Rapid decompression, e.g. of deep-sea divers, releases bubbles of nitrogen as well as oxygen and carbon dioxide. The nitrogen bubbles cause problems in the CNS and bones particularly, and in pulmonary vessels can produce functional obstruction.

Foreign bodies
Injection of foreign materials into the venous system, e.g. drug addicts, may produce embolic effects in the lungs with pulmonary hypertension.

Tumour embolism
This is sometimes seen with renal cell and bronchial carcinomas.

Pulmonary oedema

Definition
This condition is characterized by the abnormal accumulation of extravascular fluid within the lung.

Pathogenesis
The capillary wall is normally fairly permeable to water and small molecules, but not to proteins. Alveolar cells are much less permeable to all substances. Normally due to the balance between the hydrostatic pressure forcing fluid out of the capillaries and colloid osmotic pressure preventing such loss, only a small amount of fluid passes into the interstitium. This drains to the peribronchial/perivascular space, from whence it enters the lymphatic channels. If excess fluid passes out of the capillaries and the flow rate exceeds the lymphatic drainage capacity, accumulation within the peribronchial space and then the interstitium occurs. Fluid eventually passes into the alveolar spaces from whence it wells up into airways.

Aetiology
1 *Increased capillary hydrostatic pressure*: this is the commonest cause of pulmonary oedema and includes:

    (a) *Left-sided heart failure*: in myocardial infarction, aortic valve disease, mitral regurgitation and tachyarrhythmias.

    (b) *Pulmonary venous hypertension*: e.g. in mitral stenosis (see p. 71).

    (c) *Constrictive pericarditis or pericardial effusions* (see p. 61).

    (d) *Fluid overload*, e.g. excess infusion of crystalloid solutes.

2 *Increased capillary permeability*: diffuse alveolar damage (p. 386) is a very important cause of lung oedema.

3 *Decreased plasma osmotic pressure*, e.g. hypoproteinaemia due to malnutrition, nephrotic syndrome or intravenous infusion of hypotonic solutes.

4 *Lymphatic obstruction*, e.g. blockage of lymphatic channels by tumour emboli in *lymphangitis carcinomatosa*.

5 *Decreased interstitial pressure*: large mechanical forces acting on the interstitium, e.g. rapid expansion of the lung after evacuation of a large pleural effusion or pneumothorax.

6 *Unknown or uncertain mechanism*: this includes some important conditions: neurogenic pulmonary oedema after brain damage, e.g. trauma or raised intracranial pressure, haemorrhages, heroin overdose, high altitude, near-drowning.

Appearances
The lungs are heavy and congested. Fluid flows from the cut surfaces and is often seen in the large airways in fatal cases. Histologically there is filling of alveoli

with proteinaceous fluid, widening of the interstitium and congestion of capillaries.

Effects
Respiratory dysfunction, which can lead to hypoxic respiratory failure caused by a ventilation/perfusion imbalance due to filling of alveoli with fluid and airway narrowing from peribronchial fluid accumulation.

Chronic passive venous congestion

Aetiology
Chronic left heart disease, e.g. myocardial failure due to ischaemia, mitral stenosis or hypertensive heart disease (see p. 73).

Appearances
The lung is firm, fibrous and brown, with congestion of alveolar vessels, fibrous thickening of the alveolar walls, pigmented macrophages—'heart failure cells' in the alveoli and atheroma of larger vessels.

Effects
Pulmonary hypertension.

Pulmonary hypertension
This condition is fully described on pp. 94–95.

Pulmonary haemorrhage
Pulmonary haemorrhage can occur secondary to many lung disorders, e.g. pulmonary embolism and infarction, carcinoma of lung with vessel invasion, pulmonary infection, passive congestion from heart disease, diffuse alveolar damage, trauma, bleeding disorders, e.g. haemophilia, leukaemia, anticoagulant drugs and the alveolar haemorrhage syndrome.

Alveolar haemorrhage syndrome

Nature
A *rare* syndrome characterized by multiple haemorrhages in the parenchyma of both lungs. Histologically there is diffuse intra-alveolar haemorrhage.

Causes
Many of the conditions which *may* present in this way have more usual modes of presentation but include: Goodpasture's syndrome (see p. 171), systemic vasculitis (see p. 83), connective tissue diseases including rheumatoid disease and SLE (see p. 96),

idiopathic pulmonary haemosiderosis, and toxin-induced disease from penicillamine.

Diffuse alveolar damage—adult respiratory distress syndrome

Nature
An increased permeability of alveolar–capillary structures due to acute diffuse alveolar damage leading to pulmonary oedema, haemorrhage, cell necrosis and hyaline membrane formation.

It is the morphological reaction to a wide variety of major insults and underlies clinical syndromes such as the *adult respiratory distress syndrome* (ARDS) and *shock lung*.

Aetiology
1 *Septic shock*: especially Gram-negative septicaemia.
2 *Hypotensive shock*, e.g. following severe left ventricular failure, trauma–shock lung, pancreatitis, extensive burns.
3 *Tissue injury*, e.g. major trauma, pancreatitis, cardiopulmonary by-pass and other major surgical procedures.
4 *Infections*: particularly severe viral infections, e.g. influenzal pneumonia.
5 *Oxygen toxicity*: excess administered oxygen, particularly if given at positive pressure.
6 *Toxins*, e.g. paraquat poisoning or inhaled toxic gases, e.g. NO_2 (see p. 391).
7 *Aspiration*, e.g. inhalation of gastric acid (see p. 370).
8 *Others*, including near-drowning, massive blood transfusions, amniotic fluid embolism, pre-eclampsia.

Pathogenesis
There are several different mechanisms of action due to the wide range of causes. In trauma a number of factors are often present including tissue injury, sepsis, hypovolaemia and oxygen toxicity from ventilation. There is release of chemical and inflammatory mediators including leucotriene B4, complement component C5a and platelet-activating factor which causes sequestration of activated polymorphs in the lungs. These release oxygen radicals, lysosomal enzymes and arachidonic acid metabolites with damage to capillary endothelium and alveolar epithelium resulting in development of pulmonary oedema and protein leakage.

Appearances

Macroscopical

In cases dying acutely the lungs are heavy, firm, consolidated and red. There is often superadded pneumonia.

Microscopical

Acutely there is intra-alveolar and interstitial oedema, fibrin and haemorrhage. Cellular necrosis with formation of hyaline membranes occurs. In the healing phase the alveoli are lined by regenerating cuboidal type 2 pneumocytes. There is intra-alveolar and interstitial fibrous tissue formation and a slight chronic inflammatory cell infiltrate.

Effects

Acute respiratory failure

With refractory hypoxia.

Death

Occurs in approximately 50% of patients and is often due to the severity of the underlying condition, e.g. multiple burns.

Residual damage

Most of the survivors recover completely, but some have disability due to diffuse residual pulmonary scarring.

F/ENVIRONMENTAL AND OCCUPATIONAL

Asbestos-related
Silicosis
Anthracosis
Coal worker's pneumoconiosis
Rheumatoid pneumoconiosis
Man-made mineral fibres
Others

Definitions

Environmental and occupational lung disease

A wide range of pulmonary pathological reactions due to exposure to fumes, gases, irritants and dusts.

Pneumoconiosis

The non-neoplastic response of lung to inhaled mineral or organic dusts but excluding asthma, emphysema or bronchitis.

Fibre

A structure with a length to width ratio of at least 3 : 1.

Important factors in disease production

Particle size

Particles 1–5 μm reach the distal airways and are deposited in the alveolar walls. These are important in production of disease, for smaller particles usually remain in the air and are exhaled, and larger particles are retained in the upper airways. The severity of any disease produced may also depend on size, e.g. fine silica particles are more pathogenic than larger particles.

Particle shape

May be important, particularly with fibres, e.g. long thin crocidolite asbestos fibres are the most pathogenic.

Particle structure

Can be important, e.g. crystalline silica is much more fibrogenic than non-crystalline forms.

Chemical composition

This is very important. Substances range from highly irritant gases, e.g. SO_2, to inert substances, e.g. pure iron. They may also have antigenic properties, e.g. fungal spores.

Individual susceptibility

There is individual variation relevant to the development and extent of any disease for similar exposures to a given substance. This may be due to individual differences in immunological or inflammatory reactions, e.g. only a small number of exposed individuals develop farmers lung (see p. 393).

Smoking

This affects the pulmonary clearance mechanisms of all particles and can affect the 'activity' of inhaled substances, e.g. enhancement of the bronchial carcinogenicity of asbestos (see below).

Additional exposures

Pulmonary reactions may be modified by other additional substances, e.g. silica and iron produce a mixed dust fibrosis.

Asbestos-related diseases

Asbestos exposure

Asbestos is a generic term for a large number of naturally occurring magnesium silicate fibres.

The most important type commercially is now *chrysotile*—white asbestos. *Crocidolite*—blue asbestos—and *amosite*—brown asbestos—are now not used in many countries but are found as contaminants of chrysotile.

Asbestos exposure may occur in a wide range of occupations including mining, milling, production of cement products, insulation materials, brakes and clutches and the textile and construction industries. Non-industrial exposure can occur in people living near sites of production.

The effects of asbestos exposure usually take many years to become manifest, i.e. up to 30–40 years.

Heavy exposure is now relatively rare in Great Britain, but exposure is less well controlled elsewhere. The effects of lesser degrees of exposure, however, are still prevalent in Great Britain. Approximately 600 deaths per year occurred from asbestos-related diseases in the early 1980s in England and Wales.

Asbestos bodies

These are mineral fibres coated with a golden-brown glycoprotein rich in iron. They are dumb-bell-shaped and are identified in tissues as the hallmark of asbestos exposure.

Appearances

Asbestos exposure can cause a variety of changes which may either coexist or occur separately.

Asbestosis

Diffuse pulmonary fibrosis due to asbestos exposure.

Macroscopical
Slowly progressive diffuse interstitial fibrosis which starts at the lung bases where it is most marked subpleurally. This fibrosis progressively spreads centrally and eventually produces honeycomb lung (see p. 392).

Microscopical
There is inflammation and fibrous scarring of the bronchiolar walls and alveolar ducts which progressively extends to involve the alveolar septae. The presence of usually numerous asbestos bodies is the hallmark of this condition.

Pleural plaques

Macroscopical
Bilateral, well-circumscribed, irregularly shaped white raised plaques of hyaline collagen. The surface may be smooth or nodular and they are distributed over the anterior and posterolateral aspects of the *parietal* pleura and over the domes of the diaphragm.

Microscopical
Composed of dense acellular collagen lamellae with a basketweave pattern. They do not contain asbestos bodies.

Effects. Plaques do *not* produce any clinical disability but are markers of asbestos exposure.

Pleural effusion

Usually serous and may resolve or be prolonged or recurrent. May precede, by several years, the development of pleural fibrosis or mesothelioma.

Pleural fibrosis

The formation of dense bilateral fibrotic thickening of the visceral pleura over much of the lung surfaces. It occurs in association with severe asbestosis or rarely as an isolated finding. It produces 'restrictive' functional disability.

Malignant mesothelioma

This asbestos related tumour is described on p. 409.

Bronchial carcinoma

This develops in asbestosis in the areas of fibrosis, i.e. lower lobes: adenocarcinoma is the most common type.

Pathogenesis

Fibre type

The most dangerous fibres for the production of all types of asbestos-related disease are long, thin, straight and needle-shaped fibres, of which those

>8 μm long and <0.5 μm diameter are the most fibrogenic and oncogenic. Amphiboles—crocidolite, amosite and tremolite—are long and straight. They are retained by the lung and are the most important in production of disease. Crocidolite is the most dangerous. Chrysotile fibres are curly and fragment, so most do not reach the lung and those that do are cleared. Exposure to chrysotile 'dust' is associated with all types of asbestos-related disease but probably solely due to contaminant amphiboles.

Level of exposure

Severe asbestosis is due to heavy and prolonged exposure to, and inhalation of, asbestos and is dose-related. Pleural plaques, mesothelioma and diffuse pleural fibrosis may well occur with heavy asbestos exposure but can also be caused by much smaller doses, usually of amphiboles.

Malignancy

Bronchogenic carcinoma usually occurs with severe asbestosis. The risk is five times that of a non-asbestos-exposed individual with smokers having a 55 times risk. The risk of malignant mesotheliomas is not increased by smoking.

Mechanism

The exact mechanisms of oncogenesis and fibrogenesis are unclear.

Classical nodular silicosis

Exposure

This is lung disease due to inhalation of free silica (SiO_2) containing dust. Exposure occurs either in processes directly involving siliceous materials or during extraction of minerals in which the residual rock contains silica, usually as quartz.

Risk occupations include sandblasters, quarry workers, miners (through siliceous rock), foundry workers and stone masons.

Appearances

Macroscopical

Simple silicosis
There is pleural fibrosis with adhesions. Hilar lymph nodes are enlarged, pigmented and calcified. Numerous rounded grey fibrous nodules—less than 1 cm diameter—are present throughout the lungs but most marked in the upper zones and subpleurally.

Progressive massive fibrosis
Coalescence and enlargement of nodules to form masses 1 cm diameter or greater, and which can cavitate. Scarring emphysema is seen adjacent to the nodules.

Microscopical

The rounded nodules consist of concentric laminated layers of collagen containing birefringent particles of silica plus mica etc, and there is a surrounding dust-laden cellular zone. The changes are seen in relation to respiratory bronchioles and, as nodules enlarge, bronchioles, lymphatics and arterioles become obliterated by fibrosis.

Other changes

Tuberculosis and *rheumatoid pneumoconiosis* may occur (see p. 375 and p. 391).

Pathogenesis

Crystalline silica, especially quartz, is much more fibrogenic than non-crystalline forms. Particles <5 μm in diameter are more pathogenic than larger ones.

Inhaled silica is engulfed by polymorphs and macrophages with death of these cells and type 2 pneumocytes. Silica is released extracellularly. Chemo-attractant molecules from activated and dead cells result in recruitment of more inflammatory cells and re-phagocytosis of the extracellular silica. The cycle is then repeated. Secretory products from the macrophages and polymorphs include fibrogenic substances. Genetic factors and autoimmunity *may* also be important.

Results

Radiographic and clinical disease usually takes many years to develop, i.e. 20 years, and the incidence of lung cancer is probably not increased due to silica exposure. Simple silicosis is not associated with significant air flow obstruction but progressive massive fibrosis causes air flow limitation, respiratory failure and cor pulmonale. There is a 30-fold increase of tuberculosis.

Other reactions to inhaled silica

Acute silico-proteinosis
A disease of rapid onset, clinically apparent within 3 years and due to inhalation of large quantities of very fine crystalline particles. Morphologically it is similar to alveolar proteinosis (see p. 397) but with the addition of a very heavy burden of free silica.

Mixed dust fibrosis
The pulmonary response to inhaled free silica in combination with a less fibrogenic dust which modifies the tissue reaction. Examples include iron and silica in foundry work, coal dust and silica in coal mining and kaolinite, mica and silica in the ceramic industry. Clinically similar to classical silicosis but pathologically characterized by irregular stellate nodules more common in the upper lobes. The degree of fibrosis is related to the silica content and progressive massive fibrosis can occur.

Interstitial fibrosis
Diffuse interstitial fibrosis can occur in persons exposed to free silica and some less fibrogenic dusts, e.g. North Wales slate workers.

Anthracosis

Nature
The harmless accumulation of carbon dust within the lung, which occurs in all town-dwellers due to inhalation of polluted air found in industrial areas—and cigarette smokers. The black pigmented carbon dust accumulates in macrophages in the walls of bronchioles, lymphatics and lymph nodes but causes no significant clinical or pathological consequences.

Coal worker's pneumoconiosis

Nature
Pneumoconiosis due to inhalation of coal dust, which ranges from high-ranked relatively pure carbon dust with little mineral ash, e.g. anthracite, to low-ranked coal with high ash content. Certain occupations also have an increased exposure to silica, e.g. roof bolters.

Clinically significant respiratory disease is now rare in the UK due to stringent measures in decreasing occupational coal dust levels.

Appearances

Simple coal worker's pneumoconiosis—CWP

Lymphatics
These are pigmented, and lymph nodes are enlarged, firm and contain pigment-laden macrophages and fibrosis.

Macules
There are widespread centrilobular irregular impalpable macules up to 5 mm diameter, consisting of coal dust-laden macrophages in the respiratory bronchiole walls with a mild increase in collagen. Adjacent air spaces are enlarged—focal dust emphysema (see p. 381).

Nodules
Irregular palpable black nodules consisting of pigment-laden macrophages embedded in haphazardly arranged collagen. These are common in the upper lobes, subpleurally and in peribronchial regions.

Progressive massive fibrosis—PMF
The nodules are greater than 1 cm diameter and occur most commonly in the upper lobes. They are black, demarcated and irregular and cross fissures, bronchi and vessel walls. Central necrosis occurs, otherwise histological appearances are similar to the nodules of simple CWP (see above).

Emphysema
1 Focal dust emphysema (see p. 381).
2 Centrilobular destructive emphysema (see p. 378).

Other features
Diffuse interstitial fibrosis occurs in 15% of miners. Others may show silicosis (see p. 389) or rheumatoid pneumoconiosis (see p. 391).

Pathogenesis
Simple CWP is due to coal dust exposure. Transformation to PMF occurs with heavy and prolonged exposure and is more frequent with exposure to high-ranked coal. Macrophage activation is important.

Other factors implicated are tuberculosis and heavy quartz–silica exposure.

Destructive centrilobular emphysema causing COAD can be due to smoking or dust exposure, alone or both in combination.

The interstitial fibrosis is usually of unknown cause but may be due to exposure to other agents, e.g. asbestos.

Silicotic lesions are due to heavy exposures to quartz.

Results

1 *Simple CWP*: produces radiological changes and simple chronic bronchitis but is not usually associated with serious disability.

2 *Respiratory failure and cor pulmonale*: due to PMF and/or destructive emphysema.

3 *Infections*: increased in progressive lung disease.

4 *Malignancy*: exposure to coal dust does *not* cause lung cancer.

Rheumatoid pneumoconiosis— Caplan's nodules

Typical rheumatoid nodules occurring in the lungs of patients with pneumoconiosis, usually simple CWP, but can be seen in silicosis and asbestosis.

Morphologically they have the appearance of typical rheumatoid nodules (*see* p. 101) modified by rings of pigmentation.

They are rarely symptomatic but can be mistaken on X-rays for PMF lesions or tumour.

Diseases due to inhalation of man-made mineral fibres

There is no convincing evidence to suggest that the synthetic fibres of dimensions in current use have produced significant pulmonary disease.

Other occupational lung disorders

Table 20.2 illustrates a very wide range of substances that have been implicated in the production of occupational lung diseases. A very detailed clinical history is often required to identify possible aetiological agents.

G/INTERSTITIAL AND INFILTRATIVE

Honeycomb lung
  Generalized
  Localized
Fibrosing alveolitis
Extrinsic allergic bronchoalveolitis
Sarcoidosis
Pulmonary eosinophilia
Allergic angiitis
Langerhans cell granulomatosis
Other infiltrations
Alveolar proteinosis

Definitions

Conditions with bilateral diffuse pulmonary involvement by cellular or non-cellular deposits and involving the interstitium, the alveoli or both. They may or may not cause lung destruction.

Table 20.2 Examples of environmental diseases/reactions.

Pulmonary reaction	Substance/occupation
Granulomas and fibrosis	Berrylium (fluorescent light bulb manufacture)
Diffuse alveolar damage	Chemical fumes, e.g. SO_2, ammonia, cadmium (chemical industry), NO_2 (silo fillers)
Asthma	Formalin (laboratories), isocyanates, platinum (chemical industry), cotton flax
Generalized pulmonary fibrosis (diffuse/nodular)	Aluminium, kaolin (china clay workers), talc (mining, ceramics, paint industry, building), hard metal, i.e. tungsten carbide, cobalt, iron–silica (haematite miners)
Lung carcinoma	Nickel, arsenic, radon
Acute bronchiolitis	Irritant gases, acids, alkalis (chemical workers)
Simple chronic bronchitis (no COAD)	Wide variety of dust in heavy exposure
Minimal disease (dust macules)	Pure iron, titanium synthetic fibres

See text for EABA, CWP, silicosis and asbestos diseases.

Interstitial lung disorders
Disorders with widespread disease *primarily* affecting the interstitium of the lung.

Interstitial pneumonitis
An inflammatory process occurring predominantly in the interstitium and usually with associated fibrosis of variable degree.

This is a non-specific generic term and *does not* indicate an aetiology. Causes include those conditions which can give rise to *honeycomb lung* (see below) and also viral and mycoplasmal infections.

Diffuse interstitial fibrosis
Bilateral widespread fibrosis in the interstitium. When changes are severe the appearances are those of '*honeycomb lung*'. There may or may not be associated inflammatory cell infiltrate or acellular deposits. Causes include most of the conditions in this section and those of 'honeycomb lung'.

Generalized honeycomb lung

Definition
A generalized 'cystic' or 'honeycomb' appearance of the lung parenchyma and best regarded as end-stage lung resulting from a wide variety of *interstitial pulmonary diseases with fibrosis*.

Appearances

Macroscopical
The affected areas show a firm sponge-like appearance with a coarse texture due to cystic spaces up to 1–2 cm diameter with fibrous walls. The pleural surface appears nodular.

Microscopical
The cystic spaces are lined by flattened or cuboidal epithelium. The walls—interstitium—are irregular, thick and fibrous and contain hypertrophic muscle. The muscular arteries show muscle hypertrophy and fibrosis. The specific changes of the underlying disease may be present.

Aetiology

Common
Pneumoconioses, e.g. asbestosis 25%; sarcoidosis 20%; cryptogenic fibrosing alveolitis 15%; connective tissue diseases, e.g. rheumatoid disease 8%.

Less common
Diffuse alveolar damage (DAD), e.g. radiation; drug reactions, e.g. amioderone, busulphan; extrinsic allergic bronchioalveolitis (EABA), e.g. farmer's lung; chronic pulmonary venous congestion, e.g. mitral stenosis; infections, e.g. tuberculosis; histiocytosis X; graft versus host disease; recurrent gastro-oesophageal reflux and aspiration.

Results
1 *Respiratory function*: the diseases are 'restrictive' in type.
2 *Respiratory failure and cor pulmonale*: due to severe loss of alveolar capillary units. Pulmonary hypertension is due to hypoxia, fibrous obliteration of vessels and bronchopulmonary anastomoses.

Localized honeycomb change

Nature
Morphological honeycomb change restricted to a focal area of lung, which can be caused by a wide variety of conditions, e.g. post-pneumonic, tuberculosis, infarcts, irradiation and bronchiectasis.

Results
Effects are related to the area of damaged lung, e.g. recurrent infections, rather than respiratory failure.

Cryptogenic fibrosing alveolitis

Definition
A progressive chronic inflammatory disease of the lung of unknown cause which results in diffuse interstitial fibrosis and honeycomb change.

Incidence
Relatively rare with a prevalence of 3–5 cases per 10^5 population, but represents approximately 15% of diffuse interstitial fibrosis/honeycomb lung (see above).

It is usually sporadic, only rare familial forms are described.

Appearances

Macroscopical
Variable appearance depending on stage of the disease. No gross abnormality initially but changes of

honeycomb lung are seen when patients die of this disease. Changes are most severe at the lung bases and subpleurally.

Microscopical

There is marked variation throughout the lung. Diffuse infiltration of the alveolar walls (interstitium) with mononuclear inflammatory cells, i.e. plasma cells and lymphocytes with lymphoid follicle formation. Scattered macrophages, polymorphs and eosinophils are also seen. On progression there is an increasing interstitial collagen deposition until honeycomb lung develops. The alveoli are lined by cuboidal type 2 pneumocytes and contain free cells, mainly macrophages, in tissue sections but numerous polymorphs and eosinophils are found in lavage fluid.

Desquamative interstitial pneumonia is a specific histological subtype which may have an improved response to steroid therapy.

Pathogenesis

An immunologically mediated disorder of unknown cause. One theory suggests that an unidentified antigen stimulates B lymphocytes to secrete immunoglobulins which combine with antigen to form immune complexes which they bind to and activate macrophages. These secrete a wide range of cytokines, e.g. polymorph chemotactic factor, interleukin-1, fibronectin and fibroblast growth factor. Polymorphs and eosinophils are attracted to the lung and release reactive oxygen species, proteases and other toxic compounds (see p. 386) which, in combination with some of the macrophage products, produce local lung damage. Additional factors promote fibrous scarring of the damaged lung to give the characteristic changes.

Results

1 *Clinically*: a restrictive type of lung disease mostly in middle age and with progressive dyspnoea, cough, inspiratory crackles, finger clubbing, weight loss and basal mottling on chest X-ray.
2 *Respiratory dysfunction*: this is progressive, ending in *respiratory failure, cor pulmonale*.
3 *Death*: as for all diffuse end-stage interstitial fibrosis/honeycomb lung.
4 *Lung carcinoma*: increased incidence in 13% of advanced disease, usually a peripheral adenocarcinoma.

Extrinsic allergic bronchioalveolitis

Nature

An immunologically mediated interstitial granulomatous inflammation resulting from inhalation of various antigens, usually organic dusts.

Types and incidence

An important condition in which a wide variety of antigens are involved, the most important of which are:
1 *Farmer's lung*: due to inhalation of fungal spores of actinomycetes—*Mycopolysporum faeni*, present in mouldy hay.
2 *Pigeon-fanciers lung*: due to inhalation of avian protein antigen in bird droppings.
3 *Others*: include bagassosis, air conditioner lung—humidifier fever, mushroom worker's lung, malt worker's lung.

Appearances

Macroscopical

Initially the lungs appear normal but chronic exposure leads eventually to development of diffuse interstitial fibrosis progressing to honeycomb lung. Changes are most marked in the upper lobes.

Microscopical

A diffuse interstitial infiltrate of inflammatory cells including lymphocytes, plasma cells and macrophages showing a peribronchiolar accentuation. Small non-caseating granulomas similar to those found in sarcoidosis are also present. Some cases show bronchiolitis obliterans organizing pneumonia (*BOOP*).

Pathogenesis

The mechanisms are probably a combined type III immune complex hypersensitivity reaction and type IV cell-mediated delayed hypersensitivity reaction to inhaled antigen, the latter currently being considered the more important.

The disease occurs in only a small percentage of those exposed, indicating some individual susceptibility.

Dose of antigen and the effects of cigarette smoke are probably important. Precipitating antibodies in the serum and a positive skin test are useful for diagnosis.

Results

1 *Acute illness*: due to exposure to large amounts of antigen with severe dyspnoea but no permanent residual dysfunction.

2 *Diffuse pulmonary fibrosis*: due to repeated acute attacks or to chronic exposure to small quantities of antigen. Progressive diffuse interstitial pulmonary fibrosis ends in honeycomb lung and *respiratory failure*.

Sarcoidosis

Definition
A multisystem disease of unknown cause characterized by non-caseating granulomatous inflammation.

Incidence
Approximately 20 per million population in the UK, but it occurs worldwide, being more common in Africa and Asia than in Caucasians.

Slight female predominance with maximal age incidence between 20 and 40 years.

Site
Sarcoid may present in one or more organs but many organs are usually subclinically involved.

Pulmonary involvement is seen in 90% of cases and other common sites are skin, spleen, lymph node (*see* p. 266), eye (*see* p. 150), liver (*see* p. 249), bones and salivary glands.

Appearances

Microscopical
The non-caseating granuloma is the fundamental lesion of sarcoidosis and is composed of a central collection of epithelioid histiocytes and some helper T lymphocytes and occasional multinucleated giant cells of Langhans' type: outside this is a rim of suppressor T lymphocytes.

A minor degree of tissue necrosis can be seen but *there is no caseation*.

Intracellular inclusions may be seen in giant cells including asteroid and Schaumann bodies.

The granulomas heal by fibrous scarring.

Lung
Granulomas are present throughout the whole of both lungs but are most marked in the upper two-thirds. These can range from very small nodules to large masses.

Any lung structure can be the site of the granuloma formation, commonly alveolar septae, connective tissues and pleura.

The effects of the scarring depend on the extent of pulmonary involvement and on specific sites involved, e.g. blood vessels, bronchioles.

Mediastinal and hilar nodes are frequently involved.

Pathogenesis
The inciting agent, probably an antigen, is unknown but possible mechanisnms are shown in Fig. 32. Why significant fibrosis occurs in some patients but not others is unexplained.

Results
1 *Staging*: prognosis is assisted by stage, based on radiological appearances.

2 *Resolution*: more than 70% of cases resolve with minimal or no pulmonary fibrosis.

3 *Pulmonary fibrosis*: in 25% there is permanent disability due to varying degrees of diffuse interstitial fibrosis with, in severe cases, *honeycomb change* leading to *respiratory failure* and *cor pulmonale*.

4 *Death*: about 2% of patients die as a direct result of sarcoidosis.

5 *Pneumothorax*: this is rare.

6 *Large nodular lesions*: uncommon and caused by massive conglomeration of granulomas which can resemble neoplasms radiologically.

Pulmonary eosinophilia

Nature
A group of conditions characterized by a patchy pulmonary inflammatory cell infiltrate rich in eosinophils and often associated with a blood eosinophilia.

Aetiology
1 *Allergic bronchopulmonary mycosis*: Aspergillus fumigatus, Candida etc. (*see* p. 398).

2 *Helminth infections*: ascariasis—simple pulmonary eosinophilia (*see* p. 7), microfilariasis—tropical pulmonary eosinophilia, schistosomiasis (*see* p. 9).

3 *Drugs*: nitrofurantoin, aspirin, sulphonamides, penicillin, etc.

4 *Unknown*: crytogenic chronic pulmonary eosinophilia, allergic angiitis and granulomatosis—Churg–Strauss syndrome, hypereosinophilic syndrome.

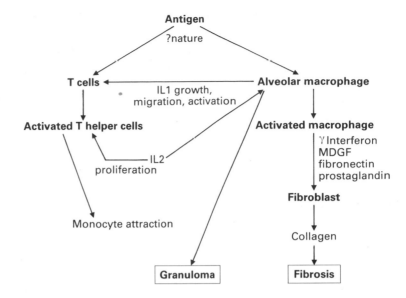

Fig. 32 Pathogenesis of sarcoidosis.

Types

Self-limiting
Some forms, e.g. helminth-induced, are self-limiting disorders with fleeting X-ray pulmonary shadows and blood eosinophilia.

Cryptogenic (chronic) pulmonary eosinophilia
Pulmonary eosinophilia when no external cause is found. There are marked systemic symptoms of appetite loss, malaise, weight loss and fever. Chronic asthma is often present. Transient pulmonary shadows are seen together with blood eosinophilia.

Allergic angiitis and granulomatosis
A rare disease with asthma, blood eosinophilia, pulmonary shadows, evidence of granuloma formation and systemic vasculitis—Churg–Strauss (see p. 396).

Appearances
There is an eosinophil infiltrate of the interstitium, bronchioles and alveolar lumina. Lesser numbers of macrophages are seen within the alveoli. Other chronic inflammatory cells are present within the interstitium.

Pathogenesis
Immunological mechanisms, probably immune complex-mediated, which may also involve mast cells and antigen–antibody reactions, are apparent. Eosinophil accumulation may dampen these reactions but release toxic substances, e.g. major basic protein and eosinophil cationic protein, which cause local damage.

Allergic angiitis and granulomatosis

Nature
This group of rare conditions all exhibit cellular infiltration of vessels—angiitis—and destruction of pulmonary parenchyma. They are diverse clinically and pathologically. The angiitis is not always inflammatory; in some it is neoplastic and the parenchymal infiltrate is not always granulomatous.

Classical Wegener's granulomatosis

Nature
A systemic clinicopathological entity characterized by necrotizing granulomatous inflammation in the upper (nose and sinuses) and lower respiratory tract (lung), a generalized focal necrotizing vasculitis (see p. 103) and segmental, usually cresentic, glomerulonephritis (see p. 171).

Antibodies to a cytoplasmic component of neutrophils (*ANCA*) is a useful diagnostic marker of this condition.

Appearances
There are multiple areas of ulceration and tissue necrosis in the upper and lower respiratory tract.

Consolidated areas in the lung often cavitate. Histologically the lesions are angiocentric with vessel necrosis/thrombosis and a giant cell, histiocytic and lymphoplasmacytic cellular infiltrate.

Clinical

This is a multisystem disease and the exact manifestations depend on the organs involved. Typically this includes chronic sinusitis, nasopharyngeal ulceration, bilateral cavitating nodular infiltrates in the lungs and renal failure.

Results

Energetic cytotoxic immunosuppressive therapy, though potentially hazardous itself, has led to long-term survival in 80% or more.

Limited Wegener's granulomatosis

Accounts for nearly half of all cases and is less aggressive. The patients have isolated pulmonary involvement as the only or major manifestation. There is no upper airways disease or renal involvement.

Other related conditions

1 Churg–Strauss syndrome: patients asthmatic (see p. 395).
2 Necrotizing sarcoidal granulomatosis.
3 Bronchocentric granulomatosis.
4 Lymphomatoid granulomatosis: a lymphoproliferative condition—non-Hodgkin's malignant lymphoma, which is angiocentric in the lung.

Histiocytosis X—Langerhans cell granulomatosis

Nature

A proliferative disorder of histiocytes and Langerhans cells, which can occur in an isolated pulmonary form or be part of a systemic histiocytosis (see p. 297). This condition was formerly called *eosinophilic granuloma*.

Appearances

Clinically presents with cough and dyspnoea and recurrent pneumothoraces are common. It is more common in females and smokers. Diffuse pulmonary linear or nodular shadows are seen radiologically.

There is a patchy but widespread bilateral, nodular, pulmonary parenchymal interstitial infiltrate of Langerhans cells, eosinophils and mononuclear in-flammatory cells which at its margin extends along alveolar septa. Fibrosis supervenes.

Course

Fifty per cent of patients stabilize and the others have slowly progressive disease from which half die, usually in respiratory failure due to diffuse interstitial fibrosis/honeycomb lung.

Lymphoid interstitial pneumonia

This is rare and characterized clinically by bilateral reticulonodular shadows on chest X-ray and progressive dyspnoea and cough.

Pathologically there is diffuse pulmonary interstitial infiltrate of mature small lymphocytes and plasma cells. Interstitial fibrosis can occur.

It may be a component of Sjögren's syndrome (see p. 103) or be associated with hyperglobulinaemia and has also been described in AIDS.

Disease progress is variable. Some patients remain stable, some develop progressive interstitial fibrosis and honeycomb lung and others develop disseminated malignant lymphoma.

Lymphangioleiomyomatosis

A rare disease in which there is a haphazard proliferation of smooth muscle through the interstitium of the lung terminating in respiratory failure. Similar changes occur in tuberose sclerosis (see p. 332).

Pulmonary alveolar microlithiasis

A rare disorder characterized by multiple calcific spherites in the lung and without detectable defects of calcium metabolism. It can cause interstitial fibrosis and respiratory failure but often little progression is seen.

Pulmonary calcification

Dystrophic

Calcification in areas of pre-existing focal abnormality, e.g. caseation and other types of tissue necrosis, fibrous scars. There is usually little pulmonary dysfunction.

Metastatic

Rare and due to disorders in calcium/phosphorus metabolism particularly in regular renal dialysis patients and in primary hyperparathyroidism (see p. 138).

There is diffuse calcification within alveolar septae, blood vessels and bronchiolar walls and diffuse interstitial fibrosis may occur. Patients are usually asymptomatic but some develop respiratory failure.

Pulmonary ossification
Focal ossification occurs in dystrophic calcification. Diffuse ossification is rare and usually due to chronic venous congestion, e.g. mitral valve disease.

Pulmonary alveolar proteinosis
A rare disorder usually in adults characterized by progressive pulmonary infiltrates, dyspnoea, cough and fever.

Affected lung is firm and yellow/tan. Histologically there is an intra-alveolar eosinophilic, granular, mucopolysaccharide–lipid material derived from type 2 pneumocytes. No inflammatory cells are seen.

There is a defect in clearance of surfactant by alveolar macrophages, either due to an intrinsic defect or suppression by excess surfactant production.

It is usually idiopathic but can be seen after silica exposure, immunological deficiencies including AIDS and underlying malignancy.

Although the disease is progressive, respiratory failure is rare: spontaneous resolution occasionally occurs.

H/MISCELLANEOUS

Immunocompromised host
AIDS
Drug-induced
Fungal diseases
Actinomycosis
Pulmonary collapse
Lipid pneumonia
Drowning

Lung disease in the immunocompromised host
Pulmonary manifestations of infective or non-infective origin are common in patients immunocompromised for whatever reason. They are most frequent and serious in AIDS (see p. 3), recipients of immunosuppressive therapy and cytotoxic agents including organ transplants (see p. 182), connective tissue diseases (see p. 96) and malignancy, particularly leukaemias and lymphomas (see p. 271).

Infections
These usually cause pneumonias.
1 *Usual organisms*: infections by the types of organisms causing pneumonias in the immunocompetent are seen more frequently and progress more rapidly. Gram-negative infections are more predominant.
2 *Mycobacteria*: tuberculosis is very common and important, as are atypical mycobacterial infections, e.g. *M. kansasii* and *M. avium intracellulare*.
3 *Fungi and parasites*: Aspergillus, Cryptococcus, Candida, Mucor, Pneumocystis and Strongyloides (see p. 399).
4 *Viruses*: cytomegalovirus and other herpes group viruses.

Non-infective
1 *Cytotoxic drugs*: diffuse alveolar damage caused by bleomycin, busulphan, etc. (see p. 386).
2 *Radiation*: alveolar damage and fibrosis following irradiation.
3 *Interstitial pneumonia*: of uncertain cause.
4 *Malignancy*: recurrent post-treatment tumour or tumour induced by immunosuppression, including Kaposi's sarcoma in AIDS, lymphoma.

Pathological findings
Pathological features, as well as the clinical and radiological changes, are often atypical. This is particularly true in infections and it is important that biopsy material is also examined microbiologically and cytologically, including special stains, notably silver preparations.

Pulmonary manifestations of acquired immunodeficiency syndrome (AIDS)

Infections

Common
Pneumocystis carinii (commonest), *Cryptococcus neoformans*, atypical mycobacterial infection, tuberculosis, CMV, pyogenic bacteria.

Less common
Aspergillus, *Mucor*, herpes simplex.

Non-infective infiltrates

Common
Diffuse alveolar damage.

Less common
Non-specific interstitial pneumonitis, lymphoid interstitial pneumonitis.

Neoplasms

Common
Kaposi's sarcoma

Less common
Lymphoma.

Drug-induced lung disease
(see Table 20.3)
Adverse reactions are important because they are avoidable, cause difficulty in differential diagnosis and can be serious.

A large number of drugs have been implicated (see Table 20.3) and can cause a wide range of pulmonary reactions. A drug cause should be considered in each type of response as the features are usually indistinguishable from naturally occurring disease. Mechanisms are poorly understood.

Fungal diseases
There is a wide geographical variability in these diseases, many of which are most commonly seen in 'opportunistic' immunosuppressive situations (see p. 397).

Aspergillus

Organism
The commonest cause of pulmonary fungal disease in the UK is usually *A. fumigatus* or *A. niger*.

Types of pulmonary disease
1 *Bronchial asthma*: exposure to high levels of spores can induce typical asthma.
2 *Extrinsic allergic bronchioalveolitis*: in farmers, malt workers, etc. (see p. 393).
3 *Allergic bronchopulmonary aspergillosis*: a clinical syndrome, usually in asthmatics, resulting from combined types I, III and IV hypersensitivities. Pathological components seen in association are:
   (a) *Eosinophilic pneumonia* (see p. 394).
   (b) *Mucoid impaction of bronchi*, i.e. mucus plugs in large bronchi.
   (c) *Bronchocentric granulomatosis*: a granulomatous infiltrate around bronchi.
   (d) *Proximal bronchiectasis*: in chronic cases.
4 *Aspergilloma*: this is a mycetoma in a pre-existing

Table 20.3 Drug-induced lung disease.

Tissue reaction	Drugs (examples)
Bronchoconstriction	Aspirin, penicillins, tartrazine, iodine-containing contrast media
Chronic interstitial pneumonitis	Amioderone, busulphan, chlorambucil, nitrofurantoin
Diffuse alveolar damage	Amioderone, cytotoxics (busulphan, methotrexate, azathioprine), gold, hydrochlorthiazide, heroin
Eosinophilic pneumonia	Sulphonamide, penicillins, tetracycline, aspirin, nitrofurantoin
Bronchiolitis obliterans	Amioderone, gold
Pulmonary haemorrhage	Anticoagulants, cytotoxics
Pulmonary hypertension	Aminorex, busulphan
Pulmonary oedema	Heroin, hydrochlorthiazide, naloxone
Pulmonary embolism	Oral contraceptives
Opportunistic infection	Immunosuppressive agents (steroids, cytotoxic drugs, cyclosporin)
Impaired ventilation	Sedative drugs (e.g. opioids, diazepam), muscle paralysing agents (e.g. succinylcholine)
Pleural disease	Penicillamine, practolol, methysergide

cavity, mostly tuberculous, by *Aspergillus*. Haemoptysis may be troublesome. Occurs in immunocompetent individuals and is non-invasive.

5 *Invasive pneumonia*: this occurs almost exclusively in immunocompromised individuals (see p. 397). Invasiveness varies from slowly progressive to fulminant pneumonic. Fungal hyphae can often be seen invading blood vessel walls and there is little or no inflammatory response. Mortality is very high.

Other fungi

1 *Cryptococcus*: *C. neoformans* is now worldwide, being very common in AIDS patients as either disseminated or more localized granulomatous inflammation.

2 *Zygomycetes*: *Mucor*, *Rhizopus* and *Absedia* are the fungi of this group which may produce lesions similar to *Aspergillus*.

3 *Candidosis*: monilial infection is common after antibiotic therapy, usually spreading from the mouth and oesophagus but remains confined to the bronchial epithelial surface except in the immunocompromised host when it may become invasive and disseminated.

4 *Histoplasmosis*: *H. capsulatum* is worldwide in distribution but heavily endemic in the central USA. In the immunocompetent it is usually a subclinical infection somewhat similar to primary tuberculosis but occasionally has a more acute pneumonic course. Dissemination often from reactivation of dormant granulomas, is frequently seen in the immunosuppressed (see p. 4).

5 *Coccidiomycosis and paracoccidioidomycosis*: the former disease caused by *C. immitis* is restricted to the Western hemisphere, largely the south-western USA, and usually manifests as a localized 'coccidioma'. The latter infection—*Paracoccidioides brasiliensis*—occurs mainly in South America, hence the synonym '*South American blastomycosis*'. This is a systemic disease with a major pulmonary component (see p. 5).

6 *North American blastomycosis*: infection by *Blastomyces dermatitidis* is predominantly a cutaneous infection and lung involvement by an isolated necrotic granuloma occurs, but is uncommon (see p. 4).

Actinomycosis

This rare infection by *Actinomyces israeli* affects the chest in 20% of cases. The pulmonary disease may be primary in 75% or secondary.

Pathologically there is localized honeycombing, usually in the lower lobes with numerous abscesses containing pus in which there are colonies of the organism—*sulphur granules*.

Pulmonary manifestations of connective tissue disorders

These conditions are fully described on pp. 96–103, but lung involvement may be prominent.

1 *Rheumatoid disease*: non-specific pleuritis or effusion, diffuse interstitial pneumonitis and fibrosis, rheumatoid nodules—Caplan's rheumatoid pneumoconiosis, bronchiolitis obliterans, vasculitis may all occur. Pulmonary hypertension, recurrent infections and effects of drug therapy are variably important (see p. 100).

2 *Systemic lupus erythematosus*: pleuritis and effusion, diffuse alveolar damage.

3 *Progressive systemic sclerosis*: diffuse interstitial pneumonitis and fibrosis leading to honeycomb lung and pulmonary hypertension is a relatively common cause of death (see p. 98). Alveolar cell carcinoma (see p. 405) occasionally complicates.

4 *Sjögren's syndrome*: atrophy of tracheobronchial glands and diffuse interstitial fibrosis/pneumonitis may occur but are not usually clinically important.

Pulmonary collapse

Definition

An airless condition of the lung which has previously been inflated. The term *atelectasis* is best restricted to failure of aeration of the lung at birth.

Causes

Compression

Extrinsic compression of the lung parenchyma by any space-occupying lesion, e.g. pneumothorax, pleural fluid, tumours, aneurysms, etc.

Obstruction

Obstruction to the lumen of bronchi or bronchioles with subsequent resorption of the air. Common causes are:

1 *Lumen*: foreign bodies; mucus, e.g. asthma; pus; aspirated material including vomit and inflammatory exudate. This is common postoperatively due to a combination of tenacious mucus, poor respiratory movements and depression of the cough reflex.

2 *Wall*: tumours and strictures of main air passages.

3 *External*: pressure from enlarged lymph nodes, e.g. tuberculosis, tumour, aneurysms and cysts.

Appearances

Collapse may be patchy and peripheral, segmental or involve the whole lung—massive collapse. Small areas have a grey–blue colour and are depressed below the surface of the surrounding normal pink and aerated lung. In *massive collapse* the lung is non-crepitant, heavy and wrinkled on the pleural surface. The cause is usually obvious.

Histologically the alveoli are airless and crowded together.

Results

1 *Resolution*: if the cause of the collapse is removed at an early stage the lung will re-expand and return to normal.
2 *Organization*: if the collapse persists there is fibrosis of the lung parenchyma—*carnification*, and later bronchiectasis.
3 *Respiratory failure and death*: can occur if massive collapse complicates underlying disease, e.g. asthma.

Lipid pneumonia

Definition

Pulmonary inflammatory reaction to lipids.

Types

Endogenous

Common and related to bronchial obstruction with infection, particularly from bronchial carcinoma.

Exogenous

From inhalation of fatty or oily substances, e.g. liquid paraffin taken as as aperient or inhaled fatty food, e.g. milk. It occurs particularly if there is oesophageal obstruction (see p. 24).

Appearances

Macroscopical

Usually involving lower lobes. The cut surface is consolidated and yellow. In more chronic cases there is a firm fibrous wall surrounding a semi-cystic mass containing droplets of oily substance which is also seen in regional lymph nodes.

Microscopical

There is replacement of the lung tissue by free fat droplets when exogenous and foam cells, foreign-body giant cells, chronic inflammatory cells and fibrous tissue.

Results

1 *Mass*: the reactions produce a mass or masses—'*paraffinomas*'.
2 *Pulmonary dysfunction*: if changes are bilateral and extensive.

Drowning and near-drowning

Immersion into water with inhalation can cause:
1 *Immediate cardiac arrest*: due to chilling effect of cold water on the skin or larynx. Alcohol may predispose to this.
2 *Asphyxia*: anoxia due to effects of water-filled lungs.
3 *Acute metabolic disturbances*: fresh water is hypotonic and inhalation leads to absorption into the blood with haemodilution, red cell lysis and hyperkalaemia causing cardiac arrest. Haemoconcentration and absorption of magnesium ions in salt water delays death for 7–9 minutes.
4 *Diffuse alveolar damage (DAD)*: very acute lung damage can occur.
5 *Near-drowning*: patients recovered from any near-drowning episode may suffer from hypothermia, systemic anoxia, DAD and pneumonia.

I/CONGENITAL AND NEONATAL

Hyaline membrane disease
Pulmonary haemorrhage
Bronchopulmonary dysplasia
Congenital abnormalities
    Tracheobronchial
    Parenchymal
Vascular

Respiratory distress in the newborn

Conditions which can cause 'respiratory distress' include hyaline membrane disease—the commonest—intraventricular/periventricular haemorrhage—from anoxia, pneumonia, transient tachypnoea of the newborn, pneumothorax and massive pulmonary haemorrhage.

Hyaline membrane disease (HMD)

Incidence
The most important cause of death in the neonatal period—25% of deaths. About 4% of all neonates and 15% of premature neonates <2500 g birthweight, develop HMD.

Predisposing factors
1 *Prematurity*: the major predisposing factor. The incidence of HMD is proportional to gestational age: occurs in 60% of neonates <28 weeks gestation and less than 5% in those >37 weeks. This is related to surfactant deficiency.
2 *Birth asphyxia*.
3 *Maternal diabetes*.
4 *Second twin*.
5 *Caesarean section*.

Appearances

Macroscopical
The lungs are expanded but firm and plum-coloured.

Microscopical
There is alveolar collapse with bronchial and bronchiolar dilatation. The bronchioles are lined by eosinophilic membrane—*hyaline membranes*—consisting of fibrin and necrotic epithelial cells. There is congestion of the alveolar septae and lymphatic space dilatation. Organizational processes are also seen if infants survive for more than 48 hours.

Pathogenesis
Surfactant deficiency is central to this condition, as identified in Fig. 33.

Results
The severity of disease varies. Possible effects include:
1 *Resolution*: after supportive treatment of variable intensity.
2 *Death*: most due to HMD *per se* occur within the first 48 hours.
3 *Pneumonia*.
4 *Interstitial emphysema/pneumothorax*.
5 *Bronchopulmonary dysplasia* (see below).
6 *Others*: the neonate is also at risk from other

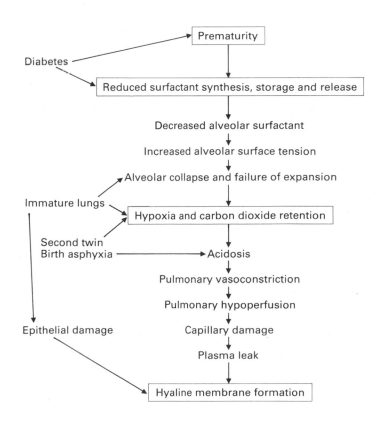

Fig. 33 Infantile respiratory distress syndrome pathogenesis.

complications of immaturity, anoxia and iatrogenic disease due to intensive therapy.

Pulmonary haemorrhage

Massive haemorrhage into the alveoli, bronchi and trachea which accounts for 10% of neonatal deaths.

Main predisposing factors are severe birth asphyxia, congenital heart disease, neonatal hypothermia, hyaline membrane disease, mechanical ventilation, fluid overload, oxygen toxicity and disseminated intravascular coagulation.

It is due to left ventricular failure from increased pulmonary capillary pressure and associated with immaturity of pulmonary capillaries.

Bronchopulmonary dysplasia

Nature
A chronic respiratory disease usually occurring in pre-term infants who have required prolonged mechanical respiratory support, and is the commonest complication of hyaline membrane disease. It is characterized by prolonged pulmonary damage and continued repair.

Appearances
The lungs are generally expanded with alternating areas of dilatation and collapse of airways.

Histologically there are residual hyaline membranes, alveolar collapse, alveolar dilatation, interstitial widening with oedema, capillary wall thickening and widespread fibrosis. Goblet cell hyperplasia, bronchial necrosis and squamous metaplasia are additional features.

Aetiology
Barotrauma from positive pressure ventilation and oxygen toxicity are causative factors.

Results
A severe disease with a 30% mortality.

Once established there is difficulty in weaning the infant from oxygen until sufficient natural lung development has occurred. Surviving infants have prolonged respiratory difficulties for 12–18 months. Persistent lung damage may occur.

Congenital abnormalities

Minor congenital abnormalities are not uncommon. Significant abnormalities are rare.

Tracheobronchial
1 *Agenesis or hypoplasia*.
2 *Fistulae*: tacheo-oesophageal or broncho-oesophageal fistulae are associated with inhalation of food into the lungs (see p. 370).
3 *Supernumerary bronchi*: abnormally distributed or supernumerary bronchi are rare and are mainly of significance to the surgeon.
4 *Bronchogenic cysts*: result from abnormal budding of developing tracheobronchial tree. They distend to form single or multiple cysts which may communicate with the bronchial tree and are lined by respiratory-type epithelium. They may remain asymptomatic, become infected or produce extrinsic bronchial compression resulting in distal pneumonia.
5 *Congenital adenomatoid malformation*: a spongy multiple cystic mass of pulmonary parenchymal tissue situated within the lung and with a rim of surrounding normal lung. Neonates present with respiratory distress due to expansion of the abnormal tissue. This requires surgery.

Parenchymal

Agenesis or hypoplasia
Often associated with other congenital abnormalities. Unilateral agenesis or hypoplasia is compatible with life but is complicated by recurrent infections.

Abnormal lobation
Increase or decrease in the number of lobes is not uncommon, and may be due to displaced normal structures, e.g. azygos vein creating the azygos lobe. They are of no functional significance.

Sequestered segments
The presence of lobes or segments separated from the normal lung with bronchi which do not communicate with the main respiratory tract. They become distended with retained secretions and often present with recurrent infection. The segment has a separate blood supply.

Vascular

Arteriovenous malformations
These are rare localized single or multiple lesions in the lung which usually present in early adult life with

dyspnoea. Complications include haemorrhage into bronchi or pleura.

Others
Rare, e.g. agenesis of pulmonary artery trunk.

J/TUMOURS

Carcinoma
Alveolar cell carcinoma
Carcinoid
Atypical carcinoid
Hamartoma
Other primary tumours
Secondary tumours
Coin lesions

Carcinoma of the bronchus

Epidemiology
Twenty-five per cent of all malignant causes of death—30 000 per year in the UK—the commonest cause of cancer in men and the second in women after breast cancer.

The overall incidence of the disease is still increasing, particularly so in women.

The average age at presentation is approximately 65 years.

Aetiological factors

Smoking
Most lung cancers are due to cigarette smoking. The condition is strongly related to the extent of smoking. This is dose-related, including the total number of cigarettes, number of puffs per cigarette, amount of inhalation of smoke, the use of filters and the length of cigarette remaining. There is a steady decline in risk if smoking stops; in light smokers this eventually equates with non-smokers after about 10 years, but there is always a slight excess risk in previously heavy smokers.

Passive smoking
Inhalation of cigarette smoke in non-smokers who live or work alongside smokers may be responsible for 5% of lung cancers.

About 10% of lung cancers occur in non-smokers.

Occupation
Exposure to certain materials increases the risk of developing carcinoma, including: asbestos, radium, uranium, chromates and nickel carbonyl.

Geography
In certain areas of the world, radioactive radon gas seeps from uranium within rocks. This may increase the local risk of developing carcinoma by 1% in non-smokers and by 10% in smokers.

There is no increase in risk of lung cancer in cities compared to rural areas after correction for the effects of smoking.

Genetic
Occasional family clustering of lung cancer occurs, but genetic factors are generally insignificant as compared to smoking.

Pulmonary fibrosis
An increased incidence of cancer is seen in patients with certain types of diffuse interstitial fibrosis, e.g. fibrosing alveolitis (see p. 392).

Focal scars occurring in association with cancers are likely to be induced by the cancer rather than vice-versa.

Tumour type and aetiology
1 Smoking is associated with all the major types of carcinoma but most strongly with squamous and oat cell types.
2 Adenocarcinomas are becoming more frequent. They are relatively more common in females, are the most common type associated with interstitial fibrosis and are the commonest type seen in non-smokers.

Appearances

Sites

Central
Seventy per cent of tumours arise in relation to the main, lobar or segmental bronchi.

Peripheral
Thirty per cent arise in the periphery of the lung, mostly in small bronchi or bronchioles. A small percentage arise from terminal bronchioles or alveolar lining cells.

Macroscopical

Bronchial

The earliest changes consist of 'warty' surface irregularity of the bronchial mucosa. Established tumours extend into the lumen as a polypoid mass with distal obstructive effects or invade through the wall into the peribronchial and parenchymal tissues. Tumour tissue is white–grey and often shows areas of haemorrhage or necrosis. Squamous tumours often cavitate.

Peripheral

Tumours form a pale mass of variable size in the peripheral lung parenchyma, usually with puckering of the pleura.

Histological types

Squamous cell carcinoma

Forty per cent of all lung carcinomas. Most are central but they can be peripheral. The tumours variably resemble normal squamous epithelium with keratin formation and intercellular bridges and they can be graded as well, moderately or poorly differentiated.

The epithelium adjacent to the invasive tumour often shows squamous metaplasia, dysplasia and carcinoma in situ.

Adenocarcinoma

Between 20% and 30%; two-thirds are located peripherally and one-third centrally.

The usual type is characterized by mucin production, tubule formation and/or papillary structures. Bronchoalveolar carcinoma is a variant (see p. 405).

Small cell carcinoma—oat cell

Twenty per cent and predominantly central. They are highly malignant and often disseminated at time of presentation. Sheets and ribbons of small oval hyperchromatic cells with scanty cytoplasm and rosette formation—oat cells. Cells may be larger with more cytoplasm—small cell intermediate. There may be considerable necrosis.

The cells show neuroendocrine differentiation as demonstrated by neurosecretory granules ultrastructurally, neural-associated enzymes, e.g. NSE, and other proteins (see p. 36).

Large cell carcinoma

Between 10% and 20% and often peripheral. Composed of large polygonal cells with vesicular nuclei and show no differentiation on light microscopy. They are probably very poorly differentiated squamous cell or adenocarcinomas.

Variants include giant cell and clear cell carcinomas.

Pathogenesis

1 Cigarette smoke contains a large number of carcinogens, e.g. polycyclic hydrocarbons and radioactive species. Other carcinogens are often occupational, e.g. asbestos.
2 The carcinogens are initiating and promoting and cause the changes in the epithelial cells.
3 The neoplasms derived from the transformed bronchial epithelial cells differentiate in different directions to produce the various histological types.
4 For squamous cell carcinoma there is a long natural history prior to invasive neoplasm, characterized initially by the development of squamous metaplasia of the respiratory epithelium due to the damaging effects of cigarette smoke. Continued exposure to carcinogen results in progressive development of epithelial dysplasia, carcinoma in situ and then invasive carcinoma.

The preinvasive phase of other types of carcinoma are poorly understood.

Molecular biology

Invasive carcinomas are associated with chromosomal abnormalities, e.g. loss of chromosome 3; oncogene abnormalities, e.g. amplification of ras oncogene; deletion of C-erb locus; and production of autocrine and paracrine factors, e.g. bombesin. The exact role of these substances is under active investigation.

Spread

Local

1 Bronchial: lumen obstruction causes pulmonary collapse, accumulation of secretions, ulcerative bronchitis, bronchiectasis, abscess or pneumonia.
2 Pleural: blood-stained effusion, empyema, chest wall invasion.
3 Superior vena cava: compression or invasion causes the superior vena caval syndrome (see p. 282).
4 Pericardium: pericarditis with haemorrhagic effusion (see p. 62).
5 Bone involvement: direct spread into ribs, sternum

and spine result in pain, hypercalcaemia and in pathological fracture.

6 *Oesophagus*: causing dysphagia or broncho-oesophageal fistula.

7 *Nerves*: spread to axilla—*Pancoast tumour*—with invasion of the brachial plexus, or cervical sympathetic chain—*Horner's syndrome*—occurs.

Lymphatic
Occurs early, with invasion of regional intrapulmonary, hilar and then extrapulmonary tracheobronchial and other mediastinal nodes. Further spread may occur to cervical, supraclavicular, axillary and more distant groups.

Nodal involvement may be massive and can be the presenting feature with caval obstruction or tracheal compression.

Blood
Widespread systemic invasion is common and metastases not uncommonly present as the first clinical manifestation. They may occur in any organ but particularly adrenals (50%), liver (30–50%), brain (20%) and bone (20%).

Transcoelomic
Multiple deposits or extensive sheets of tumour across the pleural space.

Non-metastatic systemic manifestations
Paraneoplastic syndromes are common complications of lung cancer.

Ectopic hormone production
Inappropriate secretion of hormones is common and include:

1 *Antidiuretic hormone*: causing hyponatraemia with cerebral dysfunction (see p. 125). Most commonly associated with oat cell carcinoma.

2 *ACTH*: producing metabolic and occasionally clinical Cushing's syndrome (see p. 117). Most commonly associated with oat cell carcinoma.

3 *Parathormone-like substances*: causing hypercalcaemia and most commonly associated with squamous cell carcinoma.

4 *Others*: calcitonin and gonadotrophins.

Nervous system effects
These include peripheral neuropathy, cerebellar ataxia, polymyositis, myasthenic syndromes, auto-nomic neuropathy and myelopathy.

1 *Skin*: acanthosis nigricans.

2 *Bone*: clubbing and pulmonary hypertrophic osteo-arthropathy (see p. 297).

Stage
Staging assesses the extent of tumour spread, including the assessment of distant metastatic disease (M), lymph node status (N) and extent of local spread (T). The classical TNM system may be used.

Prognosis
1 The main prognostic factors are the *stage* and *cell type*.

2 The overall 5-year survival for carcinoma of lung is between 5% and 15%.

3 *Non-small cell carcinoma*, i.e. tumours other than small cell carcinomas, are treated surgically for anticipation of cure, but 75% are inoperable at presentation and have a dismal prognosis. Of the 25% operable, 20% of these have early stage disease with a 30–50% 5-year survival. The remaining 80% have a 10–20% 5-year survival.

4 *Small (oat) cell carcinoma*: overall less than 2% of patients are alive at 5 years. These tumours are usually treated non-surgically by chemotherapy or radiotherapy. Five per cent have limited disease and 25% of these patients are alive at 5 years.

Bronchoalveolar cell carcinoma

Incidence
A rare form of adenocarcinoma of the lung—5% of cases. It occurs in both sexes equally and throughout adult life, and is peripherally located.

Appearances
Grossly these may be a single nodule, multiple nodules or a diffuse 'consolidation'. They are often bilateral due to spread via the air passages. The cut surface has a mucinous and grey appearance.

Histologically characterized by malignant glandular cells, usually mucin-producing, which spread along the surface of the alveolar walls.

Metastatic adenocarcinomas, especially from the pancreas and intestines, can produce an identical morphological appearance.

The primary tumours can show clara cell, type 2 pneumocyte or goblet cell differentiation.

Results
Solitary lesions may be surgically resected with a 75% 5-year survival but overall this is 25%.

Bronchial carcinoid—typical carcinoid

Nature
Malignant, but low-grade slowly growing tumours showing neuroendocrine differentiation. They resemble neuroendocrine tumours of carcinoid type in other sites (see p. 36).

Epidemiology
There is no association with smoking and they present in relatively young patients, often less than 40 years.

Appearances

Macroscopical
Usually central, arising from a major bronchus. They form a mucosal-covered endobronchial polypoid lesion but there is extension into peribronchial tissues.

Microscopical
Composed of nests, cords and sheets of regular uniform cells of endocrine appearance with little necrosis or mitotic activity. Ultrastructurally, dense core neurosecretory granules are seen and immunohistochemically they contain various peptide hormones, e.g. bombesin, ACTH.

Spread
There is local spread into the bronchial lumen and peribronchial tissues. About 40% have regional lymph node metastases at the time of resection. Distant metastases are unusual but described.

Results
1 *Local*:
    (a) *Bronchial spread*: causing luminal obstruction and pulmonary collapse with infection.
    (b) *Bleeding*: due to vascularity.
2 *Hormonal activity*: clinical hormonal effects are rare but carcinoid syndrome (see p. 36) and Cushing's syndrome (see p. 117) are described.

Prognosis
There is an 80% 10-year survival for resected cases.
   Metastatic disease if present, has a protracted course.

Atypical carcinoid—neuroendocrine carcinoma
A variant of the typical carcinoid, recognized histologically by areas of necrosis, increased mitotic activity and cellular pleomorphism. Prognosis is worse than a typical carcinoid—50% 5-year survival.

Bronchial hamartoma
A relatively common benign solitary peripheral lesion.
   Macroscopically forms a well-circumscribed, pale, glistening, lobulated nodule.
   Histologically contains fully mature fat, cartilage, epithelial clefts and glandular aggregates.
   These lesions grow slowly and their exact nature is uncertain, but they are not found in children and are probably not true hamartomas.

Mucous gland tumours
Tumours arising from bronchial mucous glands are rare and mostly of adenoid cystic or mucoepidermoid types. They are similar to those in salivary glands (see p. 19).

Other primary lung tumours
Other lung tumours are rare but there is a wide range of both benign and malignant types including bronchial squamous papilloma, sclerosing pneumocytoma, pulmonary blastoma, carcinosarcoma, epithelioid haemangioendothelioma.

Metastatic lung tumours
Metastatic spread of tumours to the lung is very common with the most common sites of origin being breast and kidney. Spread, e.g. from breast, intestines, pancreas, may result in widespread lymphatic permeation—*lymphangitis carcinomatosa*. This produces dyspnoea with minimal or 'interstitial' changes radiologically.

Coin lesions
The term '*coin lesion*' refers to the radiological finding of a solitary peripheral parenchymal nodule of approximately circular outline with no other specific radiological features. Causes include:

Common
Primary bronchial carcinoma; metastatic tumour; granulomatous inflammation, e.g. tuberculosis; histoplasmosis; localized pneumonia; lung abscess; hamartoma; bronchial carcinoid.

Uncommon

Other primary tumours; arteriovenous malformations; cysts; foreign bodies; mycetomas; intrapulmonary lymph node; rheumatoid nodule; Wegener's granulomatosis.

In the UK primary carcinomas account for at least 35% of cases, rising to 50% in patients older than 50 years. The incidence of malignancy in those younger than 35 years is low.

Respiratory tract—pleura

Dry pleurisy
Pleural effusion
Empyema
Haemothorax
Chylothorax
Bronchopleural fistula
Hydropneumothorax and pyopneumothorax
Pneumothorax
Tumours

Dry pleurisy

Due to inflammatory disease involving the parietal pleura. Any cause of pleural exudate (see below) can also cause dry pleurisy.

Common causes include chest infection—particularly infective exacerbations of bronchiectasis, chest trauma/rib fracture, rheumatoid arthritis, SLE, pulmonary infarction and uraemia.

Bornholm disease—epidemic myalgia—is a Coxsackie virus disease associated with dry pleurisy.

Pleural effusion

Definition

Abnormal accumulation of fluid in the pleural space. The two types are transudates and exudates.

Mechanisms

Effusions can be caused by diseases which interfere with the mechanisms that maintain the balance of entry and removal of water, electrolytes and protein into and out of the pleural cavity. These include increased intracapillary pressure, increased capillary permeability, hypoproteinaemia and impaired lymphatic drainage.

Pleural transudates

Nature

Accumulation of fluid with a low protein content within the pleural space.

Aetiology

1 *Increased hydrostatic pressure*: congestive cardiac failure, constrictive pericarditis, pericardial effusion.
2 *Decreased capillary osmotic pressure*: cirrhosis, nephrotic syndrome, malnutrition.
3 *Extension from peritoneum*: any cause of ascites, peritoneal dialysis.

Appearance

The fluid is straw-coloured, non-inflammatory and contains occasional lymphocytes and mesothelial cells. The pleural surface of the lung appears normal. Effusions are usually bilateral.

Results

1 *Pulmonary collapse*: compression of the lungs and interference with respiratory function.
2 *Resolution*: no structural alterations are seen if the cause is corrected and resorption occurs.

Pleural exudates

Nature

Accumulation of protein-rich fluid in the pleural space from leakage of capillaries.

Causes

1 *Neoplasms*: metastatic spread to pleura, mesothelioma.
2 *Infections*: pneumonia, abscess, tuberculosis, subphrenic abscess.
3 *Immune disorders*: postmyocardial infarct, rheumatoid disease, systemic lupus erythematosus, Wegener's granulomatosis.
4 *Pulmonary infarction*.
5 *Other causes*: radiation therapy, asbestos exposure, drug reactions, pancreatitis, uraemia.

Appearances

Exudates may be serous, serofibrinous, fibrinous or haemorrhagic. They are usually unilateral and consist of straw-coloured fluid containing fibrin strands. In addition to mesothelial cells and lymphocytes, polymorphs are also often present.

The surface pleura is dulled by a fibrinous exudate.

Haemorrhagic effusions are often due to neoplasia or pulmonary infarcts. In neoplastic diseases, malignant cells can often be identified within pleural fluid.

Results

1 *Pulmonary collapse*: compression of the underlying lung with decrease in respiratory function.

2 *Adhesions*: fibrous adhesions between the visceral and parietal pleura are often seen after resorption of the effusion.

3 *Pleural obliteration and fibrosis*: if the inflammatory effusion is long-standing, recurrent or very severe, there may be marked pleural fibrosis or obliteration of the pleural space.

4 *Empyema*: progession of inflammation in the underlying lung tissue may lead to empyema (see below).

Empyema

Nature
Pus within the pleural cavity.

Causes
1 *Pulmonary infection*: empyema is most commonly a complication of intrapulmonary infection, e.g. pneumonia, tuberculosis, lung abscess.

2 *Other infections*: spread from subphrenic abscess, acute mediastinitis and distant infective foci.

3 *Surgery/trauma*: as a complication of thoracic surgery or penetrating chest wall injury.

Organisms
Mixed aerobic and anaerobic organisms are common.

Gram-positive organisms, e.g. *Strep. pneumoniae* or *Staph. aureus*, are common causes of empyema complicating pulmonary parenchymal infection. Empyema secondary to surgery, trauma or oesophageal disease is usually due to Gram-negative organisms.

Appearances
Characteristically the pus is yellow or green and contains numerous polymorphs.

The pleural surface shows a fibrinous exudate.

Results
1 *Toxaemia*: systemic effects of infection are marked.

2 *Lung collapse*: compression of the lung with impaired lung function.

3 *Bronchopleural fistula*: infection ruptures into the airways and pleura resulting in fistulous communication

4 *Pleural scarring*: if the empyema is evacuated or early resolution occurs, the fibrin/granulation tissue on the pleural surface organizes with fibrous adhesions between the visceral and parietal layers. If more long-standing there is an increased deposition of granulation tissue, which heals with extensive dense pleural fibrosis or obliteration of the pleural cavity. This results in permanent encasement of the underlying lung with impaired pulmonary function and predisposition to repeated infection.

Haemothorax
Causes of bleeding into the chest include chest trauma, especially with rib fractures, pulmonary infarction and spontaneous rupture of diseased arteries, e.g. atheromatous and dissecting aortic aneurysm—usually fatal. Incomplete evacuation of blood clots results in organization and pleural fibrosis/obliteration.

Chylothorax
Accumulation of lymph in the pleural cavity is due to leakage from the thoracic duct or other major lymphatic channels. This is usually caused by malignant infiltration, surgical interference or trauma.

Bronchopleural fistula
This is a communication between the pleura and airways and causes persistent infection with respiratory dysfunction.

Hydropneumothorax and pyopneumothorax
This describes the respective presence of air and fluid, or air and pus, in the pleural space.

Pneumothorax

Nature
Air in the pleural cavity.

Aetiology

Primary spontaneous
Occurs in the absence of underlying lung disease. Most common in young males 20–40 years and is occasion-

ally bilateral and recurrent. Usually due to rupture of a pulmonary '*bleb*'—an air-filled space within the layers of the visceral pleural contiguous with the lung parenchyma.

Secondary spontaneous
Occurs in patients with evidence of underlying lung disease, most commonly emphysema, asthma, suppurative pneumonia and cystic fibrosis. Other causes include advanced pulmonary fibrosis and Langerhans cell granulomatosis (histiocytosis X) (see p. 396).

Traumatic
Occurs due to perforating injuries of the chest wall which allow air to enter the space from the outside or from the lung, following laceration of the lung substance. Pneumothorax may also occur during insertion of a chest drain, following transbronchial lung biopsies, fine needle aspirations or during aspiration of a pleural effusion.

Artificial
Refers to the deliberate introduction of air into the pleural cavity—once extensively used as a treatment for tuberculosis.

Results
1 *Lung collapse*: compression of the underlying lung occurs which if large results in *respiratory dysfunction*. If the communication seals, the pneumothorax gradually resorbs over a few weeks.
2 *Tension pneumothorax*: occurs when there is a valve-like mechanism at the site of communication between the air and the pleural cavity, allowing air to enter the cavity in inspiration but not escape in expiration. Pressure rises with progressive and massive collapse of the lung, mediastinal shift and compression of the contralateral lung producing life-threatening respiratory insufficiency.

Pleural tumours

Secondary tumours
These are by far the most common type of pleural tumour.

Primary sites of origin include lung and breast but *any* malignant tumour may spread to this site.

Mode of spread includes either direct invasion or lymphatic permeation.

Metastatic deposits produce a serosanguinous exudate, often bloodstained, which often contains malignant cells.

Benign pleural fibroma
A benign tumour of submesothelial connective tissue.

This is a well-circumscribed, localized tumour attached to the pleural surface by a pedicle and has a lobulated grey–white whorled pattern.

Microscopically there is a network of spindle fibroblast-like cells and abundant collagen fibres.

The vast majority have a benign behaviour.

The causes are not known and there is *no* association with asbestos exposure.

Malignant mesothelioma

Nature
This is a malignant primary neoplasm of the parietal or visceral pleura.

Incidence
A rather rare tumour occurring mainly in asbestos-exposed individuals and classically after a long latent period of 30–40 years (see p. 388).

Pathogenesis
This is discussed on p. 388.

Appearances

Macroscopical
A grey tumour mass which envelops and encases the whole of the lung with direct infiltration into the thoracic wall structures.

Microscopical
Three main patterns:
1 *Sarcomatoid*: composed of bundles of spindle-shaped cells.
2 *Epithelial*: composed of columnar cells forming tubules and papillae. This can be difficult to differentiate from adenocarcinoma but the cells are usually negative for neutral mucin.
3 *Mixed*: with both sarcomatoid and epithelial patterns.

Spread
Extensive local spread occurs. Distant metastases only occur late.

Effect

Recurrent or persistent pleural effusions, severe persistent chest pain and progressive restriction of chest movement.

Prognosis

Uniformly poor, with most patients dead within 2 years.

Chapter 21
Diseases of the skin

A/NON-NEOPLASTIC

Normal skin
Terminology
Types of biopsy
Inflammations
   Infections
   Non-infective inflammations
Bullous skin diseases

Normal skin

The skin consists of epidermis, dermis and subcutis together with hair follicles, sweat glands, blood vessels, lymphatics and nerves (Fig. 34). The *epidermis* is a stratified squamous epithelium with four layers:

Basal cell layer

Lies on the basement membrane. The cells are cuboidal or columnar. Basal cells divide to maintain the epithelium as cells are shed from its surface. Neuroendocrine *Merkel cells* and pigmented *melanocytes* are also present in this layer.

Prickle cell layer

The main part of the epidermis, composed of polygonal *keratinocytes* with prominent intercellular desmosomal junctions. *Langerhans cells*, which play a part in antigen presentation, are present and send dendritic processes between the keratinocytes.

Granular cell layer

A layer usually two or three cells thick, in which the cells contain basophilic keratohyaline granules.

Horny layer

The surface layer normally consisting of anucleate keratinized cells, which are constantly shed from the surface.

The junction between epidermis and dermis is convoluted and consists of downward projections of epidermis—*rete pegs*, and upward projections of dermis—*rete ridges*.

Dermis

This is a complex structure in two layers: the upper *papillary* dermis, with fine collagen and elastic fibres in the stroma and the lower *reticular* dermis, with coarser collagen and elastic fibres.

Blood vessels

Present in *superficial* and *deep* plexuses of arterioles, capillaries and venules, with associated lymphatics.

Nerves

Run through the dermis to end organs such as Paccinian and Meissner corpuscles, and send fine fibres into the epidermis, some of which connect with *Merkel cells*.

Skin-associated lymphoid tissue (SALT)

Consists of the normal resident population of T lymphocytes and macrophages of the skin, together with the Langerhans cells of the epidermis.

Sweat glands

Have a secretory coil, an excretory duct and a specialized *acrosyringium* in the epidermis. Most sweat glands are *eccrine*. The *apocrine* glands are found in the axillae and around the nipples and external genitalia. *Apoeccrine* glands develop in the axilla at puberty and are mainly responsible for the production of 'body odour'.

Hair follicles

Have a germ and matrix at their base and inner and outer root sheaths surround the growing hair shaft. The follicle has a *sebaceous gland* in its wall and an *infundibulum* which joins with the epidermis. The hair follicles follow a cycle with phases of growth (*anagen*), involution (*catagen*) and rest (*telogen*).

Subcutaneous tissue

Consists mostly of adipose tissue, divided into lobules by septae containing blood vessels.

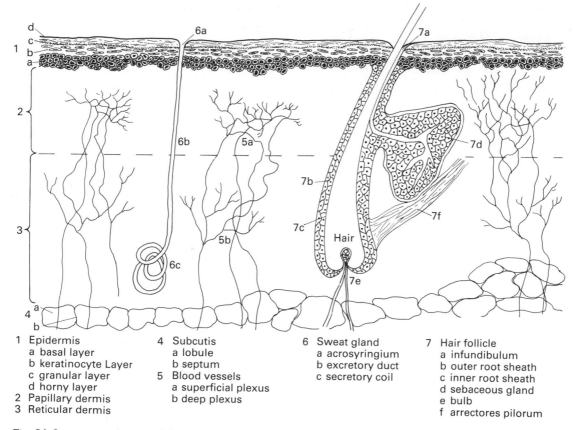

1 Epidermis
  a basal layer
  b keratinocyte Layer
  c granular layer
  d horny layer
2 Papillary dermis
3 Reticular dermis

4 Subcutis
  a lobule
  b septum
5 Blood vessels
  a superficial plexus
  b deep plexus

6 Sweat gland
  a acrosyringium
  b excretory duct
  c secretory coil

7 Hair follicle
  a infundibulum
  b outer root sheath
  c inner root sheath
  d sebaceous gland
  e bulb
  f arrectores pilorum

Fig. 34 Structures in the normal skin.

Terminology

Histopathology reports on skin biopsies may contain some of the following words, used to describe changes from the normal and mainly with reference to the epidermis.

The horny cell layer may be thickened—*hyperkeratosis*, with the normal absence of cell nuclei—*orthokeratosis*, or with persistence of the nuclei—*parakeratosis*.

The granular cell layer may be thickened—*hypergranulosis*—or reduced or even absent.

The prickle cell layer may be thickened—*acanthosis*—or atrophic. Intercellular oedema is known as *spongiosis*. If the oedema is more extensive *vesicles* may form and if they contain inflammatory cells they become *micro-abscesses*. Larger fluid-filled spaces are *bullae*, which may be intra-epidermal or sub-epidermal. Abnormal premature keratinization of cells in this layer is *dyskeratosis*.

Inflammation in which the blood vessel walls are involved and damaged is *vasculitis*. Inflammation of the subcutaneous fat is *panniculitis*.

Types of biopsy

Biopsies may be performed either to diagnose the nature of a rash or tumour, or to remove the lesion. Biopsies performed with a scalpel may be either *excisional* or *incisional*. Small *punch* biopsies are a convenient way of sampling lesions without leaving a large scar.

Superficial lesions may be scraped off with a *curette* giving a good cosmetic result but a fragmented specimen. Moles and other small benign blemishes may be *shaved* off.

Inflammations of skin

Infections

Bacterial

Infections of the skin vary according to the structures involved. *Impetigo* is a highly contagious form of infection with *Staphylococcus aureus* which forms superficial epidermal blisters. In neonates this infection can be severe, producing extensive superficial shedding of skin—*the scalded skin syndrome*. The same organism can infect hair follicles, producing *folliculitis*, which may proceed to the development of a pimple, boil or abscess.

Acne vulgaris

Acne is common at the time of puberty. Its cause is uncertain, but sex hormone levels and some foods appear to play a part. The comedone or blackhead is a hair follicle plugged with keratin and lipid. The surface lipid is oxidized to produce the black colour. Secondary infection, usually with low-grade pathogens can occur.

Hidradenitis suppurativa

The apocrine and apoeccrine glands of the axilla and anogenital regions may develop abscesses as a result of staphylococcal infection. The condition may become chronic, with scarring as well as abscesses.

Erysipelas

Streptococcal infection can produce an acute, erythematous, spreading infection, without abscess formation. The dermis is infiltrated with neutrophils.

Cellulitis

Cellulitis describes a spreading infection of the subcutaneous fat, often by *Streptococcus pyogenes*, which may progress to systemic bacteraemia. Severe infection with anaerobes can lead to necrotizing cellulitis of the scrotum—*Fournier's gangrene*, or the floor of the mouth—*Ludwig's angina*.

Necrotizing fasciitis

Deep-spreading infection of the fat, fascia and muscle, caused by anaerobic infection, can lead to extensive and life-threatening tissue necrosis. The process responds to extensive emergency surgical debridement.

Non-infective inflammatory conditions

Eczema and contact dermatitis

Dermatitis can be induced by reactions to a number of allergens and drugs. In other cases the stimulus cannot be identified. Eczema is commonly found in atopic individuals, who may also suffer from asthma or hay fever.

Microscopical

In acute reactions there is lymphocytic infiltration around superficial dermal vessels, with associated oedema. The epidermis shows both changes: exocytosis and spongiosis. Subacute lesions show the development of epidermal acanthosis and hyperkeratosis, with parakeratosis. Chronic lesions show less oedema or spongiosis and more acanthosis and hyperkeratosis—*lichen simplex*.

Psoriasis

A common condition which affects 1% of the population and shows remissions and exacerbations. In severe cases the joints as well as the skin are involved. The basic epidermal abnormality is one of increased cell turnover as a result of aberrant stimuli, the keratinocytes being otherwise normal.

Microscopical

The epidermis is hyperplastic with regular acanthosis, loss of granular layer and hyperkeratosis with the formation of parakeratotic scales. The epidermis is thinned over the dermal papillae, where inflammatory cells and oedema can form the spongiotic pustules of Kojog in the mid-epidermis and Munro's microabscesses in the cornified layer.

Lichen planus

A chronic process in which purple polygonal plaques develop on the skin, oral mucosa and genitalia, typically in middle-aged women.

Microscopical

The lesions are well circumscribed and show orthokeratotic hyperkeratosis and a band of lymphocytic infiltration in the papillary dermis, extending into the epidermis. The basal epidermis shows hydropic degeneration and the formation of keratotic eosinophilic Civatte bodies.

Lupus erythematosus

This autoimmune disease may be *systemic* (SLE), with multiple organ involvement (see p. 96) or may present as the *discoid* form (DLE) with an infiltrated erythematous 'butterfly' rash on the face.

Microscopical

Both variants have identical appearances, with hyperkeratosis, epidermal atrophy, follicular keratin plugs, basal hydropic change, and dermal lymphocytic infiltration around dermal blood vessels and appendages. Granular deposits of IgG and complement are present in the basement membrane zone, in the lesions of DLE and in both lesions and uninvolved skin in SLE.

Erythema multiforme

Usually idiopathic, although also associated with drugs, infections and autoimmune disease, this condition shows inflammatory macules, papules and target lesions with a central pale zone.

Microscopical

The characteristic epidermal feature is keratinocyte necrosis, associated with spongiosis and dyskeratosis. The dermis shows superficial oedema and vasculitis.

Granuloma annulare

Granuloma annulare occurs as small, red, firm dermal nodules, often on the hands and feet.

Microscopical

The deep dermis contains an ill-defined granuloma in which there is a peripheral palisade of macrophages arranged around a zone of degenerate or necrobiotic collagen, which is usually more eosinophilic than the uninvolved dermis. Giant cells may be present.

Vasculitis

Vasculitis presents in a number of ways, ranging from the acute leucocytoclastic vasculitis of Henoch–Schönlein purpura (see p. 84), to the necrotizing lesions of Wegener's granulomatosis (see p. 103), and including erythema nodosum.

Microscopical

All lesions have in common active inflammation and associated damage to dermal blood vessels, without which the process is not one of vasculitis. In leucocytoclastic vasculitis the affected vessels are surrounded by fragments of lysed neutrophils. Most examples show some degree of fibrin deposition in the vessel wall. In Wegener's granulomatosis there may be frank granulomatous destruction of vessels.

Erythema nodosum

This is the commonest kind of panniculitis. Most cases are idiopathic, but it is associated with many causes including infections such as β-haemolytic streptococci, deep fungal infections, leprosy, drugs, sarcoidosis, inflammatory bowel disease and underlying malignancy. The lesions occur on the shins and form tender red nodules.

Microscopical

The appearance is one of septal panniculitis without vasculitis. When the lobules rather than the septae of the subcutis are primarily inflamed the cause is more likely to be a deep fungal infection or a systemic disease such as panniculitis secondary to pancreatitis or pancreatic carcinoma.

Bullous skin diseases

Pemphigoid

Pemphigoid is the commonest of the bullous diseases, is relatively benign, and occurs in the elderly. The large vesicles and bullae rarely involve the mucous membranes.

Microscopical

The vesicles are *subepidermal and* are associated with linear deposition of IgG and complement in the epidermal basement membrane and with an inflammatory cell infiltrate including many eosinophils in the vesicle and underlying dermis.

Pemphigus

This chronic, severe and sometimes fatal disease affects the middle-aged. Large blisters are formed on the skin and in the mouth. The disease is steroid-responsive. Without therapy death is usual within a year of the onset of the disease.

Microscopical

The blisters are *intra-epidermal* and are associated with acantholysis. The blisters contain loose individual rounded-up acantholytic cells. IgG deposits are present on the prickles between the keratinocytes.

Dermatitis herpetiformis (DH)

DH occurs in young adults and is a chronic disease typified by an itchy rash with small erythematous vesicles. It is associated with the gluten-sensitive enteropathy of coeliac disease (see p. 34) but does not respond to a gluten-free diet.

Microscopical

Subepidermal micro-abscesses form at the tips of dermal papillae and contain neutrophils and eosinophils. Granular deposits of IgA are present in the micro-abscesses.

Epidermolysis bullosa aquisita (EBA)

EBA is rare and affects the skin and mucous membranes of children and adults. Blisters heal leaving scars and cysts. Microscopically it is indistinguishable from pemphigoid.

B/SKIN TUMOURS

Epidermal
  Benign
  Malignant
Melanocytic tumours
  Benign
  Malignant
Skin appendage tumours
  Hair follicle
  Sweat gland
  Sebaceous gland
Cysts
Dermal tumours
Lymphomas

Epidermal keratoses and tumours

Amongst the commonest pathological conditions are various warts, keratoses and epitheliomas, which occur more frequently with increasing age and following prolonged sun exposure.

Benign

Viral warts

Viral warts are extremely common and are a consequence of infection with one or more of the many kinds of human papilloma virus—HPV, either by direct contact or autoinoculation.

Types

1 *Common wart*: a hard papillary wart, usually of recent origin—exophytic growth.
2 *Plantar wart*: on the sole warts are forced to grow into the dermis—endophytic growth.
3 *Flat wart*: plane warts are often multiple and grow in the hands and face.
4 *Anogenital warts*: large fleshy warts around the genitalia and/or anus. May be transmitted to the sexual partner and are associated with dyskaryosis of the cervix and cervical intra-epithelial neoplasia (CIN) (see p. 211).

Microscopical

Warts show varying degrees of hyperkeratosis and papillary epidermal hyperplasia—acanthosis. There is hypergranulosis and the keratinocytes may show perinuclear vacuolization—koilocytosis. The basal layer is intact, without true dermal invasion. The dermis contains an inflammatory cell infiltrate.

Seborrhoeic wart

Also called seborrhoeic keratosis and basal cell papilloma, these are rounded, pigmented, greasy warts which occur on the trunk, face and arms of the elderly. They vary in size from a few millimetres to several centimetres and can be mistaken for melanomas. A spectrum of appearances is seen from very papillary hyperkeratotic types similar to viral warts to rounded variants similar to naevi.

Microscopical

All lesions have in common basal cell proliferation, hyperkeratosis and rounded keratin-filled horn cysts, some of which open on to the surface. A variable degree of pigmentation is present, with melanin mostly in melanophages.

Keratoacanthoma

Keratoacanthomas are warty lesions which often occur on the face of the elderly and grow rapidly, like a malignant tumour, but if left will usually involute and heal within a few months. They may be removed by curettage.

Microscopical

The lesion is radially symmetrical, with a tulip-like profile with proliferating epidermis surrounding a central keratin-filled pit. The keratinocytes are enlarged and have pale eosinophilic cytoplasm, without nuclear atypia. A small or fragmented biopsy may be difficult to distinguish from a squamous cell carcinoma.

Molluscum contagiosum

The lesions are caused by infection with a poxvirus. They are small domed papules with a central depression or umbilication. They usually heal spontaneously but AIDS patients may become heavily infected.

Microscopical

The lesions show endophytic epidermal proliferation, with the production of characteristic cells containing large viral inclusion bodies—molluscum bodies.

Premalignant lesions

Actinic keratosis

Hard scaly lesions on sun-exposed areas, especially the face, scalp and hands, of the elderly. Often curetted.

Microscopical

Hyperkeratosis with alternating columns of orthokeratosis and parakeratosis. Extreme hyperkeratosis produces a keratin or *cutaneous horn*. The prickle cell layer may be acanthotic, with a mild to moderate degree of nuclear irregularity or pleomorphism and with mitotic figures. No evidence of dermal invasion, but dermal collagen shows the homogenized appearance of solar elastosis.

Malignant

Bowen's disease

This intra-epidermal malignancy is found on sun-exposed skin and also in many other sites of squamous epithelium. It may also be caused by chronic exposure to arsenic, or may be associated with an underlying visceral malignancy. The lesions are slowly extending erythematous or scaly plaques.

Microscopical

The whole thickness of the epidermis is abnormal, with atypical keratinocytes, cellular disarray, prominent nuclear pleomorphism and large mitoses. There is no invasion through the epidermal basement membrane into the dermis.

Basal cell carcinoma

Basal cell carcinoma is the commonest kind of skin cancer. The tumours occur on sun-exposed skin in middle-aged and elderly fair-skinned people. The face is the commonest site. *Gorlin's syndrome* associates basal cell tumours in younger patients with autosomal inheritance and abnormalities of bone, nervous system, dental cysts and the eyes.

A typical tumour appears as a waxy papule, with fine telangiectatic vessels running over its surface and often with a central ulcer. The punched-out appearance of the ulcer gave rise to the older description of 'rodent ulcer'. The *morphoeic variant* forms an indurated plaque without associated ulceration.

Microscopical

Basal cell carcinoma is so called because the tumour cells resemble basal cells. The tumours are characterized by cords and nests of cells with a peripheral palisade of cells arranged with the long axis of their nuclei perpendicular to the tumour margin.

Nodular variants are well defined and easily excised. The morphoeic variant has small strands of tumour cells infiltrating widely, making complete excision difficult and local recurrence quite common. Basal cell carcinoma spreads by local invasion. Metastasis is very rare.

Squamous cell carcinoma

This tumour is also very common, particulary in the sun-exposed skin of elderly whites The tumours invade locally but only metastasize occasionally—1%—although more commonly than basal cell carcinoma. Squamous cell carcinoma may also develop in chronically inflamed lesions such as infected sinuses, burn scars and ulcers—*Marjolin's ulcer*. These tumours metastasize in 20–30% and whilst most tumours are cured by complete local excision, the later, more aggressive tumours may require lymph node dissection or adjuvant radiotherapy.

Microscopical

The tumours show malignant cells similar to keratinocytes, with cytoplasmic keratinization and intercellular prickles. Nuclear atypia and mitoses are present, with the degree of abnormality proportional to the overall degree of tumour differentiation. Well-differentiated tumours often show keratin pearls. The tumour invades the dermis and subcutaneous tissues and adjacent structures in more advanced lesions.

Basosquamous carcinoma

Some tumours show mixed appearances of basal and squamous differentiation. The squamous component predominates from a clinical point of view. The tumours are all potentially metastatic and require wide local excision to reduce the possibility of local recurrence.

Melanocytic tumours

Pigmented skin lesions are important because melanoma is a highly malignant tumour which is curable only by early diagnosis and excision.

Benign

There are several forms of benign melanocytic lesion.

Melanocytic naevi

Everybody has moles on their skin, some more than others. They develop by proliferation of naevus cells in the basal epidermis, which migrate in groups into the dermis. This growth mainly takes place during the second and third decades of life. In teenagers *compound naevi* are commonest, with both a junctional and a dermal component of naevus cells. Older *intradermal naevi* no longer have the epidermal component.

Dysplastic naevi

Occasional families show an increased rate of malignant melanoma associated with individuals who have multiple atypical pigmented lesions. The naevi are either junctional or compound and show irregular brown pigmentation and an irregular margin. Whether familial or sporadic there is an increased chance of the individual developing melanoma—*dysplastic naevus syndrome*—or *familial atypical mole and multiple melanoma syndrome* (FAMMM). The risk of melanoma in someone with one or two dysplastic naevi is the same as the risk from having red hair or freckles. Greater numbers of lesions carry a greater risk.

Microscopical

There is proliferation of junctional melanocytes with evidence of cytological atypia not amounting to the degree seen in melanoma. There is no dermal invasion.

Spitz naevus

In younger patients compound naevi, presenting as raised round pink lesions, may show features of cellular atypia, junctional proliferation and pleomorphism which mimic malignancy. Similar lesions with prominent or even heavy pigmentation have been described by Reed as *pigmented spindle cell naevi*.

Blue naevus

These common lesions form small, well-circumscribed, bluish-black nodules. The colour is due to heavy deposits of melanin that lie deep in the dermis in dendritic melanocytes arranged into loosely circumscribed bundles. *Cellular blue naevi* are more richly cellular variants, which raise the possibility of malignant change. The great majority of these lesions are benign.

Congenital melanocytic naevus

Occasionally babies are born with large hairy pigmented naevi on sites such as the trunk, face, scalp or limbs. The lesion is a form of compound naevus. There is a low rate of transformation to malignant melanoma.

Lentigo

There is a range of benign pigmented lesions from the simple freckle to the junctional naevus which show either increased degrees of pigmentation in normal basal melanocytes—*simple lentigo*, or proliferation of pigmented benign melanocytes—*junctional naevus*.

Lentigo maligna

Pigmented patches on the cheek of elderly patients develop through an intra-epidermal phase called *lentigo maligna*, which may then proceed to an invasive *lentigo maligna melanoma*. Thickness for thickness these lesions have the same prognosis as melanomas at other sites (see below).

Malignant melanoma

Melanoma is associated with sun exposure in Caucasians particularly, repeated sunburn (especially in childhood) and with the dysplastic naevus syndrome. They occur at any age but are commonest over 30 years. The incidence is increasing.

The tumours are mostly darkly pigmented, though a minority are amelanotic, and show both irregular degrees of pigmentation and an irregular margin to the tumour. Malignancy is associated with increase in size, deepening or variation in pattern of pigmentation, ulceration, bleeding or the development of satellite lesions. The majority occur on sun-exposed skin but occasionally they occur on sites such as the eye, vulva, penis or internal organs. Melanoma of the vulva is very rare in premenopausal women. Flat melanomas are called *superficial spreading*, whilst thicker tumours may be *nodular* melanomas.

Microscopical

Many different variations may be seen, often making diagnosis difficult. Usually there is evidence of epidermal invasion by single malignant cells and of dermal invasion.

Prognosis is primarily determined by the thickness of the tumour measured in millimetres from the granular layer of the overlying epidermis to the base of the tumour—*Breslow thickness* or by *Clark's levels* of invasion. Tumours less than 0.75 mm thick have a favourable prognosis and are in the *radial growth phase*. Such tumours do not appear competent for metastasis. Tumours greater than 1.75 mm thick are usually in the *vertical growth phase* and are likely to have a fatal outcome from blood-borne regional lymph node and distant metastases.

Treatment is primarily surgical. Excision biopsy for diagnosis can be followed by limited wide local excision, never more than 2 cm in radius, to reduce the chances of local recurrence. Wider local excision has no effect on prognosis. Overall prognosis gives a 5-year survival figure of about 20% and at 10 years about 10%. Metastases can appear in individual cases almost anywhere and at any time after primary treatment.

Precise individual prognosis for stage I melanoma can be determined by combining information about mitoses per square millimetre, presence or absence of tumour-infiltrating lymphocytes, Breslow thickness, anatomical site, sex of patient and histological evidence of regression.

Merkel cell carcinoma

Rapidly growing nodular tumours on the head and neck of elderly patients may show features of neuroendocrine differentiation. These primary *neuroendocrine—Merkel cell carcinomas*, must be differentiated from metastases from small cell carcinoma of the bronchus, and can themselves metastasize to regional lymph nodes or to distant sites.

Skin appendage tumours

These tumours consist of an extensive range of different entities which have in common a largely benign behaviour with cure achieved by simple local excision in most cases. The tumours may show features of sweat gland, sebaceous gland or hair follicle differentiation.

Hair follicle tumours

A common hair follicle tumour, *trichoepithelioma*, resembles basal cell carcinoma, but differs in having foci of calcification microscopically and a very low rate of local recurrence after excision. The tumours may be multiple and typically occur in the snout area of the face, around the nose and eyes.

The *trichofolliculoma* is distinguished clinically by a 'rabbit's tail' tuft of white hair. The *pilomatrixoma* is a firm nodular tumour that mimics a cyst clinically and can become very heavily calcified.

Sweat gland tumours

These tumours may show features of acrosyringium, duct or secretory coil differentiation. The *eccrine poroma* occurs as a painful nodule on the feet or hands, with features of acrosyringium. Tumours of the excretory duct occur as nodular *hidradenoma* at many sites and cystic *syringocystadenoma papilliferum* on the face and scalp and *hidradenoma papilliferum* in the vulva. A nodular tumour of the scalp may be a *cylindroma*, with columns of epithelial cells surrounded by a thick hyaline basement membrane and arranged in a jigsaw-like pattern. The *spiradenoma* is also a nodular tumour, but showing differentiation like the secretory coil.

Sebaceous gland tumours

Naevus sebaceous occurs on the scalp of children and is a malformation of hair follicles and sebaceous glands, which if not excised is likely to develop malignant change, usually in the form of basal cell carcinoma, after 30 or 40 years.

Sebaceous adenoma is rare and must be distinguished from the more common *sebaceous gland hyperplasia* seen on the face. Of the rare malignant adnexal tumours *sebaceous carcinoma* is perhaps the commonest, occurring at sites such as the eyelids.

Cysts

Cysts of various types are often seen and most have in common the fact that they are not sebaceous cysts and that the yellow material they are filled with is keratin and not sebum. The commonest are *epidermal cysts* lined by stratified squamous epithelium, with a prominent granular layer and filled with laminated keratin flakes. The *pilar cyst* is lined by epithelium similar to that seen in the inner root sheath of hair follicles, without a granular layer, and is filled with more amorphous trichilemmal keratin. The *external angular dermoid* has appendages, including sebaceous glands, in its wall and is mainly seen in children.

Dermal tumours

Dermatofibroma—histiocytoma
Dermatofibromas are common and may be mistaken for pigmented lesions. They consist of poorly circumscribed nodules of fibroblastic cells and collagen, with reactive hyperplasia and hyperpigmentation of the overlying epidermis. They are benign, possibly reactive and histiocytic rather than neoplastic, and are cured by simple excision (see p. 106).

Dermatofibrosarcoma protuberans
This alarming title describes a locally invasive tumour of low-grade malignancy. Proliferating myofibroblastic cells form a tumour nodule which may elevate the epidermis and extend into the subcutis. Adequate local excision is required to avoid local recurrence.

Haemangioma
Various forms of haemangioma occur in the skin, including cavernous and capillary forms. *Pyogenic granuloma* is a common proliferation of capillaries, producing a rounded red lesion, usually ulcerated. *Glomus tumours* form small painful bluish nodules, often on the hands or feet (see p. 90). *Angiosarcoma* is rare, but when it presents as a spreading bruise-like tumour on the face or scalp of an elderly person, is associated with a uniformly fatal outcome (see p. 256).

Kaposi's sarcoma
These tumours are usually multiple in AIDS patients and form bluish-brown plaques or nodules. Microscopically the early lesions show proliferation of small blood vessels in the dermis. Later lesions form nodules with more obvious proliferating spindle cells and intradermal haemorrhage with haemosiderin deposition (see p. 9).

The differential diagnosis includes *bacillary angiomatosis*, which has a similar clinical appearance and a microscopic appearance similar to pyogenic granuloma. Stromal collections of organisms, probably *Bartonella*, are present. The lesions regress after treatment with erythromycin.

Lymphangioma
Rarely simple, cavernous or cystic lymphangiomas may be seen in the dermis (see p. 91).

Leiomyoma
Rare dermal leiomyomas consist of multiple bundles of well-differentiated smooth muscle, derived from arrectores pilorum muscle (see p. 107).

Cutaneous lymphoma
Skin involvement by systemic lymphoma occurs in between 10% and 20% of patients with non-Hodgkin's lymphoma and to a lesser extent with Hodgkin's disease. Primary lymphomas are mainly of T-cell type. Primary cutaneous Hodgkin's disease probably does not occur. Differential diagnosis between benign and malignant lymphoid infiltrates of the skin is a problem, especially with early lesions.

Lymphocytoma cutis
Nodular lymphoid infiltration of the dermis may follow an insect bite or be idiopathic. Microscopically it may be difficult to differentiate between a reactive process and early lymphoma. The lesions show a mixed infiltrate, with lymphoid germinal centres, surrounded by T lymphocytes. When a monoclonal population of lymphocytes can be demonstrated the lesion is more likely to progress to lymphoma.

Lymphomatoid papulosis
This condition is characterized by crops of red nodular lesions which usually resolve spontaneously. Microscopically they show heavy dermal infiltration by lymphoid cells, often with a component of Reed–Sternberg-like cells and with epidermal involvement. Some cases proceed to frank lymphoma.

Cutaneous T-cell lymphoma
The tumour infiltrate usually has a T-helper cell phenotype, with spread into the epidermis—epidermotrophism. Also known as *mycosis fungoides*, the condition is characterized by hyperchromatic

intra-epidermal and dermal *mycosis cells*, with convoluted 'cerebriform' nuclei.

The *erythematous stage* has an erythematous rash with a dermal infiltrate which may not show diagnostic appearances. The disease may progress to the *plaque stage*, with heavier dermal infiltration and small collections of tumour cells in the epidermis—Pautrier's micro-abscesses. The *tumour stage* has frank tumour nodules in the skin. The disease may progress to nodal and systemic involvement. Some cases show leukaemic involvement of the blood—*Sezary's syndrome* (see p. 275).

Cutaneous B-cell lymphoma

Secondary involvement by B-cell lymphoma is much more common than primary tumours. Nodular tumours on the scalp and back of elderly people are examples of primary tumours. They have microscopic features of follicle centre cell lymphomas and have a good prognosis (see p. 272).

Index